Therapy and Prevention of Atopic Dermatitis and Psoriasis

Therapy and Prevention of Atopic Dermatitis and Psoriasis

Special Issue Editors

Masutaka Furue
Takeshi Nakahara
Gaku Tsuji

MDPI • Basel • Beijing • Wuhan • Barcelona • Belgrade • Manchester • Tokyo • Cluj • Tianjin

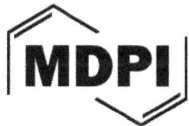

Special Issue Editors

Masutaka Furue
Kyushu University
Japan

Takeshi Nakahara
Kyushu University
Japan

Gaku Tsuji
Kyushu University Hospital
Japan

Editorial Office
MDPI
St. Alban-Anlage 66
4052 Basel, Switzerland

This is a reprint of articles from the Special Issue published online in the open access journal *International Journal of Molecular Sciences* (ISSN 1422-0067) (available at: https://www.mdpi.com/journal/ijms/special_issues/adp).

For citation purposes, cite each article independently as indicated on the article page online and as indicated below:

LastName, A.A.; LastName, B.B.; LastName, C.C. Article Title. *Journal Name* **Year**, *Article Number*, Page Range.

ISBN 978-3-03936-537-1 (Hbk)
ISBN 978-3-03936-538-8 (PDF)

© 2020 by the authors. Articles in this book are Open Access and distributed under the Creative Commons Attribution (CC BY) license, which allows users to download, copy and build upon published articles, as long as the author and publisher are properly credited, which ensures maximum dissemination and a wider impact of our publications.

The book as a whole is distributed by MDPI under the terms and conditions of the Creative Commons license CC BY-NC-ND.

Contents

About the Special Issue Editors vii

Preface to "Therapy and Prevention of Atopic Dermatitis and Psoriasis" ix

Dugarmaa Ulzii, Makiko Kido-Nakahara, Takeshi Nakahara, Gaku Tsuji, Kazuhisa Furue, Akiko Hashimoto-Hachiya and Masutaka Furue
Scratching Counteracts IL-13 Signaling by Upregulating the Decoy Receptor IL-13Rα2 in Keratinocytes
Reprinted from: *Int. J. Mol. Sci.* **2019**, *20*, 3324, doi:10.3390/ijms20133324 1

Sho Miake, Gaku Tsuji, Masaki Takemura, Akiko Hashimoto-Hachiya, Yen Hai Vu, Masutaka Furue and Takeshi Nakahara
IL-4 Augments IL-31/IL-31 Receptor Alpha Interaction Leading to Enhanced Ccl 17 and Ccl 22 Production in Dendritic Cells: Implications for Atopic Dermatitis
Reprinted from: *Int. J. Mol. Sci.* **2019**, *20*, 4053, doi:10.3390/ijms20164053 13

Sunita Keshari, Arun Balasubramaniam, Binderiya Myagmardoloonjin, Deron Raymond Herr, Indira Putri Negari and Chun-Ming Huang
Butyric Acid from Probiotic *Staphylococcus epidermidis* in the Skin Microbiome Down-Regulates the Ultraviolet-Induced Pro-Inflammatory IL-6 Cytokine via Short-Chain Fatty Acid Receptor
Reprinted from: *Int. J. Mol. Sci.* **2019**, *20*, 4477, doi:10.3390/ijms20184477 23

Hayato Nomura, Mutsumi Suganuma, Takuya Takeichi, Michihiro Kono, Yuki Isokane, Ko Sunagawa, Mina Kobashi, Satoru Sugihara, Ai Kajita, Tomoko Miyake, Yoji Hirai, Osamu Yamasaki, Masashi Akiyama and Shin Morizane
Multifaceted Analyses of Epidermal Serine Protease Activity in Patients with Atopic Dermatitis
Reprinted from: *Int. J. Mol. Sci.* **2020**, *21*, 913, doi:10.3390/ijms21030913 37

Kento Mizutani, Eri Shirakami, Masako Ichishi, Yoshiaki Matsushima, Ai Umaoka, Karin Okada, Yukie Yamaguchi, Masatoshi Watanabe, Eishin Morita and Keiichi Yamanaka
Systemic Dermatitis Model Mice Exhibit Atrophy of Visceral Adipose Tissue and Increase Stromal Cells via Skin-Derived Inflammatory Cytokines
Reprinted from: *Int. J. Mol. Sci.* **2020**, *21*, 3367, doi:10.3390/ijms21093367 49

Naoko Kanda, Toshihiko Hoashi and Hidehisa Saeki
The Roles of Sex Hormones in the Course of Atopic Dermatitis
Reprinted from: *Int. J. Mol. Sci.* **2019**, *20*, 4660, doi:10.3390/ijms20194660 63

Makoto Sugaya
The Role of Th17-Related Cytokines in Atopic Dermatitis
Reprinted from: *Int. J. Mol. Sci.* **2020**, *21*, 1314, doi:10.3390/ijms21041314 85

Risa Tamagawa-Mineoka and Norito Katoh
Atopic Dermatitis: Identification and Management of Complicating Factors
Reprinted from: *Int. J. Mol. Sci.* **2020**, *21*, 2671, doi:10.3390/ijms21082671 97

Masutaka Furue, Akiko Hashimoto-Hachiya and Gaku Tsuji
Aryl Hydrocarbon Receptor in Atopic Dermatitis and Psoriasis
Reprinted from: *Int. J. Mol. Sci.* **2019**, *20*, 5424, doi:10.3390/ijms20215424 113

Piotr Wójcik, Michał Biernacki, Adam Wroński, Wojciech Łuczaj, Georg Waeg, Neven Žarković and Elżbieta Skrzydlewska
Altered Lipid Metabolism in Blood Mononuclear Cells of Psoriatic Patients Indicates Differential Changes in Psoriasis Vulgaris and Psoriatic Arthritis
Reprinted from: *Int. J. Mol. Sci.* **2019**, *20*, 4249, doi:10.3390/ijms20174249 . . . . **131**

Koji Kamiya, Megumi Kishimoto, Junichi Sugai, Mayumi Komine and Mamitaro Ohtsuki
Risk Factors for the Development of Psoriasis
Reprinted from: *Int. J. Mol. Sci.* **2019**, *20*, 4347, doi:10.3390/ijms20184347 . . . . **149**

Marco Diani, Silvia Perego, Veronica Sansoni, Lucrezia Bertino, Marta Gomarasca, Martina Faraldi, Paolo Daniele Maria Pigatto, Giovanni Damiani, Giuseppe Banfi, Gianfranco Altomare and Giovanni Lombardi
Differences in Osteoimmunological Biomarkers Predictive of Psoriatic Arthritis among a Large Italian Cohort of Psoriatic Patients
Reprinted from: *Int. J. Mol. Sci.* **2019**, *20*, 5617, doi:10.3390/ijms20225617 . . . . **163**

Kazuhisa Furue, Takamichi Ito, Yuka Tanaka, Akiko Hashimoto-Hachiya, Masaki Takemura, Maho Murata, Makiko Kido-Nakahara, Gaku Tsuji, Takeshi Nakahara and Masutaka Furue
The EGFR-ERK/JNK-CCL20 Pathway in Scratched Keratinocytes May Underpin Koebnerization in Psoriasis Patients
Reprinted from: *Int. J. Mol. Sci.* **2020**, *21*, 434, doi:10.3390/ijms21020434 . . . . **175**

Agnieszka Owczarczyk-Saczonek, Magdalena Krajewska-Włodarczyk, Marta Kasprowicz-Furmańczyk and Waldemar Placek
Immunological Memory of Psoriatic Lesions
Reprinted from: *Int. J. Mol. Sci.* **2020**, *21*, 625, doi:10.3390/ijms21020625 . . . . **189**

Chun-Ming Shih, Chang-Cyuan Chen, Chen-Kuo Chu, Kuo-Hsien Wang, Chun-Yao Huang and Ai-Wei Lee
The Roles of Lipoprotein in Psoriasis
Reprinted from: *Int. J. Mol. Sci.* **2020**, *21*, 859, doi:10.3390/ijms21030859 . . . . **201**

Mayumi Komine
Recent Advances in Psoriasis Research; the Clue to Mysterious Relation to Gut Microbiome
Reprinted from: *Int. J. Mol. Sci.* **2020**, *21*, 2582, doi:10.3390/ijms21072582 . . . . **213**

Masutaka Furue, Kazuhisa Furue, Gaku Tsuji and Takeshi Nakahara
Interleukin-17A and Keratinocytes in Psoriasis
Reprinted from: *Int. J. Mol. Sci.* **2020**, *21*, 1275, doi:10.3390/ijms21041275 . . . . **229**

Masahiro Kamata and Yayoi Tada
Efficacy and Safety of Biologics for Psoriasis and Psoriatic Arthritis and Their Impact on Comorbidities: A Literature Review
Reprinted from: *Int. J. Mol. Sci.* **2020**, *21*, 1690, doi:10.3390/ijms21051690 . . . . **251**

About the Special Issue Editors

Masutaka Furue (Professor) Masutaka Furue graduated from the School of Medicine, at the University of Tokyo as M.D. in 1980, and received his Ph.D. from the University of Tokyo in 1986. He worked under Dr. Stephen I. Katz as a research fellow in the Dermatology Branch, National Institutes of Health, Bethesda, USA. from 1986 to 1988. He was an Associate Professor, Yamanashi Medical University from 1992 to 1995, and moved to the University of Tokyo as an Associate Professor in 1995. He has been a Chairman and Professor of the Department of Dermatology, Kyushu University since 1997. He has served as Vice Director of Kyushu University Hospital and Vice Dean of Faculty of Medical Sciences, Kyushu University. His interests are in the areas of atopic dermatitis, cutaneous neoplasms, dioxins/pollutants, and antioxidants. From 2001, he has been a chief of Yusho (dioxin intoxication) study in Japan. He was the President of many scientific meetings including the 10th International Symposium on Dendritic Cells in Fundamental and Clinical Immunology in 2008; the 108th annual meeting of the Japanese Dermatological Association in 2009; First Eastern Asia Dermatology Congress, 2010; and the 13th annual meeting of the Japanese Pressure Ulcer Society, 2011. He serves as Editor-in-Chief of the *Journal of Dermatology* (2014–2020), *Journal of Clinical Medicine* (Dermatology Section, 2020–present), *Japanese Journal of Dermatology* (2018–2020), and *Nishinihon Journal of Dermatology* (1998–present).

Takeshi Nakahara (Associate professor) Takeshi Nakahara (M.D., Ph.D.) received his M.D. in 1999 and Ph.D. in 2005 from Kyushu University, Fukuoka, Japan. He worked as a research fellow at the Memorial Sloan Kettering Cancer Center, NY, USA from 2005 to 2008. He was an Assistant Professor at Kyushu University Hospital from 2008 to 2013, and was promoted to his current position, an Associate Professor (2013–) at the Graduate school of Medical Sciences, Kyushu University. His clinical and research interests are in the field of inflammatory skin disorders, particularly atopic dermatitis, psoriasis, and urticaria.

Gaku Tsuji (Associate professor) Gaku Tsuji (M.D., Ph.D.) is a dermatologist from the Department of Dermatology, Graduate School of Medical Sciences, Kyushu University, Fukuoka, Japan. He received his Medical Doctorate in 2002 and Ph.D. in 2011 from Tottori University and Kyushu University, respectively. He worked as a research fellow at the Dermatology Branch in National Cancer Institute, National Institutes of Health (Mentor: Prof. Stephen I. Katz) from 2012 to 2014. His research interests include the role of aryl hydrocarbon receptor (AHR) in the skin, particularly AHR-mediated transcriptional networks in redox status and autophagy in human keratinocytes and fibroblasts.

Preface to "Therapy and Prevention of Atopic Dermatitis and Psoriasis"

The skin is the outermost part of the body, where various external and internal stimuli interact. The complex interface reaction is necessary for maintaining the homeostasis of the epidermal and dermal compartments, but its imbalance results in numerous types of inflammatory disorders, such as psoriasis and atopic dermatitis. The excellent therapeutic success of biological treatments stresses the pathogenic importance of TNF-α/IL-23/IL-17 axis for psoriasis, and IL-4/IL-13 signals for atopic dermatitis. Common external stimuli include ultraviolet rays, chemicals, allergens, and environmental pollutants. Some of these agents modulate psoriatic and atopic inflammation by activating the oxidative aryl hydrocarbon receptor, as well as antioxidative NRF2 transcription factors. Various cytochemokines involved in Th17 and Th2 deviation are also operative in psoriatic and atopic inflammation, respectively, by facilitating the differentiation and recruitment of pathogenic dendritic cells, T-cells, and innate lymphoid cells. In this Special Issue, we will publish cutting-edge information regarding skin inflammation, therapy, and prevention, especially related to psoriatic and atopic inflammation.

Masutaka Furue, Takeshi Nakahara, Gaku Tsuji
Special Issue Editors

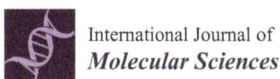

Article

Scratching Counteracts IL-13 Signaling by Upregulating the Decoy Receptor IL-13Rα2 in Keratinocytes

Dugarmaa Ulzii [1,2], Makiko Kido-Nakahara [1,*], Takeshi Nakahara [1,3], Gaku Tsuji [1,4], Kazuhisa Furue [1], Akiko Hashimoto-Hachiya [1,4] and Masutaka Furue [1,3,4]

1. Department of Dermatology, Graduate School of Medical Sciences, Kyushu University, Fukuoka 812-8582, Japan
2. Department of Dermatology, National Dermatology Center of Mongolia, Ulaanbaatar 14171, Mongolia
3. Division of Skin Surface Sensing, Graduate School of Medical Sciences, Kyushu University, Fukuoka 812-8582, Japan
4. Research and Clinical Center for Yusho and Dioxin, Kyushu University Hospital, Fukuoka 812-8582, Japan
* Correspondence: macky@dermatol.med.kyushu-u.ac.jp; Tel.: +81-92-642-5585; Fax: +81-92-642-5600

Received: 26 June 2019; Accepted: 4 July 2019; Published: 6 July 2019

Abstract: The vicious itch–scratch cycle is a cardinal feature of atopic dermatitis (AD), in which IL-13 signaling plays a dominant role. Keratinocytes express two receptors: The heterodimeric IL-4Rα/IL-13Rα1 and IL-13Rα2. The former one transduces a functional IL-13 signal, whereas the latter IL-13Rα2 works as a nonfunctional decoy receptor. To examine whether scratch injury affects the expression of IL-4Rα, IL-13Rα1, and IL-13Rα2, we scratched confluent keratinocyte sheets and examined the expression of three IL-13 receptors using quantitative real-time PCR (qRT-PCR) and immunofluorescence techniques. Scratch injuries significantly upregulated the expression of *IL13RA2* in a scratch line number-dependent manner. Scratch-induced *IL13RA2* upregulation was synergistically enhanced in the simultaneous presence of IL-13. In contrast, scratch injuries did not alter the expression of *IL4R* and *IL13RA1*, even in the presence of IL-13. Scratch-induced *IL13RA2* expression was dependent on ERK1/2 and p38 MAPK signals. The expression of IL-13Rα2 protein was indeed augmented in the scratch edge area and was also overexpressed in lichenified lesional AD skin. IL-13 inhibited the expression of involucrin, an important epidermal terminal differentiation molecule. IL-13-mediated downregulation of involucrin was attenuated in IL-13Rα2-overexpressed keratinocytes, confirming the decoy function of IL-13Rα2. Our findings indicate that scratching upregulates the expression of the IL-13 decoy receptor IL-13Rα2 and counteracts IL-13 signaling.

Keywords: scratch injury; IL-13Rα2; keratinocyte; IL-13; atopic dermatitis; IL-4Rα; IL-13Rα1; involucrin

1. Introduction

Atopic dermatitis (AD) is a common, chronic or chronically relapsing, severely pruritic, eczematous skin disease that markedly deteriorates the quality of life of afflicted patients [1–4]. Lifetime prevalence of AD is estimated to be as high as 20% in the general population [5,6]. Clinical symptoms and signs of AD are characterized by skin inflammation, barrier dysfunction (xerosis), and itching [1,7]. Severe and chronic pruritus induces unavoidable scratching, and the vicious itch–scratch cycle exacerbates and perpetuates atopic inflammation and skin barrier function [8,9].

Compounding evidence shows that acute AD lesions have a significantly greater number of T helper 2 (TH2) cells expressing interleukin-4 (IL-4) and IL-13 than normal skin or uninvolved AD skin [10]. The TH2-deviated immune response is demonstrated both in pediatric and adult AD [11,12] and is greater in chronic than in acute lesions [11,13]. IL-4 and IL-13 inhibit filaggrin (FLG) and involucrin (IVL) expression in keratinocytes, leading to deteriorated barrier function [14,15]. IL-4 and IL-13 also potentiate the neuronal pruritic signal [16]. The pathogenic importance of IL-4/IL-13 signaling in AD has been recently highlighted because its blockage by dupilumab, a specific anti-IL-4 receptor α (IL-4Rα, *IL4R*) antibody, successfully improves skin inflammation in patients with AD [17]. Notably, a more recent large-scale transcriptomic analysis revealed a specific and dominant role of IL-13 in lesional AD skin, but nearly undetectable IL-4 expression was found [18].

The IL-13 signal is regulated via a complex receptor system. In nonhematopoietic cells, IL-13 engages a heterodimeric receptor composed of IL-4Rα and IL-13Rα1 (*IL13RA1*) [19,20]. IL-13Rα1 binds IL-13 with low affinity; however, when it forms a complex with IL-4α, it binds with much higher affinity, inducing the effector functions of IL-13 [19,20]. A second receptor, IL-13Rα2 (*IL13RA2*), is closely related to IL-13Rα1. IL-13Rα2 binds IL13 with high affinity, but it lacks any significant cytoplasmic domain and does not function as a signal mediator [20]. Cells with high IL-13Rα2 expression can rapidly and efficiently deplete extracellular IL-13 [21]. Likewise, IL-13 responses are enhanced in mice lacking *IL13RA2* [22]. These studies have highlighted that IL-13Rα2 can act as a scavenger or decoy receptor of IL-13 and elicits antagonistic activity against IL-13 [20].

Epidermal keratinocytes express IL-4Rα, IL-13Rα1, and IL-13Rα2 [23,24]. However, it remains unknown whether mechanical scratching affects the expression of these three IL-13 receptors. In this study, confluent keratinocyte sheets were scratched and the expression of IL-4Rα, IL-13Rα1, and IL-13Rα2 was assessed. Unexpectedly, this in vitro scratch model showed that scratch injuries upregulated IL-13Rα2 expression in a scratch line number-dependent fashion. This is the first report that scratch injuries may be able to produce an antagonistic signal against IL-13 by upregulating IL-13Rα2 expression.

2. Results

2.1. Scratching Upregulates the Expression of IL13RA2, Which is Further Enhanced by IL-13

We first scratched confluent keratinocyte sheets in six-well culture plates with 14 scratch lines. The expression of *IL13RA2* was significantly enhanced in the scratched sheet, compared to that in the non-scratched control (Figure 1A). Notably, the gene expression of *IL4R* (Figure 1B) and *IL13RA1* (Figure 1C) was not affected by the scratch injury. The upregulation of *IL13RA2* gene expression was transient, peaking at 12 h and returning to a baseline level at 24 h (Figure 2A). The gene expression of *IL4R* (Figure 2B) and *IL13RA1* (Figure 2C) exhibited no differences over time. We next scratched the keratinocyte sheets with 7, 14, or 18 scratch lines. *IL13RA2* gene expression was significantly upregulated in a scratch line number-dependent fashion (Figure 3A). Again, *IL4R* (Figure 3B) and *IL13RA1* (Figure 3C) gene expression levels were not altered, irrespective of scratch line numbers. We next examined whether the simultaneous presence of exogenous IL-13 affected scratch-induced *IL13RA2* gene upregulation. Exogenous IL-13 itself significantly upregulated the baseline level of *IL13RA2* gene expression in non-scratched keratinocytes (Figure 4A). Notably, scratch-induced *IL13RA2* gene upregulation was significantly augmented synergistically by IL-13 in a concentration-dependent manner (Figure 4A). As shown in Figure 4B,C, graded concentrations of IL-13 did not alter the gene expression of *IL4R* and *IL13RA1* either alone or with a scratch injury.

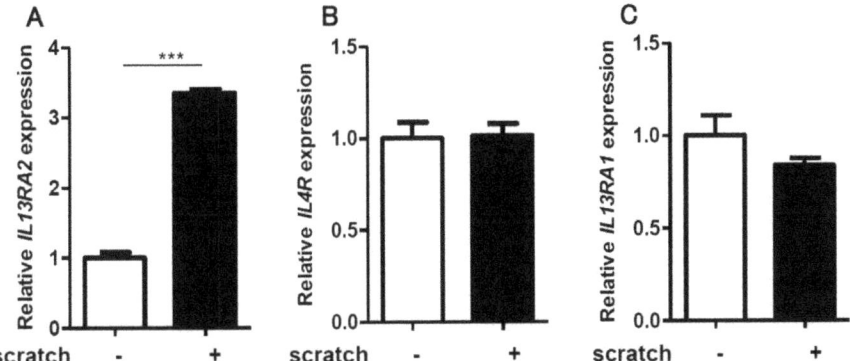

Figure 1. Scratching significantly upregulates the expression of *IL13RA2* in NHEK cells. A confluent keratinocyte culture was scratched with 14 lines, and the expression of *IL13RA2*, *IL4R*, and *IL13RA1* was analyzed by qRT-PCR and normalized to that of β-actin. Scratching significantly increased *IL13RA2* expression in NHEK cells (**A**). *IL4R* (**B**) and *IL13RA1* (**C**) expression was not altered. The cells were incubated for 6 h after scratching. Data is shown as the mean ± SEM ($n = 3$). *** $p < 0.001$.

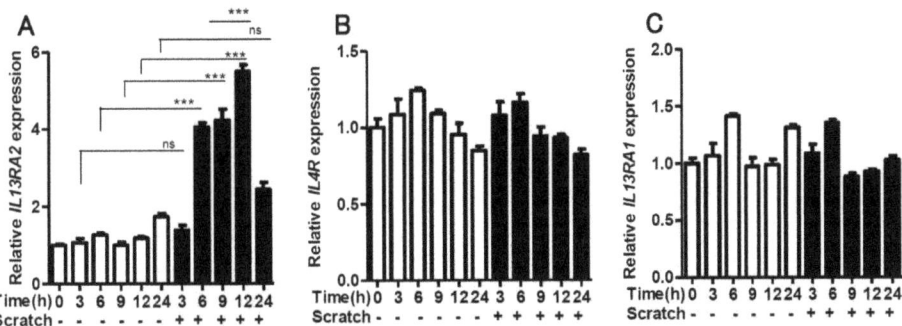

Figure 2. Time-course study for *IL13RA2* (**A**), *IL4R* (**B**), and *IL13RA1* (**C**) expression. The gene expression of *IL13RA2*, *IL4R*, and *IL13RA1* was measured with or without scratching at 0, 3, 6, 9, 12, and 24 h ($n = 3$). Data is shown as the mean ± SEM. ns: not significant. *** $p < 0.001$.

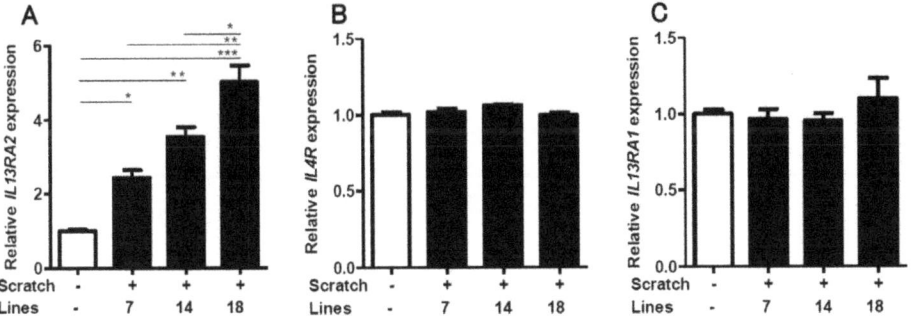

Figure 3. Scratching upregulated *IL13RA2* expression in a scratch line number-dependent manner. The keratinocyte sheet was scratched with 7, 14, and 18 scratch lines, and the gene expression of *IL13RA2* (**A**), *IL4R* (**B**), and *IL13RA1* (**C**) was measured ($n = 3$) 6 h after scratching. Data is shown as the mean ± SEM. * $p < 0.05$, ** $p < 0.01$, *** $p < 0.001$.

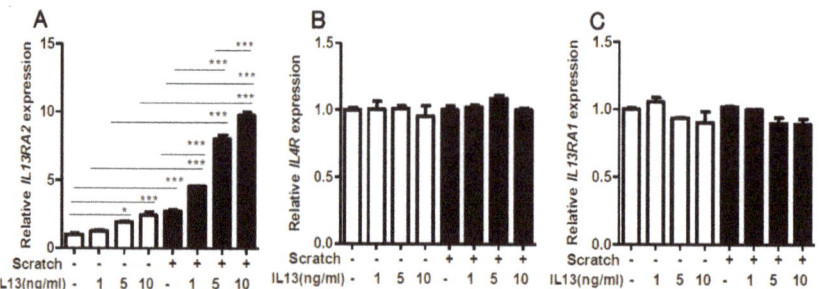

Figure 4. The effect of IL-13 on scratch-induced *IL13RA2* (**A**), *IL4R* (**B**), and *IL13RA1* (**C**) expression. Confluent keratinocyte sheets were non-scratched or scratched with 18 lines in the presence or absence of graded IL-13 concentrations (1, 5, 10 ng/mL). Cells were treated with IL-13 for 14 h before scratching and then incubated for another 6 h. Data is shown as the mean ± SEM. * $p < 0.05$, *** $p < 0.001$.

2.2. Upregulation of IL-13Rα2 Protein in a Scratched Edge Area In Vitro as well as in Lesional AD Skin

In order to determine the spatial expression of IL-13Rα2 protein in the scratched sheet, we conducted immunostaining. Immunostaining for IL-13Rα1 served as the unaffected control. The immunofluorescence intensity for IL-13Rα2 protein was significantly upregulated in the scratch edge area, compared to that in the non-scratched control (Figure 5A). The IL-13Rα2-positive signal was also slightly enhanced in the peri-edge area, but it did not reach statistical significance, compared to that in the non-scratched control (Figure 5A). In contrast, the immunofluorescence intensity for IL-13Rα1 protein was comparable among the scratch edge area, peri-edge area, and non-scratched control (Figure 5B). As a suitable anti-IL-13Rα2 antibody was unavailable, we were unable to detect IL-13Rα2 protein with western blotting.

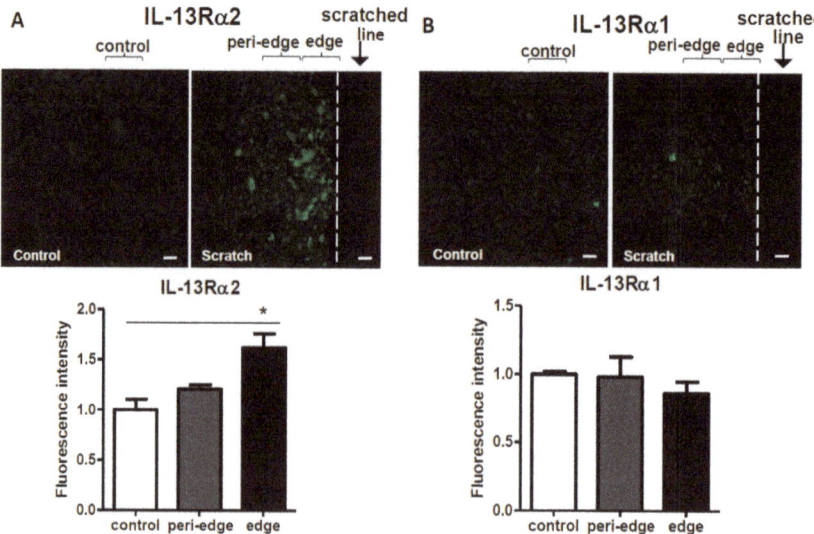

Figure 5. Immunofluorescence analysis for IL-13Rα2 (**A**) and IL-13Rα1 (**B**) proteins. Non-scratched control or scratched confluent keratinocyte sheets were immunostained with anti-IL-13Rα2 or anti-IL-13Rα1 antibodies. Data is shown as the mean ± SEM. * $p < 0.05$. Scale bar: 50 μm.

We next immunostained IL-13Rα2 protein in lichenified lesional AD skin ($n = 11$) and normal control skin ($n = 11$). In normal skin, IL-13Rα2 expression was immunodetectable, especially in the epidermal basal layer (Figure 6A). Its expression was augmented in the lesional AD epidermis, compared to that in the normal control epidermis (Figure 6A). The percentage of IL-13Rα2-positive keratinocytes was significantly increased in the lichenified AD skin, compared to that in the normal control skin (Figure 6B).

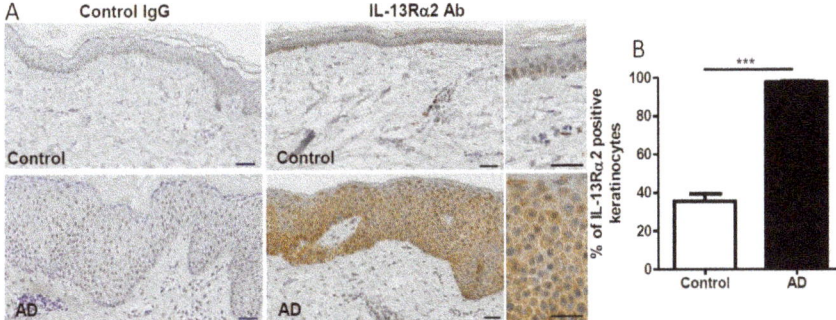

Figure 6. Immunohistochemical analysis for IL-13Rα2 expression. Control normal skin and lichenified lesional AD skin were immunostained with control IgG and anti-IL-13Rα2 antibody (**A**). The percentage of IL-13Rα2 positive keratinocytes was calculated in 11 normal skin and 11 AD skin samples (**B**). Data is shown as the mean ± SEM. *** $p < 0.001$. Scale bar: 50 μm.

2.3. Contribution of ERK1/2 and P38MAPK Activation to Scratch-Induced IL13RA2 Upregulation

We next examined the MAPK signal transduction pathways leading to scratch-induced *IL13RA2* upregulation. The scratch injury upregulated the phosphorylation of ERK1/2, JNK, and p38MAPK (Supplementary Figure S1). Correspondingly, scratch-induced *IL13RA2* upregulation was disrupted in the presence of U0126 (MEK/ERK inhibitor) and SB203580 (p38MAPK inhibitor) (Figure 7A). Interestingly, SP600125 (JNK inhibitor) did not affect scratch-induced *IL13RA2* upregulation (Figure 7A). Baseline *IL4R* expression was downregulated only by U0126 (Figure 7B). The gene expression of *IL13RA1* was stable, irrespective of these inhibitors (Figure 7C). These results suggested that ERK1/2 and p38MAPK were involved in scratch-induced *IL13RA2* upregulation.

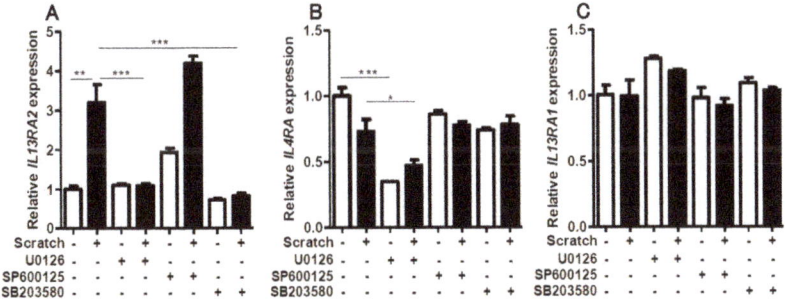

Figure 7. The effect of MAPK inhibitors on *IL13RA2* (**A**), *IL4R* (**B**), and *IL13RA1* (**C**) expression. Non-scratched and scratched confluent keratinocytes were treated with or without U0126 (MEK 1/2-ERK1/2 inhibitor), SP600125 (JNK inhibitor), and SB203580 (p38MAPK inhibitor). Data is shown as the mean ± SEM. * $p < 0.05$, ** $p < 0.01$, *** $p < 0.001$.

2.4. IL-13-Mediated IVL Downregulation is Restored in IL-13Rα2-Overexpressed HaCaT Keratinocytes

It is known that IL-13Rα2 exhibits a decoy function for IL-13 [20]. In order to examine this function, we established IL-13Rα2-Tg-HaCaT keratinocytes. The IL-13Rα2-Tg-HaCaT cells exhibited significantly higher expression of IL-13Rα2 mRNA (Figure 8A) and protein than the mock-HaCaT cells (Figure 8B and supplementary Figure S2). IL-13 is known to inhibit *IVL* and *FLG* expression in normal keratinocytes [14,15]. Likewise, IL-13 inhibited *IVL* expression in HaCaT keratinocytes (Figure 8C). However, IL-13-mediated IVL downregulation was partially, but significantly, attenuated in the IL-13Rα2-Tg-HaCaT keratinocytes (Figure 8C), suggesting that the decoy function of IL-13Rα2 was operative in keratinocytes.

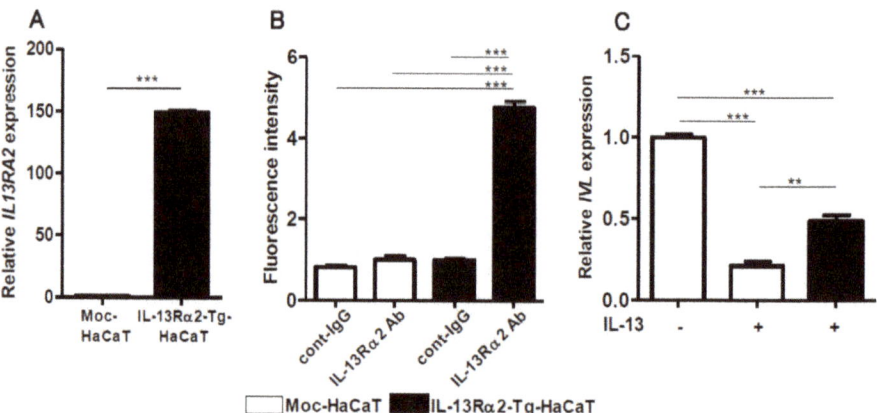

Figure 8. *IL13RA2* expression was upregulated in the IL-13Rα2-Tg-HaCaT cells more than in control Moc-HaCaT cells (**A**). Upregulated IL-13Rα2 protein expression was observed in the IL-13Rα2-Tg-HaCaT cells, compared to that in Moc-HaCaT cells (**B**). IL-13-induced *IVL* downregulation was partially restored in IL-13Rα2-Tg-HaCaT cells (**C**). ** $p < 0.01$, *** $p < 0.001$.

Intriguingly, IL-13 downregulated *FLG* expression in normal human keratinocytes, but it failed to inhibit *FLG* expression in HaCaT keratinocytes (Supplementary Figure S3). Therefore, we did not focus further on *FLG* expression.

3. Discussion

Itchiness is a specialized perception in the skin and an unpleasant sensation that elicits the desire to scratch in order to remove harmful stimuli, leading to a scratching behavior [25]. Scratching appears to exacerbate preexistent dermatitis in humans and mice [9,26], but it relieves the itching sensation [27]. Among cutaneous inflammatory skin diseases, the vicious itch–scratch cycle is particularly important in AD because it profoundly impairs the quality of life, treatment satisfaction and adherence, and socioeconomic stability of patients [28–30]. However, the subcellular biological effects caused by scratching keratinocytes remain elusive. As AD is a TH2-dominant, particularly IL-13-dominant, skin disease [18], we focused on whether a scratch injury affects the expression of three IL-13 receptors, IL-4R, IL-13Rα1, and IL-13Rα2, in keratinocytes.

In the present study, we demonstrated that the scratch injury enhanced the expression of an IL-13 decoy receptor, IL-13Rα2. Scratch-induced IL-13Rα2 upregulation was selective because no significant changes were recognized in the expression of the functional heterodimeric IL-13 receptor, IL-4R, or IL-13Rα1. Scratch-induced IL-13Rα2 upregulation was highly dependent on scratch stress because it was enhanced with more scratch lines. Moreover, immunofluorescence analysis revealed that the upregulation of IL-13Rα2 was largely confined to the scratch edge area where scratch stress was most observed. IL-13 itself enhanced IL-13Rα2 expression in keratinocytes, but this was less potent than with the scratch injury. However, strong and synergistic upregulation of IL-13Rα2 expression was observed with co-treatment of IL-13 and a scratch injury.

Historically, the in vitro scratch injury of a keratinocyte sheet has been used as a good model for wound closure in that it reflects the migratory and proliferative capacity of keratinocytes [31–33]. Therefore, no previous studies have sought to examine the scratch-mediated alteration of IL-13 receptors. The selective upregulation of IL-13Rα2 was a novel and unexpected finding. We then investigated signal transduction that led to scratch-induced IL-13Rα2 upregulation. In our experimental model, the scratch injury augmented the phosphorylation of ERK1/2, JNK, and P38 MAPK. Likewise, inhibitors for ERK1/2 and P38 MAPK, but not JNK, disrupted scratch-induced IL-13Rα2 upregulation. These results suggest a crucial role of ERK1/2 and P38 MAPK in regulating scratch-induced IL-13Rα2 upregulation.

The vicious itch–scratch cycle is one of the cardinal features of AD [9,26]. Therefore, we examined epidermal IL-13Rα2 expression in lichenified (scratched) AD lesions. IL-13Rα2 expression was significantly increased in lesional AD skin, compared to that in the normal control epidermis. To determine the functional implications of IL-13Rα2 overexpression, we finally examined whether increased IL-13Rα2 expression suppresses an IL-13-mediated event, namely, IL-13-induced *IVL* downregulation [14,15,34]. As expected, IL-13 inhibited *IVL* expression, which was significantly restored in the IL-13Rα2 overexpressed keratinocytes. Based on these results, we deduced that scratch-induced IL-13Rα2 overexpression is biologically functional and may diminish IL-13-mediated hazardous events in the epidermal inflammatory microenvironment.

Scratching may induce various biological consequences. The scratch signal exacerbates skin inflammation and conversely upregulates IL-13Rα2 expression, which may suppress excess IL-13 activity caused by the decoy function of IL-13Rα2 in keratinocytes. These fine-tuned mutually counteracting molecular events may participate in the formation of scratch-induced lichenified skin lesions.

4. Materials and Methods

4.1. Reagents and Antibodies

Recombinant human IL-13 (Peprotech, Rocky Hill, NJ, USA) was dissolved in distilled water and added to the culture medium at a final concentration of 1, 5, or 10 ng/mL. The antibodies for immunofluorescence and immunohistochemistry staining were used as follows: Anti-IL-13Rα2 mouse monoclonal antibody (Abcam, Cambridge, UK), normal mouse IgG (Santa Cruz Biotechnology, Dallas, TX, USA), and goat anti-mouse IgG conjugated with Alexa Fluor 488 dye (Thermo Fisher Scientific, Waltham, MA, USA). The antibodies for western blotting were used as follows: Anti-ERK1/2, JNK, p38 MAPK, phospho-ERK1/2 (Thr202/Tyr204), phospho-JNK (Thr183/Tyr185), and phospho-p38 MAPK (Thr180/Tyr182) rabbit monoclonal antibodies and β-actin mouse monoclonal antibody (Cell Signaling Technology, Danvers, MA, USA) as primary antibodies, and anti-mouse IgG and anti-rabbit IgG HRP-linked antibody (Cell Signaling Technology) as secondary antibodies. Signal transduction inhibitor U0126 (ERK1/2 inhibitor) was purchased from Cell Signaling Technology. SP600125 (JNK inhibitor) and SB203580 (p38 inhibitor) were obtained from Tocris Bioscience (Bristol, UK).

4.2. Cell Culture

Neonatal normal human epidermal keratinocytes (NHEKs) were purchased from Lonza (Basel, Switzerland) and cultured in KGM-Gold (Lonza), supplemented with bovine pituitary extract, recombinant human epidermal growth factor, insulin, hydrocortisone, gentamycin–amphotericin, transferrin, and epinephrine (Lonza) at 37 °C in 5% CO_2. The medium was changed every 2 days. The cells reached 70–80% confluence and were passaged three times. The third passage of cells was used in all experiments. HaCaT cells (human keratinocyte cell line) were maintained in DMEM, supplemented with 10% fetal bovine serum (FBS) and antibiotics. Cells were passaged at 70–80% confluence and used in the experiment of transfection of plasmids.

4.3. In Vitro Scratched Keratinocyte Model

To establish the in vitro scratched keratinocyte model, NHEKs were seeded into 6-well plates (Corning, NY, USA) (3.5×10^5 cells/well). Entire confluent keratinocyte sheets were scratched with 7, 14, and 18 lines, using 1000-μL tips (Greiner Bio-One, Kremsmünster, Austria), and incubated for 0, 3, 6, 9, 12, or 24 h at 37 °C in 5% CO_2 after scratching. In several assays, the scratched cell sheets were treated with IL-13 (1, 5, or 10 ng/mL, Peprotech).

4.4. Quantitative Real-Time PCR (qRT-PCR)

Total RNA was extracted from cells using RNeasy Mini Kit (Qiagen, Hilden, Germany), and cDNA was synthesized using PrimeScript RT Reagent Kit (Takara Bio, Shiga, Japan).

qRT-PCR was performed on the CFX Connect Real-Time PCR Detection System (Bio-Rad, Hercules, CA, USA), using TB Green Premix Ex Taq (Takara Bio). Denaturation was set at 95 °C for 30 s with 40 total cycles with a second step at 95 °C for 5 s. Annealing occurred at 63 °C for 30 s for *IL4R* and *IL13RA1*, and at 60 °C for 30 s for *IL13RA2* and *IVL*. The relative expression levels of *IL4R*, *IL13RA1*, *IL13RA2*, *IVL*, and *FLG* were normalized to that of β-actin.

Gene-specific primers were as follows: *IL4R* forward, 5′-CTGCTCATGGATGACGTGGT-3′; reverse, 5′-CTGGGTTTCACATGCTCGCT-3′; *IL13RA1* forward, 5′-GTCCCAGTGTAGCACCAAT GA-3′; reverse, 5′-GCTCAGGTTGTGCCAAATGC-3′; *IL13RA2* forward, 5′-GCTGGGAAGGTGA AGACCTA-3′; reverse, 5′-ACGCAAAAGCAGACCGGTTA-3′; *IVL* forward, 5′-TAACCACCCGC AGTGTCCAG-3′; reverse, 5′-ACAGATGAGACGGGCCACCTA-3′; *FLG* forward, 5′-TAACCACC CGCAGTGTCCAG-3′; reverse, 5′-ACAGATGAGACGGGCCACCTA-3′; β-actin forward, 5′-ATTGCC GACAGGATGCAGA-3′; reverse, 5′-GAGTACTTGCGCTCAGGAGGA-3′.

4.5. Immunofluorescence Analysis

Immunofluorescent analysis was performed on cell sheets cultured in 4-well slide chambers (Lab-Tek, Rochester, NY, USA) with KGM-Gold (Lonza) for 48 h, scratched using 1000-μL tips (Greine Bio-One), and incubated for 6 h at 37 °C in 5% CO_2. The cells were washed with phosphate-buffered saline 3 times for 5 min each and fixed in cold acetone for 10 min at room temperature. The cell sheets were blocked with 10% bovine serum albumin (Roche Diagnostics, Basel, Switzerland) and incubated with mouse monoclonal anti-IL13Rα2 (Abcam) or control normal mouse IgG (Santa Cruz Biotechnology). Goat anti-mouse IgG conjugated with Alexa Fluor 488 dye (Thermo Fisher Scientific) was used for the secondary antibody. The nucleus was stained with 4′,6-diamino-2-phenylindole (DAPI). Slides were then mounted with Ultra Cruz mounting medium (Santa Cruz Biotechnology) and were observed using a D-Eclipse confocal laser scanning microscope (Nikon, Tokyo, Japan). The immunofluorescence intensity was measured using ImageJ software.

4.6. Immunohistochemistry

Eleven lichenified lesional AD skin and 11 normal skin samples were embedded in paraffin by the conventional method and cut into 3-μm-thick sections. Antigen retrieval was performed using Heat Processor Solution pH 6 (Nichirei Biosciences, Tokyo, Japan) at 100 °C for 40 min, and endogenous peroxidase was blocked by incubating the sections with 3% H_2O_2 (Nichirei Biosciences). The sections were then incubated with anti-IL-13Rα2 (Abcam, 750×) antibody or control normal mouse IgG (Santa Cruz Biotechnology) for 30 min, followed by incubation with the secondary antibody, N-Histofine Simple Stain MAX-PO MULTI (Nichirei Biosciences). Immunodetection was conducted with 3,3-diaminobenzidine as the chromogen, followed by light counterstaining with hematoxylin. The number of IL-13Rα2-positive keratinocytes was counted in three high-power view areas, and the average percent positivity was calculated in each slide.

4.7. Western Blotting

Scratched or non-scratched cells were solubilized in complete Lysis-M (Roche Diagnostics, Rotkreuz, Switzerland). The cell lysates were prepared according to the standard protocol for western blotting analysis. The cell lysates were centrifuged at 14,000 rpm for 25 min and the obtained supernatants were used for analysis. The protein concentration was determined with a BCA protein assay kit (Thermo Fisher Scientific). Equal 20 µg amounts of protein were mixed with 4× LDS sample buffer (Invitrogen) and 10× sample reducing agent (Invitrogen), boiled at 70 °C for 10 min, loaded onto Bolt 4–12% Bis-Tris Plus (Thermo Fisher Scientific), and electrophoresed using Power Station III (Atto corporation, Tokyo, Japan) at 200 V and 180 mA for 25 min. The proteins were then transferred to an Immobilon PVDF Transfer Membrane (Merck, Kenilworth, NJ, USA), using Power Station III at 30 V for 1 h. Membranes were blocked with a blocking buffer, containing blocker diluent A and B, (Invitrogen) for 30 min. Membranes were probed overnight at 4 °C with the following primary antibodies: β-actin (Cell Signaling Technology), ERK1/2, JNK, p38, Phospho-ERK1/2, Phospho-JNK, and Phospho-p38 (Cell Signaling Technology).

The secondary antibodies, anti-mouse IgG HRP-linked antibody (Cell Signaling Technology) and anti-rabbit IgG HRP-linked antibody (Cell Signaling Technology), were applied at room temperature for 30 min. Visualization of protein bands was accomplished with Super Signal West Pico Chemiluminescent Substrate (Thermo Fisher Scientific), using the ChemiDoc Touch Imaging System (Bio-Rad).

4.8. Plasmid DNA and Transfection of Plasmids

Plasmids pCMV6-Entry (Mock) and *IL13RA2* (Myc-DDK-tagged), which contains a cytomegalovirus promoter, and the *IL13RA2* (NM_000640) human cDNA open reading frame clone were obtained from Origene Technologies (Rockville, MD, USA). The plasmids (1 µg) were dissolved in Amaxa P3 Primary Cell 4D-Nucleofector X Kit and were transfected into HaCaT cells using 4D-Nucleofector (Lonza, Basel, Switzerland), according to the manufacturer's protocol. Transfected cells were then selected in Dulbecco's Modified Eagle's Medium (DMEM, Sigma–Aldrich, St. Louis, MO, USA) with 5% fetal bovine serum, Modified Eagle's Medium Non-Essential Amino Acids, 10 mM HEPES, 1 mM sodium pyruvate (Thermo Fisher Scientific), and G418 disulfate aqueous solution (1500 µg/mL, Nacalai Tesque, Kyoto, Japan) for 3 weeks to obtain a stable cell line.

4.9. Statistical Analysis

All data are presented as mean ± standard error of the mean (SEM). The significance of differences between groups was assessed using Student's unpaired two-tailed *t*-test (two groups) or one-way ANOVA, followed by Bonferroni's multiple comparison test (multiple groups), using GraphPad PRISM 5 software Version 5.02 (GraphPad Software, La Jolla, CA). A *p*-value of less than 0.05 was considered statistically significant.

Supplementary Materials: Supplementary materials can be found at http://www.mdpi.com/1422-0067/20/13/3324/s1.

Author Contributions: Experimental design and interpretation of results, D.U., M.K.-N., T.N., G.T., K.F., A.H.-H. and M.F.; conducting of experiments, D.U., M.K.-N. and A.H.-H.; writing, D.U., M.K.-N., A.H.-H. and M.F.

Conflicts of Interest: The authors declare no conflict of interest.

Abbreviations

AD	atopic dermatitis
ERK	extracellular signal-regulated kinase
FLG	filaggrin
IL	interleukin
IL-4Rα	IL-4 receptor α
IL-13Rα1	IL-13 receptor α1
IL-13Rα2	IL-13 receptor α2
IVL	involucrin
JNK	c-Jun N-terminal kinase
MAPK	mitogen-activated protein kinase
MEK	mitogen-activated protein kinase kinase
NHEK	normal human epidermal keratinocyte
TH2 cell	T helper 2 cells

References

1. Bieber, T. Atopic dermatitis 2.0: From the clinical phenotype to the molecular taxonomy and stratified medicine. *Allergy* **2012**, *67*, 1475–1482. [CrossRef] [PubMed]
2. Furue, M.; Chiba, T.; Tsuji, G.; Ulzii, D.; Kido-Nakahara, M.; Nakahara, T.; Kadono, T. Atopic dermatitis: Immune deviation, barrier dysfunction, IgE autoreactivity and new therapies. *Allergol. Int.* **2017**, *66*, 398–403. [CrossRef] [PubMed]
3. Schmitt, J.; Apfelbacher, C.; Spuls, P.I.; Thomas, K.S.; Simpson, E.L.; Furue, M.; Chalmers, J.; Williams, H.C. The Harmonizing Outcome Measures for Eczema (HOME) roadmap: A methodological framework to develop core sets of outcome measurements in dermatology. *J. Invest. Dermatol.* **2015**, *135*, 24–30. [CrossRef] [PubMed]
4. Simpson, E.L.; Bruin-Weller, M.; Flohr, C.; Ardern-Jones, M.R.; Barbarot, S.; Deleuran, M.; Bieber, T.; Vestergaard, C.; Brown, S.J.; Cork, M.J.; et al. When does atopic dermatitis warrant systemic therapy? Recommendations from an expert panel of the International Eczema Council. *J. Am. Acad. Dermatol.* **2017**, *77*, 623–633. [CrossRef] [PubMed]
5. Furue, M.; Chiba, T.; Takeuchi, S. Current status of atopic dermatitis in Japan. *Asia Pac. Allergy* **2011**, *1*, 64–72. [CrossRef]
6. Williams, H.; Stewart, A.; von Mutius, E.; Cookson, W.; Anderson, H.R. International Study of Asthma and Allergies in Childhood (ISAAC) Phase One and Three Study Groups. Is eczema really on the increase worldwide? *J. Allergy Clin. Immunol.* **2008**, *121*, 947–954. [CrossRef] [PubMed]
7. Saeki, H.; Nakahara, T.; Tanaka, A.; Kabashima, K.; Sugaya, M.; Murota, H.; Ebihara, T.; Kataoka, Y.; Aihara, M.; Etoh, T.; et al. Committee for Clinical Practice Guidelines for the Management of Atopic Dermatitis of Japanese Dermatological Association. Clinical Practice Guidelines for the Management of Atopic Dermatitis 2016. *J. Dermatol.* **2016**, *43*, 1117–1145. [CrossRef]
8. Pavlis, J.; Yosipovitch, G. Management of Itch in Atopic Dermatitis. *Am. J. Clin. Dermatol.* **2018**, *19*, 319–332. [CrossRef]
9. Takeuchi, S.; Yasukawa, F.; Furue, M.; Katz, S.I. Collared mice: A model to assess the effects of scratching. *J. Dermatol. Sci.* **2010**, *57*, 44–50. [CrossRef]
10. Hamid, Q.; Boguniewicz, M.; Leung, D.Y. Differential in situ cytokine gene expression in acute versus chronic atopic dermatitis. *J. Clin. Invest.* **1994**, *94*, 870–876. [CrossRef]
11. Czarnowicki, T.; Esaki, H.; Gonzalez, J.; Malajian, D.; Shemer, A.; Noda, S.; Talasila, S.; Berry, A.; Gray, J.; Becker, L.; et al. Early pediatric atopic dermatitis shows only a cutaneous lymphocyte antigen (CLA)(+) TH2/TH1 cell imbalance, whereas adults acquire CLA(+) TH22/TC22 cell subsets. *J. Allergy Clin. Immunol.* **2015**, *136*, 941–951. [CrossRef] [PubMed]
12. Esaki, H.; Brunner, P.M.; Renert-Yuval, Y.; Czarnowicki, T.; Huynh, T.; Tran, G.; Lyon, S.; Rodriguez, G.; Immaneni, S.; Johnson, D.B.; et al. Early-onset pediatric atopic dermatitis is T(H)2 but also T(H)17 polarized in skin. *J. Allergy Clin. Immunol.* **2016**, *138*, 1639–1651. [CrossRef] [PubMed]

13. Gittler, J.K.; Shemer, A.; Suárez-Fariñas, M.; Fuentes-Duculan, J.; Gulewicz, K.J.; Wang, C.Q.; Mitsui, H.; Cardinale, I.; de Guzman Strong, C.; Krueger, J.G.; et al. Progressive activation of T(H)2/T(H)22 cytokines and selective epidermal proteins characterizes acute and chronic atopic dermatitis. *J. Allergy Clin. Immunol.* **2012**, *130*, 1344–1354. [CrossRef] [PubMed]
14. Tsuji, G.; Hashimoto-Hachiya, A.; Kiyomatsu-Oda, M.; Takemura, M.; Ohno, F.; Ito, T.; Morino-Koga, S.; Mitoma, C.; Nakahara, T.; Uchi, H.; et al. Aryl hydrocarbon receptor activation restores filaggrin expression via OVOL1 in atopic dermatitis. *Cell Death Dis.* **2017**, *8*, e2931. [CrossRef] [PubMed]
15. Van den Bogaard, E.H.; Bergboer, J.G.; Vonk-Bergers, M.; van Vlijmen-Willems, I.M.; Hato, S.V.; van der Valk, P.G.; Schröder, J.M.; Joosten, I.; Zeeuwen, P.L.; Schalkwijk, J. Coal tar induces AHR-dependent skin barrier repair in atopic dermatitis. *J. Clin. Invest.* **2013**, *123*, 917–927. [CrossRef] [PubMed]
16. Oetjen, L.K.; Mack, M.R.; Feng, J.; Whelan, T.M.; Niu, H.; Guo, C.J.; Chen, S.; Trier, A.M.; Xu, A.Z.; Tripathi, S.V.; et al. Sensory Neurons Co-opt Classical Immune Signaling Pathways to Mediate Chronic Itch. *Cell* **2017**, *171*, 217–228. [CrossRef] [PubMed]
17. Simpson, E.L.; Bieber, T.; Guttman-Yassky, E.; Beck, L.A.; Blauvelt, A.; Cork, M.J.; Silverberg, J.I.; Deleuran, M.; Kataoka, Y.; Lacour, J.P.; et al. SOLO 1 and SOLO 2 Investigators. Two Phase 3 Trials of Dupilumab versus Placebo in Atopic Dermatitis. *N. Engl. J. Med.* **2016**, *375*, 2335–2348. [CrossRef] [PubMed]
18. Tsoi, L.C.; Rodriguez, E.; Degenhardt, F.; Baurecht, H.; Wehkamp, U.; Volks, N.; Szymczak, S.; Swindell, W.R.; Sarkar, M.K.; Raja, K.; et al. Atopic dermatitis is an IL-13 dominant disease with greater molecular heterogeneity compared to psoriasis. *J. Invest. Dermatol.* **2019**, *139*, 1480–1489. [CrossRef]
19. Lumsden, R.V.; Worrell, J.C.; Boylan, D.; Walsh, S.M.; Cramton, J.; Counihan, I.; O'Beirne, S.; Medina, M.F.; Gauldie, J.; Fabre, A.; et al. Modulation of pulmonary fibrosis by IL-13Rα2. *Am. J. Physiol. Lung Cell Mol. Physiol.* **2015**, *308*, L710–L718. [CrossRef]
20. Ranasinghe, C.; Trivedi, S.; Wijesundara, D.K.; Jackson, R.J. IL-4 and IL-13 receptors: Roles in immunity and powerful vaccine adjuvants. *Cytokine Growth Factor Rev.* **2014**, *25*, 437–442. [CrossRef]
21. Kasaian, M.T.; Raible, D.; Marquette, K.; Cook, T.A.; Zhou, S.; Tan, X.Y.; Tchistiakova, L. IL-13 antibodies influence IL-13 clearance in humans by modulating scavenger activity of IL-13Rα2. *J. Immunol.* **2011**, *187*, 561–569. [CrossRef] [PubMed]
22. Wood, N.; Whitters, M.J.; Jacobson, B.A.; Witek, J.; Sypek, J.P.; Kasaian, M.; Eppihimer, M.J.; Unger, M.; Tanaka, T.; Goldman, S.J.; et al. Enhanced interleukin (IL)-13 responses in mice lacking IL-13 receptor alpha 2. *J. Exp. Med.* **2003**, *197*, 703–709. [CrossRef] [PubMed]
23. Akaiwa, M.; Yu, B.; Umeshita-Suyama, R.; Terada, N.; Suto, H.; Koga, T.; Arima, K.; Matsushita, S.; Saito, H.; Ogawa, H.; et al. Localization of human interleukin 13 receptor in non-haematopoietic cells. *Cytokine* **2001**, *13*, 75–84. [CrossRef] [PubMed]
24. Sivaprasad, U.; Warrier, M.R.; Gibson, A.M.; Chen, W.; Tabata, Y.; Bass, S.A.; Rothenberg, M.E.; Khurana Hershey, G.K. IL-13Rα2 has a protective role in a mouse model of cutaneous inflammation. *J. Immunol.* **2010**, *185*, 6802–6808. [CrossRef] [PubMed]
25. Kido-Nakahara, M.; Furue, M.; Ulzii, D.; Nakahara, T. Itch in Atopic Dermatitis. *Immunol. Allergy Clin. N. Am.* **2017**, *37*, 113–122. [CrossRef] [PubMed]
26. Li, R.; Hadi, S.; Guttman-Yassky, E. Current and emerging biologic and small molecule therapies for atopic dermatitis. *Expert. Opin. Biol. Ther.* **2019**, *19*, 367–380. [CrossRef]
27. Vierow, V.; Forster, C.; Vogelgsang, R.; Dörfler, A.; Handwerker, H.O. Cerebral Networks Linked to Itch-related Sensations Induced by Histamine and Capsaicin. *Acta. Derm. Venereol.* **2015**, *95*, 645–652. [CrossRef]
28. Furue, M.; Onozuka, D.; Takeuchi, S.; Murota, H.; Sugaya, M.; Masuda, K.; Hiragun, T.; Kaneko, S.; Saeki, H.; Shintani, Y.; et al. Poor adherence to oral and topical medication in 3096 dermatological patients as assessed by the Morisky Medication Adherence Scale-8. *Br. J. Dermatol.* **2015**, *172*, 272–275. [CrossRef]
29. Kabashima, K.; Furue, M.; Hanifin, J.M.; Pulka, G.; Wollenberg, A.; Galus, R.; Etoh, T.; Mihara, R.; Nakano, M.; Ruzicka, T. Nemolizumab in patients with moderate-to-severe atopic dermatitis: Randomized, phase II, long-term extension study. *J. Allergy Clin. Immunol.* **2018**, *142*, 1121–1130. [CrossRef]
30. Nakahara, T.; Fujita, H.; Arima, K.; Taguchi, Y.; Motoyama, S.; Furue, M. Treatment satisfaction in atopic dermatitis relates to patient-reported severity: A cross-sectional study. *Allergy* **2018**, *74*, 1179–1181. [CrossRef]
31. Morino-Koga, S.; Uchi, H.; Mitoma, C.; Wu, Z.; Kiyomatsu, M.; Fuyuno, Y.; Nagae, K.; Yasumatsu, M.; Suico, M.A.; Kai, H.; et al. 6-Formylindolo[3,2-b]Carbazole Accelerates Skin Wound Healing via Activation of ERK, but Not Aryl Hydrocarbon Receptor. *J. Invest. Dermatol.* **2017**, *137*, 2217–2226. [CrossRef] [PubMed]

32. Nasca, M.R.; O'Toole, E.A.; Palicharla, P.; West, D.P.; Woodley, D.T. Thalidomide increases human keratinocyte migration and proliferation. *J. Invest. Dermatol.* **1999**, *113*, 720–724. [PubMed]
33. Patruno, A.; Ferrone, A.; Costantini, E.; Franceschelli, S.; Pesce, M.; Speranza, L.; Amerio, P.; D'Angelo, C.; Felaco, M.; Grilli, A.; et al. Extremely low-frequency electromagnetic fields accelerates wound healing modulating MMP-9 and inflammatory cytokines. *Cell Prolif.* **2018**, *51*, e12432. [CrossRef] [PubMed]
34. Howell, M.D.; Kim, B.E.; Gao, P.; Grant, A.V.; Boguniewicz, M.; DeBenedetto, A.; Schneider, L.; Beck, L.A.; Barnes, K.C.; Leung, D.Y. Cytokine modulation of atopic dermatitis filaggrin skin expression. *J. Allergy Clin. Immunol.* **2009**, *124*, R7–R12. [CrossRef] [PubMed]

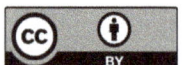

© 2019 by the authors. Licensee MDPI, Basel, Switzerland. This article is an open access article distributed under the terms and conditions of the Creative Commons Attribution (CC BY) license (http://creativecommons.org/licenses/by/4.0/).

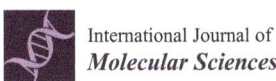

Article

IL-4 Augments IL-31/IL-31 Receptor Alpha Interaction Leading to Enhanced Ccl 17 and Ccl 22 Production in Dendritic Cells: Implications for Atopic Dermatitis

Sho Miake [1], Gaku Tsuji [1,2,*], Masaki Takemura [1], Akiko Hashimoto-Hachiya [1], Yen Hai Vu [1], Masutaka Furue [1,2,3] and Takeshi Nakahara [1,3]

1. Department of Dermatology, Graduate School of Medical Sciences, Kyushu University, Maidashi 3-1-1, Higashiku, Fukuoka 812-8582, Japan
2. Research and Clinical Center for Yusho and Dioxin, Kyushu University, Maidashi 3-1-1, Higashiku, Fukuoka 812-8582, Japan
3. Division of Skin Surface Sensing, Graduate School of Medical Sciences, Kyushu University, Maidashi 3-1-1, Higashiku, Fukuoka 812-8582, Japan
* Correspondence: gakku@dermatol.med.kyushu-u.ac.jp; Tel.: +81-92-642-5585; Fax: +81-92-642-5600

Received: 2 July 2019; Accepted: 16 August 2019; Published: 20 August 2019

Abstract: Severe pruritus is a characteristic feature of atopic dermatitis (AD) and is closely related to its activity. Recent studies have shown that IL-31 is a key determinant of pruritus in AD. Anti-IL-31 receptor alpha (IL-31RA) antibody treatment has also been reported to improve pruritus clinically, subsequently contributing to the attenuation of AD disease activity. Therefore, IL-31 has been thought to be an important cytokine for regulating pruritus and AD disease activity; however, how IL-31 is involved in the immune response in AD has remained largely unknown. Epidermal Langerhans cells (LCs) and dermal dendritic cells (DCs) derived from bone marrow cells have been reported to play a critical role in AD pathogenesis. LCs and DCs produce Ccl 17 and Ccl 22, which chemoattract Th2 cells, leading to AD development. Therefore, we aimed to clarify how IL-31/IL-31RA interaction affects Ccl 17 and Ccl 22 production. To test this, we analyzed murine bone marrow-derived DCs (BMDCs) stimulated with IL-4, an important cytokine in AD development. We found that IL-31RA expression was upregulated by IL-4 stimulation in a dose-dependent manner in BMDCs. Furthermore, IL-31 upregulates Ccl 17 and Ccl 22 production in the presence of IL-4, whereas IL-31 stimulation alone did not produce Ccl 17 and Ccl 22. These findings suggest that IL-4 mediates IL-31RA expression and IL-31/IL-31RA interaction augments Ccl 17 and Ccl 22 production in BMDCs, which promotes Th2-deviated immune response in AD. Since we previously reported that soybean tar Glyteer, an aryl hydrocarbon receptor (AHR) ligand, impairs IL-4/Stat 6 signaling in BMDCs, we examined whether Glyteer affects IL-31RA expression induced by IL-4 stimulation. Glyteer inhibited upregulation of IL-31RA expression induced by IL-4 stimulation in a dose-dependent manner. Glyteer also inhibited Ccl 17 and Ccl 22 production induced by IL-4 and IL-31 stimulation. Taken together, these findings suggest that Glyteer treatment may improve AD disease activity by impairing IL-31/IL-31RA interaction in DCs.

Keywords: IL-31; IL-31 receptor alpha; Ccl 17; Ccl 22; dendritic cell; atopic dermatitis

---

1. Introduction

Interleukin (IL)-31 is a four-helix bundle cytokine closely related to the IL-6 cytokine family [1]. It is the only known ligand for IL-31 receptor alpha (IL-31RA), which belongs to the glycoprotein 130 receptor family [2]. IL-31/IL-31RA interaction initiates signal transduction resulting in the expression of several pro-inflammatory cytokines and chemokines, which play a crucial role in inflammatory diseases relating to Th2 cytokines including IL-4 and IL-13 [3,4].

Atopic dermatitis (AD) is a chronic or chronically relapsing, eczematous, and severely pruritic skin disorder. The lesional skin of AD exhibits Th2-deviated immune reactions such as those involving IL-4, IL-5, and IL-13, which contribute to the development of this disease [5]. It has been shown that the anti-IL-4 receptor alpha (IL-4RA) antibody dupilumab causes marked and rapid improvement in AD patients [6], indicating that IL-4 plays a critical role in AD development. A recent study has also shown that anti-IL-31 receptor alpha (IL-31RA) antibody treatment using nemolizumab produced clinical improvement of pruritus, subsequently contributing to the attenuation of AD disease activity [7]. The mechanism behind this is still not fully understood, but it has been shown that IL-31RA is expressed on sensory neurons and IL-31 derived from activated T cells under Th2-skewed conditions stimulates IL-31RA on sensory nerves, resulting in severe pruritus in AD [8]. Although IL-31/IL-31RA interaction has been identified as one of the key determinants of pruritus in AD, there are limited reports regarding the effect of IL-31/IL-31RA interaction on Th2-deviated immune conditions in AD [4,9]. It has been reported that transgenic mice overexpressing IL-31 develop AD-like skin lesions with severe pruritus [10]. In addition, the neutralization of IL-31 and genetic inhibition of EPAS1, a regulator of IL-31 induction in CD4+ T cells, have been reported to ameliorate AD-like skin lesions [11]. Therefore, IL-31/IL-31RA interaction is deeply involved in AD disease activity in addition to pruritus.

Given that (1) CCL 17 and CCL 22 chemoattract Th2 cells and maintain the Th2 immune response [12,13], (2) serum CCL 17 and CCL 22 levels are closely related to the disease activity of AD [14], and (3) Langerhans cells and dermal dendritic cells (DCs) produce prominent CCL 17 and CCL 22 in the skin of AD patients [12,15], we investigated whether IL-31/IL-31RA interaction affects CCL 17 and CCL 22 production in DCs during the development of AD. To test this, we analyzed murine bone marrow-derived DCs (BMDCs) treated with IL-4, which is thought to recapitulate the conditions of skin myeloid DCs in AD.

2. Results

2.1. IL-4 Stimulation Upregulated IL-31RA Expression in BMDCs

We first examined whether IL-4 stimulation upregulated IL-31RA expression in BMDCs. We analyzed BMDCs stimulated with IL-4 (0.1, 1, and 10 ng/mL) for 24 h. Quantitative reverse-transcription (qRT-PCR) analysis revealed that IL-4 stimulation upregulated IL-31RA expression at the mRNA level in a dose-dependent manner (Figure 1a). Flow cytometry analysis of BMDCs stimulated with IL-4 (10 ng/mL) for 24 h also showed that IL-4 stimulation upregulated IL-31RA expression at the protein level (Figure 1b). We also examined expression of OSMRβ, the other subunit of IL-31 receptor; however, it was not upregulated by IL-4 stimulation at the mRNA level (Figure 1c) in BMDCs stimulated with IL-4 (0.1, 1 and 10 ng/mL) for 24 h (Figure 1c).

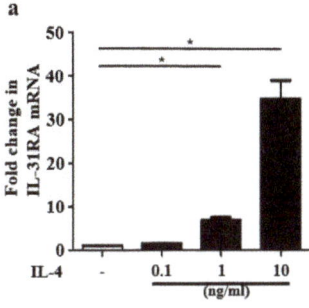
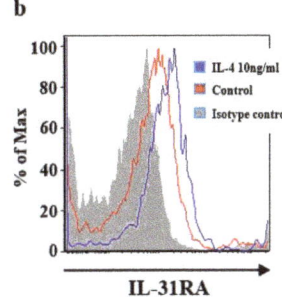
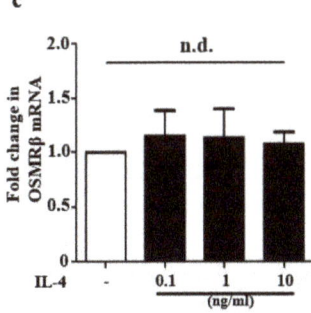

Figure 1. IL-4 stimulation upregulated IL-31RA expression in bone marrow-derived dendritic cells (BMDCs). (**a,c**) Data are expressed as mean ± standard error of the mean (S.E.M.); $n = 3$ for each group; * $p < 0.05$. Expression of IL-31RA (**a**) and OSMRβ (**c**) mRNA in BMDCs stimulated with IL-4 (0.1, 1 and 10 ng/mL) for 24 h. mRNA levels normalized for ACTB are expressed as fold induction compared with that in the control group. ACTB was utilized as a housekeeping gene. (**b**) BMDCs were treated with or without IL-4 (10 ng/mL) for 24 h. IL-31RA expression was evaluated using anti-murine IL-31RA antibody. Data are representative of experiments repeated three times with similar results.

2.2. IL-31 Stimulation Enhanced IL-4-Induced Ccl 17 and Ccl 22 Production in BMDCs

In addition to our previous report [15] describing that IL-4 stimulation induced Ccl 17 and Ccl 22 production in BMDCs, we next examined how IL-31 stimulation affects Ccl 17 and Ccl 22 production. We analyzed Ccl 17 and Ccl 22 expression in BMDCs stimulated with or without IL-4 (10 ng/mL) and IL-31 (50 and 100 ng/mL) for 24 h. qRT-PCR analysis showed that IL-31 stimulation alone (50 and 100 ng/mL) did not induce upregulation of Ccl 17 and Ccl 22 mRNA expression. Alternatively, IL-31 (50 and 100 ng/mL) with IL-4 (10 ng/mL) stimulation enhanced expression of Ccl 17 and Ccl 22 rather than IL-4 alone at the mRNA level (Figure 2a,c). ELISA analysis of the culture medium of BMDCs stimulated with IL-31 (50 and 100 ng/mL) with IL-4 (10 ng/mL) for 48 h also showed that IL-31 (50 and 100 ng/mL) with IL-4 (10 ng/mL) stimulation enhanced production of Ccl 17 and Ccl 22 rather than IL-4 alone at the protein level (Figure 2b,d). These results suggest that IL-4-induced IL-31RA upregulation is functional through IL-31/IL-31RA interaction, which leads to the enhanced production of Ccl 17 and Ccl 22 in BMDCs. Since another previous report stimulation with a high concentration (250 ng/mL) of IL-31 led to CCL22 production in human monocyte-derived DCs [16], we examined whether IL-31 stimulation (250 ng/mL) affects Ccl 22 expression. In our study, IL-31 stimulation alone (250 ng/mL) did not induce upregulation of Ccl 22 expression at the mRNA level (Figure S1a) and the protein level (Figure S1b), in BMDCs.

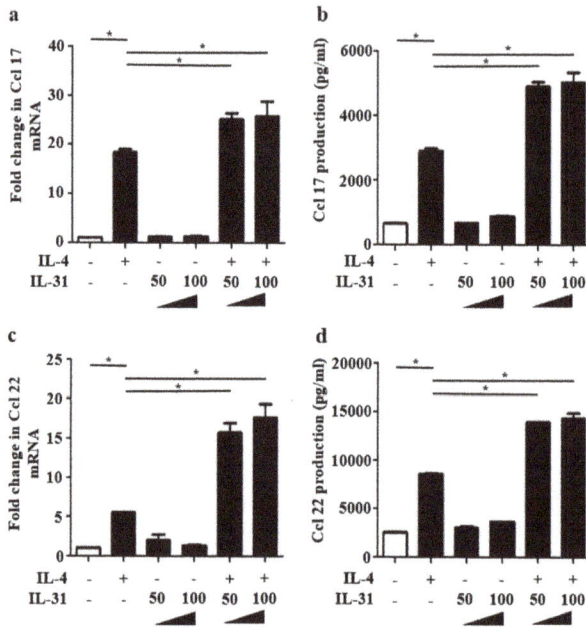

Figure 2. IL-31 stimulation enhanced IL-4-induced Ccl 17 and Ccl 22 production in BMDCs. (**a–d**) Data are expressed as mean ± standard error of the mean (S.E.M.); $n = 3$ for each group; * $p < 0.05$. Expression of Ccl 17 (a) and Ccl 22 (c) mRNA in BMDCs stimulated with or without IL-4 (10 ng/mL) and IL-31 (50 and 100 ng/mL) for 48 h and production of Ccl 17 (b) and Ccl 22 (d) in the culture supernatant were measured.

2.3. Glyteer Treatment Inhibited IL-4-Induced IL-31RA Expression in BMDCs

Since we previously reported that Glyteer treatment impairs the IL-4/STAT6 signaling pathway in BMDCs [15] and human keratinocytes [17], we examined whether Glyteer treatment also inhibits IL-31RA expression induced by IL-4 stimulation in BMDCs. We analyzed BMDCs stimulated with IL-4 (10 ng/mL) for 24 h in the presence or absence of Glyteer (10^{-5}, 10^{-6}, and 10^{-7}%). qRT-PCR analysis showed that Glyteer treatment inhibited IL-4-induced IL-31RA expression at the mRNA level in a dose-dependent manner (Figure 3a). Flow cytometry analysis of BMDCs stimulated with IL-4 (10 ng/mL) for 24 h in the presence or absence of Glyteer (10^{-5}%) also showed that IL-31RA-positive cells increased upon stimulation with IL-4 (10 ng/mL), compared with that in the control group, which was inhibited by Glyteer treatment (10^{-5}%) (around the area indicated by a white arrow).

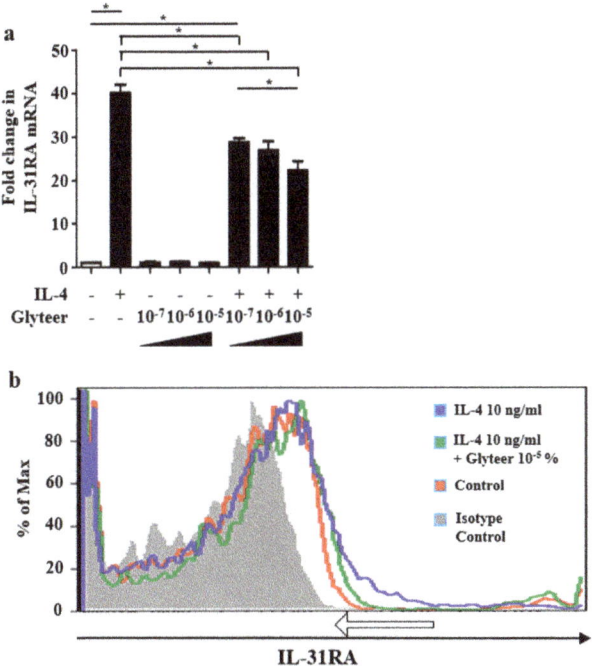

Figure 3. Glyteer impaired IL-4-induced IL-31RA expression. (**a**) Data are expressed as mean ± standard error of the mean (S.E.M.); $n = 3$ for each group; * $p < 0.05$. Expression of IL-31RA mRNA in BMDCs stimulated with or without IL-4 (10 ng/mL) and Glyteer (10^{-7}, 10^{-6} and 10^{-5}%) for 24 h. (**b**) BMDCs were treated with or without IL-4 (10 ng/mL) and Glyteer (10^{-5}%) for 24 h. IL-31RA expression was evaluated using anti-murine IL-31RA antibody. IL-31RA-positive cells increased upon stimulation with IL-4 (10 ng/mL), compared with that in the control group, which was inhibited by Glyteer treatment (10–5%) (around the area indicated by a white arrow). Data is representative of experiments repeated three times with similar results.

2.4. Glyteer Treatment Inhibited IL-4- and IL-31-Induced Ccl 17 and Ccl 22 Production in BMDCs

To further confirm the inhibitory effects of Glyteer treatment, we examined whether the enhancement of Ccl 17 and Ccl 22 production by IL-31 with IL-4 stimulation was inhibited in BMDCs. We analyzed Ccl 17 and Ccl 22 expression in BMDCs stimulated with or without IL-4 (10 ng/mL) and IL-31 (50 and 100 ng/mL) for 24 h in the presence or absence of Glyteer (10^{-5}, 10^{-6} and 10^{-7}%). qRT-PCR analysis showed that Glyteer treatment inhibited the upregulation of Ccl 17 and Ccl 22 induced by IL-4 stimulation at the mRNA level (Figure 4a,c). ELISA analysis of the culture medium of BMDCs stimulated with or without IL-4 (10 ng/mL) and IL-31 (50 and 100 ng/mL) for 48 h in the presence or absence of Glyteer (10^{-5}, 10^{-6} and 10^{-7}%) also showed that Glyteer treatment inhibited the upregulation of Ccl 17 and Ccl 22 induced by IL-4 stimulation at the protein level (Figure 4b,d). These results are already proven in our previous report [15]. Furthermore, Glyteer treatment inhibited the upregulation of Ccl 17 and Ccl 22 by IL-31 with IL-4 stimulation at the mRNA level (Figure 4a,c) and the protein level (Figure 4b,d) in a dose-dependent manner.

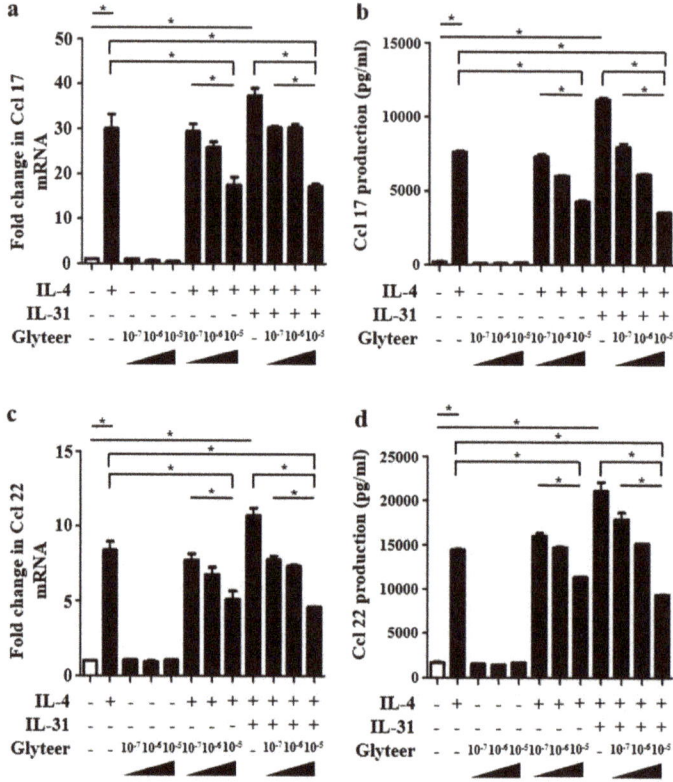

Figure 4. Glyteer impaired IL-4 with IL-31-induced Ccl 17 and Ccl 22 production in BMDCs. (**a**–**d**) Data are expressed as mean ± standard error of the mean (S.E.M.); $n = 3$ for each group; * $p < 0.05$. Expression of Ccl 17 (**a**) and Ccl 22 (**c**) mRNA in BMDCs stimulated with or without IL-4 (10 ng/mL), IL-31 (100 ng/mL), and Glyteer (10^{-7}, 10^{-6} and 10^{-5}%) for 48 h and production of Ccl 17 (**b**) and Ccl 22 (**d**) in the culture supernatant were measured.

3. Discussion

Although it has been reported that the IFN-γ/STAT1 signal mediates IL-31RA expression in DCs [16], whether Th2 cytokines such as IL-4 and IL-13 can upregulate IL-31RA expression in DCs has not been examined. Since recent studies have shown that IL-31 and its interaction with IL-31RA play a crucial role in the development of AD [7,11], clarifying the regulatory mechanism of IL-31RA expression under Th2-deviated conditions is very useful for treating AD. The present study has shown for the first time that IL-4 stimulation is capable of upregulating IL-31RA in BMDCs, which is consistent with a previous report describing that either IL-4 or IL-13 can upregulate IL-31RA via Stat6 in murine macrophages [4].

To further determine whether the IL-4-induced IL-31RA is functional, we stimulated IL-4-treated BMDCs with IL-31. This IL-31 stimulation without IL-4 treatment did not induce Ccl 17 and Ccl 22 production, indicating that the upregulation of IL-31RA expression is required for Ccl 17 and Ccl 22 production induced by IL-31, which is partially consistent with a previous report describing that CCL 17 is not produced by IL-31-stimulated human DCs [16]. Nevertheless, the IL-31 stimulation with IL-4 treatment enhanced Ccl 17 and Ccl 22 production compared with IL-4 treatment alone. These findings suggest that a Th2-prone immune condition including IL-4 treatment augments IL-31/IL-31RA interaction, which enhances Ccl 17 and Ccl 22 production and subsequently exacerbates the disease activity of AD.

The mechanism by which IL-31 stimulation enhances IL-4-induced Ccl 17 and Ccl 22 production remains incompletely understood. Several studies have reported that IL-31/IL-31RA interaction mediates STAT1/3/5 and MAP kinase activation [18,19]. Based on the evidence (1) that STAT1 activation induces CCL 17 and CCL 22 in HaCaT cells (human keratinocytes) [20], and (2) that the inhibition of MAP kinase activation reduces CCL 17 and CCL 22 production in HaCaT cells [21], multiple pathway signal transduction such as STAT1/3 and MAP kinase induced by the IL-31/IL-31RA interaction may be involved in the enhancement of Ccl 17 and Ccl 22 production by IL-31 stimulation. However, further studies are required to confirm this.

Since Glyteer inhibits IL-4-induced upregulation of IL-31 RA expression and IL-4-induced Ccl 17 and Ccl 22 production in BMDCs, the dual effects of Glyteer on IL-31RA expression and Ccl 17 and Ccl 22 production contribute to its inhibition of Ccl 17 and Ccl 22 production in AD. These findings suggest that Glyteer treatment potentiates the efficiency of nemolizumab, an IL-31 receptor α-antagonist, and dupilumab, an IL-4 receptor α-antagonist, in the treatment of AD. Nemolizumab has recently been used for the treatment of AD patients and shown to significantly improve clinical outcomes [7]. Although IL-31 is considered to be an important cytokine in the pruritus of AD, the present study revealed a new role of IL-31 in Th2-deviated immune conditions such as the production of CCL 17 and CCL 22 in AD.

In conclusion, we have demonstrated (i) that IL-31/IL-31RA interaction in dendritic cells under Th2-skewed conditions may increase the production of CCL17 and CCL22, contributing to the disease activity of AD, and (ii) that Glyteer treatment could have potential to prevent the production of CCL17 and CCL22 in AD (Figure 5). These findings should also promote our understanding of the roles of dendritic cell functions in AD.

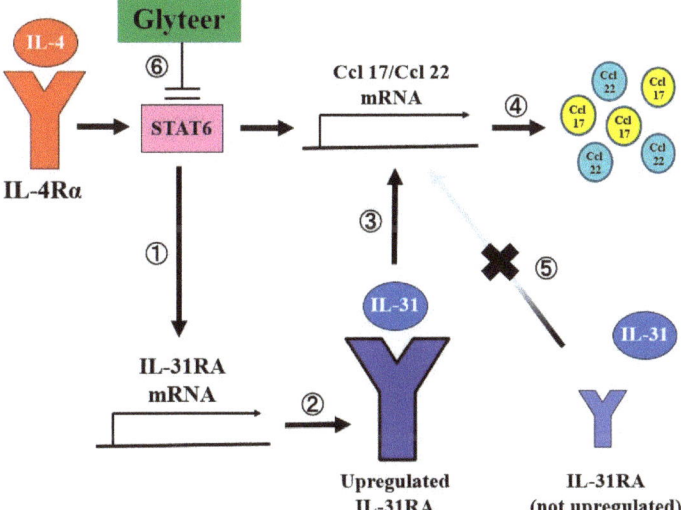

Figure 5. IL-4 augments IL-31/IL-31 RA interaction leading to enhanced Ccl 17 and Ccl 22 production in BMDCs. IL-4 induces upregulation of IL-31RA expression at the mRNA levels ① and the protein levels ②. IL-31RA expression initially upregulated by IL-4 stimulation can lead upregulation of Ccl 17 and Ccl 22 production at the mRNA levels ③ and the protein levels ④, whereas IL-31 stimulation alone without IL-31RA upregulation did not upregulate Ccl 17 and Ccl 22 production ⑤. Impairment of STAT6 signaling pathway activation by Glyteer ⑥ inhibits upregulation of IL-31RA expression and Ccl 17 and Ccl 22 production induced by IL-4 in BMDCs.

4. Materials and Methods

4.1. Reagents

DMSO was purchased from Sigma-Aldrich (St. Louis, MO, USA). Recombinant murine IL-31 and IL-4 were purchased from PeproTech (Rocky Hill, NJ, USA). Glyteer was provided by Fujinaga Pharm Co. Ltd. (Tokyo, Japan) as original sticky-liquid stock. Glyteer is generated from soybean as dry distillated tar after delipidation, which contains wide-ranged organic compounds such as polycyclic aromatic hydrocarbons. Since Glyteer is known to act as a potent AHR ligand, no farther investigations have been conducted to clarify the detailed bioactive components.

4.2. Generation of Bone Marrow-Derived DCs (BMDCs) and Cell Culture

C57BL/6J mice were housed and bred in a clean breeding facility, and the trial was approved by the animal facility of Kyushu University (A30-258-0, 20 Aug 2018–31 Mar 2020). Bone marrow cells were collected freshly from femoral and tibial bones of mice and cultured in RPMI 1640 medium (Sigma-Aldrich) containing 1 mmol/L sodium pyruvate (10 mL; Invitrogen, Waltham, MA, USA), 10 mmol/L 4-(2-hydroxyethyl)-1-piperazineethanesulfonic acid (HEPES) (10 mL; Invitrogen, Waltham, MA, USA), 1% Minimum Essential Medium Non-Essential Amino Acids (MEM NEAA) (10 mL; Invitrogen), 10% FBS (Japan Bio Serum, Fukuyama, Japan), β-mercaptoethanol (50 nmol/L; Invitrogen), 100 U/mL penicillin, and antibiotic-antimycotic 100× (5 mL; 100 mg/mL streptomycin, and 0.25 µg/mL amphotericin B; Invitrogen) with GM-CSF (10 ng/mL) (Miltenyi Biotec, Bergisch Gladbach, Germany). Medium was refreshed twice in 7 days. Non-adherent cells were collected on day 7, and cells were purified immunomagnetically by positive selection with CD11c (N418) MicroBeads (Miltenyi Biotec). Our previous study has reported that the purity of BMDCs was 95–97%, that was confirmed by flow cytometric analysis [15]. Purified BMDCs were cultured with/without stimulants such as IL-4 and IL-31, and/or Glyteer for 24 h or 48 h. Culture supernatants were collected for ELISA analysis. Cell pellets were utilized for qRT-PCR or FACS analysis. This method of generating BMDCs and cell culture matches that in our previous study [15].

4.3. Quantitative Reverse-Transcription (qRT)-PCR Analysis

Total RNA was extracted by using RNeasy® Mini Kit (Qiagen, Hilden, Germany), then reverse transcription for making cDNA was conducted by using PrimeScript™ RT reagent kit (Takara Bio, Kusatsu, Japan). qRT-PCR was performed on CFX Connect Real-time PCR Detection System (Bio-Rad, Hercules, CA, USA) using TB Green® Premix Ex Taq (Takara Bio, Kusatsu, Japan). Amplification was launched as the first step at 95 °C for 30 s, then followed by 40 cycles of qRT-PCR at 95 °C for 5 s and at 61 °C for 20 s as the second step. mRNA expression was measured with normalization by housekeeping gene using β-actin in triplicate, and the mRNA expressions were presented as the fold induction relative to the control group. Each primer sequences are shown in Table 1.

Table 1. The sequences of primers.

Gene		Sequence (5′ to 3′)
β-actin	forward	GGCTGTATTCCCCTCCATCG
	reverse	CCAGTTGGTAACAATGCCATGT
Ccl17	forward	AGGTCACTTCAGATGCTGCTC
	reverse	ACTCTCGGCCTACATTGGTG
Ccl22	forward	GACACCTGACGAGGACACA
	reverse	GCAGAGGGTGACGGATGTAG
IL-31RA	forward	CGATTGTTGTGGAAGAAGGCAA
	reverse	TACTGCTGGGTGGTGATGTTG
OSMRβ	forward	CAGGCGGGTAATCAGACCAATG
	reverse	CATGAGTAAGGGCTGGGACA

4.4. ELISA

Murine Ccl 17 and Ccl 22 ELISA Kit (R&D Systems, Minneapolis, MN, USA) was utilized to measure production of Ccl 17 and Ccl 22 following the manufacturer's protocol. Absorbance of the wells of the ELISA plate was measured using DTX 800 Multimode Detector (Beckman Coulter).

4.5. Fluorescence-Activated Cell Sorting (FACS) Analysis

LIVE/DEAD fixable dead cell staining kit (violet and near IR; Life Technologies) was used to detect dead cells. Then, BMDCs were incubated with anti-CD16/32 antibody (Becton Dickinson, Franklin Lakes, NJ, USA) for 30 min on ice. Anti-murine IL-31 RA antibody (Bioss Antibodies, Boston, MA, USA) was labeled with Zenon R-Phycoerythrin (PE) Rabbit IgG Labeling Kit (Thermo Fisher Scientific, Waltham, MA, USA), in accordance with the manufacturer's protocol. IL-31RA was stained with PE-conjugated anti-murine IL-31RA antibody. Isotype-matched antibodies were used as controls. Stained cells were analyzed on a BD Canto flow cytometer (Becton Dickinson). Stained cells were also observed using a D-Eclipse confocal laser scanning microscope (Nikon, Tokyo, Japan).

4.6. Statistical Analysis

Two-sample Student's *t* test was used for statistical evaluation of the results. A *p*-value of <0.05 was considered to show a statistically significant difference. All data are presented as mean ± standard error of the mean (S.E.M.) from three independent experiments.

Supplementary Materials: Supplementary materials can be found at http://www.mdpi.com/1422-0067/20/16/4053/s1.

Author Contributions: S.M., G.T., M.T., A.H.-H., and Y.H.V. performed the experiments. S.M., G.T., M.F. and T.N. designed the experimental protocol and wrote this manuscript.

Funding: This work was partly supported by grants from the Ministry of Health, Labor and Welfare, Japan, and JSPS KAKENHI (Grant number: JP17K10213).

Conflicts of Interest: The authors declare no conflicts of interest.

References

1. Dillon, S.R.; Sprecher, C.; Hammond, A.; Bilsborough, J.; Rosenfeld-Franklin, M.; Presnell, S.R.; Haugen, H.S.; Maurer, M.; Harder, B.; Johnston, J.; et al. Interleukin 31, a Cytokine Produced by Activated T Cells, Induces Dermatitis in Mice. *Nat. Immunol.* **2004**, *5*, 752–760. [CrossRef] [PubMed]
2. Zhang, Q.; Putheti, P.; Zhou, Q.; Liu, Q.; Gao, W. Structures and Biological Functions of IL-31 and IL-31 Receptors. *Cytokine Growth Factor Rev.* **2008**, *19*, 347–356. [CrossRef] [PubMed]
3. Stott, B.; Lavender, P.; Lehmann, S.; Pennino, D.; Durham, S.; Schmidt-Weber, C.B. Human IL-31 is Induced by IL-4 and Promotes TH2-driven Inflammation. *J. Allergy Clin. Immunol.* **2013**, *132*, 446–454.e5. [CrossRef] [PubMed]
4. Edukulla, R.; Singh, B.; Jegga, A.G.; Sontake, V.; Dillon, S.R.; Madala, S.K. Th2 Cytokines Augment IL-31/IL-31RA Interactions via STAT6-dependent IL-31RA Expression. *J. Biol. Chem.* **2015**, *290*, 13510–13520. [CrossRef] [PubMed]
5. Furue, M.; Chiba, T.; Tsuji, G.; Ulzii, D.; Kido-Nakahara, M.; Nakahara, T.; Kadono, T. Atopic Dermatitis: Immune Deviation, Barrier Dysfunction, IgE Autoreactivity and New Therapies. *Allergol. Int.* **2017**, *66*, 398–403. [CrossRef] [PubMed]
6. Simpson, E.L.; Bieber, T.; Guttman-Yassky, E.; Beck, L.A.; Blauvelt, A.; Cork, M.J.; Silverberg, J.I.; Deleuran, M.; Kataoka, Y.; Lacour, J.P.; et al. Two Phase 3 Trials of Dupilumab Versus Placebo in Atopic Dermatitis. *N. Engl. J. Med.* **2016**, *375*, 2335–2348. [CrossRef] [PubMed]
7. Ruzicka, T.; Hanifin, J.M.; Furue, M.; Pulka, G.; Mlynarczyk, I.; Wollenberg, A.; Galus, R.; Etoh, T.; Mihara, R.; Yoshida, H.; et al. Anti-Interleukin-31 Receptor A Antibody for Atopic Dermatitis. *N. Engl. J. Med.* **2017**, *376*, 826–835. [CrossRef] [PubMed]

8. Cevikbas, F.; Wang, X.; Akiyama, T.; Kempkes, C.; Savinko, T.; Antal, A.; Kukova, G.; Buhl, T.; Ikoma, A.; Buddenkotte, J.; et al. A Sensory Neuron-expressed IL-31 Receptor Mediates T Helper Cell-dependent Itch: Involvement of TRPV1 and TRPA1. *J. Allergy Clin. Immunol.* **2014**, *133*, 448–460. [CrossRef]
9. Kato, A.; Fujii, E.; Watanabe, T.; Takashima, Y.; Matsushita, H.; Furuhashi, T.; Morita, A. Distribution of IL-31 and its Receptor Expressing Cells in Skin of Atopic Dermatitis. *J. Dermatol. Sci.* **2014**, *74*, 229–235. [CrossRef]
10. Feld, M.; Garcia, R.; Buddenkotte, J.; Katayama, S.; Lewis, K.; Muirhead, G.; Hevezi, P.; Plesser, K.; Schrumpf, H.; Krjutskov, K.; et al. The Pruritus- and TH2-associated Cytokine IL-31 Promotes Growth of Sensory Nerves. *J. Allergy Clin. Immunol.* **2016**, *138*, 500–508.e24. [CrossRef]
11. Yamamura, K.; Uruno, T.; Shiraishi, A.; Tanaka, Y.; Ushijima, M.; Nakahara, T.; Watanabe, M.; Kido-Nakahara, M.; Tsuge, I.; Furue, M.; et al. The Transcription Factor EPAS1 Links DOCK8 Deficiency to Atopic Skin Inflammation via IL-31 Induction. *Nat. Commun.* **2017**, *8*, 13946. [CrossRef] [PubMed]
12. Stutte, S.; Quast, T.; Gerbitzki, N.; Savinko, T.; Novak, N.; Reifenberger, J.; Homey, B.; Kolanus, W.; Alenius, H.; Förster, I. Requirement of CCL17 for CCR7- and CXCR4-dependent Migration of Cutaneous Dendritic Cells. *Proc. Natl. Acad. Sci. USA* **2010**, *107*, 8736–8741. [CrossRef] [PubMed]
13. Kataoka, Y. Thymus and Activation-regulated Chemokine as a Clinical Biomarker in Atopic Dermatitis. *J. Dermatol.* **2014**, *41*, 221–229. [CrossRef] [PubMed]
14. Hashimoto, S.; Nakamura, K.; Oyama, N.; Kaneko, F.; Tsunemi, Y.; Saeki, H.; Tamaki, K. Macrophage-derived Chemokine (MDC)/CCL22 Produced by Monocyte Derived Dendritic Cells Reflects the Disease Activity in Patients with Atopic Dermatitis. *J. Dermatol. Sci.* **2006**, *44*, 93–99, Epub Sep 27, 2006. [CrossRef] [PubMed]
15. Takemura, M.; Nakahara, T.; Hashimoto-Hachiya, A.; Furue, M.; Tsuji, G. Glyteer, Soybean Tar, Impairs IL-4/Stat6 Signaling in Murine Bone Marrow-Derived Dendritic Cells: The Basis of Its Therapeutic Effect on Atopic Dermatitis. *Int. J. Mol. Sci.* **2018**, *19*, 1169. [CrossRef] [PubMed]
16. Horejs-Hoeck, J.; Schwarz, H.; Lamprecht, S.; Maier, E.; Hainzl, S.; Schmittner, M.; Posselt, G.; Stoecklinger, A.; Hawranek, T.; Duschl, A. Dendritic Cells Activated by IFN-γ/STAT1 Express IL-31 Receptor and Release Proinflammatory Mediators upon IL-31 Treatment. *J. Immunol.* **2012**, *188*, 5319–5326. [CrossRef] [PubMed]
17. Takei, K.; Mitoma, C.; Hashimoto-Hachiya, A.; Uchi, H.; Takahara, M.; Tsuji, G.; Kido-Nakahara, M.; Nakahara, T.; Furue, M. Antioxidant Soybean Tar Glyteer Rescues T-helper-mediated Downregulation of Filaggrin Expression via Aryl Hydrocarbon Receptor. *J. Dermatol.* **2015**, *42*, 171–180. [CrossRef]
18. Dambacher, J.; Beigel, F.; Seiderer, J.; Haller, D.; Göke, B.; Auernhammer, C.J.; Brand, S. Interleukin 31 Mediates MAP Kinase and STAT1/3 Activation in Intestinal Epithelial Cells and its Expression is Upregulated in Inflammatory Bowel Disease. *Gut* **2007**, *56*, 1257–1265. [CrossRef]
19. Kasraie, S.; Niebuhr, M.; Werfel, T. Interleukin (IL)-31 Activates Signal Transducer and Activator of Transcription (STAT)-1, STAT-5, and Extracellular Signal-regulated Kinase 1/2 and Down-regulates IL-12p40 Production in Activated Human Macrophages. *Allergy* **2013**, *68*, 739–747. [CrossRef]
20. Kwon, D.J.; Bae, Y.S.; Ju, S.M.; Goh, A.R.; Youn, G.S.; Choi, S.Y.; Park, J. Casuarinin Suppresses TARC/CCL17 and MDC/CCL22 Production via Blockade of NF-κB and STAT1 Activation in HaCaT Cells. *Biochem. Biophys. Res. Commun.* **2012**, *417*, 1254–1259. [CrossRef]
21. Yano, C.; Saeki, H.; Komine, M.; Kagami, S.; Tsunemi, Y.; Ohtsuki, M.; Nakagawa, H. Mechanism of Macrophage-Derived Chemokine/CCL22 Production by HaCaT Keratinocytes. *Ann. Dermatol.* **2015**, *27*, 152–156. [CrossRef] [PubMed]

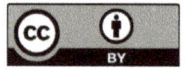

© 2019 by the authors. Licensee MDPI, Basel, Switzerland. This article is an open access article distributed under the terms and conditions of the Creative Commons Attribution (CC BY) license (http://creativecommons.org/licenses/by/4.0/).

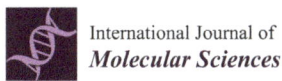

Article

Butyric Acid from Probiotic *Staphylococcus epidermidis* in the Skin Microbiome Down-Regulates the Ultraviolet-Induced Pro-Inflammatory IL-6 Cytokine via Short-Chain Fatty Acid Receptor

Sunita Keshari [1], Arun Balasubramaniam [2], Binderiya Myagmardoloonjin [2], Deron Raymond Herr [3], Indira Putri Negari [2] and Chun-Ming Huang [2,4,*]

1. Department of Life Sciences, National Central University, Taoyuan 32001, Taiwan
2. Department of Biomedical Sciences and Engineering, National Central University, Taoyuan 32001, Taiwan
3. Department of Pharmacology, National University of Singapore, Singapore 117600, Singapore
4. Department of Dermatology, School of Medicine, University of California, San Diego, CA 92093, USA
* Correspondence: chunming@ncu.edu.tw; Tel.: +886-3-422-7151 (ext. 36101); Fax: +886-3-425-3427

Received: 11 August 2019; Accepted: 9 September 2019; Published: 11 September 2019

Abstract: The glycerol fermentation of probiotic *Staphylococcus epidermidis* (*S. epidermidis*) in the skin microbiome produced butyric acid in vitro at concentrations in the millimolar range. The exposure of dorsal skin of mice to ultraviolet B (UVB) light provoked a significant increased production of pro-inflammatory interleukin (IL)-6 cytokine. Topical application of butyric acid alone or *S. epidermidis* with glycerol remarkably ameliorated the UVB-induced IL-6 production. In vivo knockdown of short-chain fatty acid receptor 2 (FFAR2) in mouse skin considerably blocked the probiotic effect of *S. epidermidis* on suppression of UVB-induced IL-6 production. These results demonstrate that butyric acid in the metabolites of fermenting skin probiotic bacteria mediates FFAR2 to modulate the production of pro-inflammatory cytokines induced by UVB.

Keywords: butyric acid; microbiome; probiotic; *S. epidermidis*; UVB

---

1. Introduction

Skin is a fundamental component of the innate immune system, providing a protective barrier against the penetration of microorganisms and preventing environmental damage to the body. Exposure to UV is known to induce clustering of specific cell-surface receptors, resulting in the activation of signal transduction pathways [1]. Prolonged exposure of ultraviolet B (UVB) with a wavelength of 280–320 nm is a significant risk factor causing chronic inflammation, DNA damage, and lipid peroxidation in the epidermis [2]. Chronic exposure to this cellular stressor commonly results in skin pathologies such as epidermal hyperplasia, erythema, and edema [3]. Within the skin epidermis, keratinocytes have been found to play a critical role in the response to photo-damage to UVB by releasing key inflammatory mediators such as interleukin (IL)-1, -6, -8, -10 and tumor necrosis factor (TNF). Among these, keratinocyte-derived IL-1 and IL-6 seem to be of particular importance [4]. Many studies have demonstrated that both human and murine keratinocytes produce these cytokines because of UV exposure [5,6]. Continuous exposure to UV results in the generation of reactive oxygen species (ROS), exposing a variety of biomolecules to oxidative stress. This leads to damage of biological structures, contributes to cellular injury, and ultimately resulting in tissue destruction [7].

The skin microbiome consists of a complex community of organisms that mediates essential physiological and pathological processes. Among these organisms, *Staphylococcus epidermidis* (*S. epidermidis*) is the predominant commensal bacterial species that colonizes normal human skin [8]. Derangement of the bacterial milieu can alter epidermal function, and thus, disrupt the local ecology of the skin [9]. This interplay of microbe and host appears to be critical for establishing homeostasis. S. epidermidis has also been shown to benefit the skin immune function by diminishing inflammation after injury [10]. Study have shown that 6-N-hydroxyaminopurine, a metabolite from S. epidermidis could selectively inhibit UV induced skin tumors in mice [11]. Additionally, studies have provided evidence that peptides and other metabolites produced from S. epidermidis, might also act as antimicrobial agents and contribute to normal defense at the epidermal interface [12,13]. In the current study, we demonstrate that butyric acid, one of the major metabolites produced by S. epidermidis fermentation, attenuates the UVB-induced production of inflammatory cytokines by interacting with cognate receptors expressed by keratinocytes. This suggests that manipulation of the S. epidermidis-butyric acid-FFAR2 axis is a potential therapeutic target to protect against skin inflammatory diseases.

2. Results

2.1. S. epidermidis Mediates Glycerol Fermentation and Acetolactate Synthase (ALS) Activity

To investigate whether S. epidermidis (ATCC 12228) can ferment glycerol, S. epidermidis (10^7 colony-forming unit (CFU) were incubated with and without glycerol (2%) in rich media with phenol red for 12 h. Uninoculated rich media containing phenol red with glycerol served as controls. Phenol red was used as an indicator to monitor bacterial fermentation. In rich media incubated with bacteria, the color of phenol red changed from red to orange because of the bacterial replication during incubation. However, in agreement with earlier results, the rich media containing bacteria along with glycerol, the phenol red color changed from red to yellow indicating the use of glycerol as a carbon source for fermentation by S. epidermidis after 12 h culture (Figure 1a) [13–15]. The color change of phenol red was quantified by measuring the optical density at 560 nm (OD_{560}) (Figure 1b). Furthermore, OD_{560nm} in rich media with S. epidermidis and glycerol was significantly lower than that in rich media with S. epidermidis alone (Figure 1a). Next, to confirm the fermentation activity of S. epidermidis using glycerol as a carbon source, we added furfural, a potent fermentation inhibitor [16], in rich media containing S. epidermidis and glycerol. Media with and without S. epidermidis, glycerol and furfural were used as controls. We did not detect any color change in the media incubated with S. epidermidis with furfural in the presence or absence of glycerol (Figure 1a). Additionally, the OD_{560nm} was comparable to the control group containing media only, or media with furfural, or media with glycerol. This indicates that the fermentation or metabolic activity of S. epidermidis might have been inhibited by furfural (Figure 1b). Microbial enzymes are found to be the major source of bacterial fermentation by catalyzing the hydrolysis of starch or peptides. Moreover, a recent study reported that acetolactate synthase (ALS) is a crucial enzyme in Staphylococcus aureus (S. aureus) which converts pyruvate into α-acetolactate, promoting the production of branched-chain amino acids (BCAA) and playing an important role in the activation of the tricarboxylic acid (TCA) cycle [17]. It also promotes anaerobic fermentation in Bacillius subtilis (B. subtilis) by converting two molecules of pyruvate to form acetolactate, functioning as a key regulatory enzyme in fermentation [18]. Reports also demonstrated that furfural exerts its inhibitory effects on microbial fermentation via interfering with the activities of enzymes in the pathways of microbial fermentation [19]. We confirmed that the ALS enzyme activity of S. epidermidis is significantly reduced when it is incubated with furfural (inhibitor) (Figure 1c). Taken together, we confirmed that S. epidermidis induced glycerol fermentation, which required furfural-sensitive ALS activity.

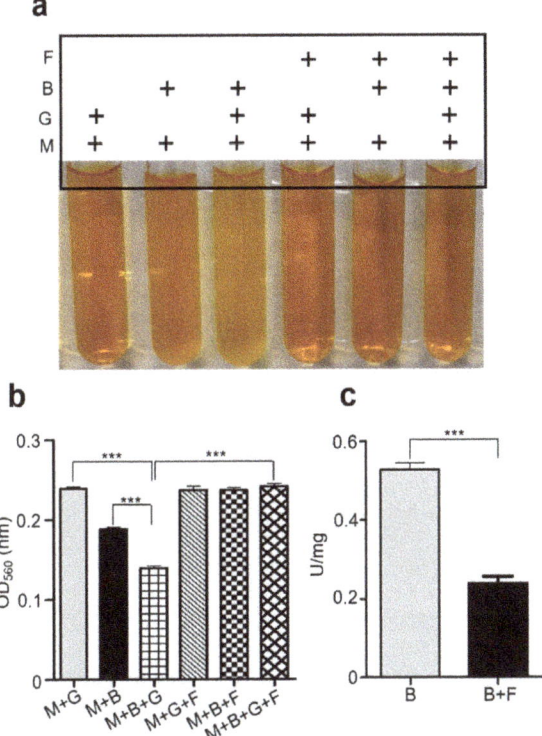

Figure 1. *S. epidermidis* mediates glycerol fermentation by ALS (acetolactate synthase) enzyme activity. (**a**) *S. epidermidis* bacteria (B) (10^7 CFU/mL) were incubated in rich media (M) containing phenol red with or without 2% glycerol (G) and in the presence and absence of fermentation inhibitor furfural (F) for 12 h. Media with glycerol (M + G), bacteria (M + B), furfural (M + F), glycerol plus furfural (M + G + F), or bacteria plus furfural (M + B + F) were taken as controls. Bacterial fermentation was indicated by the color change of phenol red to yellow (arrow). (**b**) A graph showing the OD_{560} value in all the above groups. (**c**) ALS activity by furfural. The reaction mixture containing lysates of *S. epidermidis* bacteria (B) (10^7 CFU/mL) was incubated with and without furfural (F). The activity (U/mg) of ALS in *S. epidermidis* bacteria was quantified. Data shown represent the mean ± SE of experiment performed in triplicate. *** $p < 0.001$ (two-tailed *t*-test).

2.2. Butyric Acid, a Product in Fermented Media upon Glycerol Fermentation by *S. epidermidis*

Previous studies have detected the presence of multiple short-chain fatty acids (SCFAs) such as acetic acid, butyric acid, lactic acid, and succinic in fermented media of *S. epidermidis* from glycerol fermentation [13]. Butyric acid from *S. epidermidis* was found to exert growth suppressive effects on USA300, a community-associated methicillin-resistant *S. aureus* (MRSA). Moreover, it shows potent anti-inflammatory activity in skin keratinocytes by effectively inhibiting histone deacetylase (HDAC) [20,21]. In the current study, we have screened the supernatant following glycerol fermentation of *S. epidermidis* to quantify their butyric acid producing capacity by high-performance liquid chromatography-ultraviolet (HPLC-UV) analysis. Butyric acid was detected as a sharp specific peak in the HPLC chromatogram and was determined to be at a concentration of 6 mM in the fermented media by comparison to a butyric acid standard curve (Figure 2a,b).

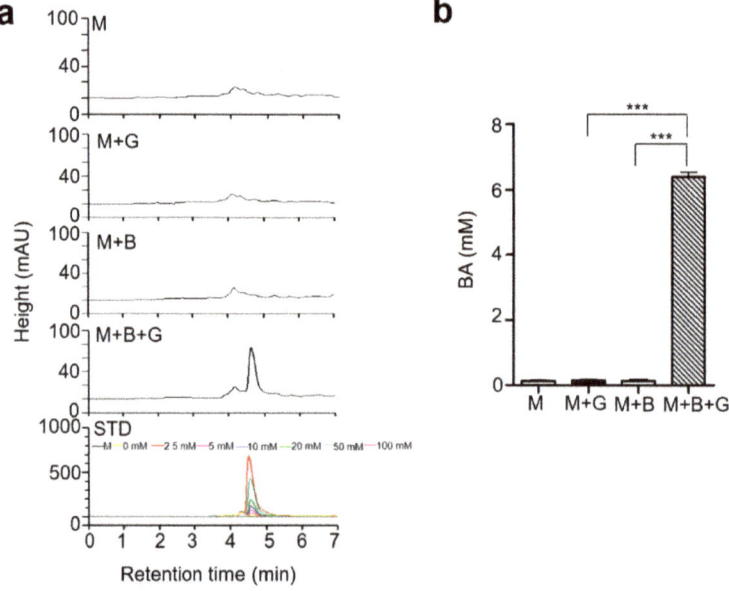

Figure 2. High-performance liquid chromatography-ultraviolet (HPLC-UV) analysis of the butyric acid. The fermented media from glycerol (G) fermentation by *S. epidermidis* bacteria (B) analyzed by HPLC. (**a**) Chromatograph of only media (M), media with glycerol (M + G), media with bacteria (M + B), and media with bacteria plus glycerol (M + B + G). The x-axis is retention time in minutes, and the y-axis is the milli-absorbance unit at 210 nm. (**b**) The concentrations of BA (butyric acid) was quantified from the height of butyric acid standard (STD) peaks. Data shown represent the mean ± SE of experiment performed in triplicate. *** $p < 0.0001$ (two-tailed *t*-test).

2.3. Mixture of S. epidermidis and Glycerol or Butyric Acid alone Inhibited UVB Induced Skin Inflammation

Exposure to prolonged UVB radiation is deleterious to human skin, which may lead to expression and secretion of pro-inflammatory cytokines such as IL-6 in human keratinocytes [22]. Furthermore, chronic UVB is responsible for epidermal hyperplasia. The dorsal skin of the Institute of Cancer Research (ICR) mice were shaved and exposed to 12 doses of UVB (195 mJ/cm^2) over 4 weeks concurrent with 4 topical applications of a mixture of *S. epidermidis* (10^7) and glycerol (2%) in phosphate-buffered saline (PBS) over the same time period. Mice topically applied with mixture of *S. epidermidis* (10^7) and glycerol (2%) in PBS with no UVB exposure were included as control. The dorsal skin of mice was photographed to measure the wound healing from 0, 16, and 30 days. Mice from all groups were sacrificed on the 30th day and skin samples were lysed to extract total protein. In mice treated with either PBS, *S. epidermidis*, or glycerol alone, variable lesions were recorded which started from edema, redness, and ulceration of the UVB exposed area and ended with thickening of the skin. However, in mice that received topical applications of *S. epidermidis* and glycerol, a comparatively lower level of erythema and ulceration were observed on UVB-exposed skin on day 16. Further improvement was noticed on day 30, signifying maximum recovery from UVB damage (Figure 3a,b) compared to non-exposed groups (Figure S1a). Upregulated levels of IL-6 and noticeable epidermal hyperplasia (as quantified by epidermal thickness) were detected in mice skin topically applied with PBS, *S. epidermidis*, or glycerol alone following UVB exposure because of an increase in the number of keratinocytes and epidermal layers. By contrast, in the *S. epidermidis* plus glycerol treated group, IL-6 levels were significantly reduced (Figure 3c) compared to non-exposed groups (Figure S1b) and the skin remained almost completely intact, showing a marked attenuation of UVB-induced skin thickening

(Figure S3a,b). This indicates that metabolites from glycerol fermentation by *S. epidermidis* might induce anti-inflammatory activity against chronic UVB radiation. To further confirm the anti-inflammatory activity of *S. epidermidis* fermentation, another group of mice were topically applied with a mixture of *S. epidermidis* and glycerol along with fermentation inhibitor, furfural. UVB irradiation-induced skin lesions, elevation of IL-6, and epidermal hyperplasia were not ameliorated upon topical application of *S. epidermidis* plus glycerol and furfural compared to control group receiving water and furfural alone (Figure 3d and Figure S3c–f). However, significant recovery from inflammation was detected in mice topically applied with a mixture of *S. epidermidis* and glycerol. This was again accompanied by a downregulated level of IL-6 and decreased epidermal thickness, confirming that glycerol fermentation from *S. epidermidis* exerts anti-inflammatory activity. In the present study, we detected the production of butyric acid in significant amount as a metabolite in the fermentation of glycerol by *S. epidermidis*. Since butyric acid has been shown to be a potent anti-inflammatory agent in skin keratinocytes and has been tested for the attenuation of different inflammatory disorders [23,24], we first investigated its role against UVB induced inflammation in human keratinocytes (CCD 1106 KERTr). The human keratinocytes were irradiated with 195 mJ/cm^2 UVB and the IL-6 production was dramatically enhanced in water control group until 12 h after irradiation. However, the addition of BA (butyric acid, 4 mM), significantly reduced the upregulated level of IL-6 (Figure S2a). As studies mentioned, both IL-6 and IL-8 undoubtedly play pivotal roles in immunologic regulation in human skin and are involved in skin inflammation in response to UV radiation [25]. We have also detected the upregulated level of IL-8 in UVB exposed keratinocytes, which further rescued upon BA treatment (Figure S2b). Further, we detected effect of BA application upon UVB exposure in vivo. Our results show that topical application of 4 mM butyric acid ameliorated UVB-induced wound formation, and wound healing was mild to significant from day 16 to day 30 (Figure S3g,h). In a similar manner, IL-6 was downregulated and epidermal hyperplasia was diminished (Figure 3e and Figure S3i,j), which was consistent with the model that butyric acid is the active glycerol fermentation metabolite by which *S. epidermidis* can inhibit UV induced inflammation in the skin.

2.4. Knocking Down Free Fatty Acid Receptor 2 (FFAR2) Inhibited Butyric Acid Mediated Attenuation of Inflammation in Chronic UVB

Most beneficial roles of SCFAs in the gastrointestinal tract (GI) are mediated by directly activating its cognate G protein-coupled receptor, GPR43 (also known as FFAR2). For example, the chemoattractant and anti-inflammatory activities of butyrate in chondrocytes are completely mediated by its binding to GPR43 [26]. The activation of FFAR2 has emerged as a potentially important mechanism by which SCFAs could directly regulate the immune cells and the process of inflammatory diseases, thus drawing much attention in recent years [27,28]. Considering the key function of FFAR2 in inflammatory processes, blocking the signaling of this receptor by a selective inhibitor could be a useful approach to evaluate the role of butyric acid in the regulation of immune function in skin during chronic UVB exposure. In the present study, FFAR2 was inhibited by via gavage feeding of FFAR2 selective antagonist GLPG0974 (0.1–1 mg/kg) 20 min prior to topical application of butyric acid followed by UVB exposure. In addition, we have also blocked FFAR2 receptor via subcutaneous injection of FFAR2 siRNA (5 μM) into the dorsal skin of ICR mice 20 min prior to topical application of butyric acid followed by UVB exposure. In both conditions of blocking FFAR2, significant wound area and redness from UVB radiation was observed (Figure S4a,b,g,h) on mice dorsal skin, which further did not recover even after topical application of butyric acid. Inflammation, as detected by upregulation of IL-6 and epidermal hyperplasia, was increased in mice upon FFAR2 inhibition and further remained unchanged even on topical application of butyric acid compared to mice applied with butyric acid alone (Figure 4a,b and Figure S4c,d,i,j). We have also confirmed the FFAR2 inhibition or gene knockdown by measuring the protein expression level of FFAR2 by Western blot analysis and mRNA relative expression by RTPCR analysis (Figure S4e,f,k,l). Our overall results demonstrate an essential role of FFAR2/GPR43 in butyrate activity in UVB-induced chronic inflammation process. Butyrate reduced pro-inflammatory mediators IL-6, by binding to its FFAR2 receptor, which further inhibits the epidermal hyperplasia in chronic UVB exposure.

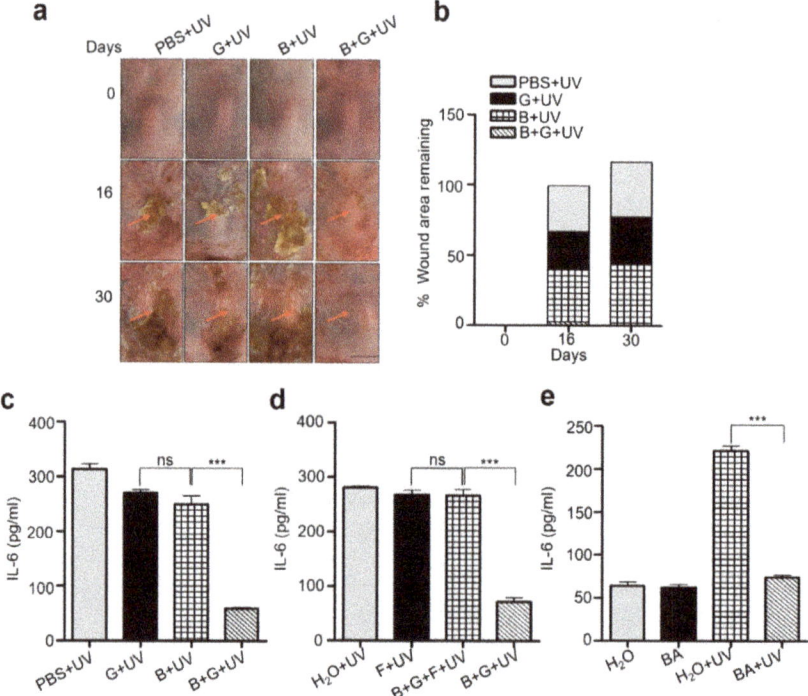

Figure 3. Attenuation of UVB induced inflammation by application of mixture of *S. epidermidis* and glycerol and its fermentation metabolite, butyric acid. (**a**) Skin morphology of ICR mice, topically applied with PBS, glycerol (G) (2%), *S. epidermidis* bacteria (B) (10^7 CFU/mL), or mixture of *S. epidermidis* bacteria plus glycerol (B + G) followed by exposure with UVB (195 mJ/cm^2) irradiation are shown at 0, 16, and 30 day. Skin lesions are indicated by red arrows. Scale bar = 5 mm. Graph (**b**) indicates percent wound area remaining of mice skin. The level of IL-6 in skin (**c**) from above all groups of ICR mice was quantified using a mouse IL-6 enzyme-linked immunosorbent assay (ELISA) kit (R&D Systems). (**d**) The IL-6 level in skin of ICR mice topically applied with H_2O, furfural (0.4%), *S. epidermidis* bacteria (B) (10^7 CFU/mL), glycerol (G) (2%) plus furfural (F) (0.4%), (B + G + F) or a mixture of *S. epidermidis* bacteria plus glycerol (B + G) followed by exposure with UVB (195 mJ/cm^2) irradiation is shown. (**e**) The IL-6 level in skin of ICR mice topically applied with H_2O and butyric acid (BA) (4 mM) followed by exposure with UVB (195 mJ/cm^2) irradiation is shown. Data are the means of three individual experiments using five mice per group. ns = non-significant. *** $p < 0.001$. (two-tailed *t*-tests).

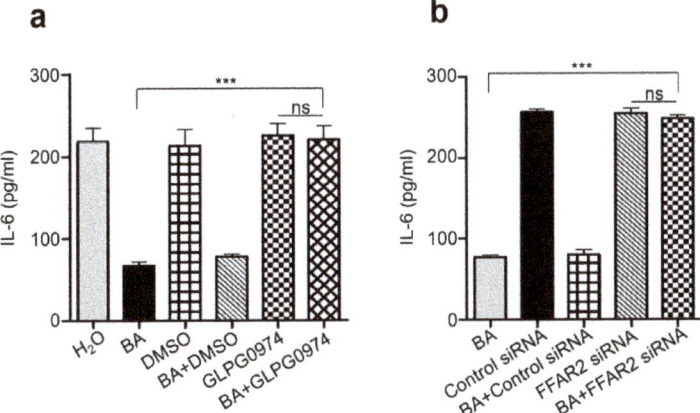

Figure 4. Blocking FFAR2 prevents the butyric acid mediated amelioration of inflammation. (**a**) The level of IL-6 in the dorsal skin of ICR mice upon gavage feeding of FFAR2 antagonist GLPG0974 dissolved in dimethyl sulfoxide (DMSO) in saline (0.01%) and topically applied butyric acid (BA) (4 mM) and was measured by ELISA. Mice fed with DMSO in saline and topically applied with H_2O were included as control. (**b**) The level of IL-6 in the dorsal skin of ICR mice subcutaneously injected with FFAR2 siRNA 10 min prior to topical application with butyric acid (BA) (4 mM) was measured by ELISA. Mice injected with scrambled or negative control siRNA and topically applied with H_2O were included as control. Data are the means of three separate experiments using five mice per group. ns = non-significant. *** $p < 0.001$. (two-tailed t-tests).

3. Discussion

Skin and its constituent epidermal keratinocytes make-up the outer most protective covering of the body, and as such, are the primary targets for solar UVB radiation. Exposure to chronic UVB radiation alters the cutaneous and systemic immune systems by causing several pathological alteration in cell signaling resulting in sunburn, erythema, inflammation, and skin carcinogenesis [29]. It primarily activates various pro-inflammatory mediators such as tumor necrosis factor-alpha (TNF-α), cyclooxygenase-2 (COX-2), and IL-6, leading to the activation of nuclear factor kappa-light-chain-enhancer of activated B cells (NF-κB) [30]. The findings from the previous studies showed that *S. epidermidis*, a commensal bacteria from human skin, could ferment glycerol into butyric acid, one of the four SCFAs detected in fermented media [13,15]. Glycerol is a major component in stratum corneum (SC) hydration with varied amount in different parts of human skin (0.7 μg/cm^2 in the cheek and 0.1 μg/cm^2 in forearm and sole). Multiple diseases characterized by xerosis and impaired epidermal barrier function, such as atopic dermatitis were improved by topical application of glycerol. Although glycerol could not penetrate deeper in SC but the SCFAs generated from glycerol fermentation by skin commensal bacteria, may modulate physiological processes such as skin barrier homeostasis and inflammation [15,31,32]. In this study, we evaluated the role of butyric acid, a major SCFA from the fermentation of glycerol by *S. epidermidis*, on chronic UVB radiation induced inflammation on ICR mice skin. The fermentation of glycerol by *S. epidermidis* was detected by change in color of phenol red from red to yellow (more acidic), which was further validated quantitatively by a significant decrease in OD_{560nm}. In addition to SCFAs, furfural is another metabolite produced by bacterial fermentation, and its accumulation has been shown to inhibit fermentation by blocking the activities of multiple enzymes involved in bacterial fermentation pathway [19,33]. We did not detect fermentation by color change or by OD_{560nm} quantification upon adding furfural to media containing *S. epidermidis* with glycerol. Furthermore, no bacterial growth was detected when furfural was added to media containing *S. epidermidis* alone, demonstrating the activity of furfural in suppressing bacterial fermentation activity. ALS is one of the major fermentation enzymes catalyzing the conversion of pyruvate to α-acetolactate which is further converted to isobutyrate and then ultimately to butyrate in subsequent pathways [34,35]. Our recent study showed, ALS activity in *S. epidermidis* was inhibited by a furfural derivative 5-methyl furfural (5MF) [14]. In the current study, we detected a significant reduction in ALS activity upon incubation of bacterial lysate with furfural. This demonstrates that ALS plays an essential role in *S. epidermidis* metabolism, triggering glycerol fermentation. We detected the production of butyric acid in fermented media by HPLC analysis on the basis of comparing the retention time and spectra with a butyric acid standard, confirming butyric acid as one of the most abundant metabolites produced from fermentation of 2% glycerol by *S. epidermidis*.

Metabolites from microbial fermentation have been under investigation as potential therapeutics against different infectious and inflammatory diseases [36]. For example, research suggested that ingestion of probiotic bacteria, *Lactobacillus johnsonii* (La1) could protect against the UVR-induced inflammation [37]. Furthermore, several lines of evidence suggest that metabolites from the fermentation of glycerol by *S. epidermidis* can inhibit the growth of pathogenic *Cutibacterium acnes* (*C. acnes*), thus, *S. epidermidis* may be an excellent probiotic for the treatment of chronic sinusitis [13,15,38]. Here we detected the probiotic effect of *S. epidermidis* in skin against UVB mediated chronic inflammation. Topical application of *S. epidermidis* or glycerol alone on ICR mice dorsal skin exposed to UVB showed noticeable erythema, ulceration, epidermal hyperplasia, and increased IL-6 levels. Following UVB exposure, increased infiltration of dermal inflammatory cells may lead to epidermal proliferation of keratinocytes and hyperplastic lesion [39,40]. A significant decrease in inflammation with attenuation of IL-6 and a reduction of epidermal thickness was observed in skin topically applied with mixture of *S. epidermidis* and glycerol, suggesting that the anti-inflammatory effect observed here is likely to be mediated through *S. epidermidis* fermentation using glycerol as a carbon source. Further, we confirmed that the anti-inflammatory activity was the result of *S. epidermidis* fermentation with the use of the fermentation inhibitor, furfural. Control mice topically applied with water or furfural alone followed by irradiation with UVB appeared to have significant ulceration, epidermal thickening, and increased IL-6. Importantly, there was no recovery from ulceration or inflammation in skin applied with a mixture of *S. epidermidis* and glycerol along with furfural. Based on these findings, we infer that a product from the fermentation of glycerol by *S. epidermidis* could inhibit inflammation from chronic UVB. Bacterial interference using live beneficial bacteria is a promising method of preventing or treating many infections. Because of the US Food and Drug Administration (FDA) restriction in use of live probiotic bacteria for cosmetics, the promotion of beneficial effects through the generation of fermentation metabolites from live probiotic bacteria has become a desirable alternative [28,29]. Consistent with a previous study [13], the current work used HPLC analysis to detect a substantial amount of butyric acid in the fermented media of *S. epidermidis* using glycerol as a carbon source. Anti-microbial, anti-inflammatory, and anti-cancer activity of butyric acid and its derivatives make it as a potential drug of choice [41,42]. It has been shown that application of both butyric acid and its co-drug could reportedly inhibit skin tumorigenesis and psoriasis-like skin inflammation [43,44]. In the current study, topical application of butyric acid markedly decreases skin ulceration and epidermal thickness from UVB exposure compared to the control mice skin applied with H_2O. In line with the anti-inflammatory activity of butyric acid, a significant reduction in IL-6 level was detected both in keratinocytes and in mice skin exposed to prolonged UVB, indicating its potential use as an agent to prevent inflammation in chronic UVB exposed skin. Reduction in level of IL-8 upon butyric acid treatment, provided new insight for the application of butyric acid against other upregulated cytokines against UVB induced inflammation.

Research demonstrated that butyrate can control immune/inflammatory reactions in the skin [42]. SCFAs exert their immunomodulatory effects via binding to its cognate receptor, GPR43 [45]. Exacerbated or unresolved inflammation was observed in GPR43-deficient ($Gpr43^{-/-}$) mice in models of colitis, arthritis, and asthma, demonstrating that SCFA-GPR43 interactions are obligatory for normal resolution of certain inflammatory responses [27]. Moreover, decreased expression of GPR43 by keratinocytes in psoriatic skin could be rescued by topical application of sodium butyrate, indicating that butyrate-GPR43 interactions might exert anti-inflammatory effects in psoriasis [46]. In our study, gavage feeding of mice with GLPG0974, an antagonist for FFAR2/GPR43 receptor, inhibited the anti-hyperplasic, anti-inflammatory effect of butyric acid. Further, topical application of butyric acid did not rescue the UVB induced skin damage and inflammatory level of IL-6 when FFAR2 receptor was knocked down by subcutaneous injection of FFAR2 siRNA. Overall, these results demonstrate that butyric acid interaction with the FFAR2 receptor is a crucial phenomenon during skin inflammation. Moreover, butyric acid-FFAR2 interactions could represent a central mechanism to account for the effect of probiotics on immune responses modulated by chronic UV radiation.

The skin microbiome plays an important role in preserving skin homeostasis. Thus, skin microbiome through fermentation activity might influence the skin immune system in a similar way to the gut under inflammatory disease conditions. A recent study demonstrated that topical application of antioxidants against UVB were found more effective than dietary supplementation because of the length of time needed to reach optimal concentrations in the skin [47]. In this current study, we determined that topical application of butyric acid, as a fermentation metabolite could act as a potent regulator of immune system during chronic UVB. Additionally, the dose of butyric acid is non-toxic to skin cells and thus may gain broad acceptance for not only therapeutics but also as an active ingredient in cosmetics with the ultimate aim of avoiding the strong effects from chronic UVB.

4. Materials and Methods

4.1. Ethics Statement

This research was conducted in strict accordance with an approved Institutional Animal Care and Use Committee (IACUC) protocol of the National Central University (NCU), Taiwan (NCU-106-016, 19 December 2017). ICR mice (8–9 week-old females; National Laboratory Animal Centre, Taipei, Taiwan) were sacrificed using dry ice in a closed box.

4.2. Chemicals

Butyric acid (Sigma), acetonitrile, H_3PO_4, ether anhydrous, formaldehyde, hydrochloric acid (HCl, 37%), sodium hydroxide (NaOH), Sodium dihydrogenphosphate (NaH_2PO_4), and phosphoric acid (H_3PO_4) were purchased from J.T.Baker, Avantor Performance Materials Taiwan Co. Ltd. DMSO and glycerol were purchased from Sigma. PBS was purchased from Gibco (Gaithersburg, MD, USA). GLPG0974 (FFAR2 inhibitor) was also obtained from Tocris Bioscience (Ellisville, MO, USA). Butyric acid was obtained from Sigma (St. Louis, MO, USA).

4.3. Bacterial Culture

S. epidermidis bacteria, from ATCC 12228 was cultured on 3% tryptic soy broth (TSB) (Sigma, St. Louis, MO, USA) agar plates overnight at 37 °C. A single colony was inoculated in 3% TSB medium (Difco, Becton Dickinson UK Ltd., Oxford, UK) and cultured at 37 °C until the logarithmic growth phase. Bacterial pellets were harvested by centrifugation at 5000× *g* for 10 min, washed with PBS, and suspended in PBS.

4.4. Fermentation of Bacteria

S. epidermidis (10^7 CFU/mL) were incubated in 10 mL rich media (10 g/L yeast extract (Biokar Diagnostics, Beauvais, France), 3 g/L TSB, 2.5 g/L K_2HPO_4, and 1.5 g/L KH_2PO_4) in the absence and presence of glycerol (2%) under aerobic conditions at 37 °C with shaking at 200 rpm. The rich media glycerol (2%) without bacteria were included as a control. The 0.002% (*w/v*) phenol red (Sigma) in rich media with glycerol (2%) acted as a fermentation indicator. A color change from red-orange to yellow indicated the occurrence of bacterial fermentation, which was detected as absorbance at 560 nm.

4.5. Inhibition of ALS Activity by Furfural

ALS (EC: 4.1. 3.18) is responsible for the conversion of pyruvate to acetolactate which can be eventually metabolized to diacetyl and 2,3-butanediol. The rate of reaction was monitored by the depletion of NADH at 340 nm during the conversion of pyruvate to 2,3-butanediol. The reaction mixture contained 70 mM sodium acetate buffer (pH 5.4), 0.17 mM thiamine pyrophosphate, and lysate (10 mg) of heat (100 °C) killed *S. epidermidis*. The reaction was started by addition of pyruvate [48] in the presence or absence of 0.4% furfural at 45 °C for 5 min. Absorbance was measured with a visible spectrophotometer at 340 nm. Values of ALS activity were expressed in enzyme as unit per mg (U/mg), in which one unit of ALS is defined as the amount of enzyme able to produce 0.1 absorbance unit per min.

4.6. Ultraviolet Light Exposure

ICR mice were exposed to chronic UVB with a ramping dose using an UV lamp (Model EB-280C, Spectronics Corp., Westbury, NY, USA). The UVB light source was set at a distance such that the dorsal surface of each mouse received 195 mJ/cm^2. Dorsal skin was exposed three times per week, followed by topical application with *S. epidermidis* (10^7) and glycerol (2%) in PBS one time per week. Whole UVB radiation and treatment was conducted for 4 weeks. Animals were photographed at 0, 16, and 30 day for measurement of wound from UVB and recovery from treatment. Animals were sacrificed 3 day following the last dose and whole skin samples, including epidermis and dermis were collected. Tissue samples (approximately 1 cm^2) were taken from similar dorso-caudal locations for histological examination. The remaining portions of the dorsal skin were used to prepare whole skin lysate for ELISA analyses. Hematoxylin and eosin (H&E) staining was performed by the Histopathology Shared Resources Core at Li-Tzung Biotechnology Inc. Quantitative measurements of skin thickness from H&E were made using ImageJ software.

4.7. Wound Measurement

To investigate the wound improvement of ICR hairless mice skin induced by UVB irradiation, the mice were transiently anesthetized using isoflurane, and the wound were measured by ImageJ software by calculating the percent of remaining wound area to the total area of skin exposed at 0, 16, and 30 day of UVB irradiation. Wounds were photographed using a USB digital microscope.

4.8. Histological Analysis

Histological analysis was performed to determine the epidermal thickness. Dorsal skin samples of the experimental groups were obtained after 4 weeks of UVB exposure, fixed with 10% formalin and embedded in paraffin. Sections were stained with H&E to examine epidermal thickness. Epidermal thickness was measured at 10× magnification using Olympus BX63 microscope (Olympus, Tokyo, Japan).

4.9. siRNA-Mediated Gene Silencing of GPR43/FFAR2

In order to silence GPR43 gene, we used the chemically-modified siRNA that targets GPR43 receptor and the siRNA negative control, which does not target any known sequence were obtained from GenePharma Co. (Shanghai, China). Their oligonucleotide sequences are siFFAR2: sense strand, 5′-CCGGUGCAGUACAAGUUAUTT-3′; anti-sense strand, 5′-AUAACUUGUACUGCACC GGTT-3′. SiControl: sense strand, 5′-UUCUCCGAACGUGUCACGUTT; anti-sense strand, 5′-ACGUGACACGUUCGGAGAATT-3′. These chemically-modified siRNAs were delivered by intradermal injection in dorsal skin of mice using a microneedle [49,50].

4.10. Drug Treatment

Selective FFAR2 antagonist GLPG0974 (0.1 or 1 mg/kg ig) was administered to ICR mice by gavage feeding [51]. GLPG0974 was dissolved in DMSO (0.01% in saline) and DMSO (0.01% in saline) was used as the vehicle control. Butyric acid (4 mM) was topically applied on dorsal skin of mice. Butyric acid was dissolved in double distilled water.

4.11. ELISA

Skin samples from ICR mice were collected after 4 weeks of UVB exposure and were then lysed with T-PER™ Tissue Protein Extraction Reagent (ThermoFisher Scientific, Waltham, MA, USA) supplemented with an ethylenediaminetetraacetic acid (EDTA)-free protease inhibitor cocktail (Sigma-Aldrich, St Louis, MO, USA). Supernatant was collected from UVB irradiated and non-irradiated human keratinocytes (CCD 1106 KERTr) with and without BA treatment. IL-6 concentration in mice skin and IL-6 and IL-8 concentration in supernatant from human keratinocytes were determined by mouse or human IL-6 and IL-8 ELISA assay kit (R&D Systems, Minneapolis, MN, USA) following previous published protocol [52].

4.12. HPLC

Media samples were vortexed and equilibrated at room temperature for 5 min. Thereafter 100 µL of concentrated HCl was added per mL of each sample, followed by a vortex-mixing step of 15 s. The samples were extracted for 20 min (by gently rolling) using 5 mL of diethyl ether. After centrifugation (5 min, 3500 rpm), the supernatant was transferred to another Pyrex extraction tube and 500 µL of a 1 M solution of NaOH was added. The samples were extracted again for 20 min, followed by a centrifugation step. The aqueous phase was transferred to an auto sampler vial and 100 µL of concentrated HCl was added. After vortex mixing, 10 µL was injected onto the HPLC–UV apparatus. The mobile phase consisted of 20 mM of NaH_2PO_4 in HPLC water (pH adjusted to 2.2 using phosphoric acid) (A) and acetonitrile (B). The UV detector was set at a wavelength of 210 nm for detection of butyric acid in sample.

4.13. Statistical Analysis

Data analysis was performed by unpaired t-test or by one-way ANOVA using GraphPad Prism® software. The *p*-values of <0.05 (*), <0.01 (**), and <0.001 (***) were considered significant. The mean ± standard error (SE) for at least three independent experiments was calculated.

Supplementary Materials: Supplementary materials can be found at http://www.mdpi.com/1422-0067/20/18/4477/s1.

Author Contributions: S.K., A.B., B.M., and I.P.N. performed the experiments. C.-M.H. designed all experiments. S.K. wrote the manuscript. S.K., C.-M.H., and D.R.H. reviewed and edited the manuscript.

Funding: This work was supported by 106/107-Landseed Hospital-NCU joint grants, National Health Research Institutes (NHRI) Grant NHRI-EX106-10607SI, and Ministry of Science and Technology (MOST) Grants 107-2314-B-008-001, 107-2622-B-008-002-CC1, and 106/107-2622-B-008-001-CC1.

Acknowledgments: We wish to thank Yu-Fen Huang, Department of Biomedical Engineering and Environmental Sciences, National Tsing Hua University, Taiwan for providing HPLC-UV analysis facility and Postdoctoral Scholar Irving Po-Jung Lai, National Central University, Taiwan for skillful help during HPLC-UV analysis.

Conflicts of Interest: The authors declare no conflict of interest.

References

1. Lopez-Camarillo, C.; Ocampo, E.A.; Casamichana, M.L.; Perez-Plasencia, C.; Alvarez-Sanchez, E.; Marchat, L.A. Protein kinases and transcription factors activation in response to UV-radiation of skin: Implications for carcinogenesis. *Int. J. Mol. Sci.* **2012**, *13*, 142–172. [CrossRef] [PubMed]
2. Armstrong, B.K.; Kricker, A. The epidemiology of UV induced skin cancer. *J. Photochem. Photobiol. B* **2001**, *63*, 8–18. [CrossRef]
3. De Fabo, E.C.; Noonan, F.P. Mechanism of immune suppression by ultraviolet irradiation in vivo. I. Evidence for the existence of a unique photoreceptor in skin and its role in photoimmunology. *J. Exp. Med.* **1983**, *158*, 84–98. [CrossRef] [PubMed]

4. Ishida, T.; Sakaguchi, I. Protection of human keratinocytes from UVB-induced inflammation using root extract of Lithospermum erythrorhizon. *Biol. Pharm. Bull.* **2007**, *30*, 928–934. [CrossRef] [PubMed]
5. Ansel, J.C.; Luger, T.A.; Green, I. The effect of in vitro and in vivo UV irradiation on the production of ETAF activity by human and murine keratinocytes. *J. Investig. Dermatol.* **1983**, *81*, 519–523. [CrossRef] [PubMed]
6. Kirnbauer, R.; Kock, A.; Neuner, P.; Forster, E.; Krutmann, J.; Urbanski, A.; Schauer, E.; Ansel, J.C.; Schwarz, T.; Luger, T.A. Regulation of epidermal cell interleukin-6 production by UV light and corticosteroids. *J. Investig. Dermatol.* **1991**, *96*, 484–489. [CrossRef]
7. Acker, T.; Fandrey, J.; Acker, H. The good, the bad and the ugly in oxygen-sensing: ROS, cytochromes and prolyl-hydroxylases. *Cardiovasc. Res.* **2006**, *71*, 195–207. [CrossRef] [PubMed]
8. Kloos, W.E.; Musselwhite, M.S. Distribution and persistence of Staphylococcus and Micrococcus species and other aerobic bacteria on human skin. *Appl. Microbiol.* **1975**, *30*, 381–385. [PubMed]
9. Sanford, J.A.; Gallo, R.L. Functions of the skin microbiota in health and disease. *Semin. Immunol.* **2013**, *25*, 370–377. [CrossRef] [PubMed]
10. Lai, Y.; Di Nardo, A.; Nakatsuji, T.; Leichtle, A.; Yang, Y.; Cogen, A.L.; Wu, Z.R.; Hooper, L.V.; Schmidt, R.R.; von Aulock, S.; et al. Commensal bacteria regulate Toll-like receptor 3-dependent inflammation after skin injury. *Nat. Med.* **2009**, *15*, 1377–1382. [CrossRef]
11. Nakatsuji, T.; Chen, T.H.; Butcher, A.M.; Trzoss, L.L.; Nam, S.-J.; Shirakawa, K.T.; Zhou, W.; Oh, J.; Otto, M.; Fenical, W.; et al. A commensal strain of *Staphylococcus epidermidis* protects against skin neoplasia. *Sci. Adv.* **2018**, *4*. [CrossRef] [PubMed]
12. Cogen, A.L.; Yamasaki, K.; Sanchez, K.M.; Dorschner, R.A.; Lai, Y.; MacLeod, D.T.; Torpey, J.W.; Otto, M.; Nizet, V.; Kim, J.E.; et al. Selective Antimicrobial Action Is Provided by Phenol-Soluble Modulins Derived from Staphylococcus epidermidis, a Normal Resident of the Skin. *J. Investig. Dermatol.* **2010**, *130*, 192–200. [CrossRef] [PubMed]
13. Wang, Y.; Kuo, S.; Shu, M.; Yu, J.; Huang, S.; Dai, A.; Two, A.; Gallo, R.L.; Huang, C.M. Staphylococcus epidermidis in the human skin microbiome mediates fermentation to inhibit the growth of Propionibacterium acnes: Implications of probiotics in acne vulgaris. *Appl. Microbiol. Biotechnol.* **2014**, *98*, 411–424. [CrossRef] [PubMed]
14. Kumar, M.; Myagmardoloonjin, B.; Keshari, S.; Negari, I.P.; Huang, C.M. 5-Methyl Furfural Reduces the Production of Malodors by Inhibiting Sodium l-Lactate Fermentation of Staphylococcus epidermidis: Implication for Deodorants Targeting the Fermenting Skin Microbiome. *Microorganisms* **2019**, *7*, 239. [CrossRef] [PubMed]
15. Yang, A.J.; Marito, S.; Yang, J.J.; Keshari, S.; Chew, C.H.; Chen, C.C.; Huang, C.M. A Microtube Array Membrane (MTAM) Encapsulated Live Fermenting Staphylococcus epidermidis as a Skin Probiotic Patch against Cutibacterium acnes. *Int. J. Mol. Sci.* **2018**, *20*, 14. [CrossRef] [PubMed]
16. Malav, M.K.; Prasad, S.; Kharia, S.K.; Kumar, S.; Sheetal, K.; Kannojiya, S. Furfural and 5-HMF: Potent fermentation inhibitors and their removal techniques. *Int. J. Curr. Microbiol. Appl. Sci.* **2017**, *6*, 2060–2066. [CrossRef]
17. Carvalho, S.M.; de Jong, A.; Kloosterman, T.G.; Kuipers, O.P.; Saraiva, L.M. The Staphylococcus aureus α-Acetolactate Synthase ALS Confers Resistance to Nitrosative Stress. *Front. Microbiol.* **2017**, *8*, 1273. [CrossRef] [PubMed]
18. Härtig, E.; Jahn, D. Regulation of the Anaerobic Metabolism in Bacillus subtilis. *Adv. Microb. Physiol.* **2012**, *61*, 195–216. [CrossRef]
19. Palmqvist, E.; Hahn-Hägerdal, B. Fermentation of lignocellulosic hydrolysates. II: Inhibitors and mechanisms of inhibition. *Bioresour. Technol.* **2000**, *33*, 25–33. [CrossRef]
20. Meijer, K.; de Vos, P.; Priebe, M.G. Butyrate and other short-chain fatty acids as modulators of immunity: What relevance for health? *Curr. Opin. Clin. Nutr. Metab. Care* **2010**, *13*, 715–721. [CrossRef] [PubMed]
21. Kao, M.S.; Huang, S.; Chang, W.L.; Hsieh, M.F.; Huang, C.J.; Gallo, R.L.; Huang, C.M. Microbiome precision editing: Using PEG as a selective fermentation initiator against methicillin-resistant Staphylococcus aureus. *Biotechnol. J.* **2017**, *12*. [CrossRef] [PubMed]
22. Xia, J.; Song, X.; Bi, Z.; Chu, W.; Wan, Y. UV-induced NF-kappaB activation and expression of IL-6 is attenuated by (-)-epigallocatechin-3-gallate in cultured human keratinocytes in vitro. *Int. J. Mol. Med.* **2005**, *16*, 943–950. [PubMed]

23. Smerdon, M.J.; Lan, S.Y.; Calza, R.E.; Reeves, R. Sodium butyrate stimulates DNA repair in UV-irradiated normal and xeroderma pigmentosum human fibroblasts. *J. Biol. Chem.* **1982**, *257*, 13441–13447. [PubMed]
24. Xiong, F.; Mou, Y.Z.; Xiang, X.Y. Inhibition of mouse B16 melanoma by sodium butyrate correlated to tumor associated macrophages differentiation suppression. *Int. J. Clin. Exp. Med.* **2015**, *8*, 4170–4174. [PubMed]
25. Yoshizumi, M.; Nakamura, T.; Kato, M.; Ishioka, T.; Kozawa, K.; Wakamatsu, K.; Kimura, H. Release of cytokines/chemokines and cell death in UVB-irradiated human keratinocytes, HaCaT. *Cell Biol. Int.* **2008**, *32*, 1405–1411. [CrossRef]
26. Pirozzi, C.; Francisco, V.; Guida, F.D.; Gomez, R.; Lago, F.; Pino, J.; Meli, R.; Gualillo, O. Butyrate Modulates Inflammation in Chondrocytes via GPR43 Receptor. *Cell Physiol. Biochem.* **2018**, *51*, 228–243. [CrossRef] [PubMed]
27. Maslowski, K.M.; Vieira, A.T.; Ng, A.; Kranich, J.; Sierro, F.; Yu, D.; Schilter, H.C.; Rolph, M.S.; Mackay, F.; Artis, D.; et al. Regulation of inflammatory responses by gut microbiota and chemoattractant receptor GPR43. *Nature* **2009**, *461*, 1282–1286. [CrossRef]
28. Masui, R.; Sasaki, M.; Funaki, Y.; Ogasawara, N.; Mizuno, M.; Iida, A.; Izawa, S.; Kondo, Y.; Ito, Y.; Tamura, Y.; et al. G protein-coupled receptor 43 moderates gut inflammation through cytokine regulation from mononuclear cells. *Inflamm. Bowel Dis.* **2013**, *19*, 2848–2856. [CrossRef] [PubMed]
29. Bode, A.M.; Dong, Z. Mitogen-activated protein kinase activation in UV-induced signal transduction. *Sci. STKE* **2003**, *2003*. [CrossRef] [PubMed]
30. Choi, K.-S.; Kundu, J.K.; Chun, K.-S.; Na, H.-K.; Surh, Y.-J. Rutin inhibits UVB radiation-induced expression of COX-2 and iNOS in hairless mouse skin: p38 MAP kinase and JNK as potential targets. *Arch. Biochem. Biophys.* **2014**, *559*, 38–45. [CrossRef] [PubMed]
31. Fluhr, J.W.; Darlenski, R.; Surber, C. Glycerol and the skin: Holistic approach to its origin and functions. *Br. J. Dermatol.* **2008**, *159*, 23–34. [CrossRef] [PubMed]
32. Lin, T.K.; Zhong, L.; Santiago, J.L. Anti-Inflammatory and Skin Barrier Repair Effects of Topical Application of Some Plant Oils. *Int. J. Mol. Sci.* **2017**, *19*, 70. [CrossRef] [PubMed]
33. Thomsen, M.H.; Thygesen, A.; Thomsen, A.B. Identification and characterization of fermentation inhibitors formed during hydrothermal treatment and following SSF of wheat straw. *Appl. Microbiol. Biotechnol.* **2009**, *83*, 447–455. [CrossRef] [PubMed]
34. Perrine, S.P.; Dover, G.H.; Daftari, P.; Walsh, C.T.; Jin, Y.; Mays, A.; Faller, D.V. Isobutyramide, an orally bioavailable butyrate analogue, stimulates fetal globin gene expression in vitro and in vivo. *Br. J. Haematol.* **1994**, *88*, 555–561. [CrossRef]
35. Vassilev, I.; Hernandez, P.A.; Batlle-Vilanova, P.; Freguia, S.; Krömer, J.O.; Keller, J.; Ledezma, P.; Virdis, B. Microbial Electrosynthesis of Isobutyric, Butyric, Caproic Acids, and Corresponding Alcohols from Carbon Dioxide. *ACS Sustain. Chem. Eng.* **2018**, *6*, 8485–8493. [CrossRef]
36. Kober, M.-M.; Bowe, W.P. The effect of probiotics on immune regulation, acne, and photoaging. *Int. J. Women's Dermatol.* **2015**, *1*, 85–89. [CrossRef]
37. Guéniche, A.; Benyacoub, J.; Buetler, T.M.; Smola, H.; Blum, S. Supplementation with oral probiotic bacteria maintains cutaneous immune homeostasis after UV exposure. *Eur. J. Dermatol.* **2006**, *16*, 511–517.
38. Cope, E.K.; Lynch, S.V. Novel microbiome-based therapeutics for chronic rhinosinusitis. *Curr. Allergy Asthma Rep.* **2015**, *15*, 9. [CrossRef]
39. Agarwal, R.; Katiyar, S.K.; Khan, S.G.; Mukhtar, H. Protection against ultraviolet B radiation-induced effects in the skin of SKH-1 hairless mice by a polyphenolic fraction isolated from green tea. *Photochem. Photobiol.* **1993**, *58*, 695–700. [CrossRef]
40. Wilgus, T.A.; Ross, M.S.; Parrett, M.L.; Oberyszyn, T.M. Topical application of a selective cyclooxygenase inhibitor suppresses UVB mediated cutaneous inflammation. *Prostaglandins Other Lipid Mediat.* **2000**, *62*, 367–384. [CrossRef]
41. Borycka-Kiciak, K.; Banasiewicz, T.; Rydzewska, G. Butyric acid—A well-known molecule revisited. *Prz. Gastroenterol.* **2017**, *12*, 83–89. [CrossRef] [PubMed]
42. Schwarz, A.; Bruhs, A.; Schwarz, T. The Short-Chain Fatty Acid Sodium Butyrate Functions as a Regulator of the Skin Immune System. *J. Investig. Dermatol.* **2017**, *137*, 855–864. [CrossRef] [PubMed]
43. Gupta, K.P.; Mehrotra, N.K. Differential effects of butyric acid on mouse skin tumorigenesis. *Biomed. Env. Sci.* **1997**, *10*, 436–441.

44. Bruhs, A.; Schwarz, T.; Schwarz, A. 325 The short chain fatty acid sodium butyrate attenuates imiquimod-induced psoriasis-like skin inflammation. *J. Investig. Dermatol.* **2017**, *137*, S248. [CrossRef]
45. Karaki, S.; Mitsui, R.; Hayashi, H.; Kato, I.; Sugiya, H.; Iwanaga, T.; Furness, J.B.; Kuwahara, A. Short-chain fatty acid receptor, GPR43, is expressed by enteroendocrine cells and mucosal mast cells in rat intestine. *Cell Tissue Res.* **2006**, *324*, 353–360. [CrossRef] [PubMed]
46. Krejner, A.; Bruhs, A.; Mrowietz, U.; Wehkamp, U.; Schwarz, T.; Schwarz, A. Decreased expression of G-protein-coupled receptors GPR43 and GPR109a in psoriatic skin can be restored by topical application of sodium butyrate. *Arch. Dermatol. Res.* **2018**, *310*, 751–758. [CrossRef] [PubMed]
47. Jurkiewicz, B.A. The Role of Free Radicals, Iron, and Antioxidants in Ultraviolet Radiation-Induced Skin Damage. Available online: https://www.healthcare.uiowa.edu/CoreFacilities/esr/education/theses/pdf/Jurkiewicz-PhD-1995.pdf (accessed on 11 August 2019).
48. Cogan, T.M.; Fitzgerald, R.J.; Doonan, S. Acetolactate synthase of Leuconostoc lactis and its regulation of acetoin production. *J. Dairy Res.* **2009**, *51*, 597–604. [CrossRef]
49. Pan, J.; Ruan, W.; Qin, M.; Long, Y.; Wan, T.; Yu, K.; Zhai, Y.; Wu, C.; Xu, Y. Intradermal delivery of STAT3 siRNA to treat melanoma via dissolving microneedles. *Sci. Rep.* **2018**, *8*, 1117. [CrossRef]
50. Dou, S.; Yao, Y.-D.; Yang, X.-Z.; Sun, T.-M.; Mao, C.-Q.; Song, E.-W.; Wang, J. Anti-Her2 single-chain antibody mediated DNMTs-siRNA delivery for targeted breast cancer therapy. *J. Control. Release* **2012**, *161*, 875–883. [CrossRef]
51. Pizzonero, M.; Dupont, S.; Babel, M.; Beaumont, S.; Bienvenu, N.; Blanque, R.; Cherel, L.; Christophe, T.; Crescenzi, B.; De Lemos, E.; et al. Discovery and optimization of an azetidine chemical series as a free fatty acid receptor 2 (FFA2) antagonist: From hit to clinic. *J. Med. Chem.* **2014**, *57*, 10044–10057. [CrossRef]
52. Keshari, S.; Sipayung, A.D.; Hsieh, C.C.; Su, L.J.; Chiang, Y.R.; Chang, H.C.; Yang, W.C.; Chuang, T.H.; Chen, C.L.; Huang, C.M. The IL-6/p-BTK/p-ERK signaling mediates the calcium phosphate-induced pruritus. *FASEB J.* **2019**. [CrossRef] [PubMed]

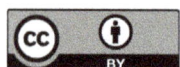

© 2019 by the authors. Licensee MDPI, Basel, Switzerland. This article is an open access article distributed under the terms and conditions of the Creative Commons Attribution (CC BY) license (http://creativecommons.org/licenses/by/4.0/).

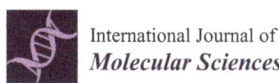

Article

Multifaceted Analyses of Epidermal Serine Protease Activity in Patients with Atopic Dermatitis

Hayato Nomura [1], Mutsumi Suganuma [2], Takuya Takeichi [2], Michihiro Kono [3], Yuki Isokane [1], Ko Sunagawa [1], Mina Kobashi [1], Satoru Sugihara [1], Ai Kajita [1], Tomoko Miyake [1], Yoji Hirai [1], Osamu Yamasaki [1], Masashi Akiyama [2] and Shin Morizane [1],*

[1] Department of Dermatology, Okayama University Graduate School of Medicine, Dentistry, and Pharmaceutical Science, 2-5-1 Shikata-cho, Kitaku, Okayama 700-8558, Japan; rsa32585@gmail.com (H.N.); pz7h9ipi@s.okayama-u.ac.jp (Y.I.); p5eh8nav@s.okayama-u.ac.jp (K.S.); x58437@gmail.com (M.K.); suginami0816@gmail.com (S.S.); gmd421029@s.okayama-u.ac.jp (A.K.); toco_my@cc.okayama-u.ac.jp (T.M.); gmd20033@s.okayama-u.ac.jp (Y.H.); yamasa-o@cc.okayama-u.ac.jp (O.Y.)
[2] Department of Dermatology, Nagoya University Graduate School of Medicine, 65 Tsurumai-cho, Showa-ku, Nagoya 466-8550, Japan; msuga@med.nagoya-u.ac.jp (M.S.); takeichi@med.nagoya-u.ac.jp (T.T.); makiyama@med.nagoya-u.ac.jp (M.A.)
[3] Department of Dermatology and Plastic Surgery, Akita University Graduate School of Medicine, Hondo 1-1-1, Akita-shi, Akita 010-8543, Japan; miro@med.akita-u.ac.jp
* Correspondence: zanemori@cc.okayama-u.ac.jp; Tel.: +81-86-235-7282

Received: 18 December 2019; Accepted: 28 January 2020; Published: 30 January 2020

Abstract: The serine proteases kallikrein-related peptidase (KLK) 5 and KLK7 cleave cell adhesion molecules in the epidermis. Aberrant epidermal serine protease activity is thought to play an important role in the pathogenesis of atopic dermatitis (AD). We collected the stratum corneum (SC) from healthy individuals ($n = 46$) and AD patients ($n = 63$) by tape stripping and then measuring the trypsin- and chymotrypsin-like serine protease activity. We also analyzed the p.D386N and p.E420K of *SPINK5* variants and loss-of-function mutations of *FLG* in the AD patients. The serine protease activity in the SC was increased not only in AD lesions but also in non-lesions of AD patients. We found, generally, that there was a positive correlation between the serine protease activity in the SC and the total serum immunoglobulin E (IgE) levels, serum thymus and activation-regulated chemokine (TARC) levels, and peripheral blood eosinophil counts. Moreover, the p.D386N or p.E420K in *SPINK5* and *FLG* mutations were not significantly associated with the SC's serine protease activity. Epidermal serine protease activity was increased even in non-lesions of AD patients. Such activity was found to correlate with a number of biomarkers of AD. Further investigations of serine proteases might provide new treatments and prophylaxis for AD.

Keywords: atopic dermatitis; serine proteases; kallikrein-related peptidases; epidermal barrier dysfunction; lympho-epithelial Kazal-type-related inhibitor (LEKTI); *SPINK5*; filaggrin

1. Introduction

Atopic dermatitis (AD) is a chronic, pruritic inflammatory skin disease that affects up to 25% of children and 2–3% of adults [1]. AD has a complex pathogenesis involving genetic, immunologic, and environmental factors which lead to a dysfunctional skin barrier and dysregulation of the immune system [1]. Aberrant epidermal serine protease activity is related to the pathogenesis of inflammatory skin diseases such as Netherton syndrome, AD, psoriasis, and rosacea [2–8]. Kallikrein-related peptidases (KLKs) are a family of 15 trypsin- or chymotrypsin-like serine proteases encoded by a cluster of protease-encoded genes (*KLK1-15*) in the human genome [9]. KLK5, a trypsin-like serine protease, and KLK7, a chymotrypsin-like serine protease, are major epidermal KLKs. These proteases have roles in the desquamation of epidermis by decomposing cell adhesion molecules such as corneodesmosin, desmoglein 1, and desmocollin 1 [10]. It has been reported that the expression and activity of several KLKs is increased in AD lesions [5,8,11]. Research suggests that KLK5 and KLK7 are particularly involved in the pathogenesis of AD. For instance, KLK5, but not KLK7, directly activates proteinase-activated receptor 2 and induces nuclear factor κB-mediated overexpression of thymic stromal lymphopoietin (TSLP) [12]. Moreover, transgenic-*KLK5* mice display cutaneous and systemic hallmarks of severe inflammation and allergy with pruritus [13]. Transgenic mice expressing human *KLK7* in epidermal keratinocytes have been found to develop pathologic skin changes with increased epidermal thickness, hyperkeratosis, dermal inflammation, and severe pruritus [14]. Our group demonstrated that Th2 cytokines increase the KLK7 expression and function in epidermal keratinocytes, suggesting an association between allergic inflammation and epidermal barrier function [15].

Serine protease activity in the skin is tightly regulated by not only KLKs but also serine protease inhibitors such as lympho-epithelial Kazal-type-related inhibitor (LEKTI), secretory leukocyte protease inhibitor (SLPI), and elafin [16]. LEKTI, encoded by the *serine protease inhibitor Kazal-type 5* (*SPINK5*) gene, is composed of 15 Kazal-type domains, all of which are capable of inhibiting serine protease activity including KLK5 and KLK7 [17,18]. Individuals with mutations of *SPINK5* develop Netherton syndrome, characterized by ichthyosis, hair abnormality, and atopic manifestations [19]. Nonsynonymous variants of *SPINK5* such as the p.D386N (c.G1156A, in exon 13) and p.E420K (c.G1258A, in exon 14) have been reported to be associated with the pathogenesis of AD [20–25]. The p.D386N variants disrupt the role of domain (D) 6 of LEKTI which suppresses the induction of TSLP by KLK5 [25]. The p.E420K variant increases the furin cleavage rate at the LEKTI linker region D6–D7 and prevents the formation of the LEKTI fragment D6D9, known to display the strongest inhibitory activity against KLK5-mediated desmoglein 1 degradation [20].

Profilaggrin is dephosphorylated and degraded to produce monomeric filaggrin in the SC and then further proteolyzed to release its component amino acids [26]. Profilaggrin, filaggrin and the amino acids each make different contributions to the epidermal structure and barrier function [26]. In 2006, loss-of-function mutations in the filaggrin gene (*FLG*) were identified as the cause of ichthyosis vulgaris [27]. The same year, it was first reported that loss-of-function genetic variants in *FLG* are predisposing factors in the context of AD [28]. In 2009, it was reported that 27% of Japanese AD patients carried *FLG* mutations [29]. To date, ten *FLG* mutations have been identified in the Japanese population [30]. Although *FLG* mutations are well known to affect epidermal barrier functions, the association between the mutations and the epidermal serine protease activity has not been investigated.

Here, we performed multifaceted analyses of epidermal serine protease activity in patients with AD. We focused particularly on the relationship between the epidermal serine protease activity and biomarkers of AD or AD-related gene variants.

2. Results

2.1. Serine Protease Activity in the SC of AD Is Increased in Both Non-Lesions and Lesions

We examined trypsin- and chymotrypsin-like serine protease activity in SC samples from normal healthy volunteers and AD patients. The activity of trypsin- and chymotrypsin-like serine proteases in the SC samples from both non-lesions and lesions of the AD patients were significantly higher than those from the healthy individuals (Figure 1A,B). The trypsin-like serine protease activity of the AD lesions was higher than that of the non-lesions (Figure 1A). A significant positive correlation between trypsin- and chymotrypsin-like serine protease activity was observed in both the non-lesions and lesions of the AD patients (Figure 1C,D).

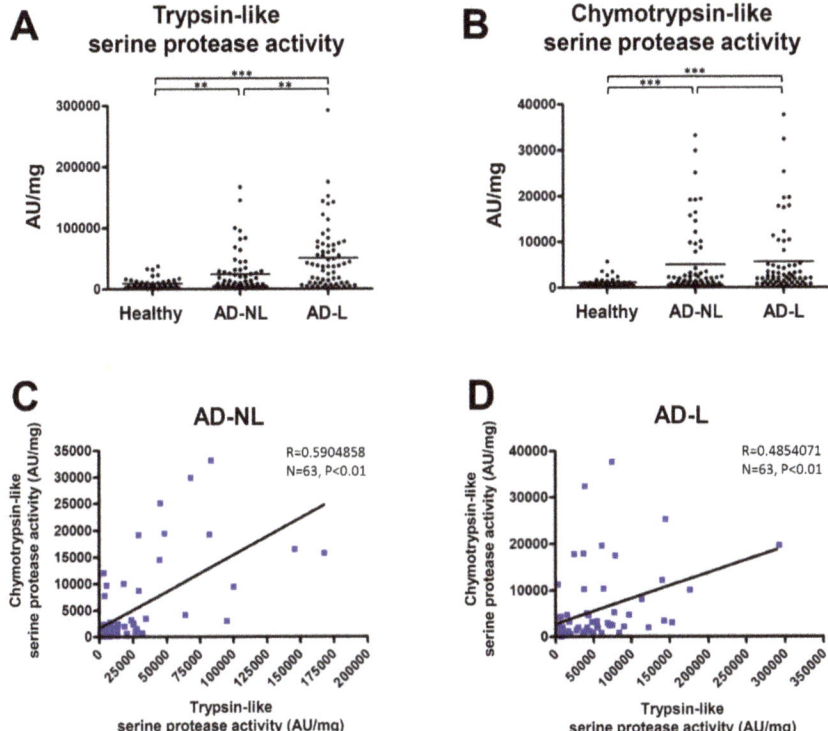

Figure 1. Serine protease activity in the stratum corneum (SC) of atopic dermatitis (AD) patients was increased in both non-lesions and lesions. (**A,B**) Trypsin- and chymotrypsin-like serine protease activity in the SC of normal healthy volunteers ($n = 46$) and both non-lesions (AD-NL) and lesions (AD-L) of AD patients ($n = 63$) were measured. ** $p < 0.01$, *** $p < 0.001$. (**C,D**) The correlations between trypsin- and chymotrypsin-like serine protease activity in the non-lesions and lesions of AD patients were analyzed by Spearman's rank correlation coefficient.

2.2. The Association between Serine Protease Activity in the SC of AD and Medical Treatments

We next analysed the association between serine protease activity in the SC in lesions of AD patients ($n = 63$) and various medical treatments. The treatments were as follows: topical corticosteroid ($n = 44$), topical tacrolimus ($n = 15$), oral antihistamine ($n = 36$), oral corticosteroid ($n = 6$) and oral cyclosporine ($n = 4$). The trypsin-like serine protease activity in the SC of patients with topical corticosteroid therapy was significantly higher than those without topical corticosteroid therapy (Figure 2A). On the other hand, the chymotrypsin-like serine protease activity in the SC was not significantly different with or without topical corticosteroid therapy (Figure 2B). Neither trypsin- and chymotrypsin-like serine protease activity in the SC was significantly different with or without topical tacrolimus, oral antihistamine, oral corticosteroid or oral cyclosporine therapies (Figure 2C–J).

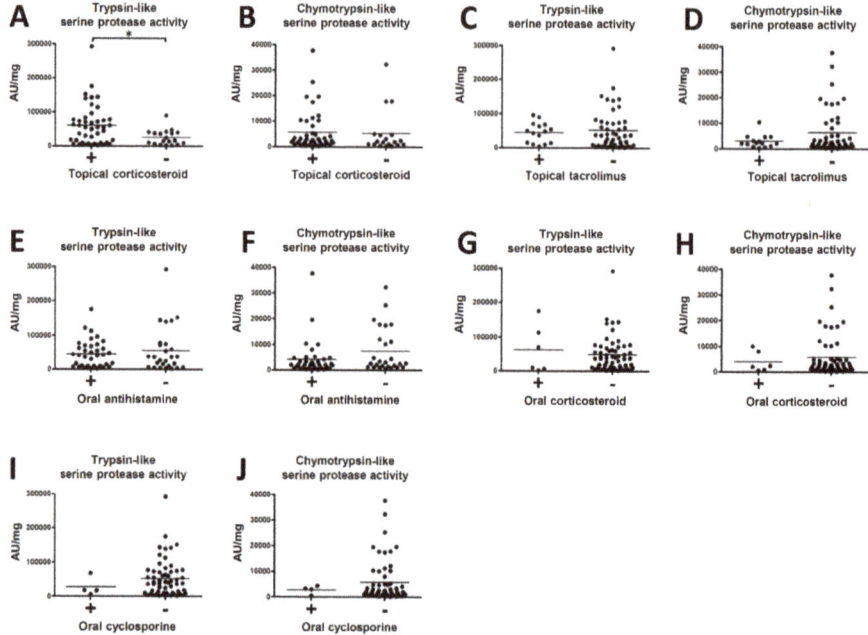

Figure 2. The association between serine protease activity in the SC in lesions of AD patients and medical treatments. Trypsin- or chymotrypsin-like serine protease activity in lesions were compared with and without topical corticosteroid (**A,B**), topical tacrolimus (**C,D**), oral antihistamine (**E,F**), oral corticosteroid (**G,H**) and oral cyclosporine therapies (**I,J**). * $p < 0.05$.

2.3. Serine Protease Activity in the SC of AD Correlate with Biomarkers of AD

We further examined the correlation between serine protease activity in the SC and the biomarkers of AD. We observed that the serum total immunoglobulin E (IgE) levels were highly correlated with the trypsin-like serine protease activity in non-lesions of the AD patients, but not with the chymotrypsin-like serine protease activity in non-lesions or the trypsin- or chymotrypsin-like serine protease activity in AD lesions (Figure 3A–D). The serum levels of thymus and activation-regulated chemokine (TARC) were highly correlated with the trypsin- or chymotrypsin-like serine protease activity in the non-lesions of the AD patients and the trypsin-like serine protease activity in AD lesions, but not with the chymotrypsin-like serine protease activity in AD lesions (Figure 3E–H). Our study found, further, that peripheral blood eosinophil counts were highly correlated with the trypsin-like serine protease activity in the non-lesions and lesions of the AD patients, but not with the chymotrypsin-like serine protease activity in the AD non-lesions or lesions (Figure 3I–L).

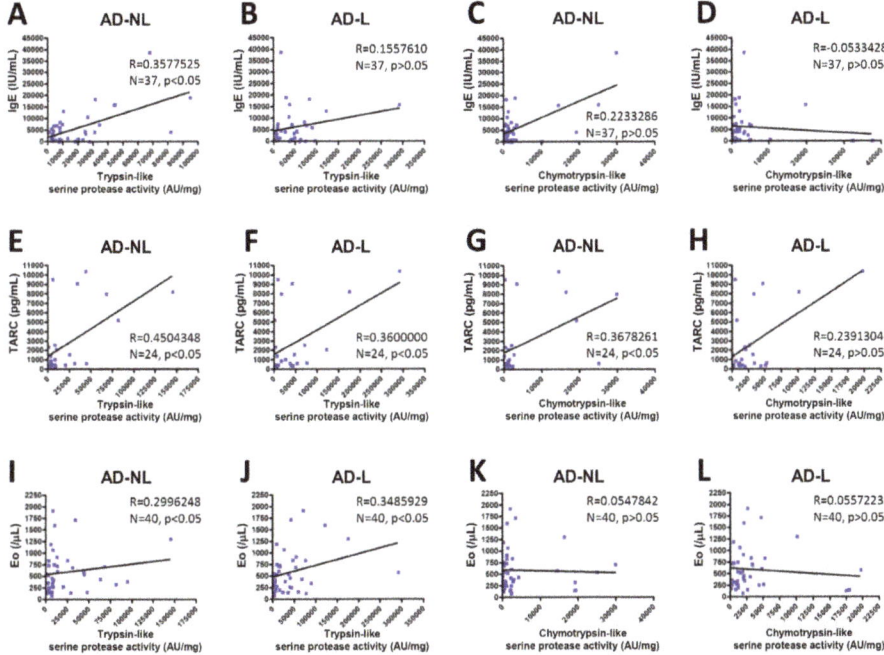

Figure 3. The correlations between serine protease activity in the SC and biomarkers of AD. The correlations between trypsin- or chymotrypsin-like serine protease activity in non-lesions (AD-NL) or lesions (AD-L) and the serum total IgE levels (**A–D**), serum TARC levels (**E–H**) and the peripheral blood eosinophil counts (Eo) (**I–L**) of the AD patients were analyzed by Spearman's rank correlation coefficient.

2.4. p.D386N and p.E420K of SPINK5 and Loss-Of-Function Mutations in FLG Do Not Affect the Serine Protease Activity in the SC

To clarify the association between serine protease activity in the SC and the AD-related gene variants, we analyzed *FLG* mutations in the AD patients. Eighteen of the 115 patients (15.7%) had one of the ten *FLG* mutations. We were able to perform protease assays with the SC samples from 61 of the AD patients. Ten of the 61 patients (16.4%) had the *FLG* mutations: p.Q1701X ($n = 1$), p.S2554X ($n = 1$), p.S2889X ($n = 4$), p.S3296X ($n = 2$) and p.K4022X ($n = 2$). We also analyzed p.D386N (c.G1156A) and p.E420K (c.G1258A) of *SPINK5* in the AD patients. In respect of p.D386N, the numbers of the genotypes were as follows: GG ($n = 21$), GA ($n = 28$), and AA ($n = 12$). For p.E420K, the numbers of the genotypes were as follows: GG ($n = 14$), GA ($n = 31$), and AA ($n = 16$). The trypsin- and chymotrypsin-like serine protease activity in the SC was not significantly different among the subgroups of p.D386N (Figure 4A,B) or p.E420K (Figure 4C,D). In addition, *FLG* mutations did not significantly affect the trypsin- or chymotrypsin-like serine protease activity of the SC in the AD patients (Figure 4E,F).

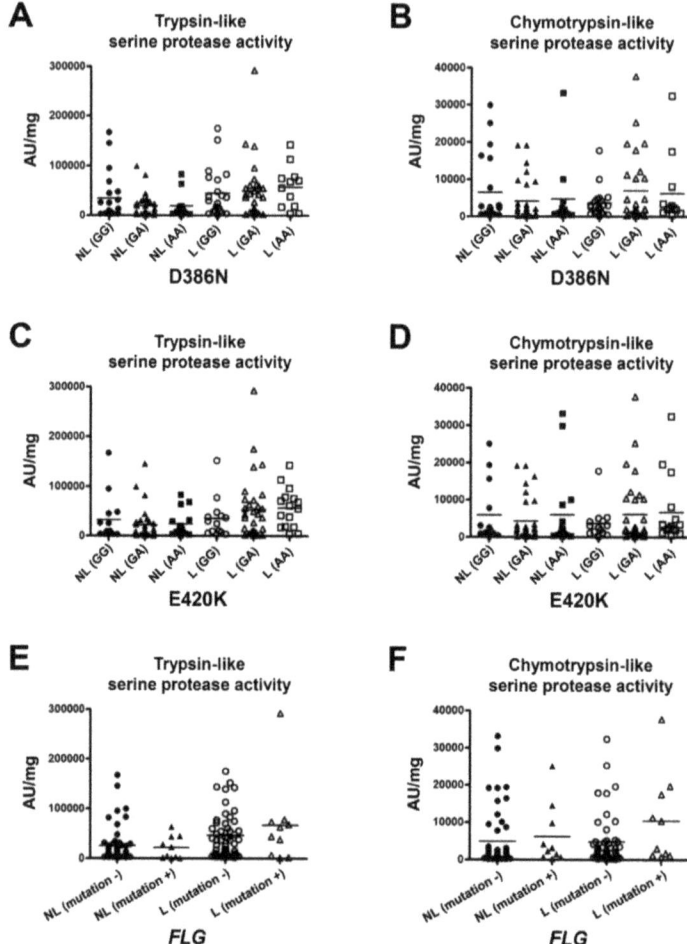

Figure 4. Serine protease activity in the SC of the subgroups of patients with the variants of the *SPINK5* gene and *FLG* gene in AD patients. Trypsin- and chymotrypsin-like serine protease activity in non-lesions and lesions was compared among the subgroups of the p.D386N (**A–B**) or p.E420K (**C–D**) of *SPINK5* and among the subgroups with or without loss-of-function mutations of *FLG* (**E–F**).

3. Discussion

It has been reported that the expression and activity of several KLKs are increased in AD lesions and trigger or enhance epidermal barrier dysfunction [5,8,11]. In this context, we examined the serine protease activity in the SC of both non-lesions and lesions of AD patients. Our findings demonstrated for the first time that serine protease activity is increased not only in lesions but also in non-lesions of AD patients.

Our results are consistent with previous reports that the quantity and activity of serine proteases are increased in AD lesions [5,8]. Our new finding that serine protease activity is also increased in non-lesions suggests two possibilities: (1) Serine protease activity may be influenced by some genetic factors; and (2) Non-lesions of AD patients have subclinical inflammation that may induce the enhancement of serine protease activity.

Considering the fact that Th2 cytokines such as interleukin (IL)-4 and IL-13 increase the expression and function of KLK7 in epidermal keratinocytes [15], the upregulation of chymotrypsin-like serine protease activity may be induced by systemic Th2 inflammation. However, the trypsin-like serine protease activity is not affected by Th2 cytokines [15]. Our present analyses showed that trypsin-like serine protease activity is also increased in both non-lesions and lesions of AD. Further analyses are needed to clarify the mechanism underlying the increase in trypsin-like serine protease activity.

We next investigated the association between serine protease activity in the SC and the content of therapy for AD. The trypsin-like serine protease activity in the SC of patients with topical corticosteroid therapy was significantly higher than those without topical corticosteroid therapy. These results suggest the possibility that patients with clinically severe AD needed to be treated with topical corticosteroid and clinically mild patients were able to be treated with topical tacrolimus or moisturizer only. Thus far, it is unknown why there is a difference between trypsin-like and chymotrypsin-like serine protease activity even though they are positively correlated (see Figure 1). Furthermore, it was unclear whether all the patients strictly took ointments or oral medicines. In addition, we did not prepare a wash-out period before collecting samples. These questions will guide future investigations.

We also investigated the correlation between serine protease activity in the SC and several biomarkers of AD. Not all serine protease activity was significantly correlated with the serum total IgE levels, serum TARC levels, or peripheral blood eosinophil counts, but there were tendencies for these to correlate positively. The absence of statistical significance in several of the comparisons might be due to the insufficiency of the sample number considered for the analysis or the technical instability of our protease assays. Serum total IgE reflects the degree of allergen sensitization [31,32]. Serum TARC is the most sensitive clinical biomarker of AD [33]. Peripheral blood eosinophil numbers also correlate roughly with disease severity [34]. Our results suggest that serine protease activity in the SC correlates with the clinical severity of AD and allergen sensitization due to epidermal barrier dysfunction.

We investigated whether nonsynonymous variants of *SPINK5* and loss-of-function mutations in *FLG* are involved in serine protease activity in the SC. p.D386N and p.E420K polymorphisms of *SPINK5* were each reported to be associated with the pathogenesis of AD [20–25]. We found, specifically, that the p.D386N variant disrupts the role of D6 of LEKTI which suppresses the induction of TSLP by KLK5 [25]. Moreover, the p.E420K substitution increases the furin cleavage rate at the LEKTI linker region D6–D7 and prevents the formation of the LEKTI fragment D6D9, known to display the strongest inhibitory activity against KLK5-mediated desmoglein 1 degradation [20]. However, our analyses revealed that p.D386N and p.E420K do not change the trypsin- or chymotrypsin-like serine protease activity of the SC in AD patients. Japanese AD patients might exhibit another genetic particularity related to serine protease activity that neutralizes the effects of p.D386N and p.E420K.

The *FLG* mutations are well known to be strongly associated with the pathogenesis of AD [28,29], but not all AD patients have *FLG* mutations. Therefore, one or more other genetic factors can be expected to be associated with the pathogenesis. We had hypothesized that AD patients without *FLG* mutations have serine proteases-related gene variants such as *SPINK5* and aberrant protease activity, but our analyses revealed that there is no significant association between these mutations and the serine protease activity in the SC. On the contrary, there was a tendency for the AD patients with *FLG* mutations to have higher serine protease activity compared to the patients without *FLG* mutations. Further analyses might clarify the association between the increase in serine protease activity and genetic factors in AD patients.

In conclusion, the results of our present analyses demonstrated for the first time that epidermal serine protease activity is increased even in non-lesions of AD patients and this activity is associated with biomarkers of AD. In addition, p.D386N and p.E420K of *SPINK5* and *FLG* mutations did not affect the serine protease activity of the SC in Japanese individuals with AD. Further investigations of epidermal serine protease activity might enable the design of new therapeutic and prophylactic drugs for the treatment of AD.

4. Subjects and Methods

4.1. Human Samples

The SC samples and blood samples were collected with written informed consent from normal healthy volunteers and patients with AD at Okayama University Hospital and its affiliated hospitals. This study was approved by the Ethics Committee of Okayama University (approval nos. 1511-012, 1605-027 and 1809-015).

4.2. Collection of the Stratum Corneum

Samples of the SC of healthy individuals were obtained from the forearms of normal healthy volunteers ($n = 46$; ages 35.0 ± 8.8 years). The SC of patients who had been diagnosed with AD based on the diagnostic criteria of Hanifin and Rajka were obtained from the upper extremities (lesions and non-lesions) ($n = 63$; ages 38.2 ± 12.8 years). Cellotape™ (Nichiban, Tokyo) was used to collect the SC samples. The 10-cm-long tape was put on and peeled from the surface of the extremities (approx. 10–20 times) until the adhesion disappeared. The tape was then stored at -20 °C until the following treatment with hexane.

The tape was soaked in 5 mL of hexane and then shaken to detach the SC from the tape's adhesive film. After the insoluble tape was removed, the solution was centrifuged at 3000 rpm for 15 min. A supernatant was subtracted and 1 mL of hexane was added. A solution was transferred to a 1.5-mL microtube and centrifuged at 15,000 rpm for 15 min. A supernatant was subtracted again and the recovered samples were air-dried. The weight was measured. The dried SC samples were mixed with 200 μL of 10 mmol/L Tris-HCl (pH 7.8) and incubated at 37 °C for 1 h on a shaker and then used in the protease assays.

4.3. Protease Assays

For the measurement of protease activity in the SC samples, 100 μL of sample solution was mixed with 100 μL of a substrate that is specific for trypsin-like serine proteases (Boc-Phe-Ser-Arg-MCA; Peptide Institute, Osaka, Japan) or chymotrypsin-like serine proteases (Suc-Leu-Leu-Val-Tyr-MCA; Peptide Institute) in 10 mmol/L Tris-HCl (pH 7.8). The final concentration of each substrate was 0.4 mmol/L. The mixture was incubated at 37 °C for 24 h and the fluorescence (excitation/emission = 380/460 nm) was then measured by a FlexStation 3 Multi-Mode Microplate Reader (Molecular Devices, Sunnyvale, CA) at the Central Research Laboratory, Okayama University Medical School. For the correction of the differences in the SC sample amounts, the value of measured fluorescence (AU) was divided by dried weight of the SC sample (mg).

4.4. Blood Examinations and Medical Treatment Histories

The patients' laboratory data were extracted from their medical records. The serum total IgE level, serum TARC level and peripheral blood eosinophil count that had been obtained at the time point closest to the patient's tape stripping were selected. We also collected the medical treatment histories of the patients such as their use of topical corticosteroid and topical tacrolimus, oral antihistamine, oral corticosteroid and oral cyclosporine.

4.5. Analysis of the SPINK5 Gene and the FLG Gene

Genomic DNA was extracted from whole blood using the Wizard Genomic DNA Purification Kit (Promega, Madison, WI, USA). For exon 13 of *SPINK5*, the 453-bp DNA was amplified with two specific primers (SPINK5-E13-FW: 5'-TTCCTATCTCTTGGCATATGATGT-3' and SPINK5-E13-RV: 5'-TGTCTCCAATCAGACAGTTTCTC-3'). For exon 14 of *SPINK5*, the 294-bp DNA was amplified with two specific primers (SPINK5-E14-FW: 5'-CAGGGTTAGGCACATCACATTC-3' and SPINK5-E14-RV: 5'-TAAGGAATGCACGTGTTCCCTG-3').

The polymerase chain reaction (PCR) products were purified using exonuclease I and shrimp alkaline phosphatase (USB, Cleveland, OH, USA) and sequenced using a BigDye Terminator v3.1 Cycle Sequencing Kit (Applied Biosystems, Foster City, CA, USA) and an ABI3100 DNA sequencer (Applied Biosystems) at the Central Research Laboratory, Okayama University Medical School.

Real-time PCR-based genotyping of FLG mutations was performed. In the present FLG mutation screening, we investigated the 10 FLG mutations as described [30]. Briefly, real-time PCR-based genotyping of the FLG mutations was performed with a TaqMan probe genotyping assay. Real-time PCR-based genotyping of the FLG mutations was performed with a TaqMan probe genotyping assay according to the manufacturer's instructions (Roche Diagnostics, Basel, Switzerland). To detect an allele of each mutation, a set of two TaqMan probes labeled with a fluorescent dye (FAM or CAL Fluor Orange 560) and a quencher dye (BHQ-1), in addition to sequence-specific forward and reverse primers, were synthesized by Biosearch Technologies (Novato, CA, USA). The sequence of assay probes/primers was as provided [30]. The real-time PCR was performed with a LightCycler 480 system II 384 plate (Roche Diagnostics) in a final volume of 5 µL. Genotyping was then performed using the endpoint genotyping analysis of the LightCycler 480 software.

4.6. Statistical Analyses

All statistical analyses were conducted with GraphPad Prism 4 ver. 4.03 software (GraphPad Software, La Jolla, CA, USA). Student's t-test was used to determine the significance of differences between pairs of groups. The correlation between serine protease activity and the blood examination results was analyzed by Spearman's rank correlation coefficient. Values of $p < 0.05$ were considered significant.

Author Contributions: Experimental design and interpretation of results: H.N., M.A., M.K. (Michihiro Kono), T.T. and S.M. Performing the experiments: H.N., Y.I., K.S., and M.S. Writing the manuscript: H.N. Review and editing the manuscript: H.N., M.K. (Mina Kobashi), S.S., A.K., T.M., Y.H., O.Y. and S.M. All authors have read and agreed to the published version of the manuscript.

Funding: This work was supported by a Grant-in-Aid for Scientific Research (C) (no. 26461658).

Conflicts of Interest: The authors declare no conflict of interest.

Abbreviations

AD	Atopic dermatitis
D	Domain
FLG	Filaggrin
IgE	Immunoglobulin E
IL	Interleukin
KLK	Kallikrein-related peptidase
LEKTI	Lympho-epithelial Kazal-type-related inhibitor
SC	Stratum corneum
SLPI	Secretory leukocyte protease inhibitor
SPINK5	Serine protease inhibitor Kazal type 5
TARC	Thymus and activation-regulated chemokine
Th	T-helper lymphocytes

References

1. Eichenfield, L.F.; Tom, W.L.; Chamlin, S.L.; Feldman, S.R.; Hanifin, J.M.; Simpson, E.L.; Berger, T.G.; Bergman, J.N.; Cohen, D.E.; Cooper, K.D.; et al. Guidelines of care for the management of atopic dermatitis: Section 1. Diagnosis and assessment of atopic dermatitis. *J. Am. Acad. Dermatol.* **2014**, *70*, 338–351. [CrossRef]
2. Chavanas, S.; Bodemer, C.; Rochat, A.; Hamel-Teillac, D.; Ali, M.; Irvine, A.D.; Bonafe, J.L.; Wilkinson, J.; Taieb, A.; Barrandon, Y.; et al. Mutations in SPINK5, encoding a serine protease inhibitor, cause Netherton syndrome. *Nat. Genet.* **2000**, *25*, 141–142. [CrossRef]

3. Descargues, P.; Deraison, C.; Bonnart, C.; Kreft, M.; Kishibe, M.; Ishida-Yamamoto, A.; Elias, P.; Barrandon, Y.; Zambruno, G.; Sonnenberg, A.; et al. Spink5-Deficient mice mimic Netherton syndrome through degradation of desmoglein 1 by epidermal protease hyperactivity. *Nat. Genet.* **2005**, *37*, 56–65. [CrossRef]
4. Komatsu, N.; Saijoh, K.; Jayakumar, A.; Clayman, G.L.; Tohyama, M.; Suga, Y.; Mizuno, Y.; Tsukamoto, K.; Taniuchi, K.; Takehara, K.; et al. Correlation between SPINK5 gene mutations and clinical manifestations in Netherton syndrome patients. *J. Investig. Dermatol.* **2008**, *128*, 1148–1159. [CrossRef] [PubMed]
5. Komatsu, N.; Saijoh, K.; Kuk, C.; Liu, A.C.; Khan, S.; Shirasaki, F.; Takehara, K.; Diamandis, E.P. Human tissue kallikrein expression in the stratum corneum and serum of atopic dermatitis patients. *Exp. Dermatol.* **2007**, *16*, 513–519. [CrossRef] [PubMed]
6. Komatsu, N.; Saijoh, K.; Kuk, C.; Shirasaki, F.; Takehara, K.; Diamandis, E.P. Aberrant human tissue kallikrein levels in the stratum corneum and serum of patients with psoriasis: Dependence on phenotype, severity and therapy. *Br. J. Dermatol.* **2007**, *156*, 875–883. [CrossRef] [PubMed]
7. Yamasaki, K.; Di Nardo, A.; Bardan, A.; Murakami, M.; Ohtake, T.; Coda, A.; Dorschner, R.A.; Bonnart, C.; Descargues, P.; Hovnanian, A.; et al. Increased serine protease activity and cathelicidin promotes skin inflammation in rosacea. *Nat. Med.* **2007**, *13*, 975–980. [CrossRef]
8. Voegeli, R.; Rawlings, A.V.; Breternitz, M.; Doppler, S.; Schreier, T.; Fluhr, J.W. Increased stratum corneum serine protease activity in acute eczematous atopic skin. *Br. J. Dermatol.* **2009**, *161*, 70–77. [CrossRef]
9. Sotiropoulou, G.; Pampalakis, G.; Diamandis, E.P. Functional roles of human kallikrein-related peptidases. *J. Biol. Chem.* **2009**, *284*, 32989–32994. [CrossRef]
10. Caubet, C.; Jonca, N.; Brattsand, M.; Guerrin, M.; Bernard, D.; Schmidt, R.; Egelrud, T.; Simon, M.; Serre, G. Degradation of corneodesmosome proteins by two serine proteases of the kallikrein family, SCTE/KLK5/hK5 and SCCE/KLK7/hK7. *J. Investig. Dermatol.* **2004**, *122*, 1235–1244. [CrossRef]
11. Morizane, S. The role of kallikrein-related peptidases in atopic dermatitis. *Acta Med. Okayama* **2019**, *73*, 1–6. [CrossRef] [PubMed]
12. Briot, A.; Deraison, C.; Lacroix, M.; Bonnart, C.; Robin, A.; Besson, C.; Dubus, P.; Hovnanian, A. Kallikrein 5 induces atopic dermatitis-like lesions through PAR2-mediated thymic stromal lymphopoietin expression in Netherton syndrome. *J. Exp. Med.* **2009**, *206*, 1135–1147. [CrossRef] [PubMed]
13. Furio, L.; de Veer, S.; Jaillet, M.; Briot, A.; Robin, A.; Deraison, C.; Hovnanian, A. Transgenic kallikrein 5 mice reproduce major cutaneous and systemic hallmarks of Netherton syndrome. *J. Exp. Med.* **2014**, *211*, 499–513. [CrossRef] [PubMed]
14. Hansson, L.; Backman, A.; Ny, A.; Edlund, M.; Ekholm, E.; Ekstrand-Hammarstrom, B.; Tornell, J.; Wallbrandt, P.; Wennbo, H.; Egelrud, T. Epidermal overexpression of stratum corneum chymotryptic enzyme in mice: A model for chronic itchy dermatitis. *J. Investig. Dermatol.* **2002**, *118*, 444–449. [CrossRef]
15. Morizane, S.; Yamasaki, K.; Kajita, A.; Ikeda, K.; Zhan, M.; Aoyama, Y.; Gallo, R.L.; Iwatsuki, K. TH2 cytokines increase kallikrein 7 expression and function in patients with atopic dermatitis. *J. Allergy Clin. Immunol.* **2012**, *130*, 259–261. [CrossRef]
16. Meyer-Hoffert, U. Reddish, scaly, and itchy: How proteases and their inhibitors contribute to inflammatory skin diseases. *Arch. Immunol. Ther. Exp.* **2009**, *57*, 345–354. [CrossRef]
17. Deraison, C.; Bonnart, C.; Lopez, F.; Besson, C.; Robinson, R.; Jayakumar, A.; Wagberg, F.; Brattsand, M.; Hachem, J.P.; Leonardsson, G.; et al. LEKTI fragments specifically inhibit KLK5, KLK7, and KLK14 and control desquamation through a pH-dependent interaction. *Mol. Biol. Cell* **2007**, *18*, 3607–3619. [CrossRef]
18. Magert, H.J.; Standker, L.; Kreutzmann, P.; Zucht, H.D.; Reinecke, M.; Sommerhoff, C.P.; Fritz, H.; Forssmann, W.G. LEKTI, a novel 15-domain type of human serine proteinase inhibitor. *J. Biol. Chem.* **1999**, *274*, 21499–21502. [CrossRef]
19. Hovnanian, A. Netherton syndrome: Skin inflammation and allergy by loss of protease inhibition. *Cell Tissue Res.* **2013**, *351*, 289–300. [CrossRef]
20. Fortugno, P.; Furio, L.; Teson, M.; Berretti, M.; El Hachem, M.; Zambruno, G.; Hovnanian, A.; D'Alessio, M. The 420K LEKTI variant alters LEKTI proteolytic activation and results in protease deregulation: Implications for atopic dermatitis. *Hum. Mol. Genet.* **2012**, *21*, 4187–4200. [CrossRef]
21. Kato, A.; Fukai, K.; Oiso, N.; Hosomi, N.; Murakami, T.; Ishii, M. Association of SPINK5 gene polymorphisms with atopic dermatitis in the Japanese population. *Br. J. Dermatol.* **2003**, *148*, 665–669. [CrossRef] [PubMed]

22. Kusunoki, T.; Okafuji, I.; Yoshioka, T.; Saito, M.; Nishikomori, R.; Heike, T.; Sugai, M.; Shimizu, A.; Nakahata, T. SPINK5 polymorphism is associated with disease severity and food allergy in children with atopic dermatitis. *J. Allergy Clin. Immunol.* **2005**, *115*, 636–638. [CrossRef] [PubMed]
23. Nishio, Y.; Noguchi, E.; Shibasaki, M.; Kamioka, M.; Ichikawa, E.; Ichikawa, K.; Umebayashi, Y.; Otsuka, F.; Arinami, T. Association between polymorphisms in the SPINK5 gene and atopic dermatitis in the Japanese. *Genes Immun.* **2003**, *4*, 515–517. [CrossRef] [PubMed]
24. Walley, A.J.; Chavanas, S.; Moffatt, M.F.; Esnouf, R.M.; Ubhi, B.; Lawrence, R.; Wong, K.; Abecasis, G.R.; Jones, E.Y.; Harper, J.I.; et al. Gene polymorphism in Netherton and common atopic disease. *Nat. Genet.* **2001**, *29*, 175–178. [CrossRef]
25. Ramesh, K.; Matta, S.A.; Chew, F.T.; Mok, Y.K. Exonic mutations associated with atopic dermatitis disrupt lympho-epithelial Kazal-type related inhibitor action and enhance its degradation. *Allergy* **2019**. [CrossRef]
26. Brown, S.J.; McLean, W.H. One remarkable molecule: Filaggrin. *J. Investig. Dermatol.* **2012**, *132*, 751–762. [CrossRef]
27. Smith, F.J.; Irvine, A.D.; Terron-Kwiatkowski, A.; Sandilands, A.; Campbell, L.E.; Zhao, Y.; Liao, H.; Evans, A.T.; Goudie, D.R.; Lewis-Jones, S.; et al. Loss-of-function mutations in the gene encoding filaggrin cause ichthyosis vulgaris. *Nat. Genet.* **2006**, *38*, 337–342. [CrossRef]
28. Palmer, C.N.; Irvine, A.D.; Terron-Kwiatkowski, A.; Zhao, Y.; Liao, H.; Lee, S.P.; Goudie, D.R.; Sandilands, A.; Campbell, L.E.; Smith, F.J.; et al. Common loss-of-function variants of the epidermal barrier protein filaggrin are a major predisposing factor for atopic dermatitis. *Nat. Genet.* **2006**, *38*, 441–446. [CrossRef]
29. Nemoto-Hasebe, I.; Akiyama, M.; Nomura, T.; Sandilands, A.; McLean, W.H.; Shimizu, H. FLG mutation p.Lys4021X in the C-terminal imperfect filaggrin repeat in Japanese patients with atopic eczema. *Br. J. Dermatol.* **2009**, *161*, 1387–1390. [CrossRef]
30. Kono, M.; Nomura, T.; Ohguchi, Y.; Mizuno, O.; Suzuki, S.; Tsujiuchi, H.; Hamajima, N.; McLean, W.H.; Shimizu, H.; Akiyama, M. Comprehensive screening for a complete set of Japanese-population-specific filaggrin gene mutations. *Allergy* **2014**, *69*, 537–540. [CrossRef]
31. Bieber, T.; D'Erme, A.M.; Akdis, C.A.; Traidl-Hoffmann, C.; Lauener, R.; Schappi, G.; Schmid-Grendelmeier, P. Clinical phenotypes and endophenotypes of atopic dermatitis: Where are we, and where should we go? *J. Allergy Clin. Immunol.* **2017**, *139*, S58–S64. [CrossRef] [PubMed]
32. Kuperstock, J.E.; Brook, C.D.; Ryan, M.W.; Platt, M.P. Correlation between the number of allergen sensitizations and immunoglobulin E: Monosensitization vs. polysensitization. *Int. Forum Allergy Rhinol.* **2017**, *7*, 385–388. [CrossRef] [PubMed]
33. Kataoka, Y. Thymus and activation-regulated chemokine as a clinical biomarker in atopic dermatitis. *J. Dermatol.* **2014**, *41*, 221–229. [CrossRef] [PubMed]
34. Simon, D.; Braathen, L.R.; Simon, H.U. Eosinophils and atopic dermatitis. *Allergy* **2004**, *59*, 561–570. [CrossRef] [PubMed]

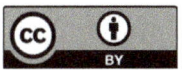

© 2020 by the authors. Licensee MDPI, Basel, Switzerland. This article is an open access article distributed under the terms and conditions of the Creative Commons Attribution (CC BY) license (http://creativecommons.org/licenses/by/4.0/).

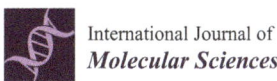

Article

Systemic Dermatitis Model Mice Exhibit Atrophy of Visceral Adipose Tissue and Increase Stromal Cells via Skin-Derived Inflammatory Cytokines

Kento Mizutani [1,†], Eri Shirakami [1,2,†], Masako Ichishi [3], Yoshiaki Matsushima [1], Ai Umaoka [1], Karin Okada [1], Yukie Yamaguchi [4], Masatoshi Watanabe [3], Eishin Morita [2] and Keiichi Yamanaka [1,*]

[1] Department of Dermatology, Graduate School of Medicine, Mie University, Mie, Tsu 514-8507, Japan; k-mizutani@clin.medic.mie-u.ac (K.M.); white818@med.shimane-u.ac.jp (E.S.); matsushima-y@clin.medi.mie-u.ac (Y.M.); ai618lovemyfamily@yahoo.co.jp (A.U.); okadakarin@clin.medic.mie-u.ac.jp (K.O.)
[2] Department of Dermatology, Faculty of Medicine, Shimane University, Shimane, Izumo 693-8501, Japan; emorita@med.shimane-u.ac.jp
[3] Department of Oncologic Pathology, Graduate School of Medicine, Mie University, Mie, Tsu 514-8507, Japan; masako-i@doc.medic.mie-u.ac.jp (M.I.); mawata@doc.medic.mie-u.ac.jp (M.W.)
[4] Department of Environmental Immuno-Dermatology, School of Medicine, Yokohama City University Graduate, Yokohama 236-0027, Japan; yui1783@yokohama-cu.ac.jp
* Correspondence: yamake@clin.medic.mie-u.ac.jp; Tel.: +81-59-231-5025; Fax: +81-59-231-5206
† These authors contributed equally to this work.

Received: 26 April 2020; Accepted: 7 May 2020; Published: 9 May 2020

Abstract: Adipose tissue (AT) is the largest endocrine organ, producing bioactive products called adipocytokines, which regulate several metabolic pathways, especially in inflammatory conditions. On the other hand, there is evidence that chronic inflammatory skin disease is closely associated with vascular sclerotic changes, cardiomegaly, and severe systemic amyloidosis in multiple organs. In psoriasis, a common chronic intractable inflammatory skin disease, several studies have shown that adipokine levels are associated with disease severity. Chronic skin disease is also associated with metabolic syndrome, including abnormal tissue remodeling; however, the mechanism is still unclear. We addressed this problem using keratin 14-specific caspase-1 overexpressing transgenic (KCASP1Tg) mice with severe erosive dermatitis from 8 weeks of age, followed by re-epithelization. The whole body and gonadal white AT (GWAT) weights were decreased. Each adipocyte was large in number, small in size and irregularly shaped; abundant inflammatory cells, including activated CD4+ or CD8+ T cells and toll-like receptor 4/CD11b-positive activated monocytes, infiltrated into the GWAT. We assumed that inflammatory cytokine production in skin lesions was the key factor for this lymphocyte/monocyte activation and AT dysregulation. We tested our hypothesis that the AT in a mouse dermatitis model shows an impaired thermogenesis ability due to systemic inflammation. After exposure to 4 °C, the mRNA expression of the thermogenic gene uncoupling protein 1 in adipocytes was elevated; however, the body temperature of the KCASP1Tg mice decreased rapidly, revealing an impaired thermogenesis ability of the AT due to atrophy. Tumor necrosis factor (TNF)-α, IL-1β and interferon (INF)-γ levels were significantly increased in KCASP1Tg mouse ear skin lesions. To investigate the direct effects of these cytokines, BL/6 wild mice were administered intraperitoneal TNF-α, IL-1β and INF-γ injections, which resulted in small adipocytes with abundant stromal cell infiltration, suggesting those cytokines have a synergistic effect on adipocytes. The systemic dermatitis model mice showed atrophy of AT and increased stromal cells. These findings were reproducible by the intraperitoneal administration of inflammatory cytokines whose production was increased in inflamed skin lesions.

Keywords: skin inflammation; cytokine; adipose tissue; adiponectin; leptin; thermogenesis

1. Introduction

Adipose tissue (AT) is the largest endocrine organ, producing bioactive products called adipocytokines, which regulate several metabolic pathways [1]. AT inflammation induces the dysregulation of adipocytokine production, which plays a critical role in the pathophysiology of atherosclerosis [2]. It is well known that obesity induces AT inflammation and contributes to vascular and AT changes, which may lead to the development of metabolic syndrome. Metabolic syndrome induces insulin resistance that causes hyperglycemia and diabetes, and causes dyslipidemia such as hypertriglyceridemia and low HDL cholesterol, which are risk factors for cardiovascular disorders [3]. In addition, obese AT causes increased angiogenesis, immune cell infiltration, the overproduction of extracellular matrix, and the increased production of pro-inflammatory adipocytokines [4]. As a result, the risks of ischemic heart disease and cerebral strokes increase.

Chronic inflammatory skin disease is also associated with metabolic syndrome [5–7]. However, the mechanism is under discussion, and the contribution of AT is still unclear. We addressed this problem by using keratin 14-specific human caspase-1 overexpressing transgenic (KCASP1Tg) mice, which are accepted as a spontaneous dermatitis model [8]. Caspase-1 is a cytoplasmic cysteine protease characterized by its ability to process the inactive pro-interleukin-1β (IL-1β) into the biologically active IL-1β [9]. IL-1β is an inflammatory cytokine that plays a key role in inflammation and keratinocyte activation. KCASP1Tg mice show severe erosive dermatitis from 8 weeks old, followed by re-epithelization and the development of parakeratotic scale-crust [8]. It was previously reported that a sustained circulating low level of IL-1α/β derived from severe dermatitis causes vascular sclerotic changes, cardiomegaly, and severe systemic amyloidosis in multiple organs [10].

In this study, we aimed to investigate the influence of chronic dermatitis in the pathological and functional changes in AT using a KCASP1Tg mouse model.

2. Results

2.1. GWAT Weight Is Decreased, and Inflammation Affects AT Atrophy

We measured whole-body and GWAT weights with a precision electronic balance to evaluate the effect of dermatitis on the AT. The whole-body and GWAT weights were significantly lower in KCASP1Tg than in wild littermate mice at 10 weeks of age (Figure 1A,B). Next, we evaluated the phenotype of adipocytes in GWAT using hematoxylin and eosin staining (HE). In KCASP1Tg mice, adipocytes were small in size and irregularly shaped compared to in wild type mice (Figure 1C). Abundant mononuclear cell infiltration compared to in control mice suggests the so-called burnout or worn out condition of the adipocytes. We performed immunohistochemical (IHC) staining to identify the stromal cells of AT such as T cells, monocytes and neutrophils. The infiltration of inflammatory cells such as lymphocytes, monocytes and neutrophils was slightly higher in KCASP1Tg mice compared to that in wild type littermates (Figure 1D).

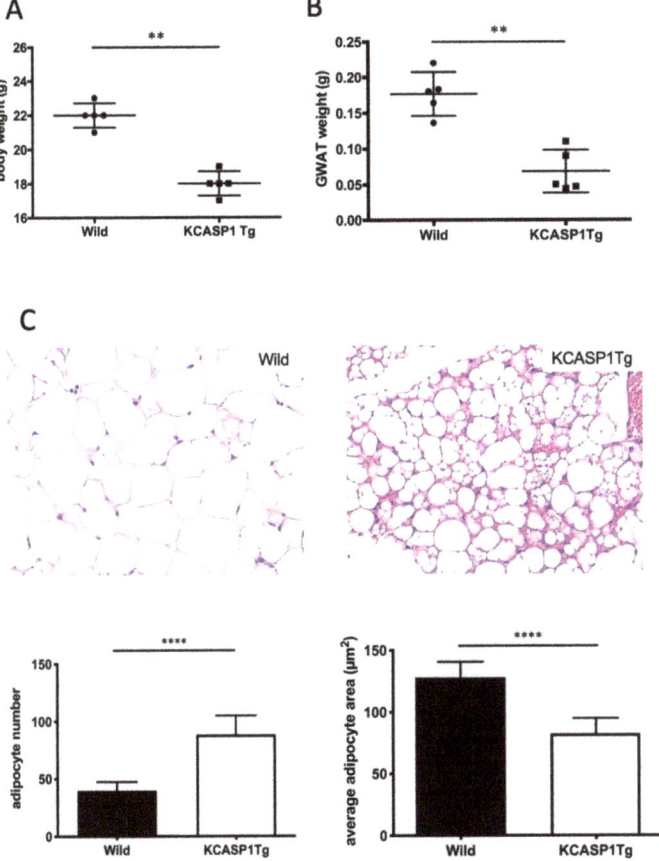

Figure 1. *Cont.*

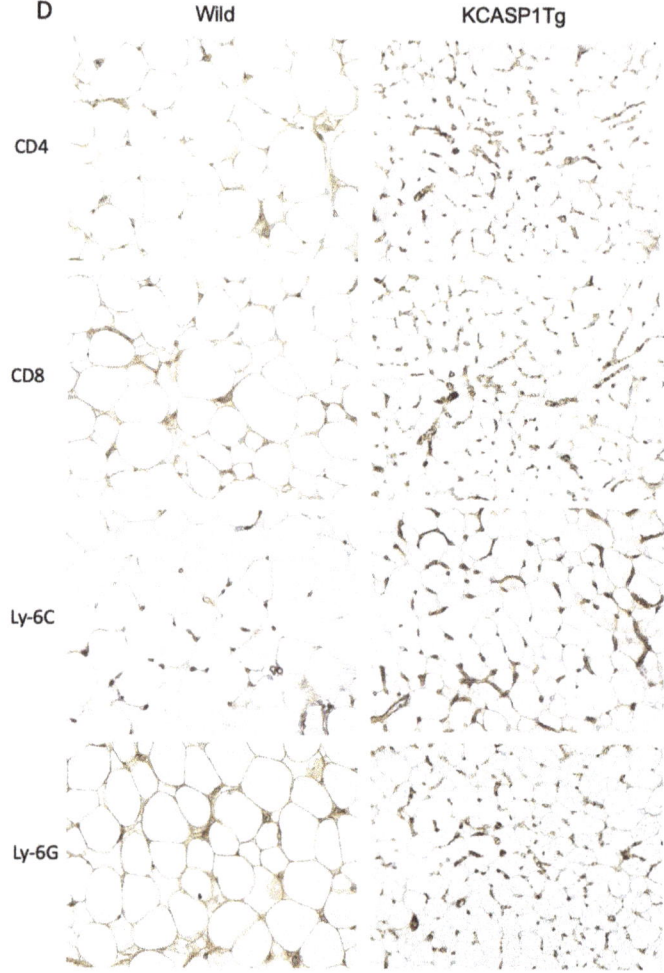

Figure 1. KCASP1Tg mice showed low gonadal white adipose tissue (GWAT) weights and degenerated adipose tissue (AT). (**A**) The whole body and (**B**) GWAT weights were decreased in KCASP1Tg compared to wild littermate mice at 10 weeks of age. (**C**) Representative photomicrographs of the hematoxylin and eosin (HE) (×400) staining of the GWAT of wild littermate and KCASP1Tg mice at 10 weeks of age. Histological sections were 3.5 μm thick. Adipocyte number and adipocyte area were measured by using ImageJ and Adiposoft (three parts of each slide, $n = 3$ in each group). Adipocytes were significantly smaller and larger in number in KCASP1Tg. (**D**) Immunohistochemical staining (×400) was performed to characterize stromal cells. Lymphocytes, monocytes and neutrophils were slightly higher in KCASP1Tg but not significantly so. ** $p < 0.01$, **** $p < 0.0001$ versus control.

2.2. Activated T Cells and Monocytes Infiltrated the AT

We assessed the number or proportion and characteristic composition of the stromal cells infiltrating the GWAT by flow cytometry. The number of infiltrated stromal cells, including lymphocytes and monocytes, was significantly increased in KCASP1Tg mice (Figure 2A). Next, we verified the characteristics of the lymphocytes and monocytes. We measured the proportion of the CD25+ T cells (Figure 2B). Activated T cells, both CD4+ and CD8+, were increased in KCASP1Tg mice (Figure 2C).

Additionally, we measured the proportion of regulatory T cells by using CD127, CD4, CD25 and Foxp3 antibodies (Figure 2D). The regulatory T cells were increased in KCASP1Tg, but there was no significant difference (Figure 2E). Finally, we measured the number of TLR4+ CD11b+ monocytes and proportion of Ly-6C+ CD11b+ monocytes TLR4+ CD11b+ monocytes were significantly increased in KCASP1Tg, and Ly-6C+ CD11b+ monocytes were also increased (Figure 2F,G).

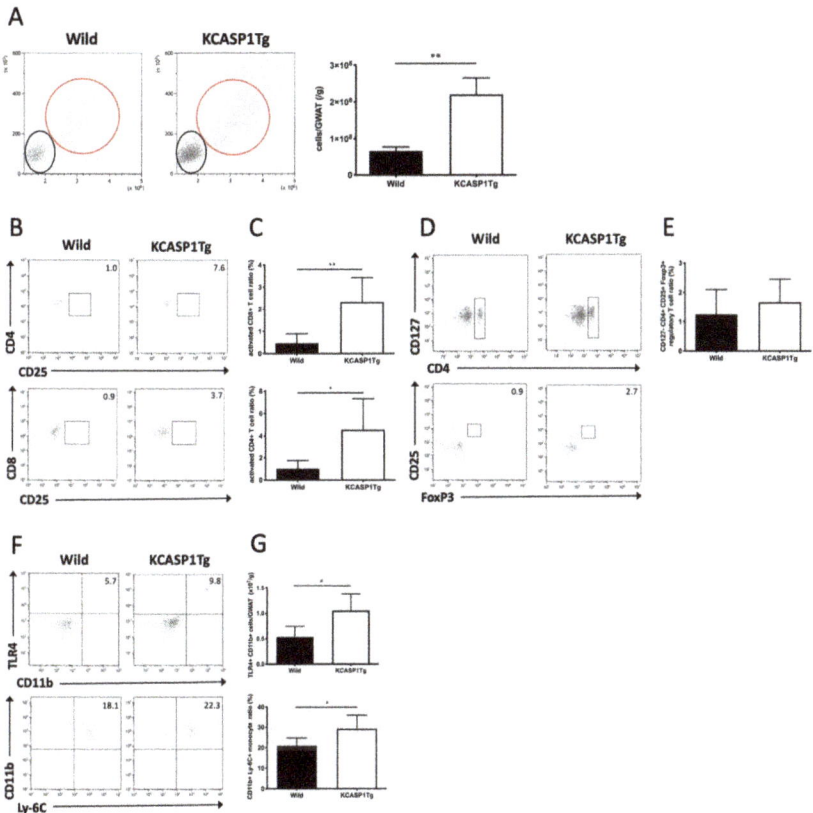

Figure 2. AT cell infiltration in KCASP1Tg mice. (A) Flow cytometric analysis of infiltrated stromal cells in GWAT. The black and red circles correspond to the lymphocyte and monocyte populations, respectively, in the left figure. Stromal cell infiltration, including lymphocytes and monocytes, was significantly increased in KCASP1Tg mice. (B,C) The population of CD25+ activated lymphocytes was measured in CD4+ or CD8+ lymphocytes. Activated T cells were significantly increased in KCASP1Tg. (D,E) The proportion of regulatory T cells in AT was measured. There was no significant difference between KCASP1Tg and wild mice. (F,G) The proportion of Ly-6C+ CD11b+ and number of TLR4+ CD11b+ activated monocytes were evaluated and increased in the AT of KCASP1Tg mice. $n = 5–6$ in each group. * $p < 0.05$, ** $p < 0.01$ versus control.

2.3. Expression of Inflammation-Related Cytokine Levels in AT

An adipocytokine is a physiologically active substance secreted from adipocytes, and the amount secreted also changes depending on the environment of the adipocytes. Representative adipocytokines such as adiponectin, TNF-α, leptin and MCP-1 were analyzed in the adipocytes of GWAT using a specific ELISA kit (Figure 3). The TNF-α level was significantly elevated in KCASP1Tg mice compared to in controls. Conversely, KCASP1Tg mice showed a lower leptin level.

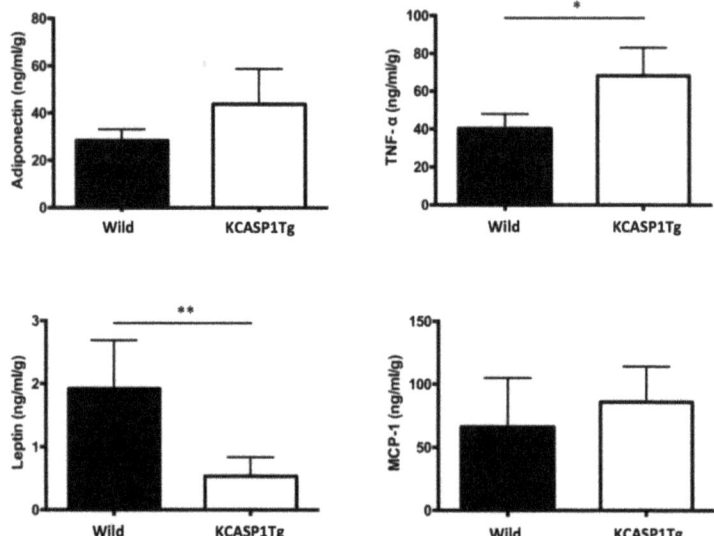

Figure 3. Adipokine expression in AT. We quantified adipocytokines such as adiponectin, TNF-α, leptin and MCP-1 from the adipocytes of GWAT by using a specific ELISA kit. The TNF-α level was elevated in KCASP1Tg mice compared to controls; conversely, the leptin level was decreased in KCASP1Tg ($n = 5$ in each group). * $p < 0.05$ and ** $p < 0.01$ versus control.

2.4. Changes in UCP1 Expression after Cold Exposure

HSP90, IL-33 and UCP-1 are deeply involved in thermogenesis in adipocytes, and their expression is increased by cold exposure or adrenergic stimulation. We investigated the heat production upon cold exposure challenge and the expression of these thermogenic genes. After 4 °C cold exposure, the mRNA expression of HSP90, IL-33 and UCP1 in adipocytes was quantified using real time-PCR. The mRNA expression of HSP90 and IL-33 was significantly decreased in KCASP1Tg mice (Figure 4A). Although the mRNA expression of UCP1 was significantly increased in KCASP1Tg mice (Figure 4A), the body temperature decreased more rapidly upon exposure to the cold environment, and the KCASP1Tg mice could not survive for a long time (Figure 4B).

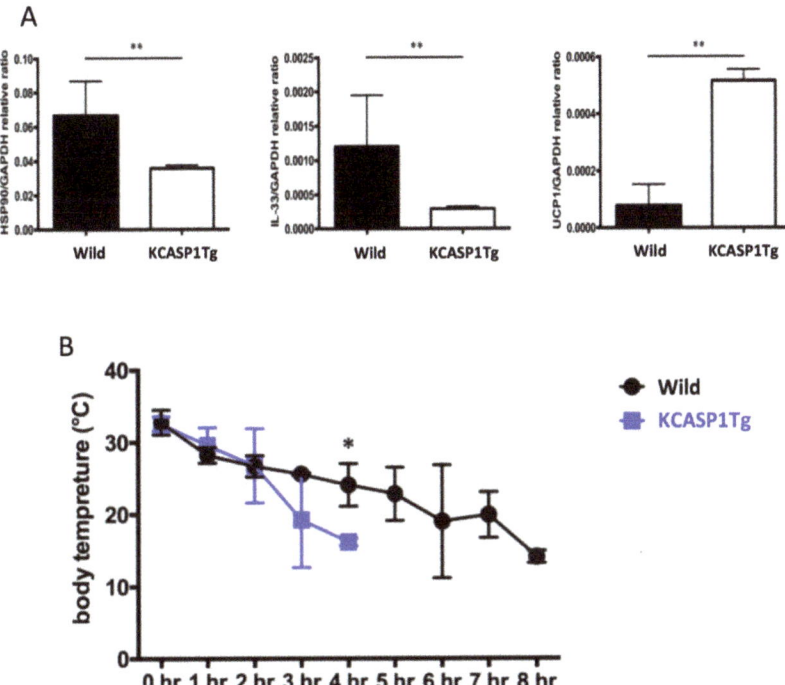

Figure 4. mRNA expression of heat-related proteins in GWAT after cold exposure. (**A**) The mRNA expression of HSP90 and IL-33 was decreased, while that of UCP1 was increased in the adipocytes of KCASP1Tg mice after exposure to 4 °C (n = 5, each group). (**B**) The body temperature of mice exposed to 4 °C was measured every 1 hour using thermal imaging camera. The body temperature of the KCASP1Tg mice decreased more rapidly in a cold environment (n = 5, each group). * $p < 0.05$, ** $p < 0.01$ versus control.

2.5. Pro-Inflammatory Cytokines Produced in Response to Dermatitis Caused AT Atrophy and Increased Activated Monocyte Infiltration In Vivo

We hypothesized that cytokines produced in inflamed skin affect AT and measured the mRNA expression levels of inflammatory cytokines in the skin of KCASP1Tg and control mice. The mRNA expression levels of TNF-α, IL-1β and IFN-γ in ear skin were measured by real-time PCR. All cytokine levels were significantly increased in KCASP1Tg mice (Figure 5A). To clarify the direct effect of skin-derived cytokines on GWAT, we treated wild-type mice by the intraperitoneal administration of inflammatory cytokines including TNF-α, IL-1β and IFN-γ. The GWATs of the TNF-α-treated wild-type mice were similar to those of KCASP1Tg mice; the adipocytes were large in number, small and irregularly shaped; IL-1β- and IFN-γ-injected mice also showed a similar trend (Figure 5B). The number of infiltrating stromal cells tended to increase in mice that were administered cytokines (Figure 5C); additionally, TLR4+ CD11b+ monocytes were significantly increased in IFN-γ treated mice (Figure 5D).

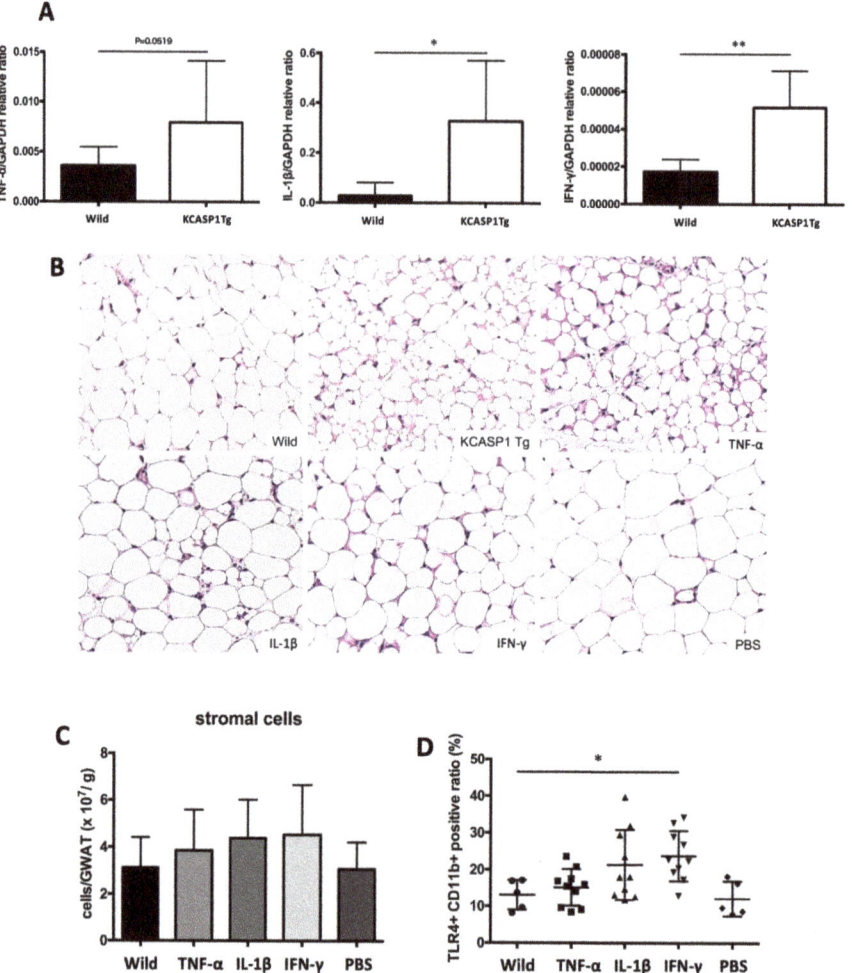

Figure 5. Production of inflammatory cytokines in the skin and the direct effect on AT. (**A**) The TNFα, IL-1β and INF-γ levels were significantly increased in KCASP1Tg mouse ear skin lesions. (**B**) Eight-week-old BL/6 wild mice were treated by intraperitoneal injections of TNF-α, IL-1β, IFN-γ (250 µg/kg body weight/each time) or PBS three times per week for two weeks. The AT of TNF-α-treated mice showed a similar appearance to that of KCASP1Tg mice; IL-1β- and IFN-γ-administrated mice also showed a similar trend; adipocytes were large in number, small and irregularly shaped (HE, ×400). (**C**,**D**) The number of infiltrating cells in GWAT was counted, and the infiltrating cells were analyzed by flowcytometry. The number of infiltrating cells in GWAT was increased in cytokine-administrated mice, while TLR4+ CD11b+ activated monocytes were significantly increased in IFN-γ-treated mice. $n = 5$ per group. * $p < 0.05$, ** $p < 0.01$ versus control.

3. Discussion

In the current study, we demonstrated that severe dermatitis induces AT atrophy accompanied by abundant lymphocyte and activated monocyte infiltration, the dysregulation of adipocytokine production and maladaptation to cold environments. We observed not only histopathological AT remodeling but also a GWAT functional change when skin is inflamed. Inflammatory skin disorders are not only skin-related but also involve systemic organ impairment. A previous study showed chronic skin inflammation induces the aberrant remodeling of vascular tissues, potentially resulting in atherosclerosis [11]. Systemic amyloidosis with functional deterioration has also been seen in inflammatory skin conditions [12]. The erupted skin of KCASP1Tg mice produces significantly higher amounts of IL-1α and β compared to normal skin, while the supernatant from skin lesions leads to a severe reduction in lipid particles in an adipocyte culture system [10]. Computed tomography imaging of KCASP1Tg mice at 6 months of age revealed a dramatic decrease in visceral fat compared to in normal controls [10]. Based on these findings, it was hypothesized that persistent dermatitis had a negative effect on visceral AT, and we investigated the state of GWAT using dermatitis model mice.

In KCASP1Tg mice, the whole body and GWAT weights were decreased compared to in wild littermate mice. Each adipocyte was small and irregularly shaped, and showed abundant inflammatory cell infiltration in GWAT. Since increased inflammatory cell infiltration and atrophy of adipocytes were observed, it was considered that AT was strongly inflamed under chronic dermatitis. The stromal cells that infiltrate into GWAT are mainly lymphocytes and monocytes, but it was difficult to quantify them by examination using immunohistochemical staining. We performed stromal cell classification using flow cytometry. It was found that lymphocytes and monocytes, which infiltrated into GWAT, were increased in KCASP1Tg mice. In the lymphocyte fraction, both CD4+ and CD8+ T cells were activated compared to in the control. Moreover, although there was no significant difference, regulatory T cells also tended to increase in the inflamed AT. The CD11b antigen is expressed when premature monocytes are activated to become differentiated monocytes and represents the best molecular marker of the macrophage lineage [13]. In monocytes, the expression of TLR4 is important in mediating inflammatory cytokine production in AT inflammation. In humans, TNF-α suppresses the expression of TLR4 on monocytes; however, IL-6 or IFN-γ mediates the upregulation of TLR4 expression [14]. The number of lymphocytes and TLR4+ CD11b+ activated monocytes was significantly higher in the AT of the KCASP1Tg mice.

AT plays an essential role in metabolic homeostasis by storing and releasing lipids and secreting bioactive proteins and peptides called adipokines, including adiponectin, leptin, MCP-1 and TNF-α in response to environmental changes. Both leptin and adiponectin are mainly produced by adipocytes. The main function of leptin seems to be to provide an afferent signal of nutritional and fat mass status to the hypothalamus, thus controlling energy fat stores and regulating appetite and body weight [15]. Leptin reduces the appetite; increased adipocyte storage leads to higher leptin production, which results in a further loss of appetite. On the other hand, adiponectin helps to repair damaged blood vessel walls, prevent arteriosclerosis, increase insulin's action and lower blood pressure. However, clinically, blood adiponectin concentration is inversely correlated to visceral fat mass; the mechanism behind this relationship has not been elucidated so far. In psoriasis, one of the most common chronic intractable inflammatory skin diseases, several studies showed that adipokine levels are associated with disease severity [16]. AT plays an important role in the development of psoriasis. Leptin induces IL-6, CXCL-1, IL-8 and MCP-1 production, which is involved in the hyperproliferation of the epidermis in psoriasis [17]. To the contrary, adiponectin is an anti-inflammatory adipocytokine, and when dermatitis is caused in adiponectin knock out mice, the expression of IL-17A, IL-17F and IL-22 increases [18]. Moreover, an increased circulating level of IL-1 has been shown to be accompanied by the local overexpression of TNF-α and IL-12/23 p40 [19], as was also seen in our model mice. However, although our model mice exhibited AT atrophy, psoriasis patients are often obese. BMI is also known to be a risk factor for developing psoriasis [20]. The lower leptin level in KCASP1Tg mice may be responsible for the upregulation of body weight. Additionally, adiponectin production from GWAT was significantly increased because adipocytes oversecrete adiponectin in chronic dermatitis. The effects of systemic dermatitis on AT in our study differ from those in psoriasis and may resemble those in erythroderma, which often results in weight loss. However, a recent report shows that psoriasis patients treated with anti-TNF-α antibodies experience weight gain [21]. If it occurs more often in patients with severe psoriasis and high improvement rates for psoriasis, it is likely that dermatitis has a considerable impact on weight loss.

We speculated that the AT in a dermatitis model shows an impaired thermogenesis ability due to systemic inflammation. After exposure to 4 °C, the mRNA expression of heat-related proteins such as HSP90, IL-33 and UCP1 in GWAT was measured. Heat shock proteins (HSPs) are primary mitigators of cell stress HSPs expression is also induced by cold exposure in brown adipose tissue [22]. It is well known that brown adipocytes play an important role in heat production in mice [23]. When white adipocytes face various stimuli such as cold exposure and adrenergic stimulation, they form beige adipocytes and induce UCP1, producing brown adipocytes [24]. This process can be induced by IL-33, which is released from various cells in response to stress and injury in adult mice and activates type 2 innate lymphocytes (ILC2) [25]. In our study, although IL-33 levels were lower in the KCASP1Tg mice, UCP1 expression was significantly increased after exposure to the 4 °C environment. Therefore, heat production occurred correctly; however, the body temperature of the KCASP1Tg mice decreased more rapidly in the cold environment, and these mice died earlier than the wild-type mice, meaning survival in a cold environment may be harder due to AT atrophy.

We assumed that increased inflammatory cytokine production in the skin lesions was the key factor for this lymphocyte/monocyte activation and AT dysregulation. In fact, TNFα, IL-1β and INF-γ levels were significantly increased in KCASP1Tg mouse ear skin lesions (Figure 5A). To investigate the direct effects of these cytokines, BL/6 wild mice were administrated intraperitoneal injections of TNF-α, IL-1β and IFN-γ, revealing small adipocytes and abundant stromal cell infiltration, suggesting those cytokines exert a synergistic effect on adipocytes (Figure 5B–D). According to our results, inflammatory cytokines whose production is increased by the eczema lesions cause AT atrophy and increased inflammatory cell infiltration in AT. We have reported, in previous studies, that the inhibition of IL-1 can prevent cerebrovascular disease [26]. In this study, we did not prove the prevention of AT damage by treating dermatitis. However, controlling dermatitis with topical corticosteroids, immunosuppressants or anti-cytokine antibodies probably reduce damage to AT. Of course, the long-term use of topical steroids can cause side effects such as skin atrophy, rosacea-like dermatitis and dermatomycosis [27,28], and immunosuppressants or anti-cytokine antibodies may cause severe infections and malignant tumors. We should realize that dermatitis causes damage to various organs and the importance of the active treatment of dermatitis.

There are only a few studies evaluating AT pathology and function in inflammatory skin disease. We found that skin-derived inflammatory cytokines led to the secretion of pro-inflammatory proteins from adipocytes. As a result, activated monocytes and lymphocytes infiltrated into the AT, which lead to AT atrophy and increased the difficulty in the metabolic adaptation to cold temperatures. Our study suggested that inflammatory skin diseases lead to organ damage and require careful attention.

4. Materials and Methods

4.1. Mouse Study

We used 8–10-week-old spontaneous dermatitis transgenic female KCASP1Tg mice, while female littermate C57BL/6 mice were used as controls. The experimental protocol was approved by the Mie University Board Committee for Animal Care and Use (Protocol #22-39-2, approved date, 1 October 2014). Eight-week-old female wild mice were also administered intraperitoneal injections of recombinant tumor necrosis factor-alpha (TNF-α), recombinant IL-1β, recombinant interferon-gamma (IFN-γ) or phosphate-buffered saline (PBS). The cytokines were diluted in PBS and 250 µg/kg of body weight each time were injected three times per week for two weeks. All the recombinant compounds were purchased from Biolegend (San Diego, CA). All the mice were sacrificed the day after the sixth injection. For the cold stimulation study, 10-week-old KCASP1Tg and littermate mice were housed, one per cage, at a temperature of 22 °C. All the mice were transferred to a 4 °C room, and body temperature was measured every hour using thermal imaging camera FLIR i5 (Extech Instruments, Waltham, MA, USA). After eight hours, all the mice were sacrificed and AT was sampled.

4.2. Tissue Sampling

Isolated adipocytes were prepared as previously reported with minor modifications [29,30]. In brief, extracted gonadal white AT (GWAT) was minced and incubated in PBS with 0.5% bovine serum albumin (BSA, Sigma-Aldrich, St. Louis, MO, USA), 10 mM $CaCl_2$, and 2 mg/mL of collagenase type II (Worthington Biochemical Corporation, Lakewood, NJ, USA) at 37 °C for 20 min at 200 rpm. The suspension was filtered through a 100-μm nylon filter and centrifuged at room temperature at 400 rpm for one minute; the floating cells (adipocytes) were then collected. The remaining suspension was further centrifuged at 1500 rpm for 10 min. The supernatant was decanted and the remaining cell pellets were resuspended with 0.5% BSA/PBS. We counted the number of viable cells based on trypan blue exclusion and diluted the cell suspensions to final concentrations of $5–10 \times 10^6$ cells/mL as adipose-infiltrated stromal cells.

4.3. Histological and Immunohistochemistry Analysis

Tissue was fixed in 10% formalin neutral buffer solution (Wako, Osaka, Japan), embedded in paraffin, cut into 3.5-μm sections and stained with hematoxylin and eosin (HE). Immunohistochemistry (IHC) was performed with primary antibodies—rabbit anti-mouse CD4 antibody (Cell Signaling Technology, Danvers, MA, USA), rabbit anti-mouse CD8a antibody (Cell Signaling Technology), rabbit anti-Ly6G antibody (Abcam, Cambridge, UK) and rat anti-Ly6C antibody (abcam)—and secondary antibodies—goat anti-rabbit immunoglobulins/biotinylated (Dako, Santa Clara, CA, USA) and simple stain MAX-PO (rat) (Nichirei Biosciences, Tokyo, Japan). The adipocytes were observed with 400× HE and counted, and the area was measured using ImageJ and Adiposoft (NIH, Bethesda, MD, USA).

4.4. Flow Cytometry Analysis

AT-infiltrating stromal cells were stained with FITC anti-mouse CD3ε antibody, PE anti-mouse CD4 antibody, PE/Cy7 anti-mouse CD25 antibody, APC anti-mouse CD8a antibody, FITC anti-mouse CD127 antibody, PerCP/Cy5.5 anti-mouse CD4 antibody, APC anti-mouse CD25 antibody (these antibodies were purchased from Biolegend, San Diego, CA, USA), PE anti-mouse/Foxp3 antibody (Invitrogen, Carlsbad, CA, USA), PE anti-mouse CD11b antibody (Biolegend), PE/Cy7 anti-mouse Ly-6C antibody (Biolegend, San Diego, CA, USA) and APC anti-toll-like receptor 4 (TLR4) antibody (Invitrogen, Waltham, MA, USA), and analyzed using an Accuri C6 (Becton, Dickinson and Company, Franklin Lakes, NJ, USA).

4.5. Real-Time Polymerase Chain Reaction (PCR)

Total RNA was extracted from ear skin and AT using TRI Reagent (Molecular Research Center, Cincinnati, OH) according to the manufacturer's protocol. The RNA concentration was measured using a NanoDrop Lite spectrophotometer (Thermo Fisher Scientific, Worsham, MA, USA) and 1 μg of total RNA was converted to cDNA using the High-Capacity RNA-to-cDNA Kit (Applied Biosystems, Foster City, CA, USA). The TaqMan Universal PCR Master Mix II with UNG (Applied Biosystems, Foster City, CA, USA) was used to measure the mRNA expression of TNF-α (Mm00443258_m1), IL-1β (Mm01336189_m1), IFN-γ (Mm01168134_m), heat shock protein 90 (HSP90, Mm00658568_gH), IL-33 (Mm00505403_m1) and uncoupling protein 1 (UCP-1, Mm01244861_m1). All probes were purchased from Applied Biosystems and glyceraldehyde-3-phosphate dehydrogenase (Mm99999915_g1) was used as the internal control. Amplification was performed in a LightCycler 96 System (Roche Diagnostics, Basel, Switzerland). The cycling parameters were as follows: 95 °C for 30 s, followed by 40 cycles of amplification at 95 °C for 5 s and 60 °C for 30 s.

4.6. Enzyme-Linked Immunosorbent Assay (ELISA)

The total protein content from adipocytes was extracted using a radioimmunoprecipitation assay buffer (Nacalai tesque, Kyoto, Japan). Adiponectin, TNF-α, leptin and monocyte chemotactic protein-1 (MCP-1) levels were measured using specific ELISA kits (R&D systems Minneapolis, MN) according to the manufacturer's protocol, and the data were normalized to GWAT weight. The absorbance was measured using MULTISKAN JX (Thermo Fisher Scientific, Worsham, MA, USA). The values were analyzed using Ascent Software for Multiskan Ascent (Thermo Fisher Scientific, Worsham, MA, USA).

4.7. Statistical Analysis

Statistical analysis was performed using the PRISM software version 8 (GraphPad, San Diego, CA, USA). The Mann–Whitney U test was used to compare variables between groups. Differences were considered significant at $p < 0.05$.

5. Conclusions

The systemic dermatitis model mice showed atrophy of AT and an increased infiltration of activated T cells and monocytes into the AT. These were reproducible by the intraperitoneal administration of inflammatory cytokines such as TNF-α, IL-1β and IFN-g, whose production was increased in inflamed skin lesions. The persistence of skin inflammation can potentially cause negative reactions in AT.

Author Contributions: K.M. and E.S. performed the experiments and wrote the paper. M.I. performed part of the histopathological analysis, and Y.M., A.U., K.O., and A.U. performed the experiments. Y.Y., M.W., E.M., and K.Y. designed and supervised the experiments. All authors have read and agreed to the published version of the manuscript.

Funding: KY (17K10241) received grant for scientific research from the Ministry of Education, Culture, Sports, Science and Technology, Japan. Other authors did not receive any financial support for the present study.

Conflicts of Interest: The authors declare no conflict of interest.

Abbreviations

AT	adipose tissue
BSA	bovine serum albumin
ELISA	enzyme-linked immunosorbent assay
KCASP1Tg	keratin 14-specific caspase-1 overexpressing transgenic mouse
GWAT	gonadal white adipose tissue
HSP90	heat shock protein 90
IL	interleukin
INF	interferon
MCP-1	monocyte chemotactic protein-1
PBS	phosphate-buffered saline
PCR	polymerase chain reaction
TLR	toll-like receptor
TNF	tumor necrosis factor
UCP	uncoupling protein 1

References

1. Scherer, P.E. Adipose tissue: From lipid storage compartment to endocrine organ. *Diabetes* **2006**, *55*, 1537–1545. [CrossRef] [PubMed]
2. Gerdes, S.; Rostami-Yazdi, M.; Mrowietz, U. Adipokines and psoriasis. *Exp. Dermatol.* **2011**, *20*, 81–87. [CrossRef] [PubMed]
3. Blaton, V. How is the metabolic syndrome related to the dyslipidemia? *EJIFCC* **2007**, *18*, 15–22. [CrossRef]
4. Suganami, T.; Ogawa, Y. Adipose tissue macrophages: Their role in adipose tissue remodeling. *J. Leukoc. Biol.* **2010**, *88*, 33–39. [CrossRef] [PubMed]

5. Caton, P.W.; Evans, E.A.; Philpott, M.P.; Hannen, R.F. Can the skin make you fat? A role for the skin in regulating adipose tissue function and whole-body glucose and lipid homeostasis. *Curr. Opin. Pharmacol.* **2017**, *37*, 59–64. [CrossRef] [PubMed]
6. Coimbra, S.; Catarino, C.; Santos-Silva, A. The triad psoriasis-obesity-adipokine profile. *J. Eur. Acad. Dermatol. Venereol.* **2016**, *30*, 1876–1885. [CrossRef] [PubMed]
7. Nakamizo, S.; Honda, T.; Adachi, A.; Nagatake, T.; Kunisawa, J.; Kitoh, A.; Otsuka, A.; Dainichi, T.; Nomura, T.; Ginhoux, F.; et al. High fat diet exacerbates murine psoriatic dermatitis by increasing the number of IL-17-producing gammadelta T cells. *Sci. Rep.* **2017**, *7*, 14076. [CrossRef] [PubMed]
8. Yamanaka, K.; Tanaka, M.; Tsutsui, H.; Kupper, T.S.; Asahi, K.; Okamura, H.; Nakanishi, K.; Suzuki, M.; Kayagaki, N.; Black, R.A.; et al. Skin-specific caspase-1-transgenic mice show cutaneous apoptosis and pre-endotoxin shock condition with a high serum level of IL-18. *J. Immunol.* **2000**, *165*, 997–1003. [CrossRef]
9. Black, R.A.; Kronheim, S.R.; Cantrell, M.; Deeley, M.C.; March, C.J.; Prickett, K.S.; Wignall, J.; Conlon, P.J.; Cosman, D.; Hopp, T.P.; et al. Generation of biologically active interleukin-1 beta by proteolytic cleavage of the inactive precursor. *J. Biol. Chem.* **1988**, *263*, 9437–9442.
10. Yamanaka, K.; Nakanishi, T.; Saito, H.; Maruyama, J.; Isoda, K.; Yokochi, A.; Imanaka-Yoshida, K.; Tsuda, K.; Kakeda, M.; Okamoto, R.; et al. Persistent release of IL-1s from skin is associated with systemic cardio-vascular disease, emaciation and systemic amyloidosis: The potential of anti-IL-1 therapy for systemic inflammatory diseases. *PLoS ONE* **2014**, *9*, e104479. [CrossRef]
11. Herrero, L.; Shapiro, H.; Nayer, A.; Lee, J.; Shoelson, S.E. Inflammation and adipose tissue macrophages in lipodystrophic mice. *Proc. Natl. Acad. Sci. USA* **2010**, *107*, 240–245. [CrossRef] [PubMed]
12. Yamanaka, K.; Okada, K.; Nakanishi, T.; Mizutani, K.; Matsushima, Y.; Kondo, M.; Habe, K.; Mizutani, H.; Seo, N. Skin inflammation leads immunoglobulin G aggregation and deposition in multiple organs. *J. Dermatol. Sci.* **2017**, *88*, 146–148. [CrossRef] [PubMed]
13. Leenen, P.J.; de Bruijn, M.F.; Voerman, J.S.; Campbell, P.A.; van Ewijk, W. Markers of mouse macrophage development detected by monoclonal antibodies. *J. Immunol. Methods* **1994**, *174*, 5–19. [CrossRef]
14. Guzzo, C.; Ayer, A.; Basta, S.; Banfield, B.W.; Gee, K. IL-27 enhances LPS-induced proinflammatory cytokine production via upregulation of TLR4 expression and signaling in human monocytes. *J. Immunol.* **2012**, *188*, 864–873. [CrossRef]
15. Schwartz, M.W.; Woods, S.C.; Porte, D.; Seeley, R.J.; Baskin, D.G. Central nervous system control of food intake. *Nature* **2000**, *404*, 661–671. [CrossRef]
16. Nakajima, H.; Nakajima, K.; Tarutani, M.; Morishige, R.; Sano, S. Kinetics of circulating Th17 cytokines and adipokines in psoriasis patients. *Arch. Dermatol. Res.* **2011**, *303*, 451–455. [CrossRef]
17. Ommen, P.; Stjernholm, T.; Kragstrup, T.; Raaby, L.; Johansen, C.; Stenderup, K.; Iversen, L.; Rosada, C. The role of leptin in psoriasis comprises a proinflammatory response by the dermal fibroblast. *Br. J. Dermatol.* **2016**, *174*, 187–190. [CrossRef]
18. Shibata, S.; Tada, Y.; Hau, C.S.; Mitsui, A.; Kamata, M.; Asano, Y.; Sugaya, M.; Kadono, T.; Masamoto, Y.; Kurokawa, M.; et al. Adiponectin regulates psoriasiform skin inflammation by suppressing IL-17 production from gammadelta-T cells. *Nat. Commun.* **2015**, *6*, 7687. [CrossRef]
19. Yu, A.P.; Tang, J.; Xie, J.; Wu, E.Q.; Gupta, S.R.; Bao, Y.; Mulani, P.M. Economic burden of psoriasis compared to the general population and stratified by disease severity. *Curr. Med. Res. Opin.* **2009**, *25*, 2429–2438. [CrossRef]
20. Budu-Aggrey, A.; Brumpton, B.; Tyrrell, J.; Watkins, S.; Modalsli, E.H.; Celis-Morales, C.; Ferguson, L.D.; Vie, G.Å.; Palmer, T.; Fritsche, L.G.; et al. Evidence of a causal relationship between body mass index and psoriasis: A mendelian randomization study. *PLoS Med.* **2019**, *16*, e1002739. [CrossRef]
21. Wu, M.-Y.; Yu, C.-L.; Yang, S.-J.; Chi, C.-C. Change in body weight and body mass index in psoriasis patients receiving biologics: A systematic review and network meta-analysis. *J. Am. Acad. Dermatol.* **2020**, *82*, 101–109. [CrossRef] [PubMed]
22. Matz, J.M.; Blake, M.J.; Tatelman, H.M.; Lavoi, K.P.; Holbrook, N.J. Characterization and regulation of cold-induced heat shock protein expression in mouse brown adipose tissue. *Am. J. Physiol. Regul. Integr. Comp. Physiol.* **1995**, *269*, R38–R47. [CrossRef] [PubMed]
23. Nedergaard, J.; Cannon, B. Brown adipose tissue as a heat-producing thermoeffector. *Handb. Clin. Neurol.* **2018**, *156*, 137–152. [CrossRef] [PubMed]
24. Wong, W. A signal to warm up to. *Sci. Signal.* **2016**, *9*, ec190. [CrossRef]

25. Mathis, D. IL-33, imprimatur of adipocyte thermogenesis. *Cell* **2016**, *166*, 794–795. [CrossRef] [PubMed]
26. Kato, S.; Matsushima, Y.; Mizutani, K.; Kawakita, F.; Fujimoto, M.; Okada, K.; Kondo, M.; Habe, K.; Suzuki, H.; Mizutani, H.; et al. The stenosis of cerebral arteries and impaired brain glucose uptake by long-lasting inflammatory cytokine release from dermatitis is rescued by Anti-IL-1 therapy. *J. Investig. Dermatol.* **2018**, *138*, 2280–2283. [CrossRef]
27. Tatu, A.L.; Ionescu, M.A.; Clatici, V.G.; Cristea, V.C. Bacillus cereus strain isolated from Demodex folliculorum in patients with topical steroid-induced rosaceiform facial dermatitis. *Bras. Dermatol.* **2016**, *91*, 676–678. [CrossRef]
28. Meena, S.; Gupta, L.K.; Khare, A.K.; Balai, M.; Mittal, A.; Mehta, S.; Bhatri, G. Topical corticosteroids abuse: A clinical study of cutaneous adverse effects. *Indian J. Dermatol.* **2017**, *62*, 675. [CrossRef]
29. Orr, J.S.; Kennedy, A.J.; Hasty, A.H. Isolation of adipose tissue immune cells. *J. Vis. Exp.* **2013**. [CrossRef]
30. Lumeng, C.N.; Deyoung, S.M.; Bodzin, J.L.; Saltiel, A.R. Increased inflammatory properties of adipose tissue macrophages recruited during diet-induced obesity. *Diabetes* **2007**, *56*, 16–23. [CrossRef]

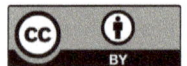

© 2020 by the authors. Licensee MDPI, Basel, Switzerland. This article is an open access article distributed under the terms and conditions of the Creative Commons Attribution (CC BY) license (http://creativecommons.org/licenses/by/4.0/).

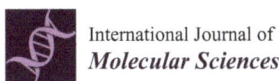

Review

The Roles of Sex Hormones in the Course of Atopic Dermatitis

Naoko Kanda [1,*], Toshihiko Hoashi [2] and Hidehisa Saeki [2]

1. Department of Dermatology, Nippon Medical School, Chiba Hokusoh Hospital, Inzai, Chiba 270-1694, Japan
2. Department of Dermatology, Nippon Medical School, Bunkyo-Ku, Tokyo 113-8602, Japan; t-hoashi@nms.ac.jp (T.H.); h-saeki@nms.ac.jp (H.S.)
* Correspondence: n-kanda@nms.ac.jp; Tel.: +81-476-99-1111; Fax: +81-476-99-1909

Received: 16 July 2019; Accepted: 18 September 2019; Published: 20 September 2019

Abstract: Atopic dermatitis (AD) is a chronic inflammatory skin disease characterized by T helper 2 cell (Th2)-shifted abnormal immunity, skin barrier impairment, and pruritus. The prevalence of AD in childhood is slightly higher in boys than in girls; after puberty, the sexual difference is reversed. The female preponderance in all generations exists in intrinsic AD with enhanced Th1 activity and nickel allergy, lacking increased serum IgE or filaggrin mutation. AD is often deteriorated before menstruation. We review the effects of sex hormones on immune responses and skin permeability barrier and propose possible hypotheses for the above phenomena. After puberty, the immune responses of patients are remarkably influenced by sex hormones. Estrogen and progesterone enhance the activities of Th2/regulatory T cell (Treg) but suppress Th1/Th17. Androgens suppress Th1/Th2/Th17 and induce Treg. The skin permeability barrier is fortified by estrogen but is impaired by progesterone and androgens. Dehydroepiandrosterone suppresses Th2 but enhances Th1. The amount of steroid sulfatase converting dehydroepiandrosterone sulfate to dehydroepiandrosterone is higher in women than in men, and thus, women might be more susceptible to the influence of dehydroepiandrosterone. The balance of modulatory effects of sex hormones on immune responses and skin barrier might regulate the course of AD.

Keywords: atopic dermatitis; estrogen; progesterone; androgen; dehydroepiandrosterone; T helper 2 cell; skin barrier

---

1. Introduction

Atopic dermatitis (AD) is a chronic inflammatory skin disease characterized by T helper 2 cell (Th2)-shifted abnormal immunity, skin barrier impairment, and pruritus (Figure 1) [1–3]. These three elements are mutually related and organize the clinicopathological features of AD. AD patients mostly show reduction of filaggrin expression partly due to mutation of this gene [1–3] and reveal decreases in water content and of ceramide synthesis in the stratum corneum (SC) [1–3]. Moreover, tight junctions (TJs) are dysfunctional in AD: the levels of zonula occludens 1 were decreased in the non-lesional sites of AD, and the levels of zonula occludens 1 and claudin-1 were decreased in the lesional sites relative to the levels in skin from healthy subjects [4]. Such impaired SC and TJ barriers allow the penetration of allergens like house dust mite, food, or pathogens, inducing sensitization to these allergens [1–3]. The AD lesional skin is infiltrated mainly by Th2 cells producing interleukin-4 (IL-4), IL-13, or IL-31 and by T22 cells producing IL-22, while chronic lesion is associated with the infiltration of Th1 cells producing interferon-γ (IFN-γ). Recently, the infiltration of Th17 cells is also noted in AD lesions [5]. Most AD patients show increased serum IgE levels and specific IgE antibodies against a variety of environmental allergens [1–3]. AD patients suffer from severe pruritus due to a variety of pruritogens like histamine, cytokines like thymic stromal lymphopoietin (TSLP), IL-31, IL-4, IL-13, or neuropeptides and abnormal extension of sensory nerves into the epidermis due to the increased expression of nerve growth factor or artemin or to the decreased expression of semaphorin 3A [2].

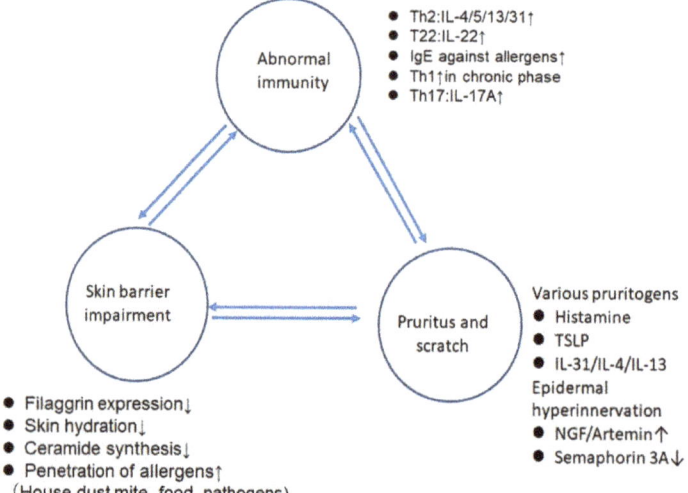

Figure 1. The three elements composing the pathogenesis of atopic dermatitis. Th2, T helper 2 cell; IL-4, interleukin-4; NGF, nerve growth factor; TSLP, thymic stromal lymphopoietin.

The prevalence of AD in childhood is slightly higher in boys than in girls: 8.7% and 5.6% for boys and girls, respectively, at <4 years old in the Netherlands [6]. After puberty, there is a slightly higher prevalence of AD in females: 5.7% and 8.1% for men and women, respectively, in Japan [7] or 6.04% and 8.01% in Europe and the USA [8]. This tendency is more remarkable in asthma, another Th2-shifted allergic disease [9]; the female:male percentage of patients was 35:65 at ages of 2 to 13 years, was inversed with 65:35 at ages of 23 to 64 years, are similar between those at ages of 14 to 22 years [10]. Adult female patients with asthma show more severe symptoms than adult male patients; the percentage of hospitalization for symptoms is 68% versus 32% in females versus males [11].

After puberty, the secretion of sex hormones from the ovary, testis, or adrenal gland is enormously increased. The immune responses or skin barrier in adolescents and adults might thus be more susceptible to influence by sex hormones compared to those in childhood. The effects of sex hormones might be related to the generation-dependent sexual difference in the prevalence of allergic diseases [12]. Interestingly, female preponderance of AD-like dermatitis possibly after puberty is detected in KFRS4/Kyo rats [13]. Dermatitis with severe pruritus initially appeared around 4 months of age, rapidly worsened from 6 to 8 months of age, and predominantly occurred in females: 100% of female versus 50% of male KFRS4/Kyo rats of 8 months old that were examined. The skin lesions were infiltrated with eosinophils, mast cells, and lymphocytes and were associated with increased plasma IgE levels and increased Th2 and Th17 cytokine mRNA levels in the skin-draining lymph nodes. Rats become sexually mature at about the sixth week but attain social maturity 5–6 months later [14], corresponding to the age with worsening dermatitis in KFRS4/Kyo rats. It is thus hypothesized that female sex hormones like estrogen or progesterone may contribute to the higher incidence of dermatitis in female KFRS4/Kyo rats.

On the other hand, female preponderance in all generations exists in intrinsic AD with enhanced Th1 activity and high incidence of nickel (Ni) allergy and without increased serum IgE values or filaggrin mutation [15]. Moreover, in female patients with AD, the disease is often deteriorated before menstruation, i.e., in the luteal phase when both estrogen and progesterone are secreted (Figure 2) [16].

These phenomena indicate that sex hormones might modulate the course of AD in the context of immune responses, skin barrier, or pruritus.

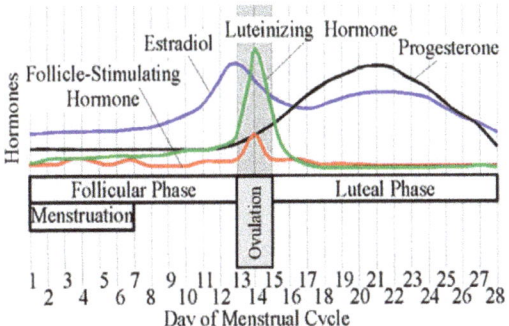

Figure 2. Menstrual cycle. Reprinted from https://commons.wikimedia.org/wiki/File:MenstrualCycle2.png. This file is licensed under the Creative Commons Attribution-Share Alike 3.0 Unported (https://creativecommons.org/licenses/by-sa/3.0/deed.en) license.

In this article, we firstly review the previous studies regarding the regulatory effects of sex hormones on the immune responses and skin barrier. We next propose hypotheses on possible hormonal regulation in the generation-dependent sexual difference in the prevalence of extrinsic AD, female preponderance of intrinsic AD, and premenstrual deterioration of AD.

2. The Effects of Sex Hormones on Immune Responses

2.1. General Tendency (Table 1)

Female hormones estrogen and progesterone mostly enhance the activities of Th2 cells and regulatory T cells (Tregs) but suppress Th1 and Th17 activities, which is favorable for the acceptance of allogeneic fetus during pregnancy [17]. Androgens like testosterone or dihydrotestosterone (DHT) are mostly immunosuppressive and suppress Th1, Th2, and Th17 activities but induce Treg activity. The magnitude of stimulation or suppression by female hormones is mostly higher than that by male hormones [18]. Generally in adolescents and adults, Th1 activities are higher in men than in women while Th2 activities are much higher in women than in men [18]. The sexual differences in Th17 or Treg activities are ambiguous. Dehydroepiandrosterone (DHEA) produced in the adrenal cortex enhances Th1 responses and shifts the balance of Th1/Th2 toward Th1-dominant immunity [19]. Females have higher amounts of steroid sulfatase converting dehydroepiandrosterone sulfate (DHEAS) to active DHEA and, thus, might be more susceptible to influence by DHEA compared to males [20]. To date, it has not been precisely examined how sex hormones regulate the activity of Th22 cells producing IL-22 alone without IL-17A.

Table 1. The effects of sex hormones on immune responses and skin barrier impairment.

Hormones	Th1	Th2	Th17	Treg	Skin Barrier Impairment
Androgen	↓	↓	↓	↑	↑
Estrogen	↑~↓	⇑	↑~↓	⇑	⇓
Progesterone	↓	⇑	↓	⇑	↑
DHEA	↑	↓	?	?	?
Total activity	F < M	F ≫ M	?	?	F < M

↑, Moderate stimulation; ⇑, strong stimulation; ↓, moderate suppression; ⇓, strong suppression; ?, ambiguous; ↑~↓, Stimulatory or inhibitory effects dependent on the concentration, tissue, or disease context; Th1, T helper 1 cell; Treg, regulatory T cell; DHEA, dehydroepiandrosterone; F, female; M, male.

2.2. Female Hormones

2.2.1. Estrogens (Table 2)

Table 2. Summary of the effects of estrogen on the activities of T helper 1 cell (Th1), Th2, Th17, and regulatory T cell (Treg).

Effects	Vivo/Vitro	Species	Th Activities	References
Adaptive Immunity				
T-bet↑	vivo	mice	Th1↑	[21] *
IFN-γ↑	vivo	mice	Th1↑	[21] *
IL-12↑	vivo	mice	Th1↑	[21] *
T-bet↓	vitro	human	Th1↓	[22] **
T-bet↓	vivo	mice	Th1↓	[23] †
IFN-γ↓	vivo	mice	Th1↓	[24] †
IFN-γ↓	vitro	mice	Th1↓	[25] §
IFN-γ↓	vitro	human	Th1↓	[22] **
IFN-γ↓	vivo	mice	Th1↓	[23] †
GATA-3↑	vivo	mice	Th2↑	[26]
GATA-3↑	vivo	mice	Th2↑	[23] †
IL-4↑	vivo	mice	Th2↑	[26]
IL-4↑	vivo	mice	Th2↑	[23] †
B cells IgM, IgE↑	vitro	mice	Th2↑	[27]
RORc↓	vivo	mice	Th17↓	[24] †
RORc↓	vitro	human	Th17↓	[28]
RORc↓	vitro/vivo	mice	Th17↓	[25]
RORγt↓	vitro	human	Th17↓	[22] **
RORγt↓	vivo	mice	Th17↓	[23] †
IL-17A↓	vitro	mice	Th17↓	[25] §
IL-17A↓	vivo	mice	Th17↓	[24] †
IL-17A↓	vitro	human	Th17↓	[22] **
IL-17A↓	vivo	mice	Th17↓	[23] †
IL-22↓	vitro	mice	Th17↓	[25] §
IL-17A↑	vivo	mice	Th17↑	[29] ‡
IL-21↑	vivo	mice	Th17↑	[29] ‡
IL-22↑	vivo	mice	Th17↑	[21] *
RORγt↑	vivo	mice	Th17↑	[21] *
RORγt↑	vivo	mice	Th17↑	[29] ‡
Foxp3↑	vitro	human	Treg↑	[28]
Foxp3↑	vitro	human	Treg↑	[30]
Foxp3↑	vivo	mice	Treg↑	[23] †
Foxp3↑	vivo/vitro	mice	Treg↑	[31]
IL-10↑	vivo	mice	Treg↑	[23] †
IL10↑	vitro	mice	Treg↑	[12]
TGF-↑	vivo	mice	Treg↑	[23] †
Foxp3↓	vitro	human	Treg↓	[22] **
IL-10↓	vitro	human	Treg↓	[22] **
Innate immunity				
Macrophage IL-10↑	vitro	human	Th2↑	[32]
Macrophage IL-1RA↑	vitro	human	Th2↑	[32]
Macrophage CD192↑	vitro	human	Th2↑	[32]
Mast cell degranulation↑	vitro	mice	Th2↑	[33]

↑, stimulation; ↓, suppression; ROR, retinoic acid receptor-related orphan nuclear receptor; Foxp3, forkhead box P3; GATA3, GATA binding protein 3; T-bet, T-box-containing protein expressed in T cells; STAT3, signal transducer and activator of transcription 3; *, Estrous level of estradiol (E2) induced the effects, pregnancy-level of E2 did not; **, Effects of polyphenolic compound delphinidin; †, Pregnancy-levels of E2; ‡, Estrogen receptor agonist diarylpropionitrile; §, 10^{-10}M E2 induced the effects, but 10^{-11}E2 did not; Effects of selective estrogen receptor modulator.

Estrogens are estrone, estradiol (E2), and estriol. E2 is produced by ovarian granulosa cells and placenta. The immunomodulatory effects of E2 are mediated mainly by intracellular estrogen receptor α (ERα) and ERβ or structurally unrelated membrane G-protein-coupled estrogen receptor 1. E2 promotes Th2 activity [26,32]: E2 at pregnancy levels of concentration enhanced the expression of GATA binding protein 3 (GATA3) and IL-4 in ovariectomized experimental autoimmune encephalomyelitis (EAE) model mice [23]. E2 also enhanced IgE production in mouse splenocytes [27].

The effects of E2 on Th1 cells are complex and depend on the concentration, tissue, or disease context: E2 at estrous levels of concentration in vivo enhanced the expression of T-box-containing protein expressed in T cell (T-bet) and IFN-γ production in female ovariectomized autoimmune thyroiditis model mice [21]. In contrast, E2 at pregnancy levels of concentration reduced the production of IL-12 and IFN-γ in phytohemagglutinin plus lipopolysaccharide (LPS)-stimulated human whole blood cells [34]. The high-dose estrogen treatment reduced the expression of IFN-γ and T-bet in EAE model mice [23]. It appears that pregnancy levels of E2 shift the Th1/Th2 balance towards Th2 profiles, inhibiting Th1 development [22,35].

Though E2 mostly suppresses Th17 activity [22,24], several studies reported the stimulatory effects of E2 on Th17 cells: E2 at estrous levels of concentration enhanced the expression of IL-21 and retinoic acid receptor-related orphan nuclear receptor γt (RORγt) in female ovariectomized autoimmune thyroiditis model mice [21]. Diarylpropionitrile, a specific agonist of ERβ and not of ERα, in vivo enhanced IL-17A, IL-21, and RORγt mRNA levels in splenocytes of experimental autoimmune thyroiditis model mice through binding of the agonist-activated ERβ to *IL-17A* and *IL-21* gene promoters [29]. In contrast, E2 at estrous levels of concentration suppressed RORc expression and IL-17A and IL-22 production in response to sperm or *Candida albicans* in female ovariectomized mice [25]. The treatment with estrogen at pregnancy levels of concentration suppressed RORγt expression and IL-17A and IL-6 production in EAE model mice [23]. E2 upregulated the expression of repressor of estrogen receptor activity (REA) and recruited REA to the estrogen response elements (EREs) on the *RORγt* promoter region, thus inhibiting RORγt expression [36].

E2 enhances the activity and/or proliferation of Tregs [28]: E2 enhanced the expression of forkhead box P3 (Foxp3) by inducing binding of the E2/ERα complex to EREs on a human *Foxp3* promoter [30]. Polanczyk et al. reported that E2 in vivo and in vitro increased Foxp3 expression and Treg number in mice [31]. Tai et al. reported that E2, at physiological doses, in vitro stimulated the conversion of CD4+CD25-T cells into CD4+CD25+T cells, which exhibited the enhanced expression of Foxp3 and IL-10 in mice [12].

Estrogen also acts on mast cells and induces IgE-mediated degranulation [33,37], indicating the stimulatory effects of E2 on allergic diseases. In Th2 hapten toluene diisocyanate (TDI)-sensitized allergic airway inflammation model mice, ERα and ERβ agonists induced IL-33 production of airway epithelial cells and eosinophil infiltration into the lung [38].

2.2.2. Progesterone (Table 3)

Progesterone is secreted by the ovarian corpus luteum and placenta and plays a major role in the establishment and maintenance of pregnancy. The effects of progesterone are mainly mediated by intracellular progesterone receptors while some rapid non-transcriptional actions are mediated by structurally unrelated membrane progesterone receptors [17].

Table 3. Summary of the effects of progesterone on the activities of T helper 1 cell (Th1), Th2, Th17, and regulatory T cell (Treg).

Effects	Vivo/Vitro	Species	Th Activities	References
Adaptive Immunity				
T-bet↓	vitro	cows	Th1↓	[39]
IFN-γ↓	vitro	cows	Th1↓	[39]
PIBF- STAT6↑	vitro	human	Th2↑	[40]
GATA3↑	vivo/vitro	mice	Th2↑	[41]
IL-4↑	ex vivo	mice	Th2↑	[42]
IL-4↑	vitro	cows	Th2↑	[39]
IL-4↑	vivo	mice	Th2↑	[42]
B cell IgE↑	vivo	mice	Th2↑	[42]
Vaginal epithelial cell TSLP↑	vivo/vitro	mice	Th2↑	[41]
STAT3 RORC CCR6 IL-23R IL-6R AHR↓	vitro	human	Th17↓	[43]
RORγt↓	vivo/vitro	mice	Th17↓	[41]
RORC↓	vitro	cows	Th17↓	[39]
IL-17A↓	vitro	human	Th17↓	[43]
IL-17A↓	vitro	cows	Th17↓	[39]
IL-17F↓	vitro	human	Th17↓	[43]
IL-21↓	vitro	human	Th17↓	[43]
CD39+ regulatory Th17↑	vivo	mice	Th17↑※	[44]
IL-17A↑	vivo	mice	Th17↑※	[44]
IL-22↑	vivo	mice	Th17↑※	[44]
IL-23↑	vivo	mice	Th17↑※	[44]
IL-6↑	vivo	mice	Th17↑※	[44]
TGF-β↑	vivo	mice	Th17↑※	[44]
Foxp3↑	vitro	mice	Treg↑	[43]
Foxp3↑	vivo/vitro	mice	Treg↑	[41]
Innate Immunity				
Airway epithelial cells Amphiregulin↑	vivo	mice		[44]

※,CD39+ regulatory Th17 cells; ↑, stimulation; ↓, suppression; ROR, retinoic acid receptor-related orphan nuclear receptor; Foxp3, forkhead box P3; GATA3, GATA binding protein 3; T-bet, T-box-containing protein expressed in T cells; STAT, signal transducer and activator of transcription; AHR, aryl hydrocarbon receptor; CCR6 CC-type chemokine receptor 6; TSLP, thymic stromal lymphopoietin; PIBF, progesterone-induced blocking factor.

Progesterone promotes Th2 activity [45]: progesterone acts on T cells and induces the secretion of progesterone-inducible blocking factor (PIBF) which binds IL-4 receptor α(IL-4Rα)/PIBFR on the cell surface and induces the Janus kinase 1 (Jak1)/signal transducer and activator of transcription 6 (STAT6) pathway to increase the production of Th2 cytokines like IL-4 or IL-10 [40]. Progesterone increased TSLP expression in vaginal epithelium and GATA-3 expression and IL-4 production in CD4+T cells in *Neisseria gonorhoeae*-infected vagina of mice [41]. Progesterone treatment increased IL-4 production in peripheral blood mononuclear cells (PBMCs) from pregnant cows [39]. The pro-Th2 effect of progesterone is consistent with the higher IL-4 and IL-10 production in PBMCs from pregnant cows with high progesterone levels than those from nonpregnant cows [39]. Progesterone treatment on ovariectomized asthma model mice increased serum IgE levels and IL-4 production in bronchoalveolar lavage cells [42], indicating the contribution of progesterone to the elicitation of allergic diseases.

In contrast, progesterone directly suppresses Th1 development in mice [46]. Progesterone treatment suppressed T-bet expression and IFN-γ production in PBMCs from pregnant cows [39]. The Th1-suppressive effect of progesterone is also consistent with the decreased IFN-γ production in PBMCs from pregnant cows compared to those from nonpregnant cows [39].

Progesterone suppresses the differentiation of Th17 cells: progesterone in vitro suppressed IL-17A, IL-17F, and IL-21 production and RORc expression in human cord blood cells under the Th17-differentiation conditions and also suppressed their STAT3 phosphorylation in response to IL-6 [43]. Progesterone suppressed RORγt expression and decreased IL-17A-producing CD4+T cell numbers in *Neisseria gonorhoeae*-infected vagina of mice [41].

Progesterone induces the differentiation of Tregs [44]: progesterone in vitro drove the allogeneic activation-induced differentiation of human cord blood naive T cells into immunosuppressive Tregs, which highly expressed FoxP3 and memory T cell marker CD45RO [43]. Progesterone increased the percentage of CD4+CD25+Foxp3+ Tregs in *Neisseria gonorhoeae*-infected vagina of mice [41]. These reports totally suggest that progesterone favors Th2/Treg activities but suppresses Th1/Th17 activities, which might be favorable for tolerance to allogeneic fetus and for maintenance of pregnancy [17].

2.3. *Androgens (Table 4)*

Table 4. Summary of the effects of androgens on the activities of T helper 1 cell (Th1), Th2, Th17, and regulatory T cell (Treg).

Effects	Vivo/Vitro	Species	Th Activities	References
Adaptive Immunity				
ptpn1↑ STAT4↓	vivo/ vitro	human and mice	Th1↓	[47]
PPARα↑	vitro/vivo	mice	Th1↓	[48]
IFN-γ↓	vitro/vivo	mice	Th1↓	[48]
IFN-γ↓	vitro	mice	Th1↓	[49]
IFN-γ↓	vitro	human	Th1↓	[50]
IL-12↓	vitro	human	Th1↓	[50]
CXCL10↓	vitro	human	Th1↓	[50]
IL-13↓	vitro	human	Th2↓	[50]
IL-4↓	vitro	human	Th2↓	[50]
IL-5↓	vitro	human	Th2↓	[50]
B cell number↓	vivo	mice	Th2↓	[51]
B cell Antigen-specific IgE production ↓	vivo	mice	Th2↓	[52]
PPARγ↓	vitro/vivo	mice	Th17↑	[48]
IL-17A↑	vitro/vivo	mice	Th17↑	[48]
IL-23R↓	vivo	mice	Th17↓	[53]
IL-23R↓	vitro	Mice	Th17↓	[54]
IL-17A↓	vitro	mice	Th17↓	[49]
IL-17A↓	vivo	mice	Th17↓	[53]
IL-17A↓	vitro	human	Th17↓	[50]
ARE-Foxp3↑	vitro	human	Treg↑	[55]
IL-10↑	vitro	human	Treg↑	[50]
Innate Immunity				
Mast cell IL-4↓	vivo	mice	Th2↓	[53]
ILC2 IL-13↓	vivo	mice	Th2↓	[53]
Basophil IL-4↓	vivo	mice	Th2↓	[53]

↑, stimulation; ↓, suppression; ROR, retinoic acid receptor-related orphan nuclear receptor; Foxp3, forkhead box P3; STAT, signal transducer and activator of transcription; ptpn1, protein tyrosine phosphatase, non-receptor type 1; PPAR peroxisome proliferator-activated receptor; ARE, androgen response element; ILC, innate lymphoid cell.

Androgens, such as dihydrotestosterone (DHT) or testosterone, are synthesized in the gonads and adrenal glands. Testosterone is the most concentrated androgen in adult male serum. DHT is present at one-tenth the concentration of testosterone though DHT is more potent than testosterone. Testosterone can be aromatized to E2 by aromatase. Androgens mainly bind intracellular androgen receptors (ARs) but also bind plasma membrane G-protein-coupled receptors [56].

Androgens are mostly immunosuppressive [51,57]. Androgens inhibit Th1 differentiation: testosterone inhibited IL-12-induced phosphorylation of STAT4 in murine CD4+T cells by inducing the expression of protein tyrosine phosphatase nonreceptor 1, which inactivates Jak2 and Tyk2 kinases [47]. DHT inhibited IFN-γ production in murine CD4+T cells by enhancing the expression of peroxisome proliferator-activated receptor α (PPARα), which represses *IFNγ* transcription [48].

Androgens inhibit Th2 differentiation: DHT treatment of bone-marrow-derived dendritic cells pulsed with *Trichuris muris* antigen reduced their Th2-priming activity with a complete ablation of IL-4, IL-10, and IL-13 production by co-cultured T cells [54]. DHT treatment of prostate stromal cells suppressed the production of IL-4, IL-5, and IL-13 production by co-cultured CD4+ T cells [50]. Gonadectomized male mice showed increased IL-13-producing innate lymphoid cell 2 (ILC2) and Th2 cells and increased serum IgE levels compared to sham-operated mice in response to house dust mite antigens [53], indicating the suppressive effects of androgens on type 2 immune responses. In male castrated phospholipase A-sensitized allergic rhinitis model mice, testosterone administration decreased the production of phospholipase A-specific IgE [52], indicating the suppressive effects of androgens on allergic rhinitis. Androgens also suppress B cell lymphopoiesis [51]: testosterone acted on bone marrow stromal cells to induce the production of transforming growth factor-β, which reduced the production of IL-7 required for B cell proliferation and differentiation [56].

Androgens suppress Th17 differentiation: male gonadectomized mice showed increased IL-17A-producing Th17 and γδT cells compared to sham-operated mice in response to house dust mite antigens [53]. The deficiency of AR signaling enhanced IL-17A production and IL-23R expression in T cells under Th17-differentiation conditions [53]. These results indicate the inhibitory effects of androgens on type 17 immune responses. Testosterone treatment of murine T cells in vitro decreased IFN-γ or IL-17 production under the Th1- or Th17-differentiation conditions, respectively [49].

On the other hand, androgens induce Tregs: androgen-activated AR bound androgen response elements on the *Foxp3* promoter and enhanced the acetylation of histone H4 on the promoter, allowing the binding of additional transcription factors, and thus enhanced the expression of Foxp3 in human T cells [55]. Danazol, an attenuated androgen, increased CD4+CD25highCD127lowFoxp3+ Tregs in patients with aplastic anemia [58].

2.4. DHEA (Table 5)

Table 5. Summary of the effects of dehydroepiandrosterone (DHEA) on the activities of T helper 1 cell (Th1), Th2, Th17, and regulatory T cell (Treg).

Effects	Vivo/Vitro	Species	Th Activities	References
Adaptive Immunity				
IFN-γ↑	vivo	mice	Th1↑	[59]
IFN-γ↑	ex vivo	mice	Th1↑	[60]
IFN-γ↑	vitro	mice	Th1↑	[19]
IL-12↑	vitro	mice	Th1↑	[10]
IFN-γ↓	vivo	mice	Th1↓	[61] *
IFN-γ↓	vivo	mice	Th1↓	[62]
IL-4↓	vivo	mice	Th2↓	[59]
IL-4↓	vitro	mice	Th2↓	[63]
IL-4↓	vitro	human	Th2↓	[64]
IL-4↓	vivo	mice	Th2↓	[61] *
IL-4↓	vivo	mice	Th2↓	[60]
IL-4↓	ex vivo	mice	Th2↓	[60]
IL-5↓	vivo	mice	Th2↓	[59]
IL-5↓	vivo	mice	Th2↓	[62]
IL-5↓	vitro	human	Th2↓	[64]
IL-5↓	ex vivo	mice	Th2↓	[60]
IL-13↓	vivo	mice	Th2↓	[59]
CCL11↓	vivo	mice	Th2↓	[59]
CCL24↓	vivo	mice	Th2↓	[59]
B cell IgE ↓	vivo	mice	Th2↓	[65]
B cell IgE ↓	vivo	mice	Th2↓	[60]
B cell IgG1↓	vivo	mice		[60]
IL-13↑	vivo	mice	Th2↑	[62]
RORC↓	vivo	mice	Th17↓	[61] *
IL-17A↓	vivo	mice	Th17↓	[61] *
IL-17A↓	vivo	mice	Th17↓	[62]
TNF-α↓	vivo	mice	Th17↓	[60]
IL-6↓	vivo	mice	Th17↓	[62]
TGFβ↓	vivo	mice	Th17↓	[62]
TNF-α↑	vitro	human	Th17↑	[66] †
IL-6↑	vitro	human	Th17↑	[66] †
IL-1β↑	vitro	human	Th17↑	[66] †
Foxp3↓	vitro	human	Treg↓	[67]
IL-10↓	vitro	mice	Treg↓	[62]
IL-10↓	vitro	mice	Treg↓	[63]
Foxp3↑	vivo	mice	Treg↑	[68] **
IL-10↑	vivo	mice	Treg↑	[61] *

Table 5. Cont.

Effects	Vivo/Vitro	Species	Th Activities	References
Innate Immunity				
Mast cell infiltration↓	vivo	mice	Th2↓	[60]
Eosinophil infiltration↓	vivo	mice	Th2↓	[59]
Eosinophil infiltration↓	vivo	mice	Th2↓	[60]
HaCat cells CCL17↓	vitro	human	Th2↓	[60]
HaCat cells CCL22↓	vitro	human	Th2↓	[60]
BEAS-2B CCL11↓	vitro	human	Th2↓	[59]
BEAS-2B CCL24↓	vitro	human	Th2↓	[59]
Ovary granulosa cell ICAM1/VCAM1↑	vivo	mice		[19]

*, Possible effects of DHEA metabolite, 5-androsten-3β,17β-diol (adiol), via estrogen receptor β (ERβ); **, Synthetic DHEA analog HE3286; †, Effects via ER; ↑, stimulation; ↓, suppression; ?, ambiguous; ROR, retinoic acid receptor-related orphan nuclear receptor; Foxp3, forkhead box P3; ICAM1, intercellular adhesion molecule 1; VCAM1, vascular cell adhesion molecule 1.

DHEAS is the most abundant steroid in human blood serum and is secreted by the adrenal cortex [69]. DHEAS is converted by steroid sulfatase to an active form, DHEA [69]. Steroid sulfatase is controlled by an X-linked gene that escapes the Lyon effect of X-inactivation; as a result, women have twice the amount of steroid sulfatase than men [70], especially in peripheral lymphoid organs [20]. The DHEA/DHEAS ratio in circulation is usually higher in women than in men [71], and under 50 years old, the plasma DHEA concentration of women is higher than that of men [72]. It is thus hypothesized that women might be more susceptible to the effects of DHEA than men [20] though the effects might be influenced by other factors such as receptor and downstream pathways. DHEA itself binds nuclear steroid hormone receptors like AR, ERα, or ERβ with lower affinities than cognate ligands. DHEA is metabolized to other steroid hormones, testosterone, DHT, or E2 (Figure 3), and these metabolites bind the corresponding steroid receptors: DHEA metabolite 5-androsten-3β,17β-diol can bind ERβ [61]. Moreover, recent studies revealed that DHEA and DHEAS act as ligands of many nuclear receptors like PPARα, pregnane X receptor, and constitutive androstanol receptor and membrane receptors like TrkA, N-methyl-D-aspartic acid receptors, or γ-amino butyric acid receptors [73]. Thus, the biological effects of DHEA depend on the levels of metabolizing enzymes and individual receptors and, thus, vary with species, tissues, or cell types.

DHEA mostly enhances Th1 differentiation: DHEA treatment enhanced IL-12 and IFN-γ production in female murine peritoneal cells in vivo and enhanced the expression of very late antigen-4 and leukocyte function-associated antigen-1 in CD4+ T cells in vitro [19]. DHEA in vivo increased the expression of vascular cell adhesion molecule-1 and intercellular adhesion molecule-1 in ovary granulosa cells of mice [19,74]. DHEA suppresses type 2 immune responses [65]: in female ovalbumin-sensitized asthma model mice, DHEA administration reduced eosinophil infiltration into the lung; serum ovalbumin-specific IgE levels; and the expression of IL-4, IL-5, and IL-13 and type 2 chemokines CC-chemokine ligand 1 (CCL1) and CCL24 in bronchoalveolar lavage fluid but increased IFN-γ production in ovalbumin-activated splenocytes [59]. DHEA reduced IL-4 production but increased IL-2 production in concanavalin A-stimulated human PBMCs [64]. In LPS-induced experimental inflammation model mice, DHEA increased the Th1/Th2 ratio in spleen T cells [63]. DHEA significantly increased Th1 cytokine levels (IL-2 and IFN-α) and decreased Th2 cytokine levels (IL-4 and IL-10) in primary cultured spleen T cells [63]. DHEA decreased Na^+K^+-ATPase activity and increased Ca^{2+} ATPase activity in T cells, which might regulate the balance of cytokine secretion [63]. Thus, DHEA enhances Th1 immune response and regulates the balance of Th1/Th2 toward Th1-dominant immunity. In AD model mice induced by topical 2,4-dinitrochlorobenzene (DNCB), oral or topical

DHEA attenuated the infiltration of eosinophils and mast cells into DNCB-challenged ear skin. In those mice, oral or topical DHEA also reduced serum IL-4 and IgE levels and reduced IL-4 and IL-5 production but increased IFN-γ production in splenocytes [60]. DHEA in vitro suppressed the production of type 2 chemokines, CCL17 and CCL22, in tumor necrosis factor-α-stimulated HaCat cells [60].

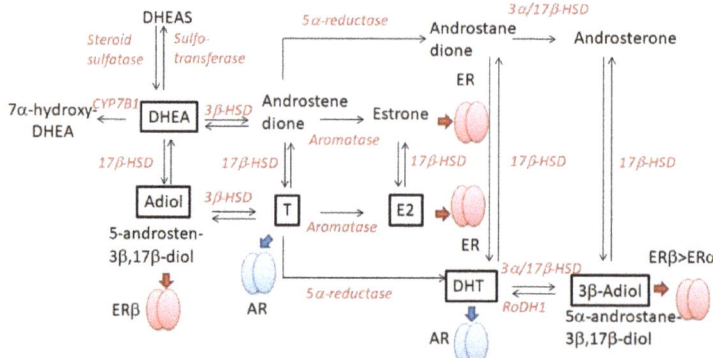

Figure 3. Dehydroepiandrosterone (DHEA) metabolizing pathway. DHEAS, dehydroepiandrosterone sulfate; DHT, dihydrotestosterone; T, testosterone; E2, estradiol; AR, androgen receptor; ER, estrogen receptor; 17β-HSD, 17β-hydroxysteroid dehydrogenase; RoDH1, retinol dehydrogenase type 1; ↓, binding to the steroid receptor described.

The effects of DHEA on Th17 and Treg are ambiguous [62] and dependent on tissue or disease context [66]: DHEA treatment increased the number of Foxp3+ Tregs in splenocytes of female ovariectomized mice [75]. In EAE model mice and human multiple sclerosis patients, DHEA directly inhibited the activity of Th17 cells, inducing IL-10-producing Tregs via ERβ activation [61]. This effect may be mediated by 5-androsten-3β,17β-diol, converted from DHEA by 17β-hydroxysteroid dehydrogenase (Figure 3). Synthetic DHEA analog HE3286 increased the frequency of CD4+CD25+Foxp3+ Tregs in spleen in collagen-induced arthritis model mice [68] though the receptors for this analog are unknown and not ERα, ERβ, or AR. In contrast, DHEA reduced the expression of Foxp3 without altering Treg frequency in PBMCs from patients co-infected with HIV and tuberculosis [67].

3. The Effects of Sex Hormones on the Skin Barrier (Table 1)

Overall, in adults, skin hydration is slightly higher in women than in men and basal transepidermal water loss (TEWL) is significantly higher in men than in women [35,76]. The epidermal permeability barrier is impaired by androgens and progesterone but is restored by E2 [77]. E2 paradoxically worsens the progesterone-induced barrier impairment [78]. The skin barrier is impaired in the luteal phase when both progesterone and estrogen are secreted [79].

The ovariectomy of female C57/BL6 mice reduced skin hydration, delayed skin permeability recovery after tape stripping, and reduced epidermal thickness; these were restored by the administration of E2 [80]. Ovariectomy also reduced the expression of desmoglein-1, involucrin, and loricrin, key constituents of corneodesmosome and cornified envelope (CE) in SC; these were restored by E2 treatment [80]. Ovariectomy of female nude mice (ICR-Foxn1nu) also reduced the expression of filaggrin and integrin β in the skin [81]. These results support that E2 strengthens the skin permeability barrier and integrity.

The castration of male mice (Sk:h1) or treatment with AR antagonist flutamide accelerated skin permeability recovery after tape stripping, and testosterone administration delayed recovery in the castrated mice [82]. Testosterone treatment of castrated mice reduced the number of lamellar bodies in the cytosol of stratum granulosum (SG) cells and decreased secreted lamellar contents at the interface of SC and SG [82]. These results support that testosterone perturbs the skin permeability barrier homeostasis. The administration of E2 in pregnant rats reduced TEWL of day-20 fetus while that was increased by DHT [77]. The administration of E2 accelerated lipid deposition and formation of lamellar unit structures in the SC of day-20 fetal epidermis in utero while these were delayed by DHT [77]. In fetal skin explants from day-17 rats, estrogen increased while DHT reduced the activity of β-glucocerebrosidase, which converts glucosylceramides to ceramides and is essential for the formation of lamellar unit structures throughout SC interstices [83]. In the same explants, estrogen accelerated while DHT delayed the expression of filaggrin and loricrin, key constituents of keratohyalin granules and CE, respectively [84]. These results indicate that E2 accelerates while androgen delays SC barrier formation.

Topical testosterone delayed skin permeability barrier recovery in male hairless mice (HR-1), and the delay was overcome by co-application of E2 [78]. Progesterone also delayed the recovery; however, the delay was paradoxically enhanced by E2 [78]. To date, the precise mechanism of how progesterone delays skin permeability barrier recovery is not elucidated; however, it is indicated that progesterone opposes the protective effect of E2 on skin permeability barrier and that the skin permeability barrier may be impaired in females in the luteal phase when both progesterone and estrogen are secreted. Muizzuddin et al. showed that the skin permeability barrier was the weakest between days 22 and 26 of the menstrual cycle, the mid-luteal phase [85]. TEWL is higher at the day of minimal estrogen/progesterone ratio (around day 26) than that at the day of maximal estrogen secretion (around day 13) [79]. It is thus hypothesized that the skin barrier might be protected by E2, which might be opposed by progesterone. The skin patch test reaction to Ni is higher at the luteal phase than that at the ovulatory phase or at the follicular phase [86], which may be due to the skin permeability barrier impairment at the luteal phase when progesterone is secreted. In the uterus of ovariectomized mice, E2 treatment increased mRNA levels of small proline-rich protein 2 (SPRR2), which was dampened by progesterone [87]. Since SPRRs are key constituents of CE in SC of the skin, further studies should elucidate if such suppressive effects of progesterone might be reproduced in the skin. In contrast, progesterone upregulated the expression of TJ proteins occludin and zona occludens 2 in the epidermis, and this effect was canceled by E2 in ovariectomized FvB mice [88]. Progesterone upregulated the expression of occludin in human gut tissues and Caco-2 cells [89]. It is thus hypothesized that the TJ barrier might be restored by progesterone but impaired by E2, opposite to the SC barrier, though confirmatory studies are required for its verification.

It is reported that oral DHEA in humans at > 60 years old improved skin hydration, epidermal thickness, sebum production, and pigmentation [90]. Such antiaging effects of DHEA are mainly generated by the enhanced collagen biosynthesis and deposition: topical DHEA increased the mRNA levels of procollagen 1/3 and heat shock protein 47, a type 1 collagen chaperone protein in human dermal fibroblasts [91]. In contrast, topical DHEA treatment reduced the expression of genes associated with the terminal differentiation and cornification of keratinocytes, corneodesmosin, claudin 8, SPRR2G, late envelope protein 7, and Jagged 1, indicating the suppression of skin barrier properties [92]. To date, the direct effects of DHEA on skin permeability barrier have not been reported and should further be examined. In the testis, DHEAS but not DHEA augmented the TJ connections between Sertoli cells by promoting the expression of claudin-3 and -5 via membrane $Gn_{\alpha 11}$-coupled receptors independent of AR [93].

4. The Effects of Sex Hormones on the Pruritus

There have been no reports that sex hormones act as pruritogens. However, E2 and/or progesterone directly or indirectly induce the secretion of Th2-related cytokines, IL-4, IL-13, IL-31, TSLP, or IL-33; these cytokines bind the corresponding receptors on C-type sensory neurons and generate an itch sensation [94]. In Th2 hapten TDI-sentitized allergic dermatitis model mice, oral or topical administration of ERα agonist propylpyrazoletriol induced TSLP and IL-33 expression in keratinocytes and promoted scratching behavior [95]; the pruritus might be caused by TSLP and IL-33. Estrogen also acted on mast cells and promoted the release of histamines [33,37], which also act as pruritogens.

In sensory neuron-keratinocyte coculture model, DHEA produced by keratinocytes promoted neurite growth possibly through the activation of TrkA [96,97], indicating the relations to abnormal neurite outgrowth into the epidermis of AD lesions. The effects of sex hormones on neurite growth should further be examined precisely.

5. Intrinsic AD

Intrinsic AD patients occupy around 10–20% of whole AD, show normal IgE values, lack IgE antibodies against environmental or food allergens, and lack barrier disruption and filaggrin gene mutation [15]. Intrinsic AD patients manifest Dennie–Morgan fold but without icthyosis vulgaris and palmar hyperlinearity and with milder severity of AD. Intrinsic AD patients show positive on patch tests to metals, especially to Ni, at a higher percentage than extrinsic AD patients, indicating the higher incidence of metal allergy [98]. Intrinsic AD patients show high Ni concentrations in serum and sweat [98,99], indicating the enhanced absorption and/or transport of Ni derived from food and sensitization with Ni in the circulation and skin. Immunologically, intrinsic AD patients show higher Th1 activity than that of extrinsic AD patients and show Th2 activity comparable to that of extrinsic AD patients [100]. Since Ni interacts with toll-like receptor 4 in addition to major histocompatibility/self-peptide complex and induces a mixed Th1 and Th2 cytokine responses [98,101–103], a considerable number of intrinsic AD patients, though not all, might show both Th1 and Th2 responses to Ni through its presentation by antigen presenting cells in the skin patch test. Thus, metals might act as the main allergens in intrinsic AD though other agents might also work in its pathogenesis. In both children or adults, the prevalence of intrinsic AD is higher in females than in males [104,105]; moreover, the prevalence of Ni allergy is higher in females than in males [106,107].

6. Possible Hypotheses on the Generation-Dependent Sexual Difference in the Prevalence of Extrinsic AD (Table 6)

It is hypothesized that prepubertal children might be mostly devoid of the influence of sex hormones considering their very low concentrations. The effects of DHEA, shifting the Th1/Th2 balance to Th1, might be more remarkably revealed in girls than in boys due to the higher levels of steroid sulfatase converting DHEAS to DHEA. Thus, both atopic asthma and extrinsic AD, Th2-shifted allergic diseases with atopic diathesis, might be more prevalent in boys than in girls. The male preponderance in childhood asthma might also involve gender-specific factors other than hormonal regulation [108]: boys have smaller airway diameters relative to lung volume (dysanapsis; [109]) and show a higher percentage of positive skin prick tests or IgE antibodies against aeroallergens than girls, indicating higher atopic diathesis in boys than in girls [110]. The higher aeroallergen sensitivities in boys may also be related to the male predominance in childhood AD [111]. Alternatively, the higher asthma incidence in boys may be because underdiagnosed and undertreated asthma patients exist among girls [112].

After puberty, the levels of sex hormones, estrogen, progesterone, testosterone, or DHT are greatly increased and individuals might thus be more greatly influenced by the immunological effects of those sex hormones than those of DHEA [18,113,114]. Women are exposed to higher levels of estrogen and progesterone promoting Th2 activity. The prevalence and severity of atopic asthma might thus become much higher in women than in men exposed to higher levels of androgens suppressing Th2 activity. The female preponderance in adult asthma may also involve other gender-specific factors [108]: the bronchial hyperresponsiveness is more frequent in women than in men; women are more likely to be exposed to indoor aeroallergens than men.

In the case of adult extrinsic AD, patients are influenced by the effects of sex hormones both on immune responses and skin barrier impairment. The Th2 shift is more prevalent in women than in men; however, skin barrier impairment is more likely to occur in men exposed to high levels of androgens perturbing skin permeability barrier. In women, skin barrier is restored by estrogen at the follicular and ovulatory phases but are disturbed by progesterone at the luteal phase. Totally, female adults might be slightly more protected from skin barrier impairment compared to male adults, considering the postmenopausal skin barrier disruption in females and its restoration by hormonal agents, including both estrogen and progesterone [115]. Thus, female adults with higher Th2 activity but slightly more protection from skin barrier impairment may show a slightly higher prevalence of extrinsic AD compared to male adults, though the sexual difference is moderate compared to strict female preponderance of adult atopic asthma. It is known that Th1 activity is enhanced in the chronic phase of AD and that Th17 cells may also be involved in the pathogenesis of AD [5], which might be more applicable to women than men since estrogen might promote Th1 and Th17 activities at estrous level of concentrations [21]. Other gender-specific factors might also be related to the moderate female preponderance of adult AD: women are more responsive to pruritogens than men, and female mice showed higher scratching counts than male mice under the stimulus of proteinase-activated receptor-2-activating peptide [116]. The involvement of sex hormones in hyperknesis or alloknesis should further be investigated.

Table 6. The generation-dependent sexual difference in the prevalence of atopic asthma and extrinsic atopic dermatitis (AD).

Atopic Asthma		Child		Adolescent–Adult		
	Atopic Diathesis		Th2 Regulation by DHEA	Th2 Regulation by Sex Hormones	Th2 Regulation by DHEA	
M	+~++		↓	↓↓by A	↓	
F	+		↓↓	↑↑↑by E, P	↓↓	
Prevalence		M > F		M ≪ F		
Extrinsic AD	Atopic Diathesis	Filaggrin Gene Mutation	Th2 Regulation by DHEA	Th2 Regulation by Sex Hormones	Th2 Regulation by DHEA	Skin Barrier Impairment by Sex Hormones
M	+~++	+ or −	↓	↓↓by A	↓	↑by A
F	+	+ or −	↓↓	↑↑↑by E, P	↓↓	↓↓by E ↑by P Totally↓
Prevalence		M > F		M < F		

↑, Stimulation; ↓, Suppression; Th2, T helper 2 cell; DHEA, dehydroepiandrosterone; F, female; M, male; A, androgen; E, estrogen; P, progesterone.

7. Possible Hypotheses on Female Preponderance of Intrinsic AD (Table 7)

We herein propose a hypothesis on female preponderance of intrinsic AD in the context of metal allergy, one possible agent of its pathogenesis. Patients with intrinsic AD are not associated with atopic diathesis, filaggrin gene mutation, or congenital skin barrier impairment and are associated with enhanced Th1 activity as well as Th2 and high incidence of Ni allergy though not in all patients. Before puberty, there is no sexual difference in the chances of Ni exposure, though in Western countries, girls are more frequently exposed to Ni due to the first pierce experiences. Th1 responses to Ni might be more remarkable in girls with higher susceptibility to DHEA promoting Th1 activity than in boys. Totally, intrinsic AD in childhood might be more prevalent in girls than in boys.

After puberty, women are more frequently exposed to Ni by wearing ornaments than men. The immune response to Ni might be gradually shifted from Th1 to Th2 since repeated elicitation with antigens alters the balance of cytokines released locally, with a shift toward Th2-dominated responses [117]. Immune responses after puberty might be more susceptible to the influence of sex hormones than of DHEA. After puberty, Th2 responses to Ni might be more remarkable in women with higher levels of estrogen and progesterone stimulating Th2 activity than men with higher levels of androgens suppressing Th2 activity. The intrinsic AD after puberty might thus become much more prevalent in women than in men. The female preponderance of intrinsic AD may also involve certain gender-dependent factors unrelated to metal allergy, which should further be identified.

Table 7. Female preponderance of intrinsic atopic dermatitis (AD).

Intrinsic AD	Child				Adolescent–Adult		
	Atopic Diathesis	Filaggrin Gene Nutation	Exposure to Ni	Stimulation of Th1 Response to Ni by DHEA	Exposure to Ni	Regulation of Th2 Response to Ni by Sex Hormones	Stimulation of Th1 Response to Ni by DHEA
M	−	−	+	↑	+	↓↓ by A	↑
F	−	−	+~++	↑↑	++	↑↑↑↑ by E, P	↑↑
Prevalence			M < F			M ≪ F	

↑, Stimulation; ↓, Suppression; Th1, T helper 1 cell; DHEA, dehydroepiandrosterone; F, female; M, male; A, androgen; E, estrogen; P, progesterone; Ni, nickel.

8. Possible Hypotheses on the Premenstrual Deterioration of AD in Females

About half of female AD patients experience premenstrual deterioration of AD symptoms [118]. The deterioration might be due to the dual effects of estrogen and progesterone on Th2 activity and skin barrier. At the luteal phase, both estrogen and progesterone are secreted and, thus, Th2-skewing effects are higher than in the other phases; moreover, the skin permeability barrier is perturbed by progesterone, especially, just prior to menstruation with minimal estrogen/progesterone ratio.

The deterioration of AD during pregnancy is also reported; 52% or 61% of female AD patients who experienced pregnancy had noticed deterioration of AD during pregnancy in the UK [119] or Korea [120], respectively. The deterioration of AD during pregnancy might also reflect the effects of extremely high concentrations of E2 and progesterone on Th2 activity and skin barrier. Moreover, the prevalence of deterioration during pregnancy was higher in intrinsic AD patients (100%) compared to that in extrinsic AD patients (47.1%) in the Korean study [120]. It is thus hypothesized that intrinsic AD patients might be more susceptible to the influence of female sex hormones compared to extrinsic AD patients.

9. Serum Hormone Concentrations in Patients with Allergic Diseases

It is reported that serum concentrations of DHEA or testosterone are lower in male AD patients compared to the reference group [64,121]. These indicate that DHEA- or testosterone-induced suppressive effects on Th2 activity are reduced in male AD patients, which might aggravate the symptoms of AD. It is also reported that serum concentrations of DHEA or DHEAS are lower in patients with asthma or chronic spontaneous urticaria compared to the reference group, irrespective of gender [122]. It is thus speculated that the reduction of Th2-suppressive effects by DHEA might accelerate the Th2 shift in these patients though confirmatory studies are needed to verify the speculation.

It is reported that prolonged physical stress with energy and sleep deprivation reduced serum DHEA levels and increased serum DHEAS levels, indicating the decrease of steroid sulfatase activity and/or increase of sulfotransferase activity by prolonged physical stress [123]. It is thus hypothesized that the reduction of DHEA levels might be one possible cause of the stress-induced exacerbation of allergic diseases.

10. Conclusions

We reviewed the effects of sex hormones related to the course of AD and focused on immune responses and skin barrier. The balance of the effects of sex hormones might up- or downregulate the prevalence and course of AD. Future studies should elucidate the effects of sex hormones on Th22 activity or pruritus, using AD model mice.

Author Contributions: N.K. is the main author in manuscript drafting; T.H. revised the bibliography and updated the figures and tables; H.S. made a critical revision of the manuscript.

Funding: This research received no external funding.

Conflicts of Interest: The authors declare no conflict of interest.

References

1. Furue, M.; Chiba, T.; Tsuji, G.; Ulzii, D.; Kido-Nakahara, M.; Nakahara, T.; Kadono, T. Atopic dermatitis: Immune deviation, barrier dysfunction, IgE autoreactivity and new therapies. *Allergol. Int.* **2017**, *66*, 398–403. [CrossRef] [PubMed]
2. Furue, M.; Ulzii, D.; Vu, Y.H.; Tsuji, G.; Kido-Nakahara, M.; Nakahara, T. Pathogenesis of Atopic Dermatitis: Current Paradigm. *Iran. J. Immunol.* **2019**, *16*, 97–107. [CrossRef] [PubMed]
3. Egawa, G.; Kabashima, K. Barrier dysfunction in the skin allergy. *Allergol. Int.* **2018**, *67*, 3–11. [CrossRef] [PubMed]
4. Yuki, T.; Tobiishi, M.; Kusaka-Kikushima, A.; Ota, Y.; Tokura, Y. Impaired tight junctions in atopic dermatitis skin and in a skin-equivalent model treated with interleukin-17. *PLoS ONE* **2016**, *11*, e0161759. [CrossRef] [PubMed]
5. Nomura, T.; Honda, T.; Kabashima, K. Multipolarity of cytokine axes in the pathogenesis of atopic dermatitis in terms of age, race, species, disease stage and biomarkers. *Int. Immunol.* **2018**, *30*, 419–428. [CrossRef] [PubMed]
6. Dirven-Meijer, P.C.; Glazenburg, E.J.; Mulder, P.G.; Oranje, A.P. Prevalence of atopic dermatitis in children younger than 4 years in a demarcated area in central Netherlands: The West Veluwe Study Group. *Br. J. Dermatol.* **2008**, *158*, 846–847. [CrossRef] [PubMed]
7. Saeki, H.; Tsunemi, Y.; Fujita, H.; Kagami, S.; Sasaki, K.; Ohmatsu, H.; Watanabe, A.; Tamaki, K. Prevalence of atopic dermatitis determined by clinical examination in Japanese adults. *J. Dermatol.* **2006**, *33*, 817–819. [CrossRef]
8. Harrop, J.; Chinn, S.; Verlato, G.; Olivieri, M.; Norback, D.; Wjst, M.; Janson, C.; Zock, J.P.; Leynaert, B.; Gislason, D.; et al. Eczema, atopy and allergen exposure in adults: A population-based study. *Clin. Exp. Allergy* **2007**, *37*, 526–535. [CrossRef]
9. Chen, W.; Mempel, M.; Schober, W.; Behrendt, H.; Ring, J. Gender difference, sex hormones, and immediate type hypersensitivity reactions. *Allergy* **2008**, *63*, 1418–1427. [CrossRef]
10. Schatz, M.; Camargo, C.A., Jr. The relationship of sex to asthma prevalence, health care utilization, and medications in a large managed care organization. *Ann. Allergy Asthma Immunol.* **2003**, *91*, 553–558. [CrossRef]
11. Schatz, M.; Clark, S.; Camargo, C.A., Jr. Sex differences in the presentation and course of asthma hospitalizations. *Chest* **2006**, *129*, 50–55. [CrossRef] [PubMed]
12. Tai, P.; Wang, J.; Jin, H.; Song, X.; Yan, J.; Kang, Y.; Zhao, L.; An, X.; Du, X.; Chen, X.; et al. Induction of regulatory T cells by physiological level estrogen. *J. Cell Physiol.* **2008**, *214*, 456–464. [CrossRef] [PubMed]
13. Kuramoto, T.; Yokoe, M.; Tanaka, D.; Yuri, A.; Nishitani, A.; Higuchi, Y.; Yoshimi, K.; Tanaka, M.; Kuwamura, M.; Hiai, H.; et al. Atopic dermatitis-like skin lesions with IgE hyperproduction and pruritus in KFRS4/Kyo rats. *J. Dermatol. Sci.* **2015**, *80*, 116–123. [CrossRef] [PubMed]
14. Sengupta, P. The laboratory rat: Relating its age with human's. *Int. J. Prev. Med.* **2013**, *4*, 624–630. [PubMed]
15. Tokura, Y. Extrinsic and intrinsic types of atopic dermatitis. *J. Dermatol. Sci.* **2010**, *58*, 1–7. [CrossRef] [PubMed]
16. Farage, M.A.; Neill, S.; MacLean, A.B. Physiological changes associated with the menstrual cycle: A review. *Obstet. Gynecol. Surv.* **2009**, *64*, 58–72. [CrossRef] [PubMed]
17. Hughes, G.C. Progesterone and autoimmune disease. *Autoimmun. Rev.* **2012**, *11*, A502–514. [CrossRef]
18. Roved, J.; Westerdahl, H.; Hasselquist, D. Sex differences in immune responses: Hormonal effects, antagonistic selection, and evolutionary consequences. *Horm. Behav.* **2017**, *88*, 95–105. [CrossRef]
19. Solano, M.E.; Sander, V.A.; Ho, H.; Motta, A.B.; Arck, P.C. Systemic inflammation, cellular influx and up-regulation of ovarian VCAM-1 expression in a mouse model of polycystic ovary syndrome (PCOS). *J. Reprod. Immunol.* **2011**, *92*, 33–44. [CrossRef]
20. Namazi, M.R. The Th1-promoting effects of dehydroepiandrosterone can provide an explanation for the stronger Th1-immune response of women. *Iran. J. Allergy Asthma Immunol.* **2009**, *8*, 65–69.

21. Xiang, Y.; Jin, Q.; Li, L.; Yang, Y.; Zhang, H.; Liu, M.; Fan, C.; Li, J.; Shan, Z.; Teng, W. Physiological low-dose oestrogen promotes the development of experimental autoimmune thyroiditis through the up-regulation of Th1/Th17 responses. *J. Reprod. Immunol.* **2018**, *126*, 23–31. [CrossRef] [PubMed]
22. Dayoub, O.; Le Lay, S.; Soleti, R.; Clere, N.; Hilairet, G.; Dubois, S.; Gagnadoux, F.; Boursier, J.; Martinez, M.C.; Andriantsitohaina, R. Estrogen receptor alpha/HDAC/NFAT axis for delphinidin effects on proliferation and differentiation of T lymphocytes from patients with cardiovascular risks. *Sci. Rep.* **2017**, *7*, 9378. [CrossRef] [PubMed]
23. Haghmorad, D.; Salehipour, Z.; Nosratabadi, R.; Rastin, M.; Kokhaei, P.; Mahmoudi, M.B.; Amini, A.A.; Mahmoudi, M. Medium-dose estrogen ameliorates experimental autoimmune encephalomyelitis in ovariectomized mice. *J. Immunotoxicol.* **2016**, *13*, 885–896. [CrossRef] [PubMed]
24. Garnier, L.; Laffont, S.; Lelu, K.; Yogev, N.; Waisman, A.; Guery, J.C. Estrogen Signaling in Bystander Foxp3(neg) CD4(+) T Cells Suppresses Cognate Th17 Differentiation in Trans and Protects from Central Nervous System Autoimmunity. *J. Immunol.* **2018**, *201*, 3218–3228. [CrossRef] [PubMed]
25. Lasarte, S.; Elsner, D.; Guia-Gonzalez, M.; Ramos-Medina, R.; Sanchez-Ramon, S.; Esponda, P.; Munoz-Fernandez, M.A.; Relloso, M. Female sex hormones regulate the Th17 immune response to sperm and Candida albicans. *Hum. Reprod.* **2013**, *28*, 3283–3291. [CrossRef] [PubMed]
26. Lambert, K.C.; Curran, E.M.; Judy, B.M.; Milligan, G.N.; Lubahn, D.B.; Estes, D.M. Estrogen receptor alpha (ERalpha) deficiency in macrophages results in increased stimulation of CD4+ T cells while 17beta-estradiol acts through ERalpha to increase IL-4 and GATA-3 expression in CD4+ T cells independent of antigen presentation. *J. Immunol.* **2005**, *175*, 5716–5723. [CrossRef] [PubMed]
27. Han, D.; Denison, M.S.; Tachibana, H.; Yamada, K. Effects of estrogenic compounds on immunoglobulin production by mouse splenocytes. *Biol. Pharm. Bull.* **2002**, *25*, 1263–1267. [CrossRef] [PubMed]
28. Iannello, A.; Rolla, S.; Maglione, A.; Ferrero, G.; Bardina, V.; Inaudi, I.; De Mercanti, S.; Novelli, F.; D'Antuono, L.; Cardaropoli, S.; et al. Pregnancy epigenetic signature in T helper 17 and T regulatory cells in multiple sclerosis. *Front. Immunol.* **2018**, *9*, 3075. [CrossRef]
29. Qin, J.; Li, L.; Jin, Q.; Guo, D.; Liu, M.; Fan, C.; Li, J.; Shan, Z.; Teng, W. Estrogen receptor beta activation stimulates the development of experimental autoimmune thyroiditis through up-regulation of Th17-type responses. *Clin. Immunol.* **2018**, *190*, 41–52. [CrossRef]
30. Adurthi, S.; Kumar, M.M.; Vinodkumar, H.S.; Mukherjee, G.; Krishnamurthy, H.; Acharya, K.K.; Bafna, U.D.; Uma, D.K.; Abhishekh, B.; Krishna, S.; et al. Oestrogen Receptor-alpha binds the FOXP3 promoter and modulates regulatory T-cell function in human cervical cancer. *Sci. Rep.* **2017**, *7*, 17289. [CrossRef]
31. Polanczyk, M.J.; Carson, B.D.; Subramanian, S.; Afentoulis, M.; Vandenbark, A.A.; Ziegler, S.F.; Offner, H. Cutting edge: Estrogen drives expansion of the CD4+CD25+ regulatory T cell compartment. *J. Immunol.* **2004**, *173*, 2227–2230. [CrossRef] [PubMed]
32. Polari, L.; Wiklund, A.; Sousa, S.; Kangas, L.; Linnanen, T.; Harkonen, P.; Maatta, J. SERMs Promote Anti-Inflammatory Signaling and Phenotype of CD14+ Cells. *Inflammation* **2018**, *41*, 1157–1171. [CrossRef] [PubMed]
33. Zaitsu, M.; Narita, S.; Lambert, K.C.; Grady, J.J.; Estes, D.M.; Curran, E.M.; Brooks, E.G.; Watson, C.S.; Goldblum, R.M.; Midoro-Horiuti, T. Estradiol activates mast cells via a non-genomic estrogen receptor-alpha and calcium influx. *Mol. Immunol.* **2007**, *44*, 1977–1985. [CrossRef] [PubMed]
34. Matalka, K.Z. The effect of estradiol, but not progesterone, on the production of cytokines in stimulated whole blood, is concentration-dependent. *Neuro Endocrinol. Lett.* **2003**, *24*, 185–191. [PubMed]
35. Polese, B.; Gridelet, V.; Araklioti, E.; Martens, H.; Perrier d'Hauterive, S.; Geenen, V. The Endocrine Milieu and CD4 T-Lymphocyte Polarization during Pregnancy. *Front. Endocrinol. (Lausanne)* **2014**, *5*, 106. [CrossRef] [PubMed]
36. Chen, R.Y.; Fan, Y.M.; Zhang, Q.; Liu, S.; Li, Q.; Ke, G.L.; Li, C.; You, Z. Estradiol inhibits Th17 cell differentiation through inhibition of RORgammaT transcription by recruiting the ERalpha/REA complex to estrogen response elements of the RORgammaT promoter. *J. Immunol.* **2015**, *194*, 4019–4028. [CrossRef] [PubMed]
37. Narita, S.; Goldblum, R.M.; Watson, C.S.; Brooks, E.G.; Estes, D.M.; Curran, E.M.; Midoro-Horiuti, T. Environmental estrogens induce mast cell degranulation and enhance IgE-mediated release of allergic mediators. *Environ. Health Perspect.* **2007**, *115*, 48–52. [CrossRef] [PubMed]

38. Watanabe, Y.; Tajiki-Nishino, R.; Tajima, H.; Fukuyama, T. Role of estrogen receptors alpha and beta in the development of allergic airway inflammation in mice: A possible involvement of interleukin 33 and eosinophils. *Toxicology* **2019**, *411*, 93–100. [CrossRef] [PubMed]
39. Maeda, Y.; Ohtsuka, H.; Tomioka, M.; Oikawa, M. Effect of progesterone on Th1/Th2/Th17 and regulatory T cell-related genes in peripheral blood mononuclear cells during pregnancy in cows. *Vet. Res. Commun.* **2013**, *37*, 43–49. [CrossRef]
40. Kozma, N.; Halasz, M.; Polgar, B.; Poehlmann, T.G.; Markert, U.R.; Palkovics, T.; Keszei, M.; Par, G.; Kiss, K.; Szeberenyi, J.; et al. Progesterone-induced blocking factor activates STAT6 via binding to a novel IL-4 receptor. *J. Immunol.* **2006**, *176*, 819–826. [CrossRef] [PubMed]
41. Xu, L.; Dong, B.; Wang, H.; Zeng, Z.; Liu, W.; Chen, N.; Chen, J.; Yang, J.; Li, D.; Duan, Y. Progesterone suppresses Th17 cell responses, and enhances the development of regulatory T cells, through thymic stromal lymphopoietin-dependent mechanisms in experimental gonococcal genital tract infection. *Microbes Infect.* **2013**, *15*, 796–805. [CrossRef] [PubMed]
42. Miyaura, H.; Iwata, M. Direct and indirect inhibition of Th1 development by progesterone and glucocorticoids. *J. Immunol.* **2002**, *168*, 1087–1094. [CrossRef] [PubMed]
43. Hall, O.J.; Limjunyawong, N.; Vermillion, M.S.; Robinson, D.P.; Wohlgemuth, N.; Pekosz, A.; Mitzner, W.; Klein, S.L. Progesterone-Based Therapy Protects Against Influenza by Promoting Lung Repair and Recovery in Females. *PLoS Pathog.* **2016**, *12*, e1005840. [CrossRef] [PubMed]
44. Mitchell, V.L.; Gershwin, L.J. Progesterone and environmental tobacco smoke act synergistically to exacerbate the development of allergic asthma in a mouse model. *Clin. Exp. Allergy* **2007**, *37*, 276–286. [CrossRef] [PubMed]
45. Lorenz, T.K.; Heiman, J.R.; Demas, G.E. Sexual activity modulates shifts in TH1/TH2 cytokine profile across the menstrual cycle: An observational study. *Fertil. Steril.* **2015**, *104*, 1513–1521. [CrossRef]
46. Lee, J.H.; Ulrich, B.; Cho, J.; Park, J.; Kim, C.H. Progesterone promotes differentiation of human cord blood fetal T cells into T regulatory cells but suppresses their differentiation into Th17 cells. *J. Immunol.* **2011**, *187*, 1778–1787. [CrossRef] [PubMed]
47. Kissick, H.T.; Sanda, M.G.; Dunn, L.K.; Pellegrini, K.L.; On, S.T.; Noel, J.K.; Arredouani, M.S. Androgens alter T-cell immunity by inhibiting T-helper 1 differentiation. *Proc. Natl. Acad. Sci. USA* **2014**, *111*, 9887–9892. [CrossRef]
48. Zhang, M.A.; Rego, D.; Moshkova, M.; Kebir, H.; Chruscinski, A.; Nguyen, H.; Akkermann, R.; Stanczyk, F.Z.; Prat, A.; Steinman, L.; et al. Peroxisome proliferator-activated receptor (PPAR)alpha and -gamma regulate IFNgamma and IL-17A production by human T cells in a sex-specific way. *Proc. Natl. Acad. Sci. USA* **2012**, *109*, 9505–9510. [CrossRef]
49. Massa, M.G.; David, C.; Jorg, S.; Berg, J.; Gisevius, B.; Hirschberg, S.; Linker, R.A.; Gold, R.; Haghikia, A. Testosterone differentially affects T cells and neurons in murine and human models of neuroinflammation and neurodegeneration. *Am. J. Pathol.* **2017**, *187*, 1613–1622. [CrossRef]
50. Vignozzi, L.; Cellai, I.; Santi, R.; Lombardelli, L.; Morelli, A.; Comeglio, P.; Filippi, S.; Logiodice, F.; Carini, M.; Nesi, G.; et al. Antiinflammatory effect of androgen receptor activation in human benign prostatic hyperplasia cells. *J. Endocrinol.* **2012**, *214*, 31–43. [CrossRef]
51. Trigunaite, A.; Dimo, J.; Jorgensen, T.N. Suppressive effects of androgens on the immune system. *Cell Immunol.* **2015**, *294*, 87–94. [CrossRef] [PubMed]
52. Yamatomo, T.; Okano, M.; Ono, T.; Nakayama, E.; Yoshino, T.; Satoskar, A.R.; Harn, D.A., Jr.; Nishizaki, K. Sex-related differences in the initiation of allergic rhinitis in mice. *Allergy* **2001**, *56*, 525–531. [CrossRef] [PubMed]
53. Fuseini, H.; Yung, J.A.; Cephus, J.Y.; Zhang, J.; Goleniewska, K.; Polosukhin, V.V.; Peebles, R.S., Jr.; Newcomb, D.C. Testosterone Decreases House Dust Mite-Induced Type 2 and IL-17A-Mediated Airway Inflammation. *J. Immunol.* **2018**, *201*, 1843–1854. [CrossRef] [PubMed]
54. Hepworth, M.R.; Hardman, M.J.; Grencis, R.K. The role of sex hormones in the development of Th2 immunity in a gender-biased model of Trichuris muris infection. *Eur. J. Immunol.* **2010**, *40*, 406–416. [CrossRef] [PubMed]
55. Walecki, M.; Eisel, F.; Klug, J.; Baal, N.; Paradowska-Dogan, A.; Wahle, E.; Hackstein, H.; Meinhardt, A.; Fijak, M. Androgen receptor modulates Foxp3 expression in CD4+CD25+Foxp3+ regulatory T-cells. *Mol. Biol. Cell* **2015**, *26*, 2845–2857. [CrossRef] [PubMed]

56. Gubbels Bupp, M.R.; Jorgensen, T.N. Androgen-Induced Immunosuppression. *Front. Immunol.* **2018**, *9*, 794. [CrossRef]
57. Fuseini, H.; Newcomb, D.C. Mechanisms Driving Gender Differences in Asthma. *Curr. Allergy Asthma Rep.* **2017**, *17*, 19. [CrossRef]
58. Khurana, H.; Malhotra, P.; Sachdeva, M.U.; Varma, N.; Bose, P.; Yanamandra, U.; Varma, S.; Khadwal, A.; Lad, D.; Prakash, G. Danazol increases T regulatory cells in patients with aplastic anemia. *Hematology* **2018**, *23*, 496–500. [CrossRef]
59. Liou, C.J.; Huang, W.C. Dehydroepiandrosterone suppresses eosinophil infiltration and airway hyperresponsiveness via modulation of chemokines and Th2 cytokines in ovalbumin-sensitized mice. *J. Clin. Immunol.* **2011**, *31*, 656–665. [CrossRef]
60. Chan, C.C.; Liou, C.J.; Xu, P.Y.; Shen, J.J.; Kuo, M.L.; Len, W.B.; Chang, L.E.; Huang, W.C. Effect of dehydroepiandrosterone on atopic dermatitis-like skin lesions induced by 1-chloro-2,4-dinitrobenzene in mouse. *J. Dermatol. Sci.* **2013**, *72*, 149–157. [CrossRef]
61. Aggelakopoulou, M.; Kourepini, E.; Paschalidis, N.; Simoes, D.C.; Kalavrizioti, D.; Dimisianos, N.; Papathanasopoulos, P.; Mouzaki, A.; Panoutsakopoulou, V. ERbeta-Dependent Direct Suppression of Human and Murine Th17 Cells and Treatment of Established Central Nervous System Autoimmunity by a Neurosteroid. *J. Immunol.* **2016**, *197*, 2598–2609. [CrossRef] [PubMed]
62. Alves, V.B.; Basso, P.J.; Nardini, V.; Silva, A.; Chica, J.E.; Cardoso, C.R. Dehydroepiandrosterone (DHEA) restrains intestinal inflammation by rendering leukocytes hyporesponsive and balancing colitogenic inflammatory responses. *Immunobiology* **2016**, *221*, 934–943. [CrossRef] [PubMed]
63. Cao, J.; Yu, L.; Zhao, J.; Ma, H. Effect of dehydroepiandrosterone on the immune function of mice in vivo and in vitro. *Mol. Immunol.* **2019**, *112*, 283–290. [CrossRef] [PubMed]
64. Tabata, N.; Tagami, H.; Terui, T. Dehydroepiandrosterone may be one of the regulators of cytokine production in atopic dermatitis. *Arch. Dermatol. Res.* **1997**, *289*, 410–414. [CrossRef] [PubMed]
65. Sudo, N.; Yu, X.N.; Kubo, C. Dehydroepiandrosterone attenuates the spontaneous elevation of serum IgE level in NC/Nga mice. *Immunol. Lett.* **2001**, *79*, 177–179. [CrossRef]
66. Frantz, M.C.; Prix, N.J.; Wichmann, M.W.; van den Engel, N.K.; Hernandez-Richter, T.; Faist, E.; Chaudry, I.H.; Jauch, K.W.; Angele, M.K. Dehydroepiandrosterone restores depressed peripheral blood mononuclear cell function following major abdominal surgery via the estrogen receptors. *Crit. Care Med.* **2005**, *33*, 1779–1786. [CrossRef] [PubMed]
67. Quiroga, M.F.; Angerami, M.T.; Santucci, N.; Ameri, D.; Francos, J.L.; Wallach, J.; Sued, O.; Cahn, P.; Salomon, H.; Bottasso, O. Dynamics of adrenal steroids are related to variations in Th1 and Treg populations during Mycobacterium tuberculosis infection in HIV positive persons. *PLoS ONE* **2012**, *7*, e33061. [CrossRef]
68. Auci, D.; Kaler, L.; Subramanian, S.; Huang, Y.; Frincke, J.; Reading, C.; Offner, H. A new orally bioavailable synthetic androstene inhibits collagen-induced arthritis in the mouse: Androstene hormones as regulators of regulatory T cells. *Ann. NY Acad. Sci.* **2007**, *1110*, 630–640. [CrossRef]
69. Sulcova, J.; Hill, M.; Hampl, R.; Starka, L. Age and sex related differences in serum levels of unconjugated dehydroepiandrosterone and its sulphate in normal subjects. *J. Endocrinol.* **1997**, *154*, 57–62. [CrossRef]
70. Muller, C.R.; Migl, B.; Traupe, H.; Ropers, H.H. X-linked steroid sulfatase: Evidence for different gene-dosage in males and females. *Hum. Genet.* **1980**, *54*, 197–199. [CrossRef]
71. Carlstrom, K.; Brody, S.; Lunell, N.O.; Lagrelius, A.; Mollerstrom, G.; Pousette, A.; Rannevik, G.; Stege, R.; von Schoultz, B. Dehydroepiandrosterone sulphate and dehydroepiandrosterone in serum: Differences related to age and sex. *Maturitas* **1988**, *10*, 297–306. [CrossRef]
72. Zumoff, B.; Rosenfeld, R.S.; Strain, G.W.; Levin, J.; Fukushima, D.K. Sex differences in the twenty-four-hour mean plasma concentrations of dehydroisoandrosterone (DHA) and dehydroisoandrosterone sulfate (DHAS) and the DHA to DHAS ratio in normal adults. *J. Clin. Endocrinol. Metab.* **1980**, *51*, 330–333. [CrossRef] [PubMed]
73. Prough, R.A.; Clark, B.J.; Klinge, C.M. Novel mechanisms for DHEA action. *J. Mol. Endocrinol.* **2016**, *56*, R139–155. [CrossRef] [PubMed]
74. Zhang, J.; Qiu, X.; Gui, Y.; Xu, Y.; Li, D.; Wang, L. Dehydroepiandrosterone improves the ovarian reserve of women with diminished ovarian reserve and is a potential regulator of the immune response in the ovaries. *Biosci. Trends* **2015**, *9*, 350–359. [CrossRef] [PubMed]

75. Qiu, X.; Gui, Y.; Xu, Y.; Li, D.; Wang, L. DHEA promotes osteoblast differentiation by regulating the expression of osteoblast-related genes and Foxp3(+) regulatory T cells. *Biosci. Trends* **2015**, *9*, 307–314. [CrossRef] [PubMed]
76. Firooz, A.; Sadr, B.; Babakoohi, S.; Sarraf-Yazdy, M.; Fanian, F.; Kazerouni-Timsar, A.; Nassiri-Kashani, M.; Naghizadeh, M.M.; Dowlati, Y. Variation of biophysical parameters of the skin with age, gender, and body region. *Sci. World J.* **2012**, *2012*, 386936. [CrossRef] [PubMed]
77. Hanley, K.; Rassner, U.; Jiang, Y.; Vansomphone, D.; Crumrine, D.; Komuves, L.; Elias, P.M.; Feingold, K.R.; Williams, M.L. Hormonal basis for the gender difference in epidermal barrier formation in the fetal rat. Acceleration by estrogen and delay by testosterone. *J. Clin. Investig.* **1996**, *97*, 2576–2584. [CrossRef]
78. Tsutsumi, M.; Denda, M. Paradoxical effects of beta-estradiol on epidermal permeability barrier homeostasis. *Br. J. Dermatol.* **2007**, *157*, 776–779. [CrossRef]
79. Harvell, J.; Hussona-Saeed, I.; Maibach, H.I. Changes in transepidermal water loss and cutaneous blood flow during the menstrual cycle. *Contact Derm.* **1992**, *27*, 294–301. [CrossRef]
80. Chen, Y.; Yokozeki, H.; Katagiri, K. Physiological and functional changes in the stratum corneum restored by oestrogen in an ovariectomized mice model of climacterium. *Exp. Dermatol.* **2017**, *26*, 394–401. [CrossRef]
81. Hung, C.F.; Chen, W.Y.; Aljuffali, I.A.; Lin, Y.K.; Shih, H.C.; Fang, J.Y. Skin aging modulates percutaneous drug absorption: The impact of ultraviolet irradiation and ovariectomy. *Age (Dordr.)* **2015**, *37*, 21. [CrossRef] [PubMed]
82. Kao, J.S.; Garg, A.; Mao-Qiang, M.; Crumrine, D.; Ghadially, R.; Feingold, K.R.; Elias, P.M. Testosterone perturbs epidermal permeability barrier homeostasis. *J. Investig. Dermatol.* **2001**, *116*, 443–451. [CrossRef] [PubMed]
83. Hanley, K.; Jiang, Y.; Holleran, W.M.; Elias, P.M.; Williams, M.L.; Feingold, K.R. Glucosylceramide metabolism is regulated during normal and hormonally stimulated epidermal barrier development in the rat. *J. Lipid Res.* **1997**, *38*, 576–584. [PubMed]
84. Komuves, L.G.; Hanley, K.; Jiang, Y.; Elias, P.M.; Williams, M.L.; Feingold, K.R. Ligands and activators of nuclear hormone receptors regulate epidermal differentiation during fetal rat skin development. *J. Investig. Dermatol.* **1998**, *111*, 429–433. [CrossRef] [PubMed]
85. Muizzuddin, N.; Marenus, K.D.; Schnittger, S.F.; Sullivan, M.; Maes, D.H. Effect of systemic hormonal cyclicity on skin. *J. Cosmet. Sci.* **2005**, *56*, 311–321. [CrossRef] [PubMed]
86. Bonamonte, D.; Foti, C.; Antelmi, A.R.; Biscozzi, A.M.; Naro, E.D.; Fanelli, M.; Loverro, G.; Angelini, G. Nickel contact allergy and menstrual cycle. *Contact derm.* **2005**, *52*, 309–313. [CrossRef]
87. Hong, S.H.; Lee, J.E.; Jeong, J.J.; Hwang, S.J.; Bae, S.N.; Choi, J.Y.; Song, H. Small proline-rich protein 2 family is a cluster of genes induced by estrogenic compounds through nuclear estrogen receptors in the mouse uterus. *Reprod. Toxicol.* **2010**, *30*, 469–476. [CrossRef]
88. Hernandez-Monge, J.; Garay, E.; Raya-Sandino, A.; Vargas-Sierra, O.; Diaz-Chavez, J.; Popoca-Cuaya, M.; Lambert, P.F.; Gonzalez-Mariscal, L.; Gariglio, P. Papillomavirus E6 oncoprotein up-regulates occludin and ZO-2 expression in ovariectomized mice epidermis. *Exp. Cell Res.* **2013**, *319*, 2588–2603. [CrossRef]
89. Zhou, Z.; Bian, C.; Luo, Z.; Guille, C.; Ogunrinde, E.; Wu, J.; Zhao, M.; Fitting, S.; Kamen, D.L.; Oates, J.C.; et al. Progesterone decreases gut permeability through upregulating occludin expression in primary human gut tissues and Caco-2 cells. *Sci. Rep.* **2019**, *9*, 8367. [CrossRef]
90. Baulieu, E.E.; Thomas, G.; Legrain, S.; Lahlou, N.; Roger, M.; Debuire, B.; Faucounau, V.; Girard, L.; Hervy, M.P.; Latour, F.; et al. Dehydroepiandrosterone (DHEA), DHEA sulfate, and aging: Contribution of the DHEAge Study to a sociobiomedical issue. *Proc. Natl. Acad. Sci. USA* **2000**, *97*, 4279–4284. [CrossRef]
91. El-Alfy, M.; Deloche, C.; Azzi, L.; Bernard, B.A.; Bernerd, F.; Coutet, J.; Chaussade, V.; Martel, C.; Leclaire, J.; Labrie, F. Skin responses to topical dehydroepiandrosterone: Implications in antiageing treatment? *Br. J. Dermatol.* **2010**, *163*, 968–976. [CrossRef] [PubMed]
92. Calvo, E.; Luu-The, V.; Morissette, J.; Martel, C.; Labrie, C.; Bernard, B.; Bernerd, F.; Deloche, C.; Chaussade, V.; Leclaire, J.; et al. Pangenomic changes induced by DHEA in the skin of postmenopausal women. *J. Steroid Biochem. Mol. Biol.* **2008**, *112*, 186–193. [CrossRef] [PubMed]
93. Papadopoulos, D.; Dietze, R.; Shihan, M.; Kirch, U.; Scheiner-Bobis, G. Dehydroepiandrosterone Sulfate Stimulates Expression of Blood-Testis-Barrier Proteins Claudin-3 and -5 and Tight Junction Formation via a Gnalpha11-Coupled Receptor in Sertoli Cells. *PLoS ONE* **2016**, *11*, e0150143. [CrossRef] [PubMed]

94. Yosipovitch, G.; Rosen, J.D.; Hashimoto, T. Itch: From mechanism to (novel) therapeutic approaches. *J. Allergy Clin. Immunol.* **2018**, *142*, 1375–1390. [CrossRef] [PubMed]
95. Watanabe, Y.; Makino, E.; Tajiki-Nishino, R.; Koyama, A.; Tajima, H.; Ishimota, M.; Fukuyama, T. Involvement of estrogen receptor alpha in pro-pruritic and pro-inflammatory responses in a mouse model of allergic dermatitis. *Toxicol. Appl. Pharmacol.* **2018**, *355*, 226–237. [CrossRef] [PubMed]
96. Ulmann, L.; Rodeau, J.L.; Danoux, L.; Contet-Audonneau, J.L.; Pauly, G.; Schlichter, R. Dehydroepiandrosterone and neurotrophins favor axonal growth in a sensory neuron-keratinocyte coculture model. *Neuroscience* **2009**, *159*, 514–525. [CrossRef]
97. Pediaditakis, I.; Iliopoulos, I.; Theologidis, I.; Delivanoglou, N.; Margioris, A.N.; Charalampopoulos, I.; Gravanis, A. Dehydroepiandrosterone: An ancestral ligand of neurotrophin receptors. *Endocrinology* **2015**, *156*, 16–23. [CrossRef]
98. Yamaguchi, H.; Kabashima-Kubo, R.; Bito, T.; Sakabe, J.; Shimauchi, T.; Ito, T.; Hirakawa, S.; Hirasawa, N.; Ogasawara, K.; Tokura, Y. High frequencies of positive nickel/cobalt patch tests and high sweat nickel concentration in patients with intrinsic atopic dermatitis. *J. Dermatol. Sci.* **2013**, *72*, 240–245. [CrossRef]
99. Hindsen, M.; Christensen, O.B.; Moller, H. Nickel levels in serum and urine in five different groups of eczema patients following oral ingestion of nickel. *Acta Derm. Venereol.* **1994**, *74*, 176–178. [CrossRef]
100. Suarez-Farinas, M.; Dhingra, N.; Gittler, J.; Shemer, A.; Cardinale, I.; de Guzman Strong, C.; Krueger, J.G.; Guttman-Yassky, E. Intrinsic atopic dermatitis shows similar TH2 and higher TH17 immune activation compared with extrinsic atopic dermatitis. *J. Allergy Clin. Immunol.* **2013**, *132*, 361–370. [CrossRef]
101. Minang, J.T.; Troye-Blomberg, M.; Lundeberg, L.; Ahlborg, N. Nickel elicits concomitant and correlated in vitro production of Th1-, Th2-type and regulatory cytokines in subjects with contact allergy to nickel. *Scand. J. Immunol.* **2005**, *62*, 289–296. [CrossRef] [PubMed]
102. Summer, B.; Stander, S.; Thomas, P. Cytokine patterns in vitro, in particular IL-5/IL-8 ratio, to detect patients with nickel contact allergy. *J. Eur. Acad. Dermatol. Venereol.* **2018**, *32*, 1542–1548. [CrossRef] [PubMed]
103. Czarnobilska, E.; Jenner, B.; Kaszuba-Zwoinska, J.; Kapusta, M.; Obtulowicz, K.; Thor, P.; Spiewak, R. Contact allergy to nickel: Patch test score correlates with IL-5, but not with IFN-gamma nickel-specific secretion by peripheral blood lymphocytes. *Ann. Agric. Environ. Med.* **2009**, *16*, 37–41. [PubMed]
104. Ott, H.; Stanzel, S.; Ocklenburg, C.; Merk, H.F.; Baron, J.M.; Lehmann, S. Total serum IgE as a parameter to differentiate between intrinsic and extrinsic atopic dermatitis in children. *Acta Derm. Venereol.* **2009**, *89*, 257–261. [CrossRef] [PubMed]
105. Kusel, M.M.; Holt, P.G.; de Klerk, N.; Sly, P.D. Support for 2 variants of eczema. *J. Allergy Clin. Immunol.* **2005**, *116*, 1067–1072. [CrossRef] [PubMed]
106. Zafrir, Y.; Trattner, A.; Hodak, E.; Eldar, O.; Lapidoth, M.; Ben Amitai, D. Patch testing in Israeli children with suspected allergic contact dermatitis: A retrospective study and literature review. *Pediatr. Dermatol.* **2018**, *35*, 76–86. [CrossRef] [PubMed]
107. Vahter, M.; Berglund, M.; Akesson, A.; Liden, C. Metals and women's health. *Environ. Res.* **2002**, *88*, 145–155. [CrossRef] [PubMed]
108. Singh, A.K.; Cydulka, R.K.; Stahmer, S.A.; Woodruff, P.G.; Camargo, C.A., Jr. Sex differences among adults presenting to the emergency department with acute asthma. Multicenter Asthma Research Collaboration Investigators. *Arch. Intern. Med.* **1999**, *159*, 1237–1243. [CrossRef]
109. Pagtakhan, R.D.; Bjelland, J.C.; Landau, L.I.; Loughlin, G.; Kaltenborn, W.; Seeley, G.; Taussig, L.M. Sex differences in growth patterns of the airways and lung parenchyma in children. *J. Appl. Physiol. Respir. Environ. Exerc. Physiol.* **1984**, *56*, 1204–1210. [CrossRef]
110. Sears, M.R.; Burrows, B.; Flannery, E.M.; Herbison, G.P.; Holdaway, M.D. Atopy in childhood. I. Gender and allergen related risks for development of hay fever and asthma. *Clin. Exp. Allergy* **1993**, *23*, 941–948. [CrossRef]
111. Mohrenschlager, M.; Schafer, T.; Huss-Marp, J.; Eberlein-Konig, B.; Weidinger, S.; Ring, J.; Behrendt, H.; Kramer, U. The course of eczema in children aged 5–7 years and its relation to atopy: Differences between boys and girls. *Br. J. Dermatol.* **2006**, *154*, 505–513. [CrossRef] [PubMed]
112. Sennhauser, F.H.; Kuhni, C.E. Prevalence of respiratory symptoms in Swiss children: Is bronchial asthma really more prevalent in boys? *Pediatr. Pulmonol.* **1995**, *19*, 161–166. [CrossRef] [PubMed]

113. Biro, F.M.; Huang, B.; Chandler, D.W.; Fassler, C.L.; Pinney, S.M. Impact of pubertal maturation and chronologic age on sex steroids in peripubertal girls. *J. Clin. Endocrinol. Metab.* **2019**, *104*, 2971–2977. [CrossRef] [PubMed]
114. Maruyama, Y.; Aoki, N.; Suzuki, Y.; Ohno, Y.; Imamura, M.; Saika, T.; Sinohara, H.; Yamamoto, T. Sex-steroid-binding plasma protein (SBP), testosterone, oestradiol and dehydroepiandrosterone (DHEA) in prepuberty and puberty. *Acta Endocrinol. (Copenh)* **1987**, *114*, 60–67. [CrossRef] [PubMed]
115. Rouskova, D.; Mittmann, K.; Schumacher, U.; Dietrich, H.; Zimmermann, T. Effectiveness, tolerability and acceptance of a low-dosed estradiol/dienogest formulation (Lafamme 1 mg/2 mg) for the treatment of menopausal complaints: A non-interventional observational study over 6 cycles of 28 days. *Gynecol. Endocrinol.* **2015**, *31*, 560–564. [CrossRef] [PubMed]
116. Yamaura, K.; Tomono, A.; Suwa, E.; Ueno, K. Sex-related differences in SLIGRL-induced pruritus in mice. *Life Sci.* **2014**, *94*, 54–57. [CrossRef] [PubMed]
117. Kitagaki, H.; Ono, N.; Hayakawa, K.; Kitazawa, T.; Watanabe, K.; Shiohara, T. Repeated elicitation of contact hypersensitivity induces a shift in cutaneous cytokine milieu from a T helper cell type 1 to a T helper cell type 2 profile. *J. Immunol.* **1997**, *159*, 2484–2491. [PubMed]
118. Raghunath, R.S.; Venables, Z.C.; Millington, G.W. The menstrual cycle and the skin. *Clin. Exp. Dermatol.* **2015**, *40*, 111–115. [CrossRef] [PubMed]
119. Kemmett, D.; Tidman, M.J. The influence of the menstrual cycle and pregnancy on atopic dermatitis. *Br. J. Dermatol.* **1991**, *125*, 59–61. [CrossRef]
120. Cho, S.; Kim, H.J.; Oh, S.H.; Park, C.O.; Jung, J.Y.; Lee, K.H. The influence of pregnancy and menstruation on the deterioration of atopic dermatitis symptoms. *Ann. Dermatol.* **2010**, *22*, 180–185. [CrossRef]
121. Ebata, T.; Itamura, R.; Aizawa, H.; Niimura, M. Serum sex hormone levels in adult patients with atopic dermatitis. *J. Dermatol.* **1996**, *23*, 603–605. [CrossRef] [PubMed]
122. Kasperska-Zajac, A.; Brzoza, Z.; Rogala, B. Dehydroepiandrosterone and dehydroepiandrosterone sulphate in atopic allergy and chronic urticaria. *Inflammation* **2008**, *31*, 141–145. [CrossRef] [PubMed]
123. Opstad, P.K. The hypothalamo-pituitary regulation of androgen secretion in young men after prolonged physical stress combined with energy and sleep deprivation. *Acta Endocrinol. (Copenh)* **1992**, *127*, 231–236. [CrossRef] [PubMed]

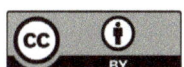

© 2019 by the authors. Licensee MDPI, Basel, Switzerland. This article is an open access article distributed under the terms and conditions of the Creative Commons Attribution (CC BY) license (http://creativecommons.org/licenses/by/4.0/).

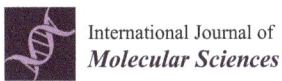

Review

The Role of Th17-Related Cytokines in Atopic Dermatitis

Makoto Sugaya

Department of Dermatology, International University of Health and Welfare, Ichikawa Hospital, 6-1-14, Kounodai, Ichikawa, Chiba 272-0827, Japan; sugayamder@iuhw.ac.jp; Tel.: +81-47-375-1111; Fax: +81-47-373-4921

Received: 25 January 2020; Accepted: 12 February 2020; Published: 15 February 2020

Abstract: T helper-17 (Th17) cells, which mainly produce IL-17, are associated with development of various autoimmune diseases such as rheumatoid arthritis, inflammatory bowel diseases, multiple sclerosis, and psoriasis. IL-17 and related cytokines are therapeutic targets of these diseases. In atopic dermatitis (AD), Th2 cytokines such as IL-4 and IL-13 are regarded to be the main player of the disease; however, Th17 cytokines are also expressed in AD skin lesions. Expression of IL-22 rather than IL-17 is predominant in AD skin, which is contrary to cytokine expression in psoriasis skin. Relatively low IL-17 expression in AD skin can induce relatively low antimicrobial peptide expression, which may be a reason why bacterial infection is frequently seen in AD patients. Failure of clinical trials for investigating the efficacy of anti-IL-12/23 p40 in AD has suggested that IL-17 expressed in skin lesions should not be the main player but a bystander responding to barrier dysfunction.

Keywords: IL-22; IL-26; subtypes of atopic dermatitis; ustekinumab; wound healing; antimicrobial peptides

---

1. Introduction

Atopic dermatitis (AD) is a chronic skin disease characterized by relapsing eczema with pruritus as a primary lesion. Most patients with AD have atopic diathesis such as family history of allergic diseases or past history of asthma, rhinitis, or conjunctivitis [1]. In Japan, AD is not a rare skin disease, whose frequency is about 10–15% until the age of forty [2]. Age-related remission is achieved in a certain proportion of patients with AD, especially when the onset is younger or the symptoms are milder [3,4]. Although some patients develop AD in their adulthood, onset of AD in elderly people is very rare. Other skin diseases such as cutaneous T-cell lymphoma (CTCL), drug eruption, and bullous diseases should be considered as a possible diagnosis. Most of all, CTCL should not be misdiagnosed with AD because immunosuppressive drugs such as cyclosporine and anti-tumor necrosis factor (TNF)-α antibody can exacerbate disease activity of CTCL [5–7]. When the diagnosis is not clear, topical steroid or ultraviolet phototherapy should be applied.

AD has significant negative social and economic impacts, substantially decreasing the quality of life of the patients and their families [8,9]. Skin conditions of AD children influence quality of life of both children and their caregivers. Pruritus, emotional distress, and sleep disturbance are big problems for them, which should be paid more attention to. It is important to induce long-term remission. Remission can be achieved by conventional treatment for mild or moderate AD, while it is very difficult for severe AD patients [3,4]. Treatment strategies consist of drug therapy with topical agents such as steroid or tacrolimus, skin care with moisturizers for dry skin, and investigation and elimination of exacerbating factors [1]. The pathogenesis of AD can be explained from the perspectives of the skin barrier, allergic inflammation, and neuroendocrine dysfunction represented by severe pruritus [10]. With regards to allergic immune responses, cytokines expressed by T helper (Th) 2 cells and group 2 innate lymphoid cells such as interleukin (IL)-4, IL-5, and IL-13 have been assumed as main players of AD [11–13]. It was also reported that Th1 cytokines like interferon (IFN)-γ were expressed in AD lesional skin [14,15]. In recent years, Th17 cytokines such as IL-17 and IL-22 were reported to be expressed in AD lesional skin [16–20]. In this review, the importance of Th17-related cytokines in pathogenesis and treatment of AD will be discussed.

2. Th17 Cells in Pathogenesis of Psoriasis

CD4+ helper T cells, upon activation, develop into different T helper cell subsets. Th17 cells, which are different from Th1 or Th2 cells, produce IL-17, IL-17F, and IL-22 as well as IL-21 [21]. Th17 cells are essential in clearing pathogens during host defense reactions. IL-17 and IL-22 are also important for chronic autoinflammatory diseases such as rheumatoid arthritis, inflammatory bowel diseases including Chron's disease and ulcerative colitis, multiple sclerosis, and psoriasis. While transforming growth factor-β and IL-6 are important for differentiation of the subset, IL-23 produced by dendritic cells activated by TNF-α is essential for its maintenance and activation. It is widely accepted that a vicious circle among TNF-α, IL-23, and IL-17 is established in psoriasis. Monoclonal antibodies against TNF-α, IL-12/23p40 subunit, IL-23p19, and IL-17 are clinically used and very effective [22–25].

IL-17 has multiple physiological functions. It activates macrophages to express TNF-α and IL-1β [26] and fibroblasts to produce IL-6, IL-8, and matrix metalloproteinases [27]. These cytokines are important for inflammatory process and tissue remodeling. It also stimulates blood endothelial cells to produce chemoattractants and express VCAM-1 and ICAM-1 in a p38 MAPK-dependent manner, which helps immune cells evade from blood to tissues [28]. Epithelial cells stimulated by IL-17 express IL-8 and granulocyte colony-stimulating factor, inducing migration and activation of neutrophils [29]. In addition, IL-17 was found to synergistically enhance TNF-α-induced production of these cytokines. IL-17 also increases production of antimicrobial peptides (AMPs), which are part of the innate immune response and are found among all classes of life [30,31]. These peptides kill bacteria, mycobacteria, enveloped viruses, and fungi. Skin-resident commensal microbes produce their own AMPs, act to enhance the normal production of AMPs by keratinocytes, and are beneficial to maintaining inflammatory homeostasis by suppressing excess cytokine release after minor epidermal injury [32]. IL-22, which is another cytokine expressed by Th17, enhances AMP production together with IL-17 [31]. This cytokine induces epidermal proliferation [33]. IL-26, an antimicrobial protein that has the ability to directly kill extracellular bacteria, is also secreted by Th17 [34]. IL-26 was more strongly expressed in lesions from the self-limited tuberculoid leprosy compared with expression in progressive lepromatous patients. IL-26 directly bound to *Mycobacterium leprae* in axenic culture and reduced bacteria viability. Thus, Th17 is important for neutrophilic infiltration, epidermal proliferation called acanthosis, and innate immune responses including enhanced production of AMPs, which are main histological findings characteristic to psoriasis.

3. Involvement of Th17-Related Cytokines in AD

3.1. Th17-Related Cytokine Expression in AD

Possible involvement of Th17 in the pathogenesis of AD has been reported by some researchers [16–20]. The percentage of IL-17-poducing CD4+ T cells in peripheral blood from AD patients was increased and associated with severity of AD [16]. There was a significant correlation between the percentages of IL-17+ and IFN-γ+ cells, although the percentage of Th17 cells was not closely related to Th1/Th2 balance. Immunohistochemically, IL-17+ cells infiltrated in the papillary dermis of AD lesional skin. There was another study showing that more IL-17-producing cells infiltrated into the site of an atopy patch test than in healthy skin [17]. IL-17 secretion was not enhanced by IL-23, IL-1β, or IL-6, but was enhanced by the *Staphylococcus aureus*-derived superantigen staphylococcal enterotoxin B. Another group, however, showed that the number of Th1 and Th17 subsets in peripheral blood from AD patients was significantly decreased, but that of the Th2 subset was similar to that of normal controls [35]. The frequency of Th17 cells showed a significant, negative correlation with serum thymus and activation-regulated chemokine (TARC) and IgE levels and the number of eosinophils. It was recently reported that the frequency of IL-13+ cells, which was correlated with IgE levels and SCORing AD (SCORAD) score, was associated with IL-22-producing T cells in severe AD patients [36]. When examining skin samples from AD, psoriasis, and healthy controls, IL-17 expression level was increased in AD skin compared to normal skin, although it was much lower than that in psoriasis skin [18]. By contrast, Th2 cells were significantly elevated in AD. Distinct IL-22-producing CD4+ and CD8+ T-cell populations were significantly increased in AD skin compared with psoriasis. IL-22-producing CD8+ T-cell frequency correlated with AD disease severity. Taken together, IL-22 rather than IL-17 is dominant in AD skin, while IL-17 is dominant in psoriasis skin.

It is a recent trend to divide various diseases into subgroups by cytokine production. Two subgroups of asthma, intrinsic and extrinsic, have been proposed [37]. Extrinsic asthma is triggered by allergens and is characterized by enhanced Th2 cytokine production. Intrinsic asthma is characterized by later onset in life, female predominance, higher degree of severity, and more frequent association to nasosinusal polyposis. This nonallergic asthma characterized by Th1 production can be objectively distinguished from allergic asthma based on negative skin tests to usual aeroallergens. Similar subgroups have been proposed for AD: intrinsic AD and extrinsic AD [38,39]. Extrinsic or allergic AD shows high total serum IgE levels and the presence of specific IgE for environmental and food allergens, whereas intrinsic or nonallergic AD exhibits normal total IgE values and the absence of specific IgE [38]. Extrinsic AD is much more common than intrinsic AD, which is approximately 20% with female predominance. The clinical features of intrinsic AD include relative late onset, milder severity, a higher frequency of metal allergy, and Dennie–Morgan folds, but no ichthyosis vulgaris or palmar hyperlinearity. The skin barrier dysfunction and filaggrin gene mutations are not a feature of intrinsic AD. The intrinsic type is characterized by the lower expression of IL-4, IL-5, and IL-13, and the higher expression of IFN-γ. In patients with intrinsic AD, Th17-related cytokines are highly expressed [39]. Positive correlations between Th17-related molecules and SCORAD scores were only found in patients with intrinsic AD, whereas only patients with extrinsic AD showed positive correlations between SCORAD scores and Th2 cytokine levels and negative correlations with keratinocyte differentiation markers such as loricrin and periplakin. Another classification of AD was proposed: Asian type and European American type. A principal component analysis using real-time PCR data clustered the Asian AD phenotype between the European American AD and psoriasis phenotypes [19]. Significantly higher Th17 and lower Th1 gene induction typified AD skin in Asian patients. Moreover, AD lesional skin in pediatric patients was reported to contain more Th17-related cytokines and AMPs than that in adult patients [20]. Taken together, it may be safely said that IL-17 expression in lesional skin of a certain group of AD patients is higher than that in normal skin. It is yet to be elucidated whether IL-17 plays a critical role in AD as it does in psoriasis.

With regards to serum levels of cytokines, it was reported that IL-22 in AD patients significantly correlated with disease activity, while IL-17 did not reflect disease burden [35].

IL-26 is another cytokine produced by Th17 cells. It was recently reported that IL-26 mRNA expression levels were elevated in AD lesional skin compared with healthy controls and that IL-26-producing cells were increased in AD lesional skin by immunohistochemistry [40]. IL-26 may play an important role for bridging between Th17 and Th2 responses, resulting in the development of AD.

3.2. AD Mouse Models and Th17-Related Cytokines

With regards to basic research, IL-17 was reported to regulate Th2 responses in the mouse AD model [41]. IL-17 triggered the production of IL-4 by Th2 cells. The lack of IL-17A reduced dermatitis and IL-4 production as well as IgE production. It is also known that IL-17 promotes the differentiation of B cells to IgE-producing plasma cells [42]. A murine epicutaneous infection model showed that *Malassezia*, which has been reported to exacerbate AD skin conditions, selectively induced IL-17-related cytokines [43]. This process is important for preventing fungal infection through the skin. Under skin barrier dysfunction mimicking AD, the presence of *Malassezia* aggravated cutaneous inflammation, which was dependent on IL-23 and IL-17. A CCR6+ Th17 subset of memory T cells specific to *Malassezia* was more frequently detected in AD skin than in healthy skin. Thus, the *Malassezia*-induced Th17 response is important not only in antifungal immunity but also in worsening skin inflammatory conditions. TNF-like weak inducer of apoptosis (TWEAK) and its receptor fibroblast growth factor (FGF) inducible 14 are highly expressed in AD skin lesions. BALB/c mice deficient in this molecule showed attenuated skin inflammation in an AD model, accompanied by less infiltration of inflammatory cells and lower local levels of proinflammatory cytokines, including TWEAK, TNF-α, and IL-17 [44]. Thus, IL-17 may be an important mediator of TWEAK-induced AD-like inflammation. The numbers of ILC3, expressing IL-17, in the skin of AD-induced mice were increased, and that neutralizing IL-17A delayed development of AD in the mouse model [45]. ILC3 induced IL-33 production by keratinocytes and fibroblasts. IL-26, another Th17 cytokine, promoted production of various cytokines such as IL-8, IL-1β, CCL20, IL-33, and β-defensin 2 by keratinocytes through phosphorylation of signal transducer and activator of transcription 1 and signal transducer and activator of transcription 3 [37]. JAK inhibitors, which are promising drugs for AD, blocked IL-26-induced cytokine production in keratinocytes. Injection of IL-26 exacerbated an oxazolone-induced AD mouse model and upregulated Th2 and Th17 cytokine expression in vivo. Thus, basic research findings also support the idea that IL-17 and its related cytokines are important in AD pathogenesis.

4. Expression of Th17 Cytokines in Other Skin Diseases

Some reports have suggested importance of IL-17 in various skin diseases other than psoriasis and AD. For example, IL-17 expression is reported to be increased in sera or lesional skin of systemic lupus erythematosus [46]. IL-17A expression was significantly increased in the involved skin and sera of systemic sclerosis patients, suggesting possible roles in the development of the disease [47,48]. Our group reported that lesional skin of mycosis fungoides (MF) and Sezary syndrome (SS), representative diseases of CTCL, contained a high amount of IL-17 and IL-22, the latter of which was dominant [49]. Serum IL-22 levels were significantly positively associated with disease activity in MF/SS. There are many clinical similarities between MF/SS and AD. Both diseases are characterized by persistent erythematous lesions with severe itch, sometimes developing to erythroderma. Bacterial, fungal, and viral infections such as impetigo contagiosum, phlegmone, tinea corporis, and herpes simplex are frequently accompanied. The number of eosinophils in peripheral blood is often increased and serum TARC level is elevated. Dominancy of IL-22 over IL-17 is seen in both diseases, which may explain clinical pictures of these diseases. Taken together, Th17 cytokine expression is widely seen in various skin diseases.

5. Clinical Trial for AD Targeting Th17 Cytokines

5.1. Clinical Effect of Ustekinumab on AD

Ustekinumab is a recombinant human IgG1 monoclonal antibody against p40, which is a common subunit of IL-12 and IL-23 [25]. This drug is used for psoriasis vulgaris and psoriatic arthritis. A previous report about four male patients with severe AD between 23 and 29 years old, whose skin eruption had been refractory to oral corticosteroids, phototherapy, and to at least two systemic drugs, showed improvement of SCORAD and itch score after treatment with 45 mg of ustekinumab injection at 0, 4 weeks, and every 12 weeks afterwards [50]. A 16-year-old woman with over a 13-year history of severe AD was also reported to show clearance of severe itch after one injection of ustekinumab 45 mg, although it had been resistant to phototherapy and systemic agents such as cyclosporine and azathioprine [51]. Complete remission was achieved with ustekinumab at the fourth week and every 12 weeks afterwards. There are, however, other reports denying efficacy of ustekinumab [52–54]. A 21-year-old man with a 7-year history of severe psoriasis refractory to conventional systemic treatments and childhood AD history was treated with ustekinumab [52]. The patient was without major respiratory symptoms and AD lesions within a period of five years before the date of starting the treatment. After an eight-month interval, ustekinumab was restarted and severe AD appeared on the neck and lower limbs. Peripheral blood eosinophilia and abnormal increase in serum IgE were also noted. The eczema lasted during 12 months of follow up after the final dose of ustekinumab, supporting the diagnosis of AD. Another group reported two psoriatic patients with high serum IgE levels, in whom ustekinumab completely improved psoriasis but paradoxically provoked or exacerbated AD-like symptoms [54]. Recently, the possibility of ustekinumab for AD was tested in clinical trials all over the world [55,56]. In the randomized, placebo-controlled, phase II study in Japan, 79 patients aged between 20 and 65 years with severe or very severe AD entered a 12-week, double-blind treatment period during which they received (1:1:1) ustekinumab 45 mg, 90 mg, or placebo subcutaneous injections at weeks 0 and 4, with follow-up until week 24 [55]. There was no significant improvement with ustekinumab treatment in least-squares mean change from baseline Eczema Area and Severity Index score at week 12. In another phase II, double-blind, placebo-controlled study, 33 patients with moderate-to-severe AD were randomly assigned to either ustekinumab ($n = 16$) or placebo ($n = 17$), with subsequent crossover at 16 weeks and last dose at 32 weeks [56]. Background therapy with mild topical steroids was allowed. Study endpoints included clinical and biopsy-based measures of tissue structure and inflammation, using protein and gene expression studies. The ustekinumab group achieved higher clinical responses at 12, 16 (the primary endpoint), and 20 weeks compared to placebo, but the difference between groups was not significant. The AD molecular profile/transcriptome showed early robust gene modulation, with sustained further improvements until 32 weeks in the initial ustekinumab group. It is still possible that a certain subset of patients with AD may particularly benefit from ustekinumab. However, it may be safely said that ustekinumab is much more effective in psoriasis than in AD.

5.2. Other Biologics and AD

There have been anecdotal case reports showing exacerbation of AD-like dermatitis after treatment with anti-IL17 antibody for psoriasis [57–59]. A 31-year-old man with severe psoriasis treated with ixekizumab presented with a one-month history of pruritic lesions [57]. The patient had no personal or family history of allergy, AD, or eczema. Treatment with ixekizumab, started 14 months before the episode, achieved an almost complete response of his skin disease. The patient developed the palms exudative erythematous plaques on the hands, the trunk, and the medial aspects of the limbs. Histologically, epidermal spongiosis with vesicle formation with dermal edema and lymphocytic perivascular infiltrate with some eosinophils were seen. Ixekizumab may suppress the expression of keratinocyte-derived AMPs, increasing the risk of bacterial and fungal infection, which can lead to the eczematous phenotype. Another group reported a 70-year-old woman with intractable psoriasis vulgaris treated with 300 mg of secukinumab [58]. Six months after the first dose of secukinumab was administered, psoriasis lesions were cleared. Blepharitis, cheilitis, and dermatitis around the nose, however, developed four days after every secukinumab injection. A common skin-resident fungus *Malassezia* may account for these skin lesions, which might be more adequately named seborrheic dermatitis-like lesions instead of AD-like eczema. Fezakinumab, an anti-IL-22 antibody, has been recently tried for treatment of AD. A randomized, double-blind, placebo-controlled trial with intravenous fezakinumab monotherapy every 2 weeks for 10 weeks, with follow-up assessments until 20 weeks, was performed for adult patients with moderate-to-severe AD [60]. At 12 weeks, the mean declines in SCORAD for the entire study population were not different between the fezakinumab arm and the placebo arm. In the severe AD patient subset, SCORAD decline was significantly stronger in the drug-treated patients than placebo-treated patients at 12 weeks. Common adverse events were upper respiratory tract infections. Although this drug significantly downregulated gene expression of multiple immune pathways including Th1, Th2, and Th17, it was clinically effective only in patients with severe AD expressing a high level of IL-22 at the baseline [61]. Taken together, biologics targeting Th17-related cytokines are not promising for the treatment of AD, except for anti-IL-22 antibody.

6. Th2 Cytokines Are Key Players in AD

If antibodies against Th17 cytokines are not useful for AD, what is the best therapeutic target? Th2-type immune responses induced by allergens such as mites and pollen are associated with worsening of AD skin conditions. Th2 immune responses including increased IL-4/IL-13 expression induce the production of IgE and TARC [62]. Serum TARC levels are useful as a marker of the disease activity of AD, which are more sensitive than serum IgE levels, lactate dehydrogenaselevels, and peripheral blood eosinophil counts [63]. Recently, thymic stromal lymphopoietin (TSLP) and periostin have been discovered to be key cytokines in Th2-dominant microenvironment [64,65]. TSLP-activated dendritic cells primed naïve T cells to produce IL-4, IL-5, IL-13, and TNF-α, while down-regulating IL-10 and IFN-γ [64]. TSLP was highly expressed by epithelial cells, especially keratinocytes from AD patients. Th2 cytokines IL-4 and IL-13 stimulated fibroblasts to produce periostin, which interacted with a functional periostin receptor on keratinocytes [65]. It induces production of proinflammatory cytokines, which consequently accelerated Th2-type immune responses. It was recently reported that the TSLP receptor was expressed by some T cell subsets from patients with Th2-dominant diseases and that TSLP directly enhanced IL-4/IL-13 production by T cells [66,67]. Taken together, these Th2-related cytokines, IL-4/IL-13, TSLP, and periostin are driving factors of a vicious circle in AD and can be good candidates for therapeutic targets. Indeed, dupilumab, a monoclonal antibody against the IL-4 receptor, is very effective for severe AD [68].

7. The Importance of Th17 Cytokines in the Skin

Skin is a border between the outer world and the body. It is important to block invasion of foreign materials such as poison and parasites. Trauma and loss of skin barrier function in diseased skin, such as in AD and psoriasis, causes a high risk of the invasion. In both conditions, mechanical stimulation can be the cause of onset. It is called the Kobner phenomenon in psoriasis. High proliferation of epidermal cells and rapid keratinization are seen in both skin conditions. Expression of K6 and K16 is increased and that of K1 and K10 is decreased [69,70]. Increased expression of cathepsin D, which modulates expression of involucrin, loricrin, and filaggrin, has been reported [71].

Cytokine expression and cellular infiltration in psoriasis lesional skin is also very similar to what is seen in cases of trauma. IL-17A, which is expressed both in wounded skin and psoriasis skin, plays important roles in wound healing, tissue regeneration, and carcinogenesis [72]. The cytokine mediates activation of EGFR, which is critical for the expansion and migration of Lrig1+ stem cells, promoting wound healing [73]. FGF2 or IL-17 deficiency resulted in impaired epithelial proliferation, increased pro-inflammatory microbiota outgrowth, and consequently worse pathology in a mouse colitis model [74]. The dysregulated microbiota in the model induced transforming growth factor-β1 expression, which in turn induced FGF2 expression mainly in regulatory T cells. Thus, microbiota-driven FGF2 and IL-17 cooperate to repair the damaged intestinal epithelium. Injury of the mucosa causes fast expansion of Th17 cells and their induction [75]. Th17 cells produce various cytokines, such as TNF-α, IL-17, and IL-22, which can promote cell survival and proliferation, and thus tissue regeneration, in several organs including the skin [72]. IL-17 promoted macrophage infiltration into wounded skin and scar formation through an indirect mechanism [76]. Depletion of macrophages with clodronate liposomes abrogated the effect of IL-17. Levels of monocyte chemotactic protein (MCP) 1, MCP2, and MCP3 were increased by IL-17 stimulation. IL-17 induced the infiltration of a specific subtype of macrophages to aggravate fibrosis through an MCP-dependent mechanism. On the other hand, Th17 cells are potentially pathogenic if not tightly controlled. Failure of these control mechanisms can result in chronic inflammatory conditions such as psoriasis.

Infiltration of neutrophils and macrophages is commonly seen, and AMP expression is increased both in wounded skin and in psoriasis skin. Vascular formation is prominent in the dermis. Taken together, it may be safely said that psoriasis is a hyperreaction to traumatic stimuli with the background of genetics, circumstances, and metabolic status (Figure 1).

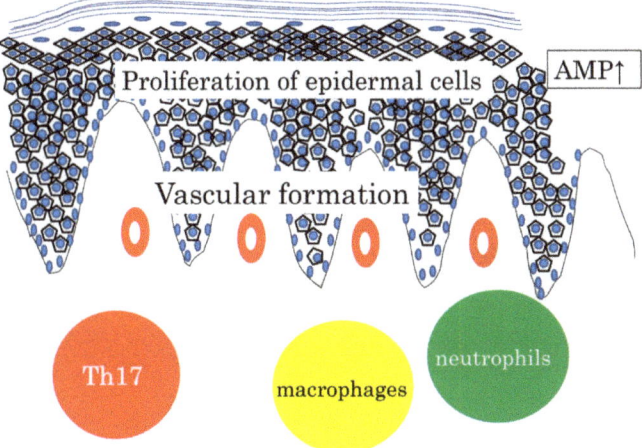

Figure 1. Proliferation of epidermal cells, AMP expression, vascular formation, and infiltration of Th17, neutrophils, and macrophages, commonly seen in wounded skin and in psoriasis skin. We sometimes experience fungal infection in patients treated with anit-IL7A or anti-IL17 receptor A antibody. Considering that Th17 cytokines are expressed in various skin diseases with barrier dysfunction and that antibodies against IL-12/IL-23p40 or IL-17A are not effective for AD, IL-17 and its related cytokine expression can be regarded as a common defense mechanism in the skin. Relatively low AMP expression leads to a higher risk of infection seen in AD and CTCL [77,78]. Targeting the Th17 cytokine has been successful for psoriasis, but may not be always the case in other skin diseases.

8. Ideal Biologics for Psoriasis, AD, and CTCL

Clinical effects of biologics are remarkable, and many diseases including skin diseases are currently treated with them. The cost of developing these agents, however, is huge and it is important to predict which molecule is promising or not. First of all, the molecule should be highly expressed in lesional skin compared to normal skin. Second, the expression of the target should be highest in the disease among various skin diseases. It is important not to block bystander cytokines. IL-22 is highly expressed in psoriasis, but its expression is lower in AD. IL-17 expression in AD is not as high as that in psoriasis. Anti-IL-22 antibody is not effective in psoriasis, and anti-IL12/23p40 or anti-IL-17A antibodies are not promising as treatment for AD. Only the anti-IL-22 antibody may be beneficial for a certain group of AD patients (Table 1). Blocking cytokines uniquely expressed in the disease is important to stop a vicious circle. Third, it would be safer to block interactions between cytokines and their receptors than targeting surface molecules. Exclusion of a certain cell type by antibody-dependent cellular cytotoxicity induced by biologics may cause unexpected severe effects. This kind of strategy targeting surface molecules should be adopted for the treatment of malignancy [79,80].

Table 1. Antibodies against Th17 and Th2-related cytokines for atopic dermatitis (AD).

Cytokines	Clinical Response	References
IL-17A	Worsening of dermatitis	[57–59]
IL-12/23p40	No effect in clinical trial	[55,56]
IL-22	Effective for some patients	[60,61]
IL-4/13	Very effective	[68]

9. Conclusions

It is true that Th17 cells infiltrate into lesional skin of AD, and Th17-related cytokines are expressed there. These cytokines have some roles in the inflammatory process of the disease. It is, however, also true that IL-17 in AD is not as important as it is in psoriasis. Expression of IL-17 and other Th17-related cytokines is widely seen in many skin diseases. My current assumption is that IL-17 expression in the skin is a defense mechanism against foreign materials invading the body.

Funding: This research received no external funding.

Conflicts of Interest: The author declares no conflict of interest.

Abbreviations

AD	atopic dermatitis
CTCL	cutaneous T-cell lymphoma
TNF	tumor necrosis factor
Th	T helper
IL	interleukin
IFN	interferon
AMPs	antimicrobial peptides
TARC	thymus and activation-regulated chemokine
SCORAD	SCORing AD
TWEAK	TNF-like weak inducer of apoptosis
FGF	fibroblast growth factor
MF	mycosis fungoides
SS	Sezary syndrome
TSLP	thymic stromal lymphopoietin
MCP	monocyte chemotactic protein

References

1. Saeki, H.; Nakahara, T.; Tanaka, A.; Kabashima, K.; Sugaya, M.; Murota, H.; Ebihara, T.; Kataoka, Y.; Aihara, M.; Etoh, T.; et al. Clinical practice guidelines for the management of atopic dermatitis. *J. Dermatol.* **2016**, *43*, 1117–1145. [CrossRef] [PubMed]
2. Saeki, H.; Oiso, N.; Honma, M.; Iizuka, H.; Kawada, A.; Tamaki, K. Prevalence of atopic dermatitis in Japanese adults and community validation of the U.K. diagnostic criteria. *J. Dermatol. Sci.* **2009**, *55*, 140–141. [CrossRef] [PubMed]
3. Williams, H.C.; Strachan, D.P. The natural history of childhood eczema: Observations from the British 1958 birth cohort study. *Br. J. Dermatol.* **1998**, *139*, 834–839. [CrossRef] [PubMed]
4. Fukiwake, N.; Furusyo, N.; Kubo, N.; Takeoka, H.; Toyoda, K.; Morita, K.; Shibata, S.; Nakahara, T.; Kido, M.; Hayashida, S.; et al. Incidence of atopic dermatitis in nursery school children—A follow-up study from 2001 to 2004, Kyushu University Ishigaki Atopic Dermatitis Study (KIDS). *Eur. J. Dermatol.* **2006**, *16*, 416–419. [PubMed]
5. Zackheim, H.S.; Koo, J.; LeBoit, P.E.; McCalmont, T.H.; Bowman, P.H.; Kashani-Sabet, M.; Jones, C.; Zehnder, J. Psoriasiform mycosis fungoides with fatal outcome after treatment with cyclosporine. *J. Am. Acad. Dermatol.* **2002**, *47*, 155–157. [CrossRef] [PubMed]
6. Miyagaki, T.; Sugaya, M. Erythrodermic cutaneous T-cell lymphoma: How to differentiate this rare disease from atopic dermatitis. *J. Dermatol. Sci.* **2011**, *64*, 1–6. [CrossRef]
7. Suga, H.; Sugaya, M.; Toyama, T.; Sumida, H.; Fujita, H.; Kogure, A.; Igarashi, A.; Sato, S. A case of mycosis fungoides with large cell transformation associated with infliximab treatment. *Acta. Derm. Venereol.* **2014**, *94*, 233–234. [CrossRef]
8. Xu, X.; van Galen, L.S.; Koh, M.J.A.; Bajpai, R.; Thng, S.; Yew, Y.W.; Ho, V.P.Y.; Alagappan, U.; Järbrink, K.S.A.; Car, J. Factors influencing quality of life in children with atopic dermatitis and their caregivers: A cross-sectional study. *Sci. Rep.* **2019**, *9*, 15990. [CrossRef]

9. Ražnatović Đurović, M.; Janković, J.; Tomić Spirić, V.; Relić, M.; Sojević Timotijević, Z.; Ćirković, A.; Đurić, S.; Janković, S. Does age influence the quality of life in children with atopic dermatitis? *PLoS ONE* **2019**, *14*, e0224618. [CrossRef]
10. Kabashima, K. New concept of the pathogenesis of atopic dermatitis: Interplay among the barrier, allergy, and pruritus as a trinity. *J. Dermatol. Sci.* **2013**, *70*, 3–11. [CrossRef]
11. Salimi, M.; Barlow, J.L.; Saunders, S.P.; Xue, L.; Gutowska-Owsiak, D.; Wang, X.; Huang, L.C.; Johnson, D.; Scanlon, S.T.; McKenzie, A.N.; et al. A role for IL-25 and IL-33-driven type-2 innate lymphoid cells in atopic dermatitis. *J. Exp. Med.* **2013**, *210*, 2939–2950. [CrossRef] [PubMed]
12. Imai, Y.; Yasuda, K.; Sakaguchi, Y.; Haneda, T.; Mizutani, H.; Yoshimoto, T.; Nakanishi, K.; Yamanishi, K. Skin-specific expression of IL-33 activates group 2 innate lymphoid cells and elicits atopic dermatitis-like inflammation in mice. *Proc. Natl. Acad. Sci. USA* **2013**, *110*, 13921–13926. [CrossRef] [PubMed]
13. Van de Veen, W.; Akdis, M. The use of biologics for immune modulation in allergic disease. *J. Clin. Invest.* **2019**, *130*, 1452–1462. [CrossRef] [PubMed]
14. Grewe, M.; Gyufko, K.; Schöpf, E.; Krutmann, J. Lesional expression of interferon-gamma in atopic eczema. *Lancet* **1994**, *343*, 25–26. [CrossRef]
15. Czarnowicki, T.; He, H.; Canter, T.; Han, J.; Lefferdink, R.; Erickson, T.; Rangel, S.; Kameyama, N.; Kim, H.J.; Pavel, A.B.; et al. Evolution of pathologic T-cell subsets in atopic dermatitis from infancy to adulthood. *J. Allergy Clin. Immunol.* **2020**, *145*, 215–228. [CrossRef] [PubMed]
16. Koga, C.; Kabashima, K.; Shiraishi, N.; Kobayashi, M.; Tokura, Y. Possible pathogenic role of Th17 cells for atopic dermatitis. *J. Invest. Dermatol.* **2008**, *128*, 2625–2630. [CrossRef] [PubMed]
17. Eyerich, K.; Pennino, D.; Scarponi, C.; Foerster, S.; Nasorri, F.; Behrendt, H.; Ring, J.; Traidl-Hoffmann, C.; Albanesi, C.; Cavani, A. IL-17 in atopic eczema: Linking allergen-specific adaptive and microbial-triggered innate immune response. *J. Allergy. Clin. Immunol.* **2009**, *123*, 59–66. [CrossRef]
18. Nograles, K.E.; Zaba, L.C.; Shemer, A.; Fuentes-Duculan, J.; Cardinale, I.; Kikuchi, T.; Ramon, M.; Bergman, R.; Krueger, J.G.; Guttman-Yassky, E. IL-22-producing "T22" T cells account for upregulated IL-22 in atopic dermatitis despite reduced IL-17-producing TH17 T cells. *J. Allergy. Clin. Immunol.* **2009**, *123*, 1244–1252. [CrossRef]
19. Noda, S.; Suárez-Fariñas, M.; Ungar, B.; Kim, S.J.; de Guzman Strong, C.; Xu, H.; Peng, X.; Estrada, Y.D.; Nakajima, S.; Honda, T.; et al. The Asian atopic dermatitis phenotype combines features of atopic dermatitis and psoriasis with increased TH17 polarization. *J. Allergy. Clin. Immunol.* **2015**, *136*, 1254–1264. [CrossRef]
20. Esaki, H.; Brunner, P.M.; Renert-Yuval, Y.; Czarnowicki, T.; Huynh, T.; Tran, G.; Lyon, S.; Rodriguez, G.; Immaneni, S.; Johnson, D.B.; et al. Early-onset pediatric atopic dermatitis is Th2 but also Th17 polarized in skin. *J. Allergy. Clin. Immunol.* **2016**, *138*, 1639–1651. [CrossRef] [PubMed]
21. Korn, T.; Bettelli, E.; Oukka, M.; Kuchroo, V.K. IL-17 and Th17 cells. *Annu. Rev. Immunol.* **2009**, *27*, 485–517. [CrossRef] [PubMed]
22. Chaudhari, U.; Romano, P.; Mulcahy, L.D.; Dooley, L.T.; Baker, D.G.; Gottlieb, A.B. Efficacy and safety of infliximab monotherapy for plaque-type psoriasis: A randomised trial. *Lancet* **2001**, *357*, 1842–1847. [CrossRef]
23. Leonardi, C.L.; Kimball, A.B.; Papp, K.A.; Yeilding, N.; Guzzo, C.; Wang, Y.; Li, S.; Dooley, L.T.; Gordon, K.B.; PHOENIX 1 study investigators. Efficacy and safety of ustekinumab, a human interleukin-12/23 monoclonal antibody, in patients with psoriasis: 76-week results from a randomised, double-blind, placebo-controlled trial (PHOENIX 1). *Lancet* **2008**, *371*, 1665–1674. [CrossRef]
24. Leonardi, C.; Matheson, R.; Zachariae, C.; Cameron, G.; Li, L.; Edson-Heredia, E.; Braun, D.; Banerjee, S. Anti-interleukin-17 monoclonal antibody ixekizumab in chronic plaque psoriasis. *N. Engl. J. Med.* **2012**, *366*, 1190–1199. [CrossRef] [PubMed]
25. Gordon, K.B.; Duffin, K.C.; Bissonnette, R.; Prinz, J.C.; Wasfi, Y.; Li, S.; Shen, Y.K.; Szapary, P.; Randazzo, B.; Reich, K. A phase 2 trial of guselkumab versus adalimumab for plaque psoriasis. *N. Engl. J. Med.* **2015**, *373*, 136–144. [CrossRef] [PubMed]
26. Jovanovic, D.V.; Di Battista, J.A.; Martel-Pelletier, J.; Jolicoeur, F.C.; He, Y.; Zhang, M.; Mineau, F.; Pelletier, J.P. IL-17 stimulates the production and expression of proinflammatory cytokines, IL-beta and TNF-alpha, by human macrophages. *J. Immunol.* **1998**, *160*, 3513–3521. [PubMed]

27. Shibata, M.; Shintaku, Y.; Matsuzaki, K.; Uematsu, S. The effect of IL-17 on the production of proinflammatory cytokines and matrix metalloproteinase-1 by human periodontal ligament fibroblasts. *Orthod. Craniofac. Res.* **2014**, *17*, 60–68. [CrossRef]
28. Roussel, L.; Houle, F.; Chan, C.; Yao, Y.; Bérubé, J.; Olivenstein, R.; Martin, J.G.; Huot, J.; Hamid, Q.; Ferri, L.; et al. IL-17 promotes p38 MAPK-dependent endothelial activation enhancing neutrophil recruitment to sites of inflammation. *J. Immunol.* **2010**, *184*, 4531–4537. [CrossRef]
29. Jones, C.E.; Chan, K. Interleukin-17stimulates the expression of interleukin-8, growth-related oncogene-alpha, and granulocyte-colony-stimulating factor by human airway epithelial cells. *Am. J. Respir. Cell. Mol. Biol.* **2002**, *26*, 748–753. [CrossRef]
30. Ganz, T. Defensins: Antimicrobial peptides of innate immunity. *Nat. Rev. Immunol.* **2003**, *3*, 710–720. [CrossRef]
31. Sonnenberg, G.F.; Fouser, L.A.; Artis, D. Border patrol: Regulation of immunity, inflammation and tissue homeostasis at barrier surfaces by IL-22. *Nat. Immunol.* **2011**, *12*, 383–390. [CrossRef] [PubMed]
32. Gallo, R.L.; Nakatsuji, T. Microbial symbiosis with the innate immune defense system of the skin. *J. Invest. Dermatol.* **2011**, *131*, 1974–1980. [CrossRef] [PubMed]
33. Boniface, K.; Bernard, F.X.; Garcia, M.; Gurney, A.L.; Lecron, J.C.; Morel, F. IL-22 inhibits epidermal differentiation and induces proinflammatory gene expression and migration of human keratinocytes. *J. Immunol.* **2005**, *174*, 3695–3702. [CrossRef] [PubMed]
34. Dang, A.T.; Teles, R.M.; Weiss, D.I.; Parvatiyar, K.; Sarno, E.N.; Ochoa, M.T.; Cheng, G.; Gilliet, M.; Bloom, B.R.; Modlin, R.L. IL-26 contributes to host defense against intracellular bacteria. *J. Clin. Investg.* **2019**, *129*, 1926–1939. [CrossRef] [PubMed]
35. Hayashida, S.; Uchi, H.; Moroi, Y.; Furue, M. Decrease in circulating Th17 cells correlates with increased levels of CCL17, IgE and eosinophils in atopic dermatitis. *J. Dermatol. Sci.* **2011**, *61*, 180–186. [CrossRef] [PubMed]
36. Czarnowicki, T.; Gonzalez, J.; Shemer, A.; Malajian, D.; Xu, H.; Zheng, X.; Khattri, S.; Gilleaudeau, P.; Sullivan-Whalen, M.; Suárez-Fariñas, M.; et al. Severe atopic dermatitis is characterized by selective expansion of circulating TH2/TC2 and TH22/TC22, but not TH17/TC17, cells within the skin-homing T-cell population. *J. Allergy. Clin. Immunol.* **2015**, *136*, 104–115. [CrossRef]
37. Romanet-Manent, S.; Charpin, D.; Magnan, A.; Lanteaume, A.; Vervloet, D.; EGEA Cooperative Group. Allergic vs nonallergic asthma: What makes the difference? *Allergy* **2002**, *57*, 607–613. [CrossRef]
38. Tokura, Y. Extrinsic and intrinsic types of atopic dermatitis. *J. Dermatol. Sci.* **2010**, *58*, 1–7. [CrossRef]
39. Suárez-Fariñas, M.; Dhingra, N.; Gittler, J.; Shemer, A.; Cardinale, I.; de Guzman Strong, C.; Krueger, J.G.; Guttman-Yassky, E. Intrinsic atopic dermatitis shows similar TH2 and higher TH17 immune activation compared with extrinsic atopic dermatitis. *J. Allergy. Clin. Immunol.* **2013**, *132*, 361–370. [CrossRef]
40. Kamijo, H.; Miyagaki, T.; Hayashi, Y.; Akatsuka, T.; Watanabe-Otobe, S.; Oka, T.; Shishido-Takahashi, N.; Suga, H.; Sugaya, M.; Sato, S. Increased IL-26 expression promotes T helper type 17- and T helper type 2-associated cytokine production by keratinocytes in atopic dermatitis. *J. Invest. Dermatol.* **2019**, in press. [CrossRef]
41. Nakajima, S.; Kitoh, A.; Egawa, G.; Natsuaki, Y.; Nakamizo, S.; Moniaga, C.S.; Otsuka, A.; Honda, T.; Hanakawa, S.; Amano, W.; et al. IL-17A as an inducer for Th2 immune responses in murine atopic dermatitis models. *J. Invest. Dermatol.* **2014**, *134*, 2122–2130. [CrossRef] [PubMed]
42. Milovanovic, M.; Drozdenko, G.; Weise, C.; Babina, M.; Worm, M. Interleukin-17A promotes IgE production in human B cells. *J. Invest. Dermatol.* **2010**, *130*, 2621–2628. [CrossRef] [PubMed]
43. Sparber, F.; De Gregorio, C.; Steckholzer, S.; Ferreira, F.M.; Dolowschiak, T.; Ruchti, F.; Kirchner, F.R.; Mertens, S.; Prinz, I.; Joller, N.; et al. The skin commensal yeast Malassezia triggers a type 17 response that coordinates anti-fungal immunity and exacerbates skin inflammation. *Cell. Host. Microbe.* **2019**, *25*, 389–403. [CrossRef] [PubMed]
44. Liu, Q.; Wang, H.; Wang, X.; Lu, M.; Tan, X.; Peng, L.; Tan, F.; Xiao, T.; Xiao, S.; Xia, Y. Experimental atopic dermatitis is dependent on the TWEAK/Fn14 signaling pathway. *Clin. Exp. Immunol.* **2020**, *199*, 56–67. [CrossRef]
45. Kim, M.H.; Jin, S.P.; Jang, S.; Choi, J.Y.; Chung, D.H.; Lee, D.H.; Kim, K.H.; Kim, H.Y. IL-17A-producing innate lymphoid cells promote skin inflammation by inducing IL-33-driven type 2 immune responses. *J. Investg. Dermatol.* **2019**, in press. [CrossRef]

46. Shen, H.H.; Fan, Y.; Wang, Y.N.; Zhao, C.N.; Zhang, Z.K.; Pan, H.F.; Wu, G.C. Elevated Circulating Interleukin-17 levels in patients with systemic lupus erythematosus: A meta-analysis. *Immunol. Invest.* **2019**, in press. [CrossRef]
47. Nakashima, T.; Jinnin, M.; Yamane, K.; Honda, N.; Kajihara, I.; Makino, T.; Masuguchi, S.; Fukushima, S.; Okamoto, Y.; Hasegawa, M.; et al. Impaired IL-17 signaling pathway contributes to the increased collagen expression in scleroderma fibroblasts. *J. Immunol.* **2012**, *188*, 3573–3583. [CrossRef]
48. Ahmed, S.; Misra, D.P.; Agarwal, V. Interleukin-17 pathways in systemic sclerosis-associated fibrosis. *Rheumatol. Int.* **2019**, *39*, 1135–1143. [CrossRef]
49. Miyagaki, T.; Sugaya, M.; Suga, H.; Kamata, M.; Ohmatsu, H.; Fujita, H.; Asano, Y.; Tada, Y.; Kadono, T.; Sato, S. IL-22, but not IL-17, dominant environment in cutaneous T-cell lymphoma. *Clin. Cancer Res.* **2011**, *17*, 7529–7538. [CrossRef]
50. Fernández-Antón Martínez, M.C.; Alfageme Roldán, F.; Ciudad Blanco, C.; Suárez Fernández, R. Ustekinumab in the treatment of severe atopic dermatitis: A preliminary report of our experience with 4 patients. *Actas Dermosifiliogr.* **2014**, *105*, 312–313. [CrossRef]
51. Agusti-Mejias, A.; Messeguer, F.; García, R.; Febrer, I. Severe refractory atopic dermatitis in an adolescent patient successfully treated with ustekinumab. *Ann. Dermatol.* **2013**, *25*, 368–370. [CrossRef] [PubMed]
52. Lis-Święty, A.; Skrzypek-Salamon, A.; Arasiewicz, H.; Brzezińska-Wcisło, L. Atopic dermatitis exacerbated with ustekinumab in a psoriatic patient with childhood history of atopy. *Allergol. Int.* **2015**, *64*, 382–383. [CrossRef] [PubMed]
53. Samorano, L.P.; Hanifin, J.M.; Simpson, E.L.; Leshem, Y.A. Inadequate response to ustekinumab in atopic dermatitis - a report of two patients. *J. Eur. Acad. Dermatol. Venereol.* **2016**, *30*, 522–523. [CrossRef] [PubMed]
54. Ishiuji, Y.; Umezawa, Y.; Asahina, A.; Fukuta, H.; Aizawa, N.; Yanaba, K.; Nakagawa, H. Exacerbation of atopic dermatitis symptoms by ustekinumab in psoriatic patients with elevated serum immunoglobulin E levels: Report of two cases. *J. Dermatol.* **2018**, *45*, 732–734. [CrossRef] [PubMed]
55. Saeki, H.; Kabashima, K.; Tokura, Y.; Murata, Y.; Shiraishi, A.; Tamamura, R.; Randazzo, B.; Imanaka, K. Efficacy and safety of ustekinumab in Japanese patients with severe atopic dermatitis: A randomized, double-blind, placebo-controlled, phase II study. *Br. J. Dermatol.* **2017**, *177*, 419–427. [CrossRef]
56. Khattri, S.; Brunner, P.M.; Garcet, S.; Finney, R.; Cohen, S.R.; Oliva, M.; Dutt, R.; Fuentes-Duculan, J.; Zheng, X.; Li, X.; et al. Efficacy and safety of ustekinumab treatment in adults with moderate-to-severe atopic dermatitis. *Exp. Dermatol.* **2017**, *26*, 28–35. [CrossRef]
57. Munera-Campos, M.; Ballesca, F.; Richarz, N.; Ferrandiz, C.; Carrascosa, J.M. Paradoxical eczematous reaction to ixekizumab. *J. Eur. Acad. Dermatol. Venereol.* **2019**, *33*, e40–e42.
58. Burlando, M.; Cozzani, E.; Russo, R.; Parodi, A. Atopic-like dermatitis after secukinumab injection: A case report. *Dermatol. Ther.* **2019**, *32*, e12751. [CrossRef]
59. Napolitano, M.; Gallo, L.; Patruno, C.; Fabbrocini, G.; Megna, M. Eczematous reaction to ixekizumab successfully treated with dupilumab. *Dermatol. Ther.* **2020**, in press. [CrossRef]
60. Guttman-Yassky, E.; Brunner, P.M.; Neumann, A.U.; Khattri, S.; Pavel, A.B.; Malik, K.; Singer, G.K.; Baum, D.; Gilleaudeau, P.; Sullivan-Whalen, M.; et al. Efficacy and safety of fezakinumab (an IL-22 monoclonal antibody) in adults with moderate-to-severe atopic dermatitis inadequately controlled by conventional treatments: A randomized, double-blind, phase 2a trial. *J. Am. Acad. Dermatol.* **2018**, *78*, 872–881. [CrossRef]
61. Brunner, P.M.; Pavel, A.B.; Khattri, S.; Leonard, A.; Malik, K.; Rose, S.; Jim On, S.; Vekaria, A.S.; Traidl-Hoffmann, C.; Singer, G.K.; et al. Baseline IL-22 expression in patients with atopic dermatitis stratifies tissue responses to fezakinumab. *J. Allergy. Clin. Immunol.* **2019**, *143*, 142–154. [CrossRef] [PubMed]
62. Furue, M.; Ulzii, D.; Vu, Y.H.; Tsuji, G.; Kido-Nakahara, M.; Nakahara, T. Pathogenesis of atopic dermatitis: CurrentpParadigm. *Iran. J. Immunol.* **2019**, *16*, 97–107. [PubMed]
63. Kakinuma, T.; Nakamura, K.; Wakugawa, M.; Mitsui, H.; Tada, Y.; Saeki, H.; Torii, H.; Asahina, A.; Onai, N.; Matsushima, K.; et al. Thymus and activation-regulated chemokine in atopic dermatitis: Serum thymus and activation-regulated chemokine level is closely related with disease activity. *J. Allergy. Clin. Immunol.* **2001**, *107*, 535–541. [CrossRef] [PubMed]
64. Soumelis, V.; Reche, P.A.; Kanzler, H.; Yuan, W.; Edward, G.; Homey, B.; Gilliet, M.; Ho, S.; Antonenko, S.; Lauerma, A.; et al. Human epithelial cells trigger dendritic cell mediated allergic inflammation by producing TSLP. *Nat. Immunol.* **2002**, *3*, 673–680. [CrossRef]

65. Masuoka, M.; Shiraishi, H.; Ohta, S.; Suzuki, S.; Arima, K.; Aoki, S.; Toda, S.; Inagaki, N.; Kurihara, Y.; Hayashida, S.; et al. Periostin promotes chronic allergic inflammation in response to Th2 cytokines. *J. Clin. Invest.* **2012**, *122*, 2590–2600. [CrossRef]
66. Tatsuno, K.; Fujiyama, T.; Yamaguchi, H.; Waki, M.; Tokura, Y. TSLP directly interacts with skin-homing Th2 Cells highly expressing its receptor to enhance IL-4 production in atopic dermatitis. *J. Investg. Dermatol.* **2015**, *135*, 3017–3024. [CrossRef]
67. Takahashi, N.; Sugaya, M.; Suga, H.; Oka, T.; Kawaguchi, M.; Miyagaki, T.; Fujita, H.; Sato, S. Thymic stromal chemokine TSLP acts through Th2 cytokine production to induce cutaneous T-cell lymphoma. *Cancer Res.* **2016**, *76*, 6241–6252. [CrossRef]
68. Blauvelt, A.; de Bruin-Weller, M.; Gooderham, M.; Cather, J.C.; Weisman, J.; Pariser, D.; Simpson, E.L.; Papp, K.A.; Hong, H.C.; Rubel, D.; et al. Long-term management of moderate-to-severe atopic dermatitis with dupilumab and concomitant topical corticosteroids (LIBERTY AD CHRONOS): A 1-year, randomised, double-blinded, placebo-controlled, phase 3 trial. *Lancet* **2017**, *389*, 2287–2303. [CrossRef]
69. Thewes, M.; Stadler, R.; Korge, B.; Mischke, D. Normal psoriatic epidermis expression of hyperproliferation-associated keratins. *Arch. Derm. Res.* **1991**, *283*, 465–471. [CrossRef]
70. Zhang, X.; Yin, M.; Zhang, L.J. Keratin 6, 16 and 17-Critical Barrier Alarmin Molecules in Skin Wounds and Psoriasis. *Cells* **2019**, *8*, E807. [CrossRef]
71. Egberts, F.; Heinrich, M.; Jensen, J.M.; Winoto-Morbach, S.; Pfeiffer, S.; Wickel, M.; Schunck, M.; Steude, J.; Saftig, P.; Proksch, E.; et al. Cathepsin D is involved in the regulation of transglutaminase 1 and epidermal differentiation. *J. Cell. Sci.* **2004**, *117*, 2295–2307. [CrossRef] [PubMed]
72. Brockmann, L.; Giannou, A.D.; Gagliani, N.; Huber, S. Regulation of Th17 cells and associated cytokines in wound healing, tissue regeneration, and carcinogenesis. *Int. J. Mol. Sci.* **2017**, *18*, E1033. [CrossRef] [PubMed]
73. Chen, X.; Cai, G.; Liu, C.; Zhao, J.; Gu, C.; Wu, L.; Hamilton, T.A.; Zhang, C.J.; Ko, J.; Zhu, L.; et al. IL-17R-EGFR axis links wound healing to tumorigenesis in Lrig1+ stem cells. *J. Exp. Med.* **2019**, *216*, 195–214.
74. Song, X.; Dai, D.; He, X.; Zhu, S.; Yao, Y.; Gao, H.; Wang, J.; Qu, F.; Qiu, J.; Wang, H.; et al. Growth factor FGF2 cooperates with interleukin-17 to repair intestinal epithelial damage. *Immunity* **2015**, *43*, 488–501. [CrossRef] [PubMed]
75. Khader, S.A.; Gaffen, S.L.; Kolls, J.K. Th17 cells at the crossroads of innate and adaptive immunity against infectious diseases at the mucosa. *Mucosal. Immunol.* **2009**, *2*, 403–411.
76. Zhang, J.; Qiao, Q.; Liu, M.; He, T.; Shi, J.; Bai, X.; Zhang, Y.; Li, Y.; Cai, W.; Han, S.; et al. IL-17 promotes scar formation by inducing macrophage infiltration. *Am. J. Pathol.* **2018**, *188*, 1693–1702. [CrossRef] [PubMed]
77. Suga, H.; Sugaya, M.; Miyagaki, T.; Ohmatsu, H.; Kawaguchi, M.; Takahashi, N.; Fujita, H.; Asano, Y.; Tada, Y.; Kadono, T.; et al. Skin barrier dysfunction and low antimicrobial peptide expression in cutaneous T-cell lymphoma. *Clin. Cancer Res.* **2014**, *20*, 4339–4348. [CrossRef]
78. Miyagaki, T.; Sugaya, M. Recent advances in atopic dermatitis and psoriasis: Genetic background, barrier function, and therapeutic targets. *J. Dermatol. Sci.* **2015**, *78*, 89–94. [CrossRef]
79. Prince, H.M.; Kim, Y.H.; Horwitz, S.M.; Dummer, R.; Scarisbrick, J.; Quaglino, P.; Zinzani, P.L.; Wolter, P.; Sanches, J.A.; Ortiz-Romero, P.L.; et al. ALCANZA study group. Brentuximab vedotin or physician's choice in CD30-positive cutaneous T-cell lymphoma (ALCANZA): An international, open-label, randomised, phase 3, multicentre trial. *Lancet* **2017**, *390*, 555–566. [CrossRef]
80. Kim, Y.H.; Bagot, M.; Pinter-Brown, L.; Rook, A.H.; Porcu, P.; Horwitz, S.M.; Whittaker, S.; Tokura, Y.; Vermeer, M.; Zinzani, P.L.; et al. MAVORIC Investigators. Mogamulizumab versus vorinostat in previously treated cutaneous T-cell lymphoma (MAVORIC): An international, open-label, randomised, controlled phase 3 trial. *Lancet Oncol.* **2018**, *19*, 1192–1204. [CrossRef]

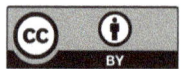

© 2020 by the author. Licensee MDPI, Basel, Switzerland. This article is an open access article distributed under the terms and conditions of the Creative Commons Attribution (CC BY) license (http://creativecommons.org/licenses/by/4.0/).

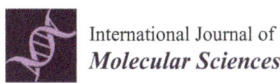

Review

Atopic Dermatitis: Identification and Management of Complicating Factors

Risa Tamagawa-Mineoka * and Norito Katoh

Department of Dermatology, Graduate School of Medical Science, Kyoto Prefectural University of Medicine, 465 Kajii-cho, Kawaramachi-Hirokoji, Kamigyo-ku, Kyoto 602-8566, Japan; nkatoh@koto.kpu-m.ac.jp
* Correspondence: risat@koto.kpu-m.ac.jp; Tel.: +81-75-251-5586

Received: 23 March 2020; Accepted: 10 April 2020; Published: 11 April 2020

Abstract: Atopic dermatitis (AD) is a chronic relapsing inflammatory skin disease, associated with impaired skin barrier function and an atopic background. Various complicating factors, such as irritants, aeroallergens, food, microbial organisms, contact allergens, sweat, and scratching can induce the development of AD symptoms. Irritants, including soap/shampoo and clothes, can cause itching and eczematous lesions. In addition, young children with AD tend to become sensitized to eggs, milk, or peanuts, while older children and adults more often become sensitized to environmental allergens, such as house dust mites (HDM), animal dander, or pollen. Serum-specific IgE levels and skin prick test reactions to food tend to show high negative predictive values and low specificity and positive predictive values for diagnosing food allergy. On the other hand, AD adult patients tend to have severe skin symptoms and exhibit high HDM-specific IgE levels. Microbial organisms, e.g., *Staphylococcus aureus* and *Malassezia furfur*, might contribute to the pathogenetic mechanisms of AD. While sweat plays a major role in maintaining skin homeostasis, it can become an aggravating factor in patients with AD. Furthermore, scratching often exacerbates eczematous lesions. Several patient-specific complicating factors are seen in most cases. The identification and management of complicating factors are important for controlling AD.

Keywords: atopic dermatitis; complicating factors; aggravating factors; triggering factors; irritants; aeroallergens; food; microbial organisms; contact allergens; sweat; scratching

1. Introduction

Atopic dermatitis (AD) is a common, chronic relapsing inflammatory, multifactorial skin disease, which is characterized by intense pruritus [1–3]. It affects up to 20% of children and 1–3% of adults [4]. The mechanisms responsible for the onset and aggravation of AD involve skin barrier dysfunction and an atopic background. In patients with AD, the functions of the intercellular lipids of the stratum corneum are impaired because of abnormal reductions in ceramide levels [5,6]. The horny cell layer, which consists of keratin and filaggrin, is structurally tough. A loss-of-function mutation in filaggrin and filaggrin deficiency related to inflammation have been observed in patients with AD [7,8]. A reduction in skin barrier function might allow stimuli and allergens to penetrate the skin more easily. Interleukin (IL)-33, IL-25, and thymic stromal lymphopoietin (TSLP), which are released from epidermal keratinocytes upon exposure to proteases, allergens, infections, or tissue damage, induce type-2 immune reactions, leading to the induction of allergen-specific IgE antibody production.

With regard to the treatment of AD, topical corticosteroids and topical calcineurin inhibitors are the main treatments for inflammation, whereas the topical application of moisturizers is used to treat cutaneous barrier dysfunction [1,2,9]. Systemic treatment, e.g., oral cyclosporin and UV irradiation, is an option for severe refractory cases [1,2,10]. Several patient-specific complicating factors are seen in most cases. It is important to identify such factors and establish strategies to combat them. This review concisely discusses the identification and management of the complicating factors of AD.

2. Irritants

Skin barrier function is impaired in patients with AD. Therefore, there is a tendency for itching and eczematous lesions to develop after AD patients come into contact with irritants (Table 1). To prevent this, AD patients should cleanse their skin gently to get rid of any dirt. Regarding the pH of the corneal layer, a subacidic state is considered healthy. A barrier-dependent increase in pH, e.g., due to the use of neutral-to-alkaline soaps, leads to a reduction in skin barrier function [11]. Soaps and shampoos that contain non-irritant ingredients can be used instead. Furthermore, residual soap and shampoo can induce irritant dermatitis. Therefore, it is important to fully wash away soap/shampoo. Synthetic fabrics and wool also tend to produce itching and irritate the skin [1,2,12–14]. A previous study has shown that the irritative capacity of synthetic shirts is significantly higher in patients with AD, while cotton shirts are tolerated best [12]. Thus, AD patients should select non-irritating clothes.

Table 1. Management of irritants.

Irritants	Management	References
Scrubbing the body	Wash the body gently without using nylon towels	[1,2]
Soap and shampoo	Use non-irritating soap and shampoo	[1,2,7]
Irritating clothes (e.g., wool-based clothes)	Choose suitable non-irritating clothes (e.g., cotton clothes)	[1,2,8,9]
Hair	Tie hair up	[1]
Saliva (during infancy)	Wash away or wipe off	[1]

3. Aeroallergens

3.1. House Dust Mites (HDM)

Aeroallergens, such as HDM, animal dander, and pollen, can lead to the exacerbation of AD. HDM is one of the main allergens blamed for household dust allergies [15]. The most frequently responsible mites are *Dermatophagoides pteronyssinus* (European house dust mite) and *D. farinae* (American house dust mite), which produce various allergens in their bodies and feces. Currently, there are >30 defined mite allergens (Table 2) [16]. It is considered that the most clinically important allergens are Der p 1 and Der p 2 from *D. Pteronyssinus* and Der f 1 and Der f 2 from *D. farinae*. The HDM allergen Der p 1 is found at concentrations of 0.05–0.2 ng/m^3 in inhalable indoor air [17].

Table 2. Representative allergens derived from *D. Pteronyssinus* and *D. farina* [16].

Allergen	Biochemical Name	Molecular Weight (kDa)
Der p 1/Der f 1	Cysteine protease	24 and 27
Der p 2/Der f 2	NPC2 family	15
Der p 3/Der f 3	Trypsin	31 and 29
Der p 4/Der f 4	Alpha-amylase	60 and 57.9
Der p 5/Der f 5	Unknown	14 and 15.5
Der p 6/Der f 6	Chymotrypsin	25
Der p 7/Der f 7	Bactericidal permeability-increasing like protein	26, 30, and 31
Der p 8/Der f 8	Glutathione S-transferase	27 and 32
Der p 9	Collagenolytic serine protease	29
Der p 10/Der f 10	Tropomyosin	36 and 37

Patients with AD frequently exhibit high total serum IgE levels and environmental allergen-specific IgE. In addition, skin prick testing and atopic patch testing (APT) produce positive reactions to these allergens in AD patients [18–20]. APT has been used to test for delayed-type hypersensitivity/eczematous reactions. Langerhans cells from AD patients have been shown to have an increased capacity to present HDM allergen antigens to T cells via the high affinity receptor for IgE (FcεRI) [21,22], suggesting that IgE-mediated delayed-type hypersensitivity reactions to HDM allergens are associated with the pathogenesis of AD [23–25]. It has been reported that AD patients that experience delayed-type hypersensitivity reactions tend to have severe skin symptoms and exhibit high total IgE levels and HDM-specific IgE levels [17]. In addition, the positivity rate of patch tests performed with HDM antigens was found to be significantly higher in patients that mainly had eczema lesions on exposed areas, such as the hands, forearms, head, and neck, than in patients who also had eczema lesions on non-exposed areas [26].

Even when a patient's serum levels of HDM-specific IgE are increased and strong reactions to HDM are seen during skin tests, whether exposure to HDM is considered to be an aggravating factor in that case should be determined based on the patient's episodes and symptoms [1]. For example, it should be clarified whether the patient develops symptoms of immediate-type hypersensitivity reactions, i.e., wheals, conjunctival or rhinitis symptoms, or asthma attacks, when they are in environments containing large amounts of HDM. Regarding the involvement of delayed-type hypersensitivity reactions in AD, if a patient experiences periods in which their skin symptoms improve or worsen due to changes in their living environment, e.g., due to moving house, travelling, or hospitalization, mites should be considered to be a potential aggravating factor, and the anti-mite measures described below are recommended [1].

Measures that can reduce HDM levels include the use of wood flooring, floor cleaning, vacuum cleaning bedclothes, drying bedclothes in the sun, and the removal of sofas made of cloth and stuffed toys [1,2,14]. While AD lesions were improved by HDM avoidance based on such measures [27,28], reductions in HDM levels had no effect on skin symptoms [29]. The effects of HDM allergen immunotherapy on AD lesions have been investigated by several groups [30,31]. Ridolo et al. reported that the treatment of AD with the causative aeroallergen can be used as an add-on therapy in selected patients who are non-responsive to conventional therapy [30].

3.2. Animal Dander

In most modern cities, cats and dogs are often present in houses, and some individuals become allergic to proteins found in cat or dog dander. Cats are the second most common source of indoor environmental allergens after HDM. Cat allergens are found at high levels (20 ng/m^3) [32]. Ten cat allergens have been identified. The major allergen responsible for symptoms is Fel d 1, a secretoglobin [33].

Čelakovská et al. reported that persistent AD lesions occurred more often in patients that had become sensitized to animal dander or HDM [34]. In addition, IgE sensitization to animal dander or HDM might increase the risk of patients developing asthma or rhinitis [34]. In patients with cat allergies, allergen immunotherapy has been performed with cat dander extract, which was effective at treating cat allergy symptoms, especially respiratory symptoms [35]. In addition, weaker skin test reactions to the cat extract were seen in the treated group than in the placebo group [35].

3.3. Pollen

Pollen grains, which represent a small fraction of the viable biological particles present in the air, are important aeroallergens in the outdoor environment. Airborne pollen can exacerbate AD lesions [36–38]. In a previous study, pronounced eczema flare-ups occurred on exposed rather than covered areas of skin. Epicutaneous patch testing with pollen allergen extract induced eczematous lesions in patients with AD [36,37]. In grass pollen-exposed subjects, the serum levels of chemokine (C-C motif) ligand 17 (CCL17), CCL22, and IL-4 were significantly increased [30]. The preventative measures that can be used against pollen allergies include brushing pollen off clothes, washing your face when arriving home, wearing glasses and masks, and using air conditioning with pollen filters (Table 3) [1,2,14].

Table 3. Evaluation and management of aeroallergens.

Allergen	Evaluation	Management	References
HDM	Serum-specific IgE antibody levels Skin prick testing and patch testing Evaluating changes in skin symptoms caused by environmental changes (e.g., trips, hospitalization, or moving house)	Ventilation Cleaning room Cleaning bedclothes with a vacuum cleaner, drying them in the sun, and washing sheets Encasing mattresses and bedding to protect patients from mites	[1,2,14]
Animal dander	Serum-specific IgE antibody levels Asking the patient about experiences involving the worsening of skin symptoms due to contact with animals	Giving up pets Washing pets Prohibiting pets in the bedroom	[1,2,14]
Pollen	Serum-specific IgE antibody levels Skin prick testing and patch testing Asking the patient about experiences involving the worsening of skin symptoms on exposed areas during a period of pollen scattering	Brushing pollen off clothes and washing face when arriving home Using protective glasses and masks Using air conditioning with pollen filters	[1,2,14]

4. Food

4.1. Blood and Skin Tests

Food allergens might contribute to the pathogenetic mechanisms of AD, especially during infancy. Serum-specific IgE levels and skin prick test results exhibit high negative predictive values (95%) and low specificity and positive predictive values (40–60%) for diagnosing food hypersensitivity [14,39–41]. These findings indicate that negative test results are helpful for ruling out food allergies; however, positive results only signify sensitization and need to be assessed in combination with clinical findings. Therefore, the effects of food allergens should be evaluated based on the results of oral food challenges, which should be performed after causative food elimination in addition to obtaining a detailed medical history and evaluating the patient's serum-specific IgE antibody levels and skin test results [1,2,14].

4.2. Allergen-Free Diet for Pregnant/Lactating Women

A systematic review of randomized controlled studies that examined the use of allergen-free diets in pregnant/lactating women has been reported [42]. Dietary restrictions involving allergen elimination in pregnant and lactating women did not prevent the onset of AD in infants. Therefore, dietary restrictions in pregnant and lactating women are not needed to prevent the onset of AD in their children [1].

4.3. Percutaneous Sensitization in Food Allergy

Lack et al. performed an epidemiological survey of peanut allergies and detected a significant relationship between peanut allergies and the application of skincare preparations containing peanut oil in children [43]. Based on these findings, the dual-allergen exposure hypothesis, which suggests that oral allergen intake induces immunotolerance, whereas allergen exposure via skin with decreased barrier function induces sensitization, has been proposed [44]. Since the proposal of this hypothesis, allergies caused by percutaneous sensitization, in which sensitization is established by the skin coming into contact with foods, has attracted attention as a mechanism that might be responsible for food allergies.

5. Microbial Organisms

5.1. Staphylococcus Aureus

Staphylococcus aureus is frequently detected in AD lesions. Kong et al. reported that the frequency of *Staphylococcus* sequences, particularly *S. aureus*, increased during disease flare-ups and was correlated with the severity of skin symptoms in children with AD [45]. In addition, Simpson et al. demonstrated that AD patients that had been colonized with *S. aureus* had higher levels of type-2 biomarkers (higher blood eosinophil counts and serum levels of total IgE, CCL17, and periostin) and exhibited greater allergen sensitization than both non-colonized AD patients and non-atopic, non-colonized control individuals [46]. Huang et al. investigated the effects of suppressing *S. aureus* growth with sodium hypochlorite (bleach) baths [47]. The AD patients that received bleach baths displayed significantly greater reductions in disease severity compared with the control subjects.

5.2. Malassezia Furfur

The characteristic distribution of AD skin lesions, which often affect the head and neck, implies that an association exists between the exacerbation of AD and cutaneous microflora, such as *Malassezia furfur*. Reactivity to *Malassezia* allergens, which was measured based on serum-specific IgE levels, positive skin prick tests, and positive patch tests, was found to be increased in AD patients with head and neck dermatitis [48–50]. It has been reported that oral [51] and topical antifungal drugs [52] are effective against AD. Taken together with the findings of previous studies into *S. aureus* and *M. furfur*, further research is required to fully understand the relationship between the microbial organisms found on the skin and the clinical symptoms of AD [1].

6. Contact Allergens

6.1. Contact Allergy

Allergic contact dermatitis is a delayed-type hypersensitivity reaction to small environmental chemicals, i.e., haptens or prehaptens, that come into contact with the skin. Contact allergies can cause refractory eczematous lesions in patients with AD. In particular, if an AD patient displays an atypical distribution of eczematous lesions, they might be suffering from a contact allergy. According to previous studies, the frequency of contact allergies in AD patients ranges from 26% to 54% [53]. The most common contact allergens are metals, topical drugs, fragrance, and rubber accelerators [53–55] (Table 4). In a previous study, the avoidance of products containing allergenic substances markedly or partially improved eczematous lesions in two-thirds of AD patients that exhibited positive patch test reactions [53]. With regard to nickel and cosmetics, females become sensitized to them more often than males, probably because of their greater use of cosmetics and jewelry, especially among females with pierced ears.

6.2. Intrinsic AD

AD can be categorized into the IgE-high, extrinsic type and the IgE-normal, intrinsic type [56]. Extrinsic AD is the classical type, which displays a high prevalence and is associated with elevated IgE levels and skin barrier dysfunction due to decreased filaggrin expression. On the other hand, the incidence of intrinsic AD, which predominantly affects females, is approximately 20%. It has been shown that the percentage of interferon-γ-producing Th1 cells in the peripheral blood is significantly higher in intrinsic AD patients than in extrinsic AD patients [57]. Interestingly, patients with intrinsic AD displayed a higher proportion of positive patch test reactions to metals than those with extrinsic AD, and a metal-free diet partially ameliorated skin symptoms in patients with intrinsic AD, but not those with extrinsic AD [53,58]. Furthermore, Yamaguchi et al. reported that the concentration of nickel in sweat was higher in intrinsic AD patients than in extrinsic AD patients and was inversely correlated with serum IgE levels [58]. These findings suggest that metal allergies are a potential cause of intrinsic AD.

Table 4. Representative contact allergens in AD patients.

Contact Allergens	Details of Contents	References
Metals	Nickel sulfate Cobalt chloride Potassium dichromate	[53–55]
Fragrances	Fragrance mix *Myroxylon pereirae* (Balsam of Peru)	[53–55]
Preservatives	Paraben mix Thiomersal	[53,54]
Rubber accelerators	Mercapto mix Thiuram mix Dithiocarbamate mix	[53,54]
Topical drugs	Steroids Antibiotics Moisturizer Eye drops	[53–55]
Cosmetics		[53]
Other chemicals	Lanolin	[53,55]

7. Sweating

7.1. The Function and Composition of Sweat

Sweat includes natural moisturizing factors (e.g., lactate, urea, and electrolytes, free amino acids, and pyrrolidone carboxylic acid), antimicrobial peptides (e.g., dermcidin, β-defensins, and cathelicidin), IgA, sodium bicarbonate, pyruvic acid, proteases, and protease inhibitors, and contributes to skin homeostasis, including temperature regulation, skin moisture regulation, and immune functions [59,60]. Several previous studies have reported that the composition of sweat was changed in patients with AD [61–63]. Liebke et al. found that the sodium concentration of sweat was significantly higher in children with AD than in healthy children [61]. Moreover, Sugawara et al. showed that patients with AD had significantly reduced levels of sodium, potassium, lactate, urea, and pyrrolidone carboxylic acid in their sweat than healthy controls [62]. These findings suggest that impaired sweating might reduce the levels of natural moisturizing factors and cause dry skin in patients with AD. It is considered that patients with AD are at higher risk of skin infections and *S. aureus* colonization. Rieg et al. found that patients with AD displayed significantly lower levels of dermcidin-derived antimicrobial peptides in their sweat than healthy controls [63]. Furthermore, the skin bacterial count after physical exercise-induced sweating was lower in the AD patients than in the healthy subjects [63]. Imayama et al. demonstrated that AD patients had lower secretory IgA levels in their sweat than healthy controls [64]. These findings suggest that decreased levels of antimicrobial peptides and IgA in sweat might lead to increased susceptibility to skin infections in patients with AD.

7.2. Decreased Sweating in AD Patients

Patients with AD often sweat significantly less than healthy individuals [65–67]. Several possible mechanisms have been suggested to be responsible for the decreased sweating seen in patients with AD [59,60]. It has previously been reported that horny plugs or mucopolysaccharides were seen in the openings of the sweat ducts in conditions involving sweat retention [68,69]. With regard to sweat-gland functions, acetylcholine-induced sweating responses were reduced in AD patients compared with those seen in healthy controls, and histamine suppressed acetylcholine-induced sweating via H1 receptor-mediated signaling [70,71]. Furthermore, sweat leakage into the surrounding tissues was observed in patients with AD. The leakage of sweat, as demonstrated by sweat gland-specific dermcidin expression in the dermis around the sweat ducts and glands, was specifically detected in the skin of AD patients [72]. Interestingly, the expression of claudin-3, which acts as a component of the tight junctions between the luminal cells throughout the sweat gland, was significantly reduced in patients with AD compared with that observed in healthy individuals [71]. The reductions in sweating induced via these mechanisms might cause skin dryness and increase patients' susceptibility to infection, resulting in the exacerbation of the symptoms of AD.

7.3. Sweat Allergies

While sweat is important for maintaining homeostasis, it is likely to induce pruritus in patients with AD. Hide et al. reported that intradermal tests with autologous sweat induced positive reactions in many patients with AD [73]. In addition, it has been reported that patients with AD exhibited positive reactions to sweat antigens in a histamine release test [73]. Interestingly, Hiragun et al. found that MGL_1304, a fungal protein derived from *Malassezia globosa*, is a major antigen in human sweat, and recombinant MGL_1304 induced histamine release from basophils in most AD patients [74]. Patients with AD might develop immediate-type hypersensitivity reactions to sweat antigens, leading to exacerbated itching and irritation in response to sweating. These findings suggest that mast cells might react to sweat that leaks from weak sweat ducts and glands in patients with AD.

7.4. Measures for Sweating

It is not necessary to avoid sweating because sweating is important for skin homeostasis. However, leaving excess sweat on the skin surface can induce itching in patients with AD. Several studies have shown that taking a shower after sweating is effective at relieving symptoms [75,76]. Therefore, if excess sweat remains on the skin surface, it can be washed away or wiped off [1].

8. Scratching Behavior

8.1. Scratching-Induced Aggravation of AD Lesions

Patients with AD often scratch their skin, resulting in further skin damage, which can lead to the exacerbation of eczematous lesions. It has been hypothesized that IL-33, IL-25, and TSLP, which are released from epidermal keratinocytes, act as endogenous "danger signals" or "alarmins" that alert the immune system to tissue damage [77]. It has been shown that the serum levels of IL-33 were higher in AD patients than in healthy individuals [78]. In addition, the patients' serum IL-33 levels were correlated with their excoriation scores [78]. These findings suggest that tissue injuries caused by scratching of the skin might result in increased release of keratinocyte-derived cytokines, including IL-33, from damaged cells in patients with AD. Moreover, several previous studies have suggested that endogenous molecules that are released from tissues or cells by skin damage, including scratching, stimulate immune reactions in allergic dermatitis [79–81]. Therefore, scratching contributes to the exacerbation of eczematous lesions in AD.

8.2. Factors Influencing Scratching Behavior

Scratching can be caused by various itching-related and non-itching-related factors (Table 5). Itching signals are transmitted from the periphery to the brain via the dorsal horn by primary sensory neurons and spinothalamic tract neurons, and itching is induced by various mediators [77,82,83]. At the periphery, histamine acts as a pruritogen. Several type-2 cytokines, such as IL-4, IL-13, and IL-31, also directly activate sensory neurons [77,84–87]. Targeting the IL-31 pathway has been shown to be effective in patients with AD [84]. IL-4 and IL-13 are cytokines that are central to the pathogenesis of atopic disease and are primarily produced by Th2 cells [77]. Dupilumab is a human monoclonal antibody that is directed against the α-subunit of the IL-4 receptor. It blocks signaling from both IL-4 and IL-13 [85]. The administration of dupilumab resulted in significant improvements in inflammation and pruritus in AD patients [86]. Moreover, the epithelium-derived cytokine TSLP, which is deeply involved in the development of inflammatory responses in AD [77], acts directly on a subset of primary sensory neurons and induces itching [87].

Table 5. Major factors influencing scratching in AD.

Factors	Details of Contents	References
Inflammatory mediators	Amines (histamine, serotonin)	[13,88]
	Cytokines (IL-4, IL-13, IL-31, IL-33, and TSLP)	[77,82,83]
	Proteases (kallikreins, tryptase, endogenous/exogenous proteases)	[89,90]
	Neuropeptides (substance P)	[91,92]
	Neurotrophic factors (nerve growth factor, artemin)	[82,93]
	Neurotransmitters (acetylcholine)	[94]
Environmental factors	Temperature, humidity, dry environments	[83]
	Psychological stress	[1,83]
	Habitual scratching	[1]

In addition to these mediators, proteases (e.g., kallikreins, tryptase, endogenous/exogenous proteases) [89,90], neuropeptides (e.g., substance P) [91,92], and neurotrophic factors (nerve growth factor (NGF), artemin) [82,83,93] are considered to contribute to pruritus. Moreover, it has been reported that abnormal elongation of the sensory nerves into the epidermis occurs in the skin of AD patients [82]. In a mouse model of dry skin-induced itching, the expression of NGF was found to be elevated in the skin, and the number of intradermal nerve fibers increased [95]. On the other hand, semaphorins are a class of secreted membrane proteins, which function as axonal growth cone guidance molecules [82]. Semaphorin 3A is the first member of the semaphorin family that has been shown to cause growth cone collapse in neurons [96]. Semaphorin 3A regulates NGF-induced sprouting of sensory afferents in the spinal cord [97]. The abnormal elongation of the sensory nerves seen in AD is considered to be caused by an imbalance in the levels of nerve elongation factors, such as NGF, and nerve-repulsion factors, such as semaphorin 3A [82]. Such abnormal extension of the sensory nerves into the epidermis might lead to mechanical itching-induced dysesthesia, in which abnormal sensory states are induced by light cutaneous stimuli (alloknesis) [77,83]. In addition, patients with AD can experience strong itching in response to normal itch-evoking stimuli (hyperknesis) [77,83]. Non-itching sensations, such as heat and pain, can also be experienced as itching by patients with AD [83].

The micro-opioid (beta-endorphin/micro-opioid receptor) and kappa-opioid (dynorphin A (DynA)/kappa-opioid receptor) systems are involved in the regulation of pruritus in the central nervous system. It has been reported that the micro-opioid and kappa-opioid systems are present in the human epidermis [98], suggesting that these systems might be responsible for peripheral pruritus. Kumagai et al. suggested that the micro-opioid system is itch-inducible, while the kappa-opioid system is itch-suppressive [99]. Interestingly, Tominaga et al. reported that the kappa-opioid system was downregulated in the epidermises of AD patients [100], indicating that patients with AD might experience itching due to the downregulation of the itch-suppressive system.

Patients with AD often scratch their skin in response to factors that are not related to itching. With regard to psychological aspects, it is known that the itching symptoms of AD patients can be worsened by stress and can be improved by stress management and behavioral modification [1]. Moreover, a vicious cycle of itching, scratching, and damaged skin might lead to scratching mainly out of habit instead of due to itching (habitual scratching). Thus, it is important to consider the possible involvement of such non-itching-related factors in addition to suppressing inflammation and pruritus in order to control the scratching behavior of AD patients.

9. Other Factors

9.1. Psychological Stressors

Emotional stress can increase not only itching but also the inflammation via the release of inflammatory mediators in AD patients [101,102]. The patients with AD had higher anxiety levels than healthy individuals, and those with a stronger trait anxiety than state anxiety showed elevated serum IgE levels and Th2 shifting [101]. Moreover, psychological variables affect serum levels of interferon-γ and IL-4 more in the patients with AD than healthy individuals [102]. These findings suggest that psychological stressors might affect the immunological reactions in the patients with AD.

9.2. Circadian Rhythms

Clinical symptoms in patients with allergic diseases including AD often depend on diurnal variations [103]. An intrinsic daily physiological rhythm called circadian rhythm is thought to affect the immune system. Several experimental studies have demonstrated that mutation in the circadian clock genes greatly affects immune responses [104–106]. Immune tolerance development is closely associated with the onset of immunological disorders. It has been shown that exposure to constant light impairs circadian rhythms, leading to the disturbance of tolerance induction [107]. Therefore, constant light environments such as lighting conditions at home in our night-active modern society may affect the development of AD.

10. Conclusions

Various aggravating factors, including both allergic and non-allergic factors, have been suggested to influence the course of AD. To identify factors that are specific to individual patients, it is important to consider whether the degree of eczematous lesions is affected by environmental changes, oral food challenges, or the avoidance of contact with suspected causative substances. In addition, we need to establish treatment strategies that take patients' lifestyles into account. Furthermore, it is not necessary for AD patients to avoid sweating because it is important for skin homeostasis. However, leaving excess sweat on the skin can induce skin symptoms; therefore, sweat should be washed away or wiped off. Moreover, scratching leads to further skin damage, resulting in the exacerbation of eczematous lesions. It is important to consider clinical factors that might influencing scratching behavior (e.g., inflammation, stress, and habitual scratching). Future studies will contribute to the elucidation of the pathogenetic mechanism of AD, leading to improvements in the management of complicating factors.

Author Contributions: R.T.-M. wrote the first draft. N.K. reviewed the draft. R.T-M. finalized the article, and both authors approved the submission of the article. All authors have read and agreed to the published version of the manuscript.

Funding: This research received no external funding.

Conflicts of Interest: R.T.-M. has no conflict of interest to declare. N.K. has received honoraria and research grants (to the Department of Dermatology, Kyoto Prefectural University of Medicine) from AbbVie, Lilly, LEO Pharma, Maruho, Mitsubishi Tanabe, Kyowa Kirin, Taiho, Regeneron, and Sanofi.

References

1. Katoh, N.; Ohya, Y.; Ikeda, M.; Ebihara, T.; Katayama, I.; Saeki, H.; Shimojo, N.; Tanaka, A.; Nakahara, T.; Nagao, M.; et al. Clinical practice guidelines for the management of atopic dermatitis 2018. *J. Dermatol.* **2019**, *46*, 1053–1101. [CrossRef] [PubMed]
2. Ring, J.; Alomar, A.; Bieber, T.; Deleuran, M.; Fink-Wagner, A.; Gelmetti, C.; Gieler, U.; Lipozencic, J.; Luger, T.; Oranje, A.P.; et al. Guidelines for treatment of atopic eczema (atopic dermatitis) Part I. *J. Eur. Acad. Dermatol. Venereol.* **2012**, *26*, 1045–1060. [CrossRef] [PubMed]
3. Eichenfield, L.F.; Tom, W.L.; Chamlin, S.L.; Feldman, S.R.; Hanifin, J.M.; Simpson, E.L.; Berger, T.G.; Bergman, J.N.; Cohen, D.E.; Cooper, K.D.; et al. Guidelines of care for the management of atopic dermatitis:

Section 1 diagnosis and assessment of atopic dermatitis. *J. Am. Acad. Dermatol.* **2014**, *70*, 338–351. [CrossRef] [PubMed]
4. Williams, H.C. Atopic dermatitis. In *The Epidemiology, Causes and Prevention of Atopic Eczema*; Williams, H.C., Ed.; Cambridge University Press: Cambridge, UK, 2000.
5. Elias, P.M. Stratum corneum defensive functions: An integrated view. *J. Gen. Intern Med.* **2005**, *125*, 183–200. [CrossRef] [PubMed]
6. Melnik, B.; Hollmann, J.; Plewig, G. Decreased stratum corneum ceramides in atopic individuals–a pathobiochemical factor in xerosis? *Br. J. Dermatol.* **1988**, *119*, 547–549. [CrossRef] [PubMed]
7. Cabanillas, B.; Novak, N. Atopic dermatitis and filaggrin. *Curr. Opin. Immunol.* **2016**, *42*, 1–8. [CrossRef]
8. Kono, M.; Nomura, T.; Ohguchi, Y.; Mizuno, O.; Suzuki, S.; Tsujiuchi, H.; Hamajima, N.; McLean, W.H.; Shimizu, H.; Akiyama, M. Comprehensive screening for a complete set of Japanese-population-specific filaggrin gene mutations. *Allergy* **2014**, *69*, 537–540. [CrossRef]
9. Eichenfield, L.F.; Tom, W.L.; Berger, T.G.; Krol, A.; Paller, A.S.; Schwarzenberger, K.; Bergman, J.N.; Chamlin, S.L.; Cohen, D.E.; Cooper, K.D.; et al. Guidelines of care for the management of atopic dermatitis: Section Management and treatment of atopic dermatitis with topical therapies. *J. Am. Acad. Dermatol.* **2014**, *71*, 116–132. [CrossRef]
10. Sidbury, R.; Davis, D.M.; Cohen, D.E.; Cordoro, K.M.; Berger, T.G.; Bergman, J.N.; Chamlin, S.L.; Cooper, K.D.; Feldman, S.R.; Hanifin, J.M.; et al. Guidelines of care for the management of atopic dermatitis: Section 3. Management and treatment with phototherapy and systemic agents. *J. Am. Acad. Dermatol.* **2014**, *71*, 327–349. [CrossRef]
11. Elias, P.M.; Hatano, Y.; Williams, M.L. Basis for the barrier abnormality in atopic dermatitis: Outside-inside-outside pathogenic mechanisms. *J. Allergy Clin. Immunol.* **2008**, *121*, 1337–13343. [CrossRef]
12. Diepgen, T.L.; Stäbler, A.; Hornstein, O.P. Textile intolerance in atopic eczema -a controlled clinical study. *Z. Hautkr.* **1990**, *65*, 907–910. [PubMed]
13. Wahlgren, C.F.; Hägermark, O.; Bergström, R. Patients' perception of itch induced by histamine, compound 48/80 and wool fibres in atopic dermatitis. *Acta. Derm. Venereol.* **1991**, *71*, 488–494. [PubMed]
14. Sidbury, R.; Tom, W.L.; Bergman, J.N.; Cooper, K.D.; Silverman, R.A.; Berger, T.G.; Chamlin, S.L.; Cohen, D.E.; Cordoro, K.M.; Davis, D.M. Guidelines of care for the management of atopic dermatitis: Section 4. *J. Am. Acad. Dermatol.* **2014**, *71*, 1218–1233. [CrossRef] [PubMed]
15. Thomas, W.R. Hierarchy and molecular properties of house dust mite allergens. *Allergol. Int.* **2015**, *64*, 304–311. [CrossRef] [PubMed]
16. Allergen Nomenclature. WHO/IUIS Allergen Nomenclature Sub-Committee. Available online: www.allergen.org/ (accessed on 15 August 2019).
17. Tovey, E.R.; Willenborg, C.M.; Crisafulli, D.A.; Rimmer, J.; Marks, G.B. Marks most personal exposure to house dust mite aeroallergen occurs during the day. *PLoS ONE* **2013**, *8*, e69900. [CrossRef] [PubMed]
18. Darsow, U.; Vieluf, D.; Ring, J. Evaluating the relevance of aeroallergen sensitization in atopic eczema with the atopy patch test: A randomized, double-blind multicenter study. Atopy Patch Test Study Group. *J. Am. Acad. Dermatol.* **1999**, *40*, 187–193. [CrossRef]
19. Darsow, U.; Laifaoui, J.; Kerschenlohr, K.; Wollenberg, A.; Przybilla, B.; Wüthrich, B.; Borelli, S., Jr.; Giusti, F.; Seidenari, S.; Drzimalla, K.; et al. The prevalence of positive reactions in the atopy patch test with aeroallergens and food allergens in subjects with atopic eczema: A European multicenter study. *Allergy* **2004**, *59*, 1318–1325. [CrossRef]
20. Katoh, N.; Hirano, S.; Suehiro, M.; Masuda, K.; Kishimoto, S. The characteristics of patients with atopic dermatitis demonstrating a positive reaction in a scratch test after 48 hours against house dust mite antigen. *J. Dermatol.* **2004**, *31*, 720–726. [CrossRef]
21. Bruijnzeel-Koomen, C.; van Wicker, D.; Toonstra, J.; Bruijnzeel, P. The presence of IgE molecules on epidermal Langerhans cells from patients with atopic dermatitis. *Arch. Dermatol. Res.* **1986**, *278*, 199–205. [CrossRef]
22. Mudde, G.C.; van Reijsen, F.C.; Boland, G.J.; de Gast, G.C.; Bruijnzeel, P.L.; Bruijnzeel-Koomen, C.A. Allergen presentation by epidermal Langerhans' cells from patients with atopic dermatitis is mediated by IgE. *Immunology* **1990**, *69*, 335–341.
23. Bieber, T.; de la Salle, H.; Wollenberg, A. Human epidermal Langerhans cells express the high affinity receptor for immunoglobulin E (FcεRI). *J. Exp. Med.* **1992**, *175*, 1285–1290. [CrossRef] [PubMed]

24. Wang, B.; Rieger, A.; Kilgus, O. Epidermal Langerhans cells from normal human skin bind monomeric IgE via FcεRI. *J. Exp. Med.* **1992**, *175*, 1353–1365. [CrossRef] [PubMed]
25. Jürgens, M.L.; Wollenberg, A.; Hanau, D.; de la Salle, H.; Bieber, T. Activation of human epidermal Langerhans cells by engagement of the high affinity receptor for IgE, FcεRI. *J. Immunol.* **1995**, *155*, 5184–5189. [PubMed]
26. Darsow, U.; Vieluf, D.; Ring, J. The atopy patch test: An increased rate of reactivity in patients who have an air-exposed pattern of atopic eczema. *Br. J. Dermatol.* **1996**, *135*, 182–186. [CrossRef]
27. Ricci, G.; Patrizi, A.; Specchia, F.; Menna, L.; Bottau, P.; D'Angelo, V.; Masi, M. Effect of house dust mite avoidance measures in children with atopic dermatitis. *Br. J. Dermatol.* **2000**, *143*, 379–384. [CrossRef]
28. Oosting, A.J.; de Bruin-Weller, M.S.; Terreehorst, I.; Tempels-Pavlica, Z.; Aalberse, R.C.; de Monchy, J.G.; van Wijk, R.G.; Bruijnzeel-Koomen, C.A. Effect of mattress encasings on atopic dermatitis outcome measures in a double-blind, placebo-controlled study: The Dutch mite avoidance study. *J. Allergy. Clin. Immunol.* **2002**, *110*, 500–506. [CrossRef]
29. Gutgesell, C.; Heise, S.; Seubert, S.; Seubert, A.; Domhof, S.; Brunner, E.; Neumann, C. Double-blind placebo-controlled house dust mite control measures in adult patients with atopic dermatitis. *Br. J. Dermatol.* **2001**, *145*, 70–74. [CrossRef]
30. Ridolo, E.; Martignago, I.; Galeazzo Riario-Sforza, G.; Incorvaia, C. Allergen immunotherapy in atopic dermatitis. *Expert Rev. Clin. Immunol.* **2018**, *14*, 61–68. [CrossRef]
31. Bussmann, C.; Böckenhoff, A.; Henke, H.; Werfel, T.; Novak, N. Does allergen-specific immunotherapy represent a therapeutic option for patients with atopic dermatitis? *J. Allergy Clin. Immunol.* **2006**, *118*, 1292–1298. [CrossRef]
32. Thomas, W.R. Innate affairs of allergens. *Clin. Exp. Allergy* **2013**, *43*, 152–163. [CrossRef]
33. Bonnet, B.; Messaoudi, K.; Jacomet, F.; Michaud, E.; Fauquert, J.L.; Caillaud, D.; Evrard, B. An update on molecular cat allergens: Fel d 1 and what else? Chapter 1: Fel d 1, the major cat allergen. *Allergy Asthma. Clin. Immunol.* **2018**, *14*, 14. [CrossRef] [PubMed]
34. Čelakovská, J.; Ettlerová, K.; Ettler, K.; Vaněčková, J.; Bukač, J. Sensitization to aeroallergens in atopic dermatitis patients: Association with concomitant allergic diseases. *J. Eur. Acad. Dermatol. Venereol.* **2015**, *29*, 1500–1505. [CrossRef] [PubMed]
35. Alvarez-Cuesta, E.; Berges-Gimeno, P.; González-Mancebo, E.; Mancebo, E.G.; Fernández-Caldas, E.; Cuesta-Herranz, J.; Casanovas, M. Sublingual immunotherapy with a standardized cat dander extract: Evaluation of efficacy in a double blind placebo controlled study. *Allergy* **2007**, *62*, 810–817. [CrossRef] [PubMed]
36. Yokozeki, H.; Takayama, K.; Katayama, I.; Nishioka, K. Japanese cedar pollen as an exacerbation factor in atopic dermatitis: Results of atopy patch testing and histological examination. *Acta. Derm. Venereol.* **2006**, *86*, 148–151.
37. Darsow, U.; Behrendt, H.; Ring, J. Gramineae pollen as trigger factors of atopic eczema: Evaluation of diagnostic measures using the atopy patch test. *Br. J. Dermatol.* **1997**, *137*, 201–207. [CrossRef]
38. Werfel, T.; Heratizadeh, A.; Niebuhr, M.; Kapp, A.; Roesner, L.M.; Karch, A.; Erpenbeck, V.J.; Lösche, C.; Jung, T.; Krug, N. Exacerbation of atopic dermatitis on grass pollen exposure in an environmental challenge chamber. *J. Allergy Clin. Immunol.* **2015**, *136*, 96–103. [CrossRef]
39. Bock, S.A.; Lee, W.Y.; Remigio, L.; Holst, A.; May, C.D. Appraisal of skin tests with food extracts for diagnosis of food hypersensitivity. *Clin. Allergy* **1978**, *8*, 559–564. [CrossRef]
40. Sampson, H.A.; Albergo, R. Comparison of results of skin tests, RAST, and double-blind, placebo-controlled food challenges in children with atopic dermatitis. *J. Allergy Clin. Immunol.* **1984**, *74*, 26–33. [CrossRef]
41. Lemon-Mule, H.; Nowak-Wegrzyn, A.; Berin, C.; Knight, A.K. Pathophysiology of food-induced anaphylaxis. *Curr. Allergy Asthma. Rep.* **2008**, *8*, 201–208. [CrossRef]
42. Kramer, M.S.; Kakuma, R. Maternal dietary antigen avoidance during pregnancy or lactation, or both, for preventing or treating atopic disease in the child. *Cochrane Database Syst. Rev.* **2012**, *9*, CD000133. [CrossRef] [PubMed]
43. Lack, G.; Fox, D.; Northstone, K.; Golding, J. Avon Longitudinal Study of Parents and Children Study Team. Factors associated with the development of peanut allergy in childfood. *N Engl. J. Med.* **2003**, *348*, 977–985. [CrossRef] [PubMed]
44. Lack, G. Epidemiologic risks for food allergy. *J. Allergy Clin. Immunol.* **2008**, *129*, 1187–1197. [CrossRef] [PubMed]

45. Kong, H.H.; Oh, J.; Deming, C.; Conlan, S.; Grice, E.A.; Beatson, M.A.; Nomicos, E.; Polley, E.C.; Komarow, H.D.; NISC Comparative Sequence Program; et al. Temporal shifts in the skin microbiome associated with disease flares and treatment in children with atopic dermatitis. *Genome. Res.* **2012**, *22*, 850–859. [CrossRef] [PubMed]
46. Simpson, E.L.; Villarreal, M.; Jepson, B.; Rafaels, N.; David, G.; Hanifin, J.; Taylor, P.; Boguniewicz, M.; Yoshida, T.; De Benedetto, A.; et al. Patients with atopic dermatitis colonized with Staphylococcus aureus have a distinct phenotype and endotype. *J. Investig. Dermatol.* **2018**, *138*, 2224–2233. [CrossRef] [PubMed]
47. Huang, J.T.; Abrams, M.; Tlougan, B.; Rademaker, A.; Paller, A.S. Treatment of staphylococcus aureus colonization in atopic dermatitis decreases disease severity. *Pediatrics* **2009**, *123*, e808–e814. [CrossRef] [PubMed]
48. Johansson, C.; Sandström, M.H.; Bartosik, J.; Särnhult, T.; Christiansen, J.; Zargari, A.; Bäck, O.; Wahlgren, C.F.; Faergemann, J.; Scheynius, A.; et al. Atopy patch test reactions to Malassezia allergens differentiate subgroups of atopic dermatitis patients. *Br. J. Dermatol.* **2003**, *148*, 479–488. [CrossRef]
49. Kim, T.Y.; Jang, I.G.; Park, Y.M.; Kim, H.O.; Kim, C.W. Head and neck dermatitis: The role of Malassezia furfur, topical steroid use and environmental factors in its causation. *Clin. Exp. Dermatol.* **1999**, *24*, 226–231. [CrossRef]
50. Johansson, C.; Eshaghi, H.; Linder, M.T.; Jakobson, E.; Scheynius, A. Positive atopy patch test reaction to Malassezia furfur in atopic dermatitis correlates with a T helper 2-like peripheral blood mononuclear cells response. *J. Investig. Dermatol.* **2002**, *118*, 1044–1051. [CrossRef]
51. Takechi, M. Minimum effective dosage in the treatment of chronic atopic dermatitis with itraconazole. *J. Int. Med. Res.* **2005**, *33*, 2732–2783. [CrossRef]
52. Mayser, P.; Kupfer, J.; Nemetz, D.; Schäfer, U.; Nilles, M.; Hort, W.; Gieler, U. Treatment of head and neck dermatitis with ciclopiroxolamine cream-results of a double-blind, placebo-controlled study. *Skin. Pharmacol. Physiol.* **2006**, *19*, 1531–1558. [CrossRef]
53. Tamagawa-Mineoka, R.; Masuda, K.; Ueda, S.; Nakamura, N.; Hotta, E.; Hattori, J.; Minamiyama, R.; Yamazaki, A.; Katoh, N. Contact sensitivity in patients with recalcitrant atopic dermatitis. *J. Dermatol.* **2015**, *42*, 720–722. [CrossRef] [PubMed]
54. Thyssen, J.P.; Johansen, J.D.; Linneberg, A.; Menné, T.; Engkilde, K. The association between contact sensitization and atopic disease by linkage of a clinical database and a nationwide patient registry. *Allergy* **2012**, *67*, 1157–1164. [CrossRef] [PubMed]
55. Giordano-Labadie, F.; Rance, F.; Pellegrin, F.; Bazex, J.; Dutau, G.; Schwarze, H.P. Frequency of contact allergy in children with atopic dermatitis: Results of a prospective study of 137 cases. *Contact Dermatitis* **1999**, *40*, 192–195. [CrossRef] [PubMed]
56. Tokura, Y. Extrinsic and intrinsic types of atopic dermatitis. *J. Dermatol. Sci.* **2010**, *58*, 1–7. [CrossRef] [PubMed]
57. Kabashima-Kubo, R.; Nakamura, M.; Sakabe, J.; Sugita, K.; Hino, R.; Mori, T.; Kobayashi, M.; Bito, T.; Kabashima, K.; Ogasawara, K.; et al. A group of atopic dermatitis without IgE elevation or barrier impairment shows a high Th1 frequency: Possible immunological state of the intrinsic type. *J. Dermatol. Sci.* **2012**, *67*, 37–43. [CrossRef] [PubMed]
58. Yamaguchi, H.; Kabashima-Kubo, R.; Bito, T.; Sakabe, J.; Shimauchi, T.; Ito, T.; Hirakawa, S.; Hirasawa, N.; Ogasawara, K.; Tokura, Y. High frequencies of positive nickel/cobalt patch tests and high sweat nickel concentration in patients with intrinsic atopic dermatitis. *J. Dermatol. Sci.* **2013**, *72*, 240–245. [CrossRef] [PubMed]
59. Murota, H.; Yamaga, K.; Ono, E.; Katayama, I. Sweat in the pathogenesis of atopic dermatitis. *Allergol. Int.* **2018**, *67*, 455–459. [CrossRef]
60. Shelmire, J.B., Jr. Some interrelations between sebum, sweat and the skin surface. *J. Investig. Dermatol.* **1959**, *32*, 471–472. [CrossRef]
61. Liebke, C.; Wahn, U.; Niggemann, B. Sweat electrolyte concentrations in children with atopic dermatitis. *Lancet* **1997**, *350*, 1678–1679. [CrossRef]
62. Sugawara, T.; Kikuchi, K.; Tagami, H.; Aiba, S.; Sakai, S. Decreased lactate and potassium levels in natural moisturizing factor from the stratum corneum of mild atopic dermatitis patients are involved with the reduced hydration state. *J. Dermatol. Sci.* **2012**, *66*, 154–159. [CrossRef]

63. Rieg, S.; Steffen, H.; Seeber, S.; Humeny, A.; Kalbacher, H.; Dietz, K.; Garbe, C.; Schittek, B. Deficiency of dermcidin-derived antimicrobial peptides in sweat of patients with atopic dermatitis correlates with an impaired innate defense of human skin in vivo. *J. Immunol.* **2005**, *174*, 8003–8010. [CrossRef] [PubMed]
64. Imayama, S.; Shimozono, Y.; Hoashi, M.; Yasumoto, S.; Ohta, S.; Yoneyama, K.; Hori, Y. Reduced secretion of IgA to skin surface of patients with atopic dermatitis. *J. Allergy Clin. Immunol.* **1994**, *94*, 195–200. [CrossRef] [PubMed]
65. Eishi, K.; Lee, J.B.; Bae, S.J.; Takenaka, M.; Katayama, I. Impaired sweating function in adult atopic dermatitis: Results of the quantitative sudomotor axon reflex test. *Br. J. Dermatol.* **2002**, *147*, 683–688. [CrossRef] [PubMed]
66. Kijima, A.; Murota, H.; Matsui, S.; Takahashi, A.; Kimura, A.; Kitaba, S.; Lee, J.B.; Katayama, I. Abnormal axon reflex-mediated sweating correlates with high state of anxiety in atopic dermatitis. *Allergol. Int.* **2012**, *61*, 469–473. [CrossRef] [PubMed]
67. Takahashi, A.; Murota, H.; Matsui, S.; Kijima, A.; Kitaba, S.; Lee, J.B.; Katayama, I. Decreased sudomotor function is involved in the formation of atopic eczema in the cubital fossa. *Allergol. Int.* **2013**, *62*, 473–478. [CrossRef] [PubMed]
68. Sulzberger, M.B.; Herrmann, F.; Zak, F.G. Studies of sweating; preliminary report with particular emphasis of a sweat retention syndrome. *J. Investig. Dermatol.* **1947**, *9*, 221–242. [CrossRef]
69. Papa, C.M.; Kligman, A.M. Mechanisms of eccrine anidrosis. I. High level blockade. *J. Investig. Dermatol.* **1966**, *47*, 1–9. [CrossRef]
70. Murota, H.; Matsui, S.; Ono, E.; Kijima, A.; Kikuta, J.; Ishii, M.; Katayama, I. Sweat, the driving force behind normal skin: An emerging perspective on functional biology and regulatory mechanisms. *J. Dermatol. Sci.* **2015**, *77*, 3–10. [CrossRef]
71. Matsui, S.; Murota, H.; Takahashi, A.; Yang, L.; Lee, J.B.; Omiya, K.; Ohmi, M.; Kikuta, J.; Ishii, M.; Katayama, I. Dynamic Analysis of Histamine-Mediated Attenuation of Acetylcholine-Induced Sweating via GSK3β Activation. *J. Investig. Dermatol.* **2014**, *134*, 326–334. [CrossRef]
72. Shiohara, T.; Doi, T.; Hayakawa, J. Defective sweating responses in atopic dermatitis. *Curr. Probl. Dermatol.* **2011**, *41*, 68–79.
73. Hide, M.; Tanaka, T.; Yamamura, Y.; Koro, O.; Yamamoto, S. IgE-mediated hypersensitivity against human sweat antigen in patients with atopic dermatitis. *Acta. Derm. Venereol.* **2002**, *82*, 335–340. [CrossRef] [PubMed]
74. Hiragun, T.; Ishii, K.; Hiragun, M.; Suzuki, H.; Kan, T.; Mihara, S.; Yanase, Y.; Bartels, J.; Schröder, J.M.; Hide, M. Fungal protein MGL_1304 in sweat is an allergen for atopic dermatitis patients. *J. Allergy Clin. Immunol.* **2013**, *132*, 608–615. [CrossRef]
75. Murota, H.; Takahashi, A.; Nishioka, M.; Matsui, S.; Terao, M.; Kitaba, S.; Katayama, I. Showering reduces atopic dermatitis in elementary school students. *Eur. J. Dermatol.* **2010**, *20*, 4104–4111. [CrossRef] [PubMed]
76. Mochizuki, H.; Muramatsu, R.; Tadaki, H.; Mizuno, T.; Arakawa, H.; Morikawa, A. Effects of skin care with shower therapy on children with atopic dermatitis in elementary schools. *Pediatr. Dermatol.* **2009**, *26*, 223–225. [CrossRef] [PubMed]
77. Kabashima, K. New concept of the pathogenesis of atopic dermatitis: Interplay among the barrier, allergy, and pruritus as a trinity. *J. Dermatol. Sci.* **2013**, *70*, 3–11. [CrossRef] [PubMed]
78. Tamagawa-Mineoka, R.; Okuzawa, Y.; Masuda, K.; Katoh, N. Increased serum levels of interleukin 33 in patients with atopic dermatitis. *J. Am. Acad. Dermatol.* **2014**, *70*, 882–888. [CrossRef] [PubMed]
79. Nakamura, N.; Tamagawa-Mineoka, R.; Ueta, M.; Kinoshita, S.; Katoh, N. Toll-like receptor 3 increases allergic and irritant contact dermatitis. *J. Investig. Dermatol.* **2015**, *135*, 411–417. [CrossRef]
80. Yoon, J.; Leyva-Castillo, J.M.; Wang, G.; Galand, C.; Oyoshi, M.K.; Kumar, L.; Hoff, S.; He, R.; Chervonsky, A.; Oppenheim, J.J.; et al. IL-23 induced in keratinocytes by endogenous TLR4 ligands polarizes dendritic cells to drive IL-22 responses to skin immunization. *J. Exp. Med.* **2016**, *213*, 2147–2166. [CrossRef]
81. Bernard, J.J.; Cowing-Zitron, C.; Nakatsuji, T.; Muehleisen, B.; Muto, J.; Borkowski, A.W.; Martinez, L.; Greidinger, E.L.; Yu, B.D.; Gallo, R.L. Ultraviolet radiation damages self noncoding RNA and is detected by TLR3. *Nat. Med.* **2012**, *18*, 1286–1290. [CrossRef]
82. Tominaga, M.; Takamori, K. Itch and nerve fibers with special reference to atopic dermatitis: Therapeutic implications. *J. Dermatol.* **2014**, *41*, 205–212. [CrossRef]

83. Murota, H.; Katayama, I. Exacerbating factors of itch in atopic dermatitis. *Allergol. Int.* **2017**, *66*, 8–13. [CrossRef] [PubMed]
84. Meng, J.; Moriyama, M.; Feld, M.; Buddenkotte, J.; Buhl, T.; Szöllösi, A.; Zhang, J.; Miller, P.; Ghetti, A.; Fischer, M.; et al. New mechanism underlying IL-31–induced atopic dermatitis. *J. Allergy Clin. Immunol.* **2018**, *141*, 1677–1689. [CrossRef] [PubMed]
85. Gooderham, M.J.; Hong, H.C.; Eshtiaghi, P.; Papp, K.A. Dupilumab: A review of its use in the treatment of atopic dermatitis. *J. Am. Acad. Dermatol.* **2018**, *78*, S28–S36. [CrossRef]
86. Uchida, H.; Kamata, M.; Mizukawa, I.; Watanabe, A.; Agematsu, A.; Nagata, M.; Fukaya, S.; Hayashi, K.; Fukuyasu, A.; Tanaka, T.; et al. Real-world effectiveness and safety of dupilumab for the treatment of atopic dermatitis in Japanese patients: A single-centre retrospective study. *Br. J. Dermatol.* **2019**, *181*, 1083–1085. [CrossRef] [PubMed]
87. Wilson, S.R.; Thé, L.; Batia, L.M.; Beattie, K.; Katibah, G.E.; McClain, S.P.; Pellegrino, M.; Estandian, D.M.; Bautista, D.M. The epithelial cell-derived atopic dermatitis cytokine TSLP activates neurons to induce itch. *Cell* **2013**, *155*, 285–295. [CrossRef]
88. Bautista, D.M.; Wilson, S.R.; Hoon, M.A. Why we scratch an itch: The molecules, cells and circuits of itch. *Nat. Neurosci.* **2014**, *17*, 175–182. [CrossRef]
89. Steinhoff, M.; Neisius, U.; Ikoma, A.; Fartasch, M.; Heyer, G.; Skov, P.S.; Luger, T.A.; Schmelz, M. Proteinase-activated receptor-2 mediates itch: A novel pathway for pruritus in human skin. *J. Neurosci.* **2003**, *23*, 6176–6180. [CrossRef]
90. Kempkes, C.; Buddenkotte, J.; Cevikbas, F.; Buhl, T.; Steinhoff, M. Role of PAR-2 in Neuroimmune Communication and Itch. In *Itch: Mechanisms and Treatment*; Carstens, E., Akiyama, T., Eds.; CRC Press/Taylor & Francis: Boca Raton, FL, USA, 2014.
91. Hon, K.L.; Lam, M.C.; Wong, K.Y.; Leung, T.F.; Ng, P.C. Pathophysiology of nocturnal scratching in childhood atopic dermatitis: The role of brain-derived neurotrophic factor and substance P. *Br. J. Dermatol.* **2007**, *157*, 922–925. [CrossRef]
92. Heyer, G.; Hornstein, O.P.; Handwerker, H.O. Reactions to intradermally injected substance P and topically applied mustard oil in atopic dermatitis patients. *Acta. Derm. Venereol.* **1991**, *71*, 291–295.
93. Murota, H.; Izumi, M.; Abd El-Latif, M.I.; Nishioka, M.; Terao, M.; Tani, M.; Matsui, S.; Sano, S.; Katayama, I. Artemin causes hypersensitivity to warm sensation, mimicking warmth-provoked pruritus in atopic dermatitis. *J. Allergy. Clin. Immunol.* **2012**, *130*, 671–682. [CrossRef]
94. Heyer, G.; Vogelgsang, M.; Hornstein, O.P. Acetylcholine is an inducer of itching in patients with atopic eczema. *J. Dermatol.* **1997**, *24*, 621–625.
95. Tominaga, M.; Ozawa, S.; Tengara, S.; Ogawa, H.; Takamori, K. Intraepidermal nerve fibers increase in dry skin of acetone-treated mice. *J. Dermatol. Sci.* **2007**, *48*, 103–111.
96. Fujisawa, H. Discovery of semaphorin receptors, neuropilin and plexin, and their functions in neural development. *J. Neurobiol.* **2004**, *59*, 24–33. [CrossRef] [PubMed]
97. Tang, X.Q.; Tanelian, D.L.; Smith, G.M. Semaphorin 3A inhibits nerve growth factor-induced sprouting of nociceptive afferents in adult rat spinal cord. *J. Neurosci.* **2004**, *24*, 819–827. [CrossRef] [PubMed]
98. Bigliardi, P.L.; Bigliardi-Qi, M.; Buechner, S.; Rufli, T. Expression of mu-opiate receptor in human epidermis and keratinocytes. *J. Investig. Dermatol.* **1998**, *111*, 297–301. [CrossRef] [PubMed]
99. Kumagai, H.; Ebata, T.; Takamori, K.; Muramatsu, T.; Nakamoto, H.; Suzuki, H. Effect of a novel kappa-receptor agonist, nalfurafine hydrochloride, on severe itch in 337 haemodialysis patients: A Phase III, randomized, double-blind, placebo-controlled study. *Nephrol. Dial. Transplant.* **2010**, *25*, 1251–1257. [CrossRef] [PubMed]
100. Tominaga, M.; Ogawa, H.; Takamori, K. Possible roles of epidermal opioid systems in pruritus of atopic dermatitis. *J. Investig. Dermatol.* **2007**, *127*, 2228–2235. [CrossRef] [PubMed]
101. Hashizume, H.; Horibe, T.; Ohshima, A.; Ito, T.; Yagi, H.; Takigawa, M. Anxiety accelerates T-helper 2-tilted immune responses in patients with atopic dermatitis. *Br. J. Dermatol.* **2005**, *152*, 1161–1164. [CrossRef]
102. Hashiro, M.; Okumura, M. The relationship between the psychological and immunological state in patients with atopic dermatitis. *J. Dermatol. Sci.* **1998**, *16*, 231–235. [CrossRef]
103. Smolensky, M.H.; Portaluppi, F.; Manfredini, R.; Hermida, R.C.; Tiseo, R.; Sackett-Lundeen, L.L.; Haus, E.L. Diurnal and twenty-four hour patterning of human diseases: Acute and chronic common and uncommon medical conditions. *Sleep Med. Rev.* **2015**, *21*, 12–22. [CrossRef]

104. Hashiramoto, A.; Yamane, T.; Tsumiyama, K.; Yoshida, K.; Komai, K.; Yamada, H.; Yamazaki, F.; Doi, M.; Okamura, H.; Shiozawa, S. Mammalian clock gene Cryptochrome regulates arthritis via proinflammatory cytokine TNF-alpha. *J. Immunol.* **2010**, *184*, 1560–1565. [CrossRef]
105. Nakamura, Y.; Harama, D.; Shimokawa, N.; Hara, M.; Suzuki, R.; Tahara, Y.; Ishimaru, K.; Katoh, R.; Okumura, K.; Ogawa, H.; et al. Circadian clock gene Period2 regulates a time-of-day-dependent variation in cutaneous anaphylactic reaction. *J. Allergy Clin. Immunol.* **2011**, *127*, 1038–1045. [CrossRef] [PubMed]
106. Takita, E.; Yokota, S.; Tahara, Y.; Hirao, A.; Aoki, N.; Nakamura, Y.; Nakao, A.; Shibata, S. Biological clock dysfunction exacerbates contact hypersensitivity in mice. *Br. J. Dermatol.* **2013**, *168*, 39–46. [CrossRef] [PubMed]
107. Mizutani, H.; Tamagawa-Mineoka, R.; Minami, Y.; Yagita, K.; Katoh, N. Constant light exposure impairs immune tolerance development in mice. *J. Dermatol. Sci.* **2017**, *86*, 63–70. [CrossRef] [PubMed]

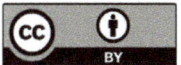

© 2020 by the authors. Licensee MDPI, Basel, Switzerland. This article is an open access article distributed under the terms and conditions of the Creative Commons Attribution (CC BY) license (http://creativecommons.org/licenses/by/4.0/).

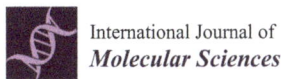

Review

Aryl Hydrocarbon Receptor in Atopic Dermatitis and Psoriasis

Masutaka Furue [1,2,3,*], Akiko Hashimoto-Hachiya [1,2] and Gaku Tsuji [1,2]

[1] Department of Dermatology, Graduate School of Medical Sciences, Kyushu University, Maidashi 3-1-1, Higashiku, Fukuoka 812-8582, Japan; ahachi@dermatol.med.kyushu-u.ac.jp (A.H.-H.); gakku@dermatol.med.kyushu-u.ac.jp (G.T.)
[2] Research and Clinical Center for Yusho and Dioxin, Kyushu University, Maidashi 3-1-1, Higashiku, Fukuoka 812-8582, Japan
[3] Division of Skin Surface Sensing, Graduate School of Medical Sciences, Kyushu University, Maidashi 3-1-1, Higashiku, Fukuoka 812-8582, Japan
* Correspondence: furue@dermatol.med.kyushu-u.ac.jp; Tel.: +81-92-642-5581; Fax: +81-92-642-5600

Received: 15 October 2019; Accepted: 25 October 2019; Published: 31 October 2019

Abstract: The aryl hydrocarbon receptor (AHR)/AHR-nuclear translocator (ARNT) system is a sensitive sensor for small molecular, xenobiotic chemicals of exogenous and endogenous origin, including dioxins, phytochemicals, microbial bioproducts, and tryptophan photoproducts. AHR/ARNT are abundantly expressed in the skin. Once activated, the AHR/ARNT axis strengthens skin barrier functions and accelerates epidermal terminal differentiation by upregulating filaggrin expression. In addition, AHR activation induces oxidative stress. However, some AHR ligands simultaneously activate the nuclear factor-erythroid 2-related factor-2 (NRF2) transcription factor, which is a master switch of antioxidative enzymes that neutralizes oxidative stress. The immunoregulatory system governing T-helper 17/22 (Th17/22) and T regulatory cells (Treg) is also regulated by the AHR system. Notably, AHR agonists, such as tapinarof, are currently used as therapeutic agents in psoriasis and atopic dermatitis. In this review, we summarize recent topics on AHR related to atopic dermatitis and psoriasis.

Keywords: aryl hydrocarbon receptor (AHR); aryl hydrocarbon receptor-nuclear translocator (ARNT); nuclear factor-erythroid 2-related factor-2 (NRF2); atopic dermatitis; psoriasis; tapinarof; filaggrin; skin barrier; Th17; Th22; Treg; reactive oxygen species; antioxidants

1. Introduction

The skin is the outermost surface of the body and is vulnerable to a myriad of external chemicals and internal substances. To maintain homeostasis, skin cells, including keratinocytes, sebocytes, fibroblasts, dendritic cells, and other immune cells, express several chemical sensors, such as aryl hydrocarbon receptor (AHR), pregnane X receptor, constitutive androstane receptor, and peroxisome proliferator-activated receptors [1–4]. Among these chemical receptors, AHR has gained special attention because it plays a crucial role in photoaging, epidermal differentiation, and immunomodulation [2,3,5–7].

AHR, also called dioxin receptor, binds to environmental polyaromatic hydrocarbons and dioxins with high affinity and induces oxidative stress by generating abundant reactive oxygen species (ROS) [5–7]. Additionally, AHR is a promiscuous receptor and is activated by a plethora of exogenous and endogenous ligands, such as photo-induced chromophores, phytochemicals, and microbial bioproducts [8–12]. Many AHR ligands exert antioxidative activity by activating antioxidative transcription factor nuclear factor-erythroid 2-related factor-2 (NRF2) [10,13]. Medicinal coal tar and soybean tar Glyteer activate both AHR and NRF2 and have been used to treat inflammatory skin diseases, such as atopic dermatitis (AD) and psoriasis [14,15].

AD and psoriasis are common inflammatory skin diseases. An excellent therapeutic response to biologics indicates a pivotal pathogenic role of interleukin (IL)-4/IL-13 signaling in AD [16,17] and the tumor necrosis factor (TNF)-α/IL-23/IL-17A axis in psoriasis [18,19]. Although distinct signaling pathways operate in developing full-blown AD and psoriasis, 81% of dysregulated genes in AD are shared with those in psoriasis in skin lesions [20]. Notably, recent phase II, randomized dose-finding studies have demonstrated that topical application of the natural AHR agonist tapinarof is efficacious and well tolerated in patients with AD and psoriasis [21,22].

The purpose of this article is to summarize the diverse action of AHR signaling in balancing skin homeostasis and to elucidate the fundamental mechanisms of therapeutic AHR potentials in the treatment of AD and psoriasis.

2. AHR Signaling and Modulation of Oxidative and Antioxidative Balance

AHR is a ligand-activated transcription factor [7]. In the absence of ligands, AHR resides in the cytoplasm where it forms a protein complex with heat shock protein 90 (HSP90), hepatitis B virus X-associated protein 2 (XAP-2), and p23 [23,24]. After ligand binding, AHR dissociates from the cytoplasmic complex and a nuclear translocation site of AHR is exposed. Then, AHR is translocated into the nucleus where AHR dimerizes with AHR-nuclear translocator (ARNT), binds DNA responsive elements called xenobiotic responsive elements (XREs), and upregulates the transcription of target genes, such as phase I metabolizing enzyme cytochrome P450 (CYP) members (i.e., *CYP1A1*, *CYP1A2*, and *CYP1B1*) [7,25–29].

Hazardous dioxins such as 2,3,7,8,-tetrachlorodibenzo-p-dioxin (TCDD) activate AHR and upregulate CYP1A1, CYP1A2, and CYP1B1 expression [5,30,31]. Human keratinocytes abundantly express CYP1A1 and to a lesser extent CYP1B1 but not CYP1A2 [32]. CYP1A1 attempts to metabolize TCDD but the continuous efforts of CYP1A1 are unsuccessful because TCDD is structurally stable [33]. The metabolizing process by CYP1A1 generates excessive amounts of ROS and induces oxidative damage in the cell [5,30,31] (Figure 1). To demonstrate these findings, TCDD-induced ROS production was inhibited in AHR-silenced or CYP1A1-silenced cells [30]. As CYP1B1 silencing did not affect TCDD-induced ROS generation, the AHR-CYP1A1 axis is likely to be crucial for generating cellular oxidative stress by hazardous dioxins [30]. A chemical carcinogen β-naphthoflavone also activates CYP1A1 and CYP1A2 via AHR activation in mice [34]. β-Naphthoflavone induces mitochondrial ROS generation. However, this activation is attenuated by an AHR inhibitor or CYP1A1/1A2 silencing [34]. AHR-CYP1A1-mediated oxidative stress is responsible at least in part for the production of proinflammatory cytokines, such as interleukin (IL)-1, IL-6, and IL-8 [35,36].

To survive during oxidative stress, antioxidative machinery is simultaneously activated after AHR activation in the cells. Ligation of AHR also activates antioxidative transcription factor NRF2 and upregulates the expression of phase II antioxidative enzymes (i.e., glutathione S-transferases, heme oxygenase 1 (HMOX1), NAD(P)H dehydrogenase, quinone 1 (NQO1), glutathione S-transferases, and uridine 5′-diphospho-glucuronosyltransferases [13,14,25,26,37–40]. In contrast to proinflammatory consequences after AHR-CYP1A1-ROS induction, the AHR-NRF2 axis is likely to be anti-inflammatory and reduces the production of proinflammatory cytokines [13,39,41]. Many salubrious antioxidative phytochemical extracts (i.e., artichoke (*Cynara scolymus*) in Mediterranean regions, *Opuntia ficus-indica* in Latin America, and *Houttuynia cordata* in Asia) activate the AHR-NRF2 system and upregulate the expression of antioxidative enzymes [13,37,38]. Dioxins activate the AHR-NRF2 battery [40,42,43], however, their powerful AHR-CYP1A1 activation may induce far more oxidative stress that cannot be extinguished by the AHR-NRF2 antioxidative system. Alternatively, salubrious phytochemical AHR ligands stimulate the AHR-NRF2 axis more strongly than the AHR-CYP1A1-ROS pathway and exert antioxidative action [10].

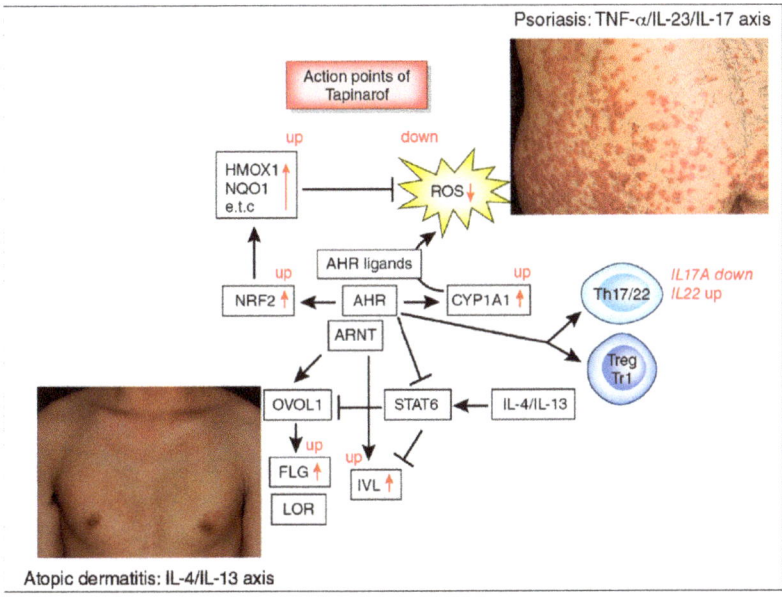

Figure 1. Aryl hydrocarbon receptor (AHR) signal and action points of tapinarof (red words and arrows). AHR is a promiscuous chemical sensor that is activated by various oxidative and antioxidative ligands. Once activated, cytoplasmic AHR translocates into the nucleus where it heterodimerizes with an AHR-nuclear translocator (ARNT) and then induces the transcription of AHR-responsive genes such as cytochrome P450 1A1 (CYP1A1). CYP1A1 degrades AHR ligands. Some ligands such as dioxins are chemically stable and long-lived. Therefore, CYP1A1 generates high amounts of reactive oxygen species (ROS) after sustained efforts to degrade them. Some antioxidative AHR ligands activate nuclear factor-erythroid 2-related factor-2 (NRF2) transcription factor, which upregulates gene expression of various antioxidative enzymes, such as heme oxygenase 1 (HMOX1), NAD(P)H dehydrogenase, and quinone 1 (NQO1), and these antioxidative enzymes neutralize ROS. AHR/ARNT signaling also activates OVO-like 1 (OVOL1) transcription factor and upregulates the expression of filaggrin (FLG) and loricrin (LOR). AHR upregulates the expression of involucrin (IVL) in an OVOL1-independent manner. Therefore, AHR/ARNT signaling accelerates epidermal terminal differentiation and enhances the repair of barrier disruption. Interleukin (IL)-4 and IL-13 activate signal transducer and activator of transcription 6 (STAT6) and inhibit the OVOL1/FLG, OVOL1/LOR, and AHR/IVL axes. However, suitable AHR activation can inhibit the IL-4/IL-13-mediated STAT6 activation and restore the expression of FLG, LOR, and IVL. Regarding immune response, AHR signaling affects T-helper (Th17) differentiation and is essential for IL-22 production. AHR ligation (especially by high concentrations of ligands) induces the differentiation of regulatory cell populations, Treg and Tr1 cells. Tapinarof is an antioxidative AHR ligand and upregulates CYP1A1 expression. Topical tapinarof is efficacious in psoriasis and atopic dermatitis. Current studies demonstrate that tapinarof activates NRF2/antioxidative signaling and reduces oxidative stress. Tapinarof also upregulates FLG and IVL expression. Tapinarof downregulates IL-17A production and increases IL-22 production.

3. AHR and Epidermal Terminal Differentiation

The mammalian epidermis protects the body against injuries from external and environmental factors by providing a barrier-forming cornified layer. Epidermal terminal differentiation or cornified envelope maturation is accomplished by sequential cross-linking of ceramides and various terminal differentiation proteins, such as involucrin (IVL), loricrin (LOR), and filaggrin (FLG) by transglutaminase-1; the majority of these skin barrier-forming proteins map to chromosome 1q21 [44,45].

Notably, activation of the AHR-ARNT axis accelerates epidermal terminal differentiation by coordinately upregulating the production of a series of skin barrier-forming proteins in vivo [46] and in vitro [3,44,47,48]. In parallel, both *Ahr*-deficient and *Ahr*-transgenic mice reveal an abnormality in keratinization [49,50]. Severe abnormalities in keratinization are also observed in *Arnt*-deficient mice [51,52].

Both oxidative and antioxidative ligands for AHR can accelerate epidermal terminal differentiation [3,12,44,47,48]. Slow-metabolizing dioxins induce strong and sustained AHR activation, which results in exaggerated keratinization of keratinocytes and sebocytes and the development of chloracne [2,53]. In contrast, mild and transient AHR activation by antioxidative phytochemical or endogenous AHR ligands are effective in maintaining healthy barrier-intact skin [3,10,54].

Sunlight, especially UVB, generates tryptophan photoderivatives such as formylindolo[3,2-b]carbazole (FICZ), which is a high-affinity ligand for AHR that upregulates CYP1A1 expression [8,55–57]. Compared with slow-metabolizing TCDD, FICZ is rapidly metabolized by CYP1A1 [8,55,56]. Similar to other AHR ligands, FICZ upregulates filaggrin via AHR signaling [57–59]. Although an erythematogenic dose of UVB is harmful through a variety of mechanisms, exposure to a suberythematous dose of UVB prior to tape-stripping results in significantly accelerated barrier recovery rates [60]. Physiological low-dose UVB exposure may be beneficial for skin barrier protection by FICZ-AHR/ARNT-mediated upregulation of filaggrin and other barrier-related proteins [57–59] (Figure 1). In this context, topical application of FICZ significantly attenuated transepidermal water loss and dermatitis score in a murine mite-induced dermatitis model [58].

Mechanisms regarding how AHR signaling accelerates keratinocyte differentiation are not fully understood. Kennedy et al. points to an essential role of ROS production in this regulation [47]. We have demonstrated that AHR signaling upregulates the expression of OVO-like 1 (OVOL1) transcription factor and activates its cytoplasmic to nuclear translocation [3,59,61,62]. Both filaggrin and loricrin are under the control of the AHR-OVOL1 pathway, whereas AHR-mediated involucrin upregulation is independent of OVOL1 [63].

IL-4/IL-13 signaling downregulates the expression of filaggrin, loricrin, and involucrin via signal transducer and activator of transcription 6 (STAT6) activation, impairing the epidermal terminal differentiation and barrier dysfunction [14,15,37,44,61,64,65]. IL-4/IL-13 signaling is likely to impair the cytoplasmic to nuclear translocation of OVOL1, which interferes with the AHR-OVOL1-filaggrin axis [59,61]. Notably, IL-4/IL-13 signaling reciprocally enhances the protein expression of AHR and to a lesser extent ARNT in keratinocytes (Figure 2). Similar results were observed in murine B cells [66]. The implication of IL-4/IL-13-mediated AHR upregulation remains elusive. In addition, IL-4/IL-13-mediated STAT6 activation stimulates keratinocyte to produce periostin, which induces IL-24 production in keratinocytes [67]. IL-24 reduces the filaggrin expression via STAT3 activation [67]. AHR ligands, such as coal tar, Glyteer and FICZ, activate the AHR/ARNT pathway, block the IL-4/IL-13-mediated STAT6 activation, induce the entry of OVOL1 into the nuclei, and restore barrier dysfunction [15,59,61,68].

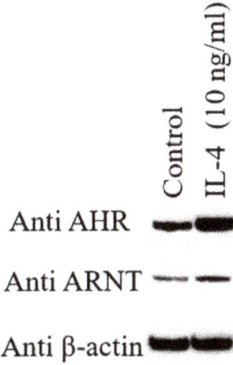

Figure 2. Human epidermal keratinocytes are stimulated with 10 ng/mL of IL-4 augments the protein expression of aryl hydrocarbon receptor (AHR) and AHR-nuclear translocator (ARNT) compared with untreated control by Western blot analysis.

4. AHR and Immune Modulation

As a crucial chemosensor, AHR activity modulates immune function. AHR and its immunological significance are best characterized in intestinal immunology [28,29,69,70]. *Ahr*-deficient mice have an inherent weak gut barrier [71–73]. In this context, genome-wide association studies have identified AHR as a susceptibility locus in inflammatory bowel diseases [74]. Indeed, the expression of AHR is reduced in the lesioned intestine in inflammatory bowel diseases [75]. This finding may be strongly related to the fact that the intestinal tract is a rich source of AHR ligands derived from dietary materials and microbial bioproducts [69,76].

Early research on AHR-mediated immune modulation was based on toxicological approaches using dioxins [77]. Dioxin-exposed rodents exhibit waste syndrome, dose-dependent thymic involution, depletion of other lymphoid organs, and reduced circulating lymphocyte counts [77]. Antibody production by B cells is also inhibited by toxic doses of dioxins [77]. However, extensive attention by immunologists has recently been focused on the physiological function of AHR in immune regulation [29,69,70,76].

Ligation of AHR by TCDD and endogenous or natural compounds preferentially affects differentiation and propagation of T-helper 17 (Th17) and T regulatory (Treg) cells [29,69,70]. Tryptophan is an essential amino acid and is thought to produce various candidates for endogenous AHR ligands by different metabolic processes. These metabolic pathways include kynurenine production by indoleamine 2,3-dioxygenase and tryptophan 2,3-dioxygenase, FICZ by UVB exposure, and indole derivatives by bacterial degradation [29,69,70]. Dietary materials such as *Brasicca* contain glucosinolate glucobrassicin, which is metabolized to produce indolo-[3,2-b]-carbazole (ICZ) [29]. The major metabolic pathway of tryptophan is the kynurenine pathway, however, the binding capacity of kynurenine to AHR is very low compared to FICZ and ICZ [29].

In murine CD4$^+$ cells, AHR is highly expressed in Th17 cells, not detectable in Th1 and Th2 cells, and marginally expressed in Treg cells [78]. In addition, Lin-Sca$^+$ and Sca$^-$ progenitor cells in bone marrow, double negative (CD4$^-$ and CD8$^-$) cells in the thymus, innate lymphoid cell type 3 (ILC3) cells, dendritic cells, γδ T cells, and Langerhans cells express high levels of AHR [28,29]. In *Ahr*-deficient mice, *T-bet* and *Ifng* expression in Th1, *Gata3* and *Il4* expression in Th2, and RORγt (*Rorc*) and *Il17a/Il17f* expression in Th17 cells are not significantly affected. However, *Il22* expression in Th17 cells is almost completely abrogated in *Ahr*-deficient mice [78]. FICZ upregulates *Il17a*, *Il17f*, and *Il22* expression in Th17 cells. The expression of AHR is detected in human Th17 cells at higher levels than in Th1 cells and FICZ upregulates the *IL17A*, *IL17F*, and *IL22* expression in Th17 cells [78]. Flowcytometric analysis also revealed that FICZ enhances Th17 differentiation and IL-22 production [69]. In a murine

Th17-mediated experimental autoimmune encephalomyelitis model, injection of FICZ accelerated disease onset whereas it was delayed in *Ahr*-deficient mice. Treg cells were unaffected in this model [78]. In contrast, TCDD treatment increased the number of Treg cells, which exhibited an immunosuppressive function in a murine graft-versus-host disease model [79]. The TCDD-induced increase in Treg number was abrogated in *Ahr*-deficient mice [79]. These studies suggest that prolonged activation of AHR by TCDD may potentiate Treg cell deviation, but transient AHR activation may shift the immune response toward Th17 and more strongly to Th22 cell differentiation (Figure 1).

Th17 and ILC3 cells express high levels of AHR, IL-17, and IL-22 and are crucial for intestinal protective immunity against commensal and pathogenic microbiota [80]. In contrast to the abovementioned experimental autoimmune encephalomyelitis model in which AHR ligation enhances IL-17 and IL-22 production, *Ahr*-deficiency augments Th17 cell differentiation in the intestinal tract where large amounts of dietary- and microbiota-derived AHR ligands are present [80]. In *Ahr*-deficient mice, the amount of microbiota is significantly increased, which is likely to promote Th17 differentiation. Alternatively, *Ahr*-deficient mice exhibit IL-22 reduction, which is consistently found in an experimental autoimmune encephalomyelitis model. Notably, IL-22 supplementation to *Ahr*-deficient mice normalizes the expansion of the microbiota and reduces Th17 deviation, demonstrating that IL-22 is protective against intestinal infection [80]. In addition, ILC3s produce larger amounts of IL-22 than Th17 cells after AHR ligation [80].

In the gut, heterogenous cell populations exist in Foxp3$^+$ Treg cells depending on the expression of neuropilin (Nrp1) and RORγt. Nrp1 is a surface marker to distinguish thymus-derived Tregs (Nrp1$^+$ tTregs) versus peripherally derived Tregs (Nrp1$^-$ pTregs) [70]. In the small and large intestines, all Nrp1$^+$ RORγt$^-$, Nrp1$^-$ RORγt$^+$ and Nrp1$^-$ RORγt$^-$ Treg subpopulations express high levels of AHR [70]. *Ahr* deficiency in these Treg cells induces a significant decrease of Nrp1$^-$ RORγt$^+$ and Nrp1$^-$ RORγt$^-$, but not Nrp1$^+$ RORγt$^-$, Treg subpopulations in the intestine, whereas those in the spleen and mesenteric lymph nodes are not affected [70]. In contrast, AHR activation by FICZ injection preferentially enhances the Nrp1$^-$ RORγt$^-$ Treg subpopulation. High-throughput RNA sequencing revealed that *Ccr6*, *Gpr15*, *Itgae*, *Rgs9*, and *Gzma* genes important for Treg homing and functions in the gut are downregulated in *Ahr*-deficient Tregs while Th1-associated genes *Ifng*, *Ccl5*, and *Tbx21* are upregulated. Moreover, these AHR-expressing Treg cells inhibit T cell-induced wasting disease and colitis [70].

As described above, AHR ligation induces the CYP1A1 production, which efficiently degrades AHR ligands [28,29]. Therefore, constitutive overexpression of CYP1A1 in mice depletes the reservoir of natural AHR ligands, generating a quasi *Ahr*-deficient state [76]. Th17 cells from *Ahr*-deficient mice do not produce IL-22. In parallel, *Cyp1a1*-overexpressed Th17 cells show a reduced IL-22 production [76]. Both *Ahr*-deficient and *Cyp1a1*-overexpressed mice exhibit loss of ILC3 in the small and large intestines. IL-22 derived from ILC3 and Th17 cells is essential in the defense against *Citrobacter rodentium*. Thus, *C. rodentium*-induced colitis becomes life-threatening both in *Ahr*-deficient and *Cyp1a1*-overexpressed mice [76]. Although AHR ligation upregulates CYP1A1, CYP1B1, and CYP1A2 expression, CYP1B1 and CYP1A2 are not crucial for degrading AHR ligands [76]. FICZ-mediated Th17 differentiation and IL-22 production is achieved by extremely low concentrations of FICZ in *Cyp1a1*-deficient CD4$^+$ cells [69]. Furthermore, FICZ promotes IL-17A$^+$ IL-22$^+$, but not IL-17$^+$ IL-22$^-$, cell differentiation [69].

Although AHR ligation tends to affect Th17 and Treg cell differentiation, outcomes are inconsistent in different experimental systems. The dose and the duration of AHR activation by high-affinity AHR ligands are likely the primary factors that explain the fate of T cell differentiation [81]. To this end, Ehrlich et al. examined the effects of low and high doses of four high-affinity AHR ligands (TCDD, FICZ, 2-(1H-Indol-3-ylcarbonyl)-4-thiazolecarboxylic acid (ITE), and 11-Chloro-7H-benzo[de]benzo[4,5]imidazo[2,1-a]isoquinolin-7-one (11-Cl-BBQ)) on CD4$^+$ T cell differentiation using a parent-into-F1 alloresponse mouse model. Intraperitoneal injection of high doses of all agents induced the production of IL-10 producing, Foxp3$^+$ type 1 regulatory T cells (Tr1 cells) on day 2, and increased Foxp3+ Tregs on day 10 in conjunction with suppression of the alloresponse. Alternatively, low doses of the ligands, even when given daily, did not induce Tregs nor alter the alloresponse, but instead increased the percentage of CD4+ cells that produce IL-17 [81]. In summary, accumulating evidence suggests that AHR ligation stimulates Th17 cells to differentiate into Th17/22 cells. AHR ligands may also enhance the regulatory cell population especially in high doses.

5. AHR and Atopic Dermatitis

AD is a common and heterogenous eczematous skin disorder characterized by Th2-deviated skin inflammation, barrier disruption, and chronic pruritus [17,82,83]. Frequent relapse with intense pruritus deteriorates quality of life and decreases treatment satisfaction of the afflicted patients [84–88]. The lifetime incidence of AD is as high as 20% in the general population [89]. Skin barrier dysfunction is associated with the reduced production of terminal differentiation molecules such as filaggrin [15,51]. Abnormal skin barrier integrity also causes an increased colonization of microbes such as *Staphylococcus aureus*, which further exacerbate Th2-deviated skin inflammation [90,91]. In addition, some autoimmune diseases are comorbid with AD [92].

Investigation on *AHR* gene polymorphism reveals that *AHR* rs10249788 and rs2066853 polymorphisms are found in patients with AD, psoriasis, and healthy controls, but no significant differences were detected in genotype or allele frequencies between the three groups [93]. However, the *AHR* rs2066853 (AG + AA) or rs10249788 (CT + TT) genotypes are a risk factor for severe dry skin phenotype and the combined rs10249788 (CT + TT) and rs2066853 (AG + AA) genotypes lead to a higher risk for severe dry skin in Chinese patients with AD [93]. rs10249788 exists in the AHR promoter region where nuclear factor 1C (NF1C) binds and suppresses the transcription and protein expression of AHR [94]. Notably, NF1C prefers to associate with the C allele compared to the T allele at rs10249788. Thus, subjects with the rs10249788 (CC) allele express less AHR than those with the rs10249788 (TT) allele [94]. In fact, AHR mRNA levels for the TT genotype are 1.7-fold higher than those for the CC genotype [95]. No significant differences were obtained in AHR production between the CC and CT genotypes [95]. In parallel with increased levels of AHR, cells with the TT genotype express significantly higher levels of CYP1A1, IL-24, and IL-1β [95]. It is intriguing that IL-24 downregulates the filaggrin expression via STAT3 activation [67].

Immunohistological and real time PCR studies for AHR have been reported in AD [96,97]. Hong et al. showed an increased expression of both AHR and ARNT without CYP1A1 induction in the lesioned skin of AD compared with normal control skin [96]. Alternatively, Kim et al. demonstrated an increased expression of ARNT and CYP1A1 but not AHR in the lesional skin of AD [97]. As the Th2-deviated milieu potently reduces filaggrin and other barrier-related molecules, the upregulation of AHR/ARNT may be compensatory to attenuate the Th2-mediated filaggrin reduction. A recent study by Yu et al. demonstrated the possibility that the Th2-deviated milieu decreases the production of endogenous AHR ligand such as indole-3-aldehyde by commensal skin microbiota [98]. These findings collectively suggest that most AHR likely lack physiological ligands in the Th2-prone milieu in AD. Therefore, rapid-metabolizing AHR ligands, such as FICZ and indole-3-aldehyde, appropriately activate the AHR/ARNT/FLG axis and may be beneficial in treating AD [58,98]. However, vigorous and long-lasting activation of the AHR/ARNT/FLG axis by slow-metabolizing dioxins and environmental pollutants may exacerbate barrier dysfunction and aggravate AD [96,99].

Although the pathogenic implication of AHR and its gene polymorphism in AD remain elusive, recent clinical trials using topical AHR ligand tapinarof have reported its efficacy for AD [100–102]. Tapinarof (5-[(E)-2-phenylethenyl]-2-[propan-2-yl] benzene-1, 3-diol, WBI-1001, GSK2894512 or bentivimod) is a naturally derived (but is now a fully synthetic) hydroxylated stilbene produced by bacterial symbionts of entomopathogenic nematodes [100–103]. Tapinarof is a high affinity AHR ligand with antioxidative activity via NRF2 activation and a ROS-scavenging structure [102] (Figure 1). Tapinarof has gained increased attention because its topical application is efficacious for patients with AD in clinical trials [21,100,104]. Tapinarof activates the AHR/CYP1A1 axis and augments the expression of filaggrin and involucrin [102]. Even in barrier-disrupted AD patients, systemic absorption of topical tapinarof is limited and likely decreases during the treatment course in parallel with treatment success that restores the barrier dysfunction [104]. In general, topical tapinarof is tolerable but frequent adverse events include headaches and folliculitis [104].

In an early clinical trial, patients with AD affecting 3–20% of their body surface area (BSA) and with an Investigator's Global Assessment (IGA; 0: clear, 1: almost clear, 2: mild, 3: moderate, 4: severe, 5: very severe) of 2–4 were randomized (1:1:1) to receive a placebo ($n = 51$), topical tapinarof 0.5% ($n = 50$) or 1% ($n = 47$) in a cream formulation applied twice daily for six weeks [100]. There was a decrease of 1.3 (43%; $p < 0.001$; 95% confidence interval (CI) −1.2 to −0.5) and 1.8 (56.3%; $p < 0.001$; 95% CI −1.6 to −0.9) in IGA at day 42 in the topical tapinarof 0.5% and 1% groups, respectively, compared with a decrease of 0.5 (14.7%) in the placebo group. At day 42, improvement in Eczema Area and Severity Index (EASI) score was 68.9% ($p < 0.001$) and 76.3% ($p < 0.001$) for tapinarof 0.5% and 1%, respectively, compared with 23.3% for placebo. Improvement in pruritus severity score at day 42 was 29.8% ($p < 0.001$) and 66.9% ($p < 0.001$) for tapinarof 0.5% and 1%, respectively, compared with 9.5% for placebo [100]. Adverse events included headaches (placebo: 0%; 0.5% tapinarof: 8%; 1% tapinarof: 14%), migraines (placebo: 0%; 0.5% tapinarof: 4%; 1% tapinarof: 3%), folliculitis (placebo: 0%; 0.5% tapinarof: 6%; 1% tapinarof: 8%), and contact dermatitis (placebo: 0%; 0.5% tapinarof: 3%: 1% tapinarof: 5%) [100].

A phase II, double-blind, vehicle-controlled, randomized, six-arm trial (1:1:1:1:1:1) in patients aged 12 to 65 years, with BSA involvement of at least 5% to 35% and an IGA score of 3 or higher (moderate to severe) at baseline was performed. Primary end points included an IGA score of clear or almost clear (0 or 1) and a minimum two-grade improvement (treatment success) at week 12 [21]. The rates of treatment success with topical tapinarof cream at week 12 were 53% (1% twice daily, $n = 40$), 46% (1% once daily, $n = 41$), 37% (0.5% twice daily, $n = 43$), 34% (0.5% once daily, $n = 41$), 24% (vehicle twice daily, $n = 42$), and 28% (vehicle once daily, $n = 40$). The rate with tapinarof 1% twice daily (53%) was statistically significantly higher than the rate with vehicle twice daily (24%). Notably, treatment success was maintained for four weeks after the end of tapinarof treatment. The proportion of patients achieving EASI75 (75% or greater improvement in EASI) score reduction at week 12 was significantly higher in the groups treated with 1% tapinarof (60% and 51% for twice daily and once daily, respectively) than with vehicle (26% and 25% in the groups receiving vehicle twice daily and once daily, respectively) [21]. Headaches (e.g., 10% (1% twice daily), 2% (0.5% twice daily), and 0% (0.5% twice daily)) and folliculitis (e.g., 10% (1% twice daily), 7% (0.5% twice daily), and 0% (0.5% twice daily)) were again frequent adverse events [21].

In a murine dermatitis model, topically applied FICZ activated AHR and significantly reduced the dermatitis score and histological inflammation with a decrease of *Il22* gene expression in chronic mite antigen-induced dermatitis [58]. In addition, topical FICZ restored the dermatitis-induced filaggrin downregulation [58]. CCL17 and CCL22 are crucial chemokines to recruit Th2 cells [68]. IL-4/IL-13 stimulates dendritic cells to produce CCL17 and CCL22 via STAT6 activation and contributes to the recruitment of Th2 cells in the lesional skin of AD [68]. Soybean tar Glyteer inhibits the IL-4/IL-13-mediated STAT6 activation and subsequent production of CCL17 and CCL22 in dendritic cells [68]. In addition, pruritogenic Th2 cytokine IL-31 synergistically upregulates the IL-4/IL-13-mediated CCL17 and CCL22 production in dendritic cells because IL-4/IL-13 increase IL-31 receptor A (IL31RA) expression [105]. Glyteer again attenuates the IL-4/IL-13-mediated IL31RA upregulation and subsequent CCL17 and CCL22 production by inhibiting STAT6 activation [105]. It is known that coal tar inhibits STAT6 activation via the NRF2-antioxidative pathway [15]. Ligation of AHR by FICZ also reduces the expression of type 1 IgE Fc receptor in Langerhans cells [106].

Although antioxidative AHR ligands are therapeutic for dermatitis, exaggerated activation of AHR by genetic manipulation in transgenic mice or by dioxin treatment induces itchy dermatitis most likely due to an abnormally accelerated keratinization process, epidermal acanthosis, elongation of nerve fibers, and production of pruritogenic artemin [47,99,107]. Therefore, extreme activation of AHR is deleterious for skin. In parallel, ovalbumin-induced delayed hypersensitivity is enhanced by topical benzopyrene with upregulation of IL-5, IL-13, and IL-17 expression in lymph node cells [96].

Since FICZ is an endogenous UVB photoproduct [8], the barrier-protecting effects of FICZ may explain, at least in part, why UVB phototherapy is efficacious for the treatment of AD and psoriasis [108,109].

6. AHR and Psoriasis

Psoriasis is an (auto)immune-mediated disease that manifests as widespread desquamative erythema [110,111]. Males are twice as likely to be affected than females [112,113]. The cosmetic disfigurement associated with psoriasis profoundly impairs the patients' quality of life, treatment satisfaction and adherence, and socioeconomic stability [114,115]. The autoimmune nature of psoriasis is exemplified by its high comorbidity with psoriatic arthritis [110,116–118] and other autoimmune diseases including autoimmune bullous diseases [119–124]. Psoriasis is also comorbid with cardiovascular diseases, metabolic diseases, and renal disorders, which represent a condition called inflammatory skin march [111,125–129]. The excellent therapeutic efficacy of anti-TNF-α/IL-23/IL-17A biologics for psoriasis point to the central role of the TNF-α/IL-23/IL-17A axis in its pathogenesis [18,19,130–134] Additionally, genetic and environmental factors are known to be involved in its pathogenesis [135,136].

As AHR predominantly regulates the immune balance of Th17/22 and Treg cells [28,29,69,70], AHR is expected to play a significant role in psoriasis [102]. In an imiquimod-induced psoriasis model, *AhR* deficiency exacerbates skin inflammation with upregulated gene expression of *Il22*, *Il17a*, and *Il23* [137]. The intensity of delayed type-hypersensitivity is also enhanced in *Ahr*-deficient mice [137]. However, further experiments demonstrated that *Ahr*-deficiency in nonhematopoietic cells, including keratinocytes, but not in hematopoietic cells, was likely responsible for the exacerbation of inflammation [137]. Notably, intraperitoneal injection of FICZ ameliorated the imiquimod-induced psoriasis-like inflammation. Tapinarof and FICZ also reduced the imiquimod-induced psoriasiform skin inflammation by inhibiting *Il17a*, *Il17f*, *Il19*, *Il22*, *Il23a*, and *Il1b* gene expression [102]. The therapeutic action of tapinarof and FICZ was AHR-dependent because it was not observed in *Ahr*-deficient mice [102]. In an ex vivo activation assay of skin-resident immunocompetent cells using normal human skin, tapinarof inhibited the expression of *IL17A* message approximately 50% but increased the *IL22* expression [102,138] (Figure 1). In mice, IL-22 is produced from Th17, $\gamma\delta$T, ILC3, and CD4$^-$CD8$^-$TCRβ^+ cells [139]. AHR was required for IL-22 production by Th17, but not by the three other cell types, in the imiquimod-treated ears [139]. Although imiquimod-induced skin inflammation is popular as a psoriasis model, attention should be paid because imiquimod is degraded by CYP1A1 so the efficacy of AHR agonists may partly rely on this effect in the imiquimod model [140].

Immunohistological and real time PCR studies have demonstrated that the expression of AHR and ARNT is upregulated in the lesional skin of psoriasis, whereas CYP1A1 expression was significantly decreased compared to normal controls [97]. In contrast, serum levels of both AHR and CYP1A1 are elevated in patients with psoriasis compared to normal controls [141]. Further studies are warranted to investigate these controversial data.

In parallel with its preclinical studies, topical tapinarof is efficacious in the treatment of psoriasis. In a randomized, double-blind, placebo-controlled phase II trial, 61 patients with 1–10% BSA covered with plaque psoriasis and a PGA of 2–4 were randomized (2:1) to receive either 1% tapinarof cream or placebo, applied twice daily for 12 weeks [142]. At week 12, the improvement in PGA was 62.8% for patients treated with tapinarof compared with 13.0% for patients randomized to placebo ($p < 0.0001$). The proportion of patients who achieved a PGA of clear or almost clear was significantly higher with tapinarof treatment (67.5%) compared with placebo (4.8%, $p < 0.0001$) [142]. In another double-blind, vehicle-controlled, randomized six-arm trial (1:1:1:1:1:1) in adults with psoriasis with body surface involvement ≥ 1% and ≤ 15% and PGA score ≥ 2 at baseline, treatment success defined by PGA 0 or 1 and a two-grade improvement at week 12 was significantly higher in the tapinarof groups (65% (1% twice daily), 56% (1% once daily), 46% (0.5% twice daily), and 36% (0.5% once daily)) than vehicle groups (11% (twice daily) and 5% (once daily)); this was maintained for four weeks post-treatment [22]. The most commonly (≥5%) reported adverse events that emerged after treatment were folliculitis (19/152, 13% tapinarof groups and 1/75, 1% vehicle groups) and contact dermatitis (12/152, 8% only in the tapinarof groups) [22]. These preclinical and clinical studies reinforce that AHR ligand tapinarof is efficacious in the treatment of psoriasis and atopic dermatitis. In 2019, tapinarof (1% benvitimod cream) was officially approved by the Chinese government for medical use for psoriasis after successful Chinese clinical trials [103]. Overall, why topical and systemic AHR ligands reduce psoriatic inflammation by inhibiting IL-17 and IL-22 in vivo while the same ligands upregulate the expression of IL-17 and IL-22 in vitro is still unknown.

7. Conclusions

Humans empirically utilize natural antioxidative resources to keep their skin healthy, including coal tar, *Galactomyces* fermentation filtrate, *Opuntia ficus-indica* in Latin America, Artichoke in Mediterranean regions, and *Houttuynia cordata* and *Artemisia princeps* in Asia [12,13,15,37,38,62]. These agents are potent AHR ligands which activate the AHR-ARNT system and enhance the terminal differentiation of epidermal keratinocytes [12,13,15,37,38,62]. They also exert antioxidative action via AHR-NRF2 activation [12,13,15,37,38]. The study of the signal transduction mechanisms of the AHR/ARNT system has demonstrated that this system is also deeply involved in immune regulation especially in Th17/22 and Treg maturation [28,29]. A selective AHR agonist, tapinarof is currently being studied because this medicinal agent improves both psoriasis and AD in which different pathomechanisms operate (the TNF-α/IL-23/IL-17 axis in psoriasis and IL-4/IL-13 signaling in AD). Further mechanistic approaches are warranted to develop new drugs targeting the AHR system.

Author Contributions: M.F. wrote the first draft. A.H.-H. and G.T. reviewed the draft. M.F. finalized the article, and all authors approved the submission of the article.

Funding: This work was partly supported by grants from The Ministry of Health, Labour, and Welfare in Japan (H30-Shokuhin-Shitei-005) and The Leading Advanced Projects for Medical Innovation in Japan (LEAP).

Conflicts of Interest: The authors have no conflict of interest. The funders had no role in the design of the study; in the collection, analyses, or interpretation of data; in the writing of the manuscript, or in the decision to publish the results.

References

1. Furue, K.; Mitoma, C.; Tsuji, G.; Furue, M. Protective role of peroxisome proliferator-activated receptor α agonists in skin barrier and inflammation. *Immunobiology* **2018**, *223*, 327–330. [CrossRef] [PubMed]
2. Furue, M.; Fuyuno, Y.; Mitoma, C.; Uchi, H.; Tsuji, G. Therapeutic agents with AHR inhibiting and NRF2 activating activity for managing chloracne. *Antioxidants (Basel)* **2018**, *7*, 90. [CrossRef]
3. Furue, M.; Hashimoto-Hachiya, A.; Tsuji, G. Antioxidative phytochemicals accelerate epidermal terminal differentiation via the AHR-OVOL1 pathway: Implications for atopic dermatitis. *Acta Derm. Venereol.* **2018**, *98*, 918–923. [CrossRef] [PubMed]
4. Omiecinski, C.J.; Vanden Heuvel, J.P.; Perdew, G.H.; Peters, J.M. Xenobiotic metabolism, disposition, and regulation by receptors: From biochemical phenomenon to predictors of major toxicities. *Toxicol. Sci.* **2011**, *120*, S49–S75. [CrossRef] [PubMed]
5. Esser, C.; Bargen, I.; Weighardt, H.; Haarmann-Stemmann, T.; Krutmann, J. Functions of the aryl 1002 hydrocarbon receptor in the skin. *Semin. Immunopathol.* **2013**, *35*, 677–691. [CrossRef]
6. Furue, M.; Takahara, M.; Nakahara, T.; Uchi, H. Role of AhR/ARNT system in skin homeostasis. *Arch. Dermatol. Res.* **2014**, *306*, 769–779. [CrossRef]
7. Mimura, J.; Fujii-Kuriyama, Y. Functional role of AhR in the expression of toxic effects by TCDD. *Biochim. Biophys. Acta* **2003**, *1619*, 263–268. [CrossRef]

8. Fritsche, E.; Schäfer, C.; Calles, C.; Bernsmann, T.; Bernshausen, T.; Wurm, M.; Hübenthal, U.; Cline, J.E.; Hajimiragha, H.; Schroeder, P.; et al. Lightening up the UV response by identification of the aryl hydrocarbon receptor as a cytoplasmatic target for ultraviolet B radiation. *Proc. Natl. Acad. Sci. USA* **2007**, *104*, 8851–8856. [CrossRef]
9. Rannug, A.; Rannug, U.; Rosenkranz, H.S.; Winqvist, L.; Westerholm, R.; Agurell, E.; Grafström, A.K. Certain photooxidized derivatives of tryptophan bind with very high affinity to the Ah receptor and are likely to be endogenous signal substances. *J. Biol. Chem.* **1987**, *262*, 15422–15427.
10. Furue, M.; Uchi, H.; Mitoma, C.; Hashimoto-Hachiya, A.; Chiba, T.; Ito, T.; Nakahara, T.; Tsuji, G. Antioxidants for healthy skin: The emerging role of aryl hydrocarbon receptors and nuclear factor-erythroid 2-related factor-2. *Nutrients* **2017**, *9*, 223. [CrossRef]
11. Magiatis, P.; Pappas, P.; Gaitanis, G.; Mexia, N.; Melliou, E.; Galanou, M.; Vlachos, C.; Stathopoulou, K.; Skaltsounis, A.L.; Marselos, M.; et al. Malassezia yeasts produce a collection of exceptionally potent activators of the Ah (dioxin) receptor detected in diseased human skin. *J. Investig. Dermatol.* **2013**, *133*, 2023–2030. [CrossRef] [PubMed]
12. Takei, K.; Mitoma, C.; Hashimoto-Hachiya, A.; Takahara, M.; Tsuji, G.; Nakahara, T.; Furue, M. Galactomyces fermentation filtrate prevents T helper 2-mediated reduction of filaggrin in an aryl hydrocarbon receptor-dependent manner. *Clin. Exp. Dermatol.* **2015**, *40*, 786–793. [CrossRef] [PubMed]
13. Takei, K.; Hashimoto-Hachiya, A.; Takahara, M.; Tsuji, G.; Nakahara, T.; Furue, M. Cynaropicrin attenuates UVB-induced oxidative stress via the AhR-Nrf2-Nqo1 pathway. *Toxicol. Lett.* **2015**, *234*, 74–80. [CrossRef] [PubMed]
14. Takei, K.; Mitoma, C.; Hashimoto-Hachiya, A.; Uchi, H.; Takahara, M.; Tsuji, G.; Kido-Nakahara, M.; Nakahara, T.; Furue, M. Antioxidant soybean tar Glyteer rescues T-helper-mediated downregulation of filaggrin expression via aryl hydrocarbon receptor. *J. Dermatol.* **2015**, *42*, 171–180. [CrossRef]
15. Van den Bogaard, E.H.; Bergboer, J.G.; Vonk-Bergers, M.; van Vlijmen-Willems, I.M.; Hato, S.V.; van der Valk, P.G.; Schröder, J.M.; Joosten, I.; Zeeuwen, P.L.; Schalkwijk, J. Coal tar induces AHR-dependent skin barrier repair in atopic dermatitis. *J. Clin. Investig.* **2013**, *123*, 917–927. [CrossRef]
16. Simpson, E.L.; Bieber, T.; Guttman-Yassky, E.; Beck, L.A.; Blauvelt, A.; Cork, M.J.; Silverberg, J.I.; Deleuran, M.; Kataoka, Y.; Lacour, J.P.; et al. Two Phase 3 Trials of dupilumab versus placebo in atopic dermatitis. *N. Engl. J. Med.* **2016**, *375*, 2335–2348. [CrossRef]
17. Furue, M.; Ulzii, D.; Vu, Y.H.; Tsuji, G.; Kido-Nakahara, M.; Nakahara, T. Pathogenesis of atopic dermatitis: Current paradigm. *Iran. J. Immunol.* **2019**, *16*, 97–107.
18. Furue, K.; Ito, T.; Furue, M. Differential efficacy of biologic treatments targeting the TNF-α/IL-23/IL-17 axis in psoriasis and psoriatic arthritis. *Cytokine* **2018**, *111*, 182–188. [CrossRef]
19. Furue, K.; Ito, T.; Tsuji, G.; Kadono, T.; Furue, M. Psoriasis and the TNF/IL23/IL17 axis. *G. Ital. Dermatol. Venereol.* **2019**, *154*, 418–424. [CrossRef]
20. Tsoi, L.C.; Rodriguez, E.; Degenhardt, F.; Baurecht, H.; Wehkamp, U.; Volks, N.; Szymczak, S.; Swindell, W.R.; Sarkar, M.K.; Raja, K.; et al. Atopic dermatitis is an IL-13-dominant disease with greater molecular heterogeneity compared to psoriasis. *J. Investig. Dermatol.* **2019**, *139*, 1480–1489. [CrossRef]
21. Peppers, J.; Paller, A.S.; Maeda-Chubachi, T.; Wu, S.; Robbins, K.; Gallagher, K.; Kraus, J.E. A phase 2, randomized dose-finding study of tapinarof (GSK2894512 cream) for the treatment of atopic dermatitis. *J. Am. Acad. Dermatol.* **2019**, *80*, 89–98. [CrossRef] [PubMed]
22. Robbins, K.; Bissonnette, R.; Maeda-Chubachi, T.; Ye, L.; Peppers, J.; Gallagher, K.; Kraus, J.E. Phase 2, randomized dose-finding study of tapinarof (GSK2894512 cream) for the treatment of plaque psoriasis. *J. Am. Acad. Dermatol.* **2019**, *80*, 714–721. [CrossRef] [PubMed]
23. Kazlauskas, A.; Sundström, S.; Poellinger, L.; Pongratz, I. The hsp90 chaperone complex regulates intracellular localization of the dioxin receptor. *Mol. Cell. Biol.* **2001**, *21*, 2594–2607. [CrossRef] [PubMed]
24. Lees, M.J.; Peet, D.J.; Whitelaw, M.L. Defining the role for XAP2 in stabilization of the dioxin receptor. *J. Biol. Chem.* **2003**, *278*, 35878–35888. [CrossRef]
25. Hayes, J.D.; McMahon, M. Molecular basis for the contribution of the antioxidant responsive element to cancer chemoprevention. *Cancer Lett.* **2001**, *174*, 103–113. [CrossRef]
26. Miao, W.; Hu, L.; Scrivens, P.J.; Batist, G. Transcriptional regulation of NF-E2 p45-related factor (NRF2) expression by the aryl hydrocarbon receptor-xenobiotic response element signaling pathway: Direct cross-talk between phase I and II drug-metabolizing enzymes. *J. Biol. Chem.* **2005**, *280*, 20340–20348. [CrossRef]

27. Esser, C.; Rannug, A. The aryl hydrocarbon receptor in barrier organ physiology, immunology, and toxicology. *Pharmacol. Rev.* **2015**, *67*, 259–279. [CrossRef]
28. Esser, C. The aryl hydrocarbon receptor in immunity: Tools and potential. *Methods Mol. Biol.* **2016**, *1371*, 239–257.
29. Stockinger, B.; Di Meglio, P.; Gialitakis, M.; Duarte, J.H. The aryl hydrocarbon receptor: Multitasking in the immune system. *Annu. Rev. Immunol.* **2014**, *32*, 403–432. [CrossRef]
30. Kopf, P.G.; Walker, M.K. 2,3,7,8-tetrachlorodibenzo-p-dioxin increases reactive oxygen species production in human endothelial cells via induction of cytochrome P4501A. *Toxicol. Appl. Pharmacol.* **2010**, *245*, 91–99. [CrossRef]
31. Denison, M.S.; Soshilov, A.A.; He, G.; DeGroot, D.E.; Zhao, B. Exactly the same but different: Promiscuity and diversity in the molecular mechanisms of action of the aryl hydrocarbon (dioxin) receptor. *Toxicol. Sci.* **2011**, *124*, 1–22. [CrossRef] [PubMed]
32. Baron, J.M.; Höller, D.; Schiffer, R.; Frankenberg, S.; Neis, M.; Merk, H.F.; Jugert, F.K. Expression of multiple cytochrome p450 enzymes and multidrug resistance-associated transport proteins in human skin keratinocytes. *J. Investig. Dermatol.* **2001**, *116*, 541–548. [CrossRef] [PubMed]
33. Inui, H.; Itoh, T.; Yamamoto, K.; Ikushiro, S.; Sakaki, T. Mammalian cytochrome P450-dependent metabolism of polychlorinated dibenzo-p-dioxins and coplanar polychlorinated biphenyls. *Int. J. Mol. Sci.* **2014**, *15*, 14044–14057. [CrossRef] [PubMed]
34. Anandasadagopan, S.K.; Singh, N.M.; Raza, H.; Bansal, S.; Selvaraj, V.; Singh, S.; Chowdhury, A.R.; Leu, N.A.; Avadhani, N.G. β-Naphthoflavone-induced mitochondrial respiratory damage in Cyp1 knockout mouse and in cell culture systems: Attenuation by resveratrol treatment. *Oxid. Med. Cell Longev.* **2017**, *2017*, 5213186. [CrossRef]
35. Tanaka, Y.; Uchi, H.; Hashimoto-Hachiya, A.; Furue, M. Tryptophan photoproduct FICZ upregulates IL1A, IL1B, and IL6 expression via oxidative stress in keratinocytes. *Oxid. Med. Cell. Longev.* **2018**, *2018*, 9298052. [CrossRef]
36. Tsuji, G.; Takahara, M.; Uchi, H.; Takeuchi, S.; Mitoma, C.; Moroi, Y.; Furue, M. An environmental contaminant, benzo(a)pyrene, induces oxidative stress-mediated interleukin-8 production in human keratinocytes via the aryl hydrocarbon receptor signaling pathway. *J. Dermatol. Sci.* **2011**, *62*, 42–49. [CrossRef]
37. Nakahara, T.; Mitoma, C.; Hashimoto-Hachiya, A.; Takahara, M.; Tsuji, G.; Uchi, H.; Yan, X.; Hachisuka, J.; Chiba, T.; Esaki, H.; et al. Antioxidant *Opuntia ficus-indica* extract activates AHR-NRF2 signaling and upregulates filaggrin and loricrin expression in human keratinocytes. *J. Med. Food* **2015**, *18*, 1143–1149. [CrossRef]
38. Doi, K.; Mitoma, C.; Nakahara, T.; Uchi, H.; Hashimoto-Hachiya, A.; Takahara, M.; Tsuji, G.; Nakahara, M.; Furue, M. Antioxidant Houttuynia cordata extract upregulates filaggrin expression in an aryl hydrocarbon-dependent manner. *Fukuoka Igaku Zasshi* **2014**, *105*, 205–213.
39. Tsuji, G.; Takahara, M.; Uchi, H.; Matsuda, T.; Chiba, T.; Takeuchi, S.; Yasukawa, F.; Moroi, Y.; Furue, M. Identification of ketoconazole as an AhR-Nrf2 activator in cultured human keratinocytes: The basis of its anti-inflammatory effect. *J. Investig. Dermatol.* **2012**, *132*, 59–68. [CrossRef]
40. Yeager, R.L.; Reisman, S.A.; Aleksunes, L.M.; Klaassen, C.D. Introducing the "TCDD-inducible AhR-Nrf2 gene battery". *Toxicol. Sci.* **2009**, *111*, 238–246. [CrossRef]
41. Wang, K.; Lv, Q.; Miao, Y.M.; Qiao, S.M.; Dai, Y.; Wei, Z.F. Cardamonin, a natural flavone, alleviates inflammatory bowel disease by the inhibition of NLRP3 inflammasome activation via an AhR/Nrf2/NQO1 pathway. *Biochem. Pharmacol.* **2018**, *155*, 494–509. [CrossRef] [PubMed]
42. Ma, Q.; Kinneer, K.; Bi, Y.; Chan, J.Y.; Kan, Y.W. Induction of murine NAD(P)H:quinone oxidoreductase by 2,3,7,8-tetrachlorodibenzo-p-dioxin requires the CNC (cap 'n' collar) basic leucine zipper transcription factor Nrf2 (nuclear factor erythroid 2-related factor 2): Cross-interaction between AhR (aryl hydrocarbon receptor) and Nrf2 signal transduction. *Biochem. J.* **2004**, *377*, 205–213. [PubMed]
43. Noda, S.; Harada, N.; Hida, A.; Fujii-Kuriyama, Y.; Motohashi, H.; Yamamoto, M. Gene expression of detoxifying enzymes in AhR and Nrf2 compound null mutant mouse. *Biochem. Biophys. Res. Commun.* **2003**, *303*, 105–111. [CrossRef]
44. Furue, M.; Tsuji, G.; Mitoma, C.; Nakahara, T.; Chiba, T.; Morino-Koga, S.; Uchi, H. Gene regulation of filaggrin and other skin barrier proteins via aryl hydrocarbon receptor. *J. Dermatol. Sci.* **2015**, *80*, 83–88. [CrossRef] [PubMed]

45. Kypriotou, M.; Huber, M.; Hohl, D. The human epidermal differentiation complex: Cornified envelope precursors, S100 proteins and the 'fused genes' family. *Exp. Dermatol.* **2012**, *21*, 643–649. [CrossRef] [PubMed]
46. Loertscher, J.A.; Lin, T.M.; Peterson, R.E.; Allen-Hoffmann, B.L. In utero exposure to 2,3,7,8-tetrachlorodibenzo-p-dioxin causes accelerated terminal differentiation in fetal mouse skin. *Toxicol. Sci.* **2002**, *68*, 465–472. [CrossRef]
47. Kennedy, L.H.; Sutter, C.H.; Leon Carrion, S.; Tran, Q.T.; Bodreddigari, S.; Kensicki, E.; Mohney, R.P.; Sutter, T.R. 2,3,7,8-Tetrachlorodibenzo-p-dioxin-mediated production of reactive oxygen species is an essential step in the mechanism of action to accelerate human keratinocyte differentiation. *Toxicol. Sci.* **2013**, *132*, 235–249. [CrossRef]
48. Sutter, C.H.; Bodreddigari, S.; Campion, C.; Wible, R.S.; Sutter, T.R. 2,3,7,8-Tetrachlorodibenzo-p-dioxin increases the expression of genes in the human epidermal differentiation complex and accelerates epidermal barrier formation. *Toxicol. Sci.* **2011**, *124*, 128–137. [CrossRef]
49. Fernandez-Salguero, P.M.; Ward, J.M.; Sundberg, J.P.; Gonzalez, F.J. Lesions of aryl-hydrocarbon receptor-deficient mice. *Vet. Pathol.* **1997**, *34*, 605–614. [CrossRef]
50. Tauchi, M.; Hida, A.; Negishi, T.; Katsuoka, F.; Noda, S.; Mimura, J.; Hosoya, T.; Yanaka, A.; Aburatani, H.; Fujii-Kuriyama, Y.; et al. Constitutive expression of aryl hydrocarbon receptor in keratinocytes causes inflammatory skin lesions. *Mol. Cell. Biol.* **2005**, *25*, 9360–9368. [CrossRef]
51. Geng, S.; Mezentsev, A.; Kalachikov, S.; Raith, K.; Roop, D.R.; Panteleyev, A.A. Targeted ablation of Arnt in mouse epidermis results in profound defects in desquamation and epidermal barrier function. *J. Cell Sci.* **2006**, *119*, 4901–4912. [CrossRef] [PubMed]
52. Takagi, S.; Tojo, H.; Tomita, S.; Sano, S.; Itami, S.; Hara, M.; Inoue, S.; Horie, K.; Kondoh, G.; Hosokawa, K.; et al. Alteration of the 4-sphingenine scaffolds of ceramides in keratinocyte-specific Arnt-deficient mice affects skin barrier function. *J. Clin. Investig.* **2003**, *112*, 1372–1382. [CrossRef]
53. Ju, Q.; Fimmel, S.; Hinz, N.; Stahlmann, R.; Xia, L.; Zouboulis, C.C. 2,3,7,8-Tetrachlorodibenzo-p-dioxin alters sebaceous gland cell differentiation in vitro. *Exp. Dermatol.* **2011**, *20*, 320–325. [CrossRef] [PubMed]
54. Lin, Y.K.; Leu, Y.L.; Yang, S.H.; Chen, H.W.; Wang, C.T.; Pang, J.H. Anti-psoriatic effects of indigo naturalis on the proliferation and differentiation of keratinocytes with indirubin as the active component. *J. Dermatol. Sci.* **2009**, *54*, 168–174. [CrossRef] [PubMed]
55. Rannug, A.; Rannug, U. The tryptophan derivative 6-formylindolo[3,2-b]carbazole, FICZ, a dynamic mediator of endogenous aryl hydrocarbon receptor signaling, balances cell growth and differentiation. *Crit. Rev. Toxicol.* **2018**, *48*, 555–574. [CrossRef]
56. Wincent, E.; Amini, N.; Luecke, S.; Glatt, H.; Bergman, J.; Crescenzi, C.; Rannug, A.; Rannug, U. The suggested physiologic aryl hydrocarbon receptor activator and cytochrome P4501 substrate 6-formylindolo[3,2-b]carbazole is present in humans. *J. Biol. Chem.* **2009**, *284*, 2690–2696. [CrossRef]
57. Furue, M.; Uchi, H.; Mitoma, C.; Hashimoto-Hachiya, A.; Tanaka, Y.; Ito, T.; Tsuji, G. Implications of tryptophan photoproduct FICZ in oxidative stress and terminal differentiation of keratinocytes. *G. Ital. Dermatol. Venereol.* **2019**, *154*, 37–41. [CrossRef]
58. Kiyomatsu-Oda, M.; Uchi, H.; Morino-Koga, S.; Furue, M. Protective role of 6-formylindolo[3,2-b]carbazole (FICZ), an endogenous ligand for arylhydrocarbon receptor, in chronic mite-induced dermatitis. *J. Dermatol. Sci.* **2018**, *90*, 284–294. [CrossRef]
59. Tsuji, G.; Ito, T.; Chiba, T.; Mitoma, C.; Nakahara, T.; Uchi, H.; Furue, M. The role of the OVOL1-OVOL2 axis in normal and diseased human skin. *J. Dermatol. Sci.* **2018**, *90*, 227–231. [CrossRef]
60. Hong, S.P.; Kim, M.J.; Jung, M.Y.; Jeon, H.; Goo, J.; Ahn, S.K.; Lee, S.H.; Elias, P.M.; Choi, E.H. Biopositive effects of low-dose UVB on epidermis: Coordinate upregulation of antimicrobial peptides and permeability barrier reinforcement. *J. Investig. Dermatol.* **2008**, *128*, 2880–2887. [CrossRef]
61. Tsuji, G.; Hashimoto-Hachiya, A.; Kiyomatsu-Oda, M.; Takemura, M.; Ohno, F.; Ito, T.; Morino-Koga, S.; Mitoma, C.; Nakahara, T.; Uchi, H.; et al. Aryl hydrocarbon receptor activation restores filaggrin expression via OVOL1 in atopic dermatitis. *Cell Death Dis.* **2017**, *8*, e2931. [CrossRef]
62. Hirano, A.; Goto, M.; Mitsui, T.; Hashimoto-Hachiya, A.; Tsuji, G.; Furue, M. Antioxidant *Artemisia princeps* extract enhances the expression of filaggrin and loricrin via the AHR/OVOL1 pathway. *Int. J. Mol. Sci.* **2017**, *18*, 1948. [CrossRef]

63. Hashimoto-Hachiya, A.; Tsuji, G.; Murai, M.; Yan, X.; Furue, M. Upregulation of FLG, LOR, and IVL expression by *Rhodiola crenulata* root extract via aryl hydrocarbon receptor: Differential involvement of OVOL. *Int. J. Mol. Sci.* **2018**, *19*, 1654. [CrossRef]
64. Van den Bogaard, E.H.; Podolsky, M.A.; Smits, J.P.; Cui, X.; John, C.; Gowda, K.; Desai, D.; Amin, S.G.; Schalkwijk, J.; Perdew, G.H.; et al. Genetic and pharmacological analysis identifies a physiological role for the AHR in epidermal differentiation. *J. Investig. Dermatol.* **2015**, *135*, 1320–1328. [CrossRef]
65. Zhang, W.; Sakai, T.; Matsuda-Hirose, H.; Goto, M.; Yamate, T.; Hatano, Y. Cutaneous permeability barrier function in signal transducer and activator of transcription 6-deficient mice is superior to that in wild-type mice. *J. Dermatol. Sci.* **2018**, *92*, 54–61. [CrossRef]
66. Tanaka, G.; Kanaji, S.; Hirano, A.; Arima, K.; Shinagawa, A.; Goda, C.; Yasunaga, S.; Ikizawa, K.; Yanagihara, Y.; Kubo, M.; et al. Induction and activation of the aryl hydrocarbon receptor by IL-4 in B cells. *Int. Immunol.* **2005**, *17*, 797–805. [CrossRef]
67. Mitamura, Y.; Nunomura, S.; Nanri, Y.; Ogawa, M.; Yoshihara, T.; Masuoka, M.; Tsuji, G.; Nakahara, T.; Hashimoto-Hachiya, A.; Conway, S.J.; et al. The IL-13/periostin/IL-24 pathway causes epidermal barrier dysfunction in allergic skin inflammation. *Allergy* **2018**, *73*, 1881–1891. [CrossRef] [PubMed]
68. Takemura, M.; Nakahara, T.; Hashimoto-Hachiya, A.; Furue, M.; Tsuji, G. Glyteer, soybean tar, impairs IL-4/Stat6 signaling in murine bone marrow-derived dendritic cells: The basis of its therapeutic effect on atopic dermatitis. *Int. J. Mol. Sci.* **2018**, *19*, 1169. [CrossRef]
69. Schiering, C.; Vonk, A.; Das, S.; Stockinger, B.; Wincent, E. Cytochrome P4501-inhibiting chemicals amplify aryl hydrocarbon receptor activation and IL-22 production in T helper 17 cells. *Biochem. Pharmacol.* **2018**, *151*, 47–58. [CrossRef] [PubMed]
70. Ye, J.; Qiu, J.; Bostick, J.W.; Ueda, A.; Schjerven, H.; Li, S.; Jobin, C.; Chen, Z.E.; Zhou, L. The aryl hydrocarbon receptor preferentially marks and promotes gut regulatory T cells. *Cell Rep.* **2017**, *21*, 2277–2290. [CrossRef] [PubMed]
71. Kiss, E.A.; Vonarbourg, C.; Kopfmann, S.; Hobeika, E.; Finke, D.; Esser, C.; Diefenbach, A. Natural aryl hydrocarbon receptor ligands control organogenesis of intestinal lymphoid follicles. *Science* **2011**, *334*, 1561–1565. [CrossRef] [PubMed]
72. Lee, J.S.; Cella, M.; McDonald, K.G.; Garlanda, C.; Kennedy, G.D.; Nukaya, M.; Mantovani, A.; Kopan, R.; Bradfield, C.A.; Newberry, R.D.; et al. AHR drives the development of gut ILC22 cells and postnatal lymphoid tissues via pathways dependent on and independent of Notch. *Nat. Immunol.* **2011**, *13*, 144–151. [CrossRef] [PubMed]
73. Qiu, J.; Heller, J.J.; Guo, X.; Chen, Z.M.; Fish, K.; Fu, Y.X.; Zhou, L. The aryl hydrocarbon receptor regulates gut immunity through modulation of innate lymphoid cells. *Immunity* **2012**, *36*, 92–104. [CrossRef] [PubMed]
74. Liu, J.Z.; van Sommeren, S.; Huang, H.; Ng, S.C.; Alberts, R.; Takahashi, A.; Ripke, S.; Lee, J.C.; Jostins, L.; Shah, T.; et al. Association analyses identify 38 susceptibility loci for inflammatory bowel disease and highlight shared genetic risk across populations. *Nat. Genet.* **2015**, *47*, 979–986. [CrossRef]
75. Monteleone, I.; Rizzo, A.; Sarra, M.; Sica, G.; Sileri, P.; Biancone, L.; MacDonald, T.T.; Pallone, F.; Monteleone, G. Aryl hydrocarbon receptor-induced signals up-regulate IL-22 production and inhibit inflammation in the gastrointestinal tract. *Gastroenterology* **2011**, *141*, 237–248. [CrossRef]
76. Schiering, C.; Wincent, E.; Metidji, A.; Iseppon, A.; Li, Y.; Potocnik, A.J.; Omenetti, S.; Henderson, C.J.; Wolf, C.R.; Nebert, D.W.; et al. Feedback control of AHR signalling regulates intestinal immunity. *Nature* **2017**, *542*, 242–245. [CrossRef]
77. Holsapple, M.P.; Morris, D.L.; Wood, S.C.; Snyder, N.K. 2,3,7,8-tetrachlorodibenzo-p-dioxin-induced changes in immunocompetence: Possible mechanisms. *Annu. Rev. Pharmacol. Toxicol.* **1991**, *31*, 73–100. [CrossRef]
78. Veldhoen, M.; Hirota, K.; Westendorf, A.M.; Buer, J.; Dumoutier, L.; Renauld, J.C.; Stockinger, B. The aryl hydrocarbon receptor links TH17-cell-mediated autoimmunity to environmental toxins. *Nature* **2008**, *453*, 106–109. [CrossRef]
79. Funatake, C.J.; Marshall, N.B.; Steppan, L.B.; Mourich, D.V.; Kerkvliet, N.I. Cutting edge: Activation of the aryl hydrocarbon receptor by 2,3,7,8-tetrachlorodibenzo-p-dioxin generates a population of CD4+ CD25+ cells with characteristics of regulatory T cells. *J. Immunol.* **2005**, *175*, 4184–4188. [CrossRef]
80. Qiu, J.; Guo, X.; Chen, Z.M.; He, L.; Sonnenberg, G.F.; Artis, D.; Fu, Y.X.; Zhou, L. Group 3 innate lymphoid cells inhibit T-cell-mediated intestinal inflammation through aryl hydrocarbon receptor signaling and regulation of microflora. *Immunity* **2013**, *39*, 386–399. [CrossRef]

81. Ehrlich, A.K.; Pennington, J.M.; Bisson, W.H.; Kolluri, S.K.; Kerkvliet, N.I. TCDD, FICZ, and other high affinity AhR ligands dose-dependently determine the fate of CD4+ T cell differentiation. *Toxicol. Sci.* **2018**, *161*, 310–320. [CrossRef] [PubMed]
82. Furue, M.; Chiba, T.; Tsuji, G.; Ulzii, D.; Kido-Nakahara, M.; Nakahara, T.; Kadono, T. Atopic dermatitis: Immune deviation, barrier dysfunction, IgE autoreactivity and new therapies. *Allergol. Int.* **2017**, *66*, 398–403. [CrossRef] [PubMed]
83. Seo, E.; Yoon, J.; Jung, S.; Lee, J.; Lee, B.H.; Yu, J. Phenotypes of atopic dermatitis identified by cluster analysis in early childhood. *J. Dermatol.* **2019**, *46*, 117–123. [CrossRef]
84. Arima, K.; Gupta, S.; Gadkari, A.; Hiragun, T.; Kono, T.; Katayama, I.; Demiya, S.; Eckert, L. Burden of atopic dermatitis in Japanese adults: Analysis of data from the 2013 National Health and Wellness Survey. *J. Dermatol.* **2018**, *45*, 390–396. [CrossRef]
85. Igarashi, A.; Fujita, H.; Arima, K.; Inoue, T.; Dorey, J.; Fukushima, A.; Taguchi, Y. Health-care resource use and current treatment of adult atopic dermatitis patients in Japan: A retrospective claims database analysis. *J. Dermatol.* **2019**, *46*, 652–661. [CrossRef]
86. Jung, H.J.; Bae, J.Y.; Kim, J.E.; Na, C.H.; Park, G.H.; Bae, Y.I.; Shin, M.K.; Lee, Y.B.; Lee, U.H.; Jang, Y.H.; et al. Survey of disease awareness, treatment behavior and treatment satisfaction in patients with atopic dermatitis in Korea: A multicenter study. *J. Dermatol.* **2018**, *45*, 1172–1180. [CrossRef]
87. Komura, Y.; Kogure, T.; Kawahara, K.; Yokozeki, H. Economic assessment of actual prescription of drugs for treatment of atopic dermatitis: Differences between dermatology and pediatrics in large-scale receipt data. *J. Dermatol.* **2018**, *45*, 165–174. [CrossRef]
88. Takeuchi, S.; Oba, J.; Esaki, H.; Furue, M. Non-corticosteroid adherence and itch severity influence perception of itch in atopic dermatitis. *J. Dermatol.* **2018**, *45*, 158–164. [CrossRef]
89. Williams, H.; Stewart, A.; von Mutius, E.; Cookson, W.; Anderson, H.R. Is eczema really on the increase worldwide? *J. Allergy Clin. Immunol.* **2008**, *121*, 947–954. [CrossRef] [PubMed]
90. Furue, M.; Iida, K.; Imaji, M.; Nakahara, T. Microbiome analysis of forehead skin in patients with atopic dermatitis and healthy subjects: Implication of *Staphylococcus* and *Corynebacterium*. *J. Dermatol.* **2018**, *45*, 876–877. [CrossRef]
91. Iwamoto, K.; Moriwaki, M.; Miyake, R.; Hide, M. Staphylococcus aureus in atopic dermatitis: Strain-specific cell wall proteins and skin immunity. *Allergol. Int.* **2019**, *68*, 309–315. [CrossRef] [PubMed]
92. Furue, M.; Kadono, T. "Inflammatory skin march" in atopic dermatitis and psoriasis. *Inflamm. Res.* **2017**, *66*, 833–842. [CrossRef] [PubMed]
93. Li, Z.Z.; Zhong, W.L.; Hu, H.; Chen, X.F.; Zhang, W.; Huang, H.Y.; Yu, B.; Dou, X. Aryl hydrocarbon receptor polymorphisms are associated with dry skin phenotypes in Chinese patients with atopic dermatitis. *Clin. Exp. Dermatol.* **2019**, *44*, 613–619. [CrossRef] [PubMed]
94. Li, D.; Takao, T.; Tsunematsu, R.; Morokuma, S.; Fukushima, K.; Kobayashi, H.; Saito, T.; Furue, M.; Wake, N.; Asanoma, K. Inhibition of AHR transcription by NF1C is affected by a single-nucleotide polymorphism, and is involved in suppression of human uterine endometrial cancer. *Oncogene* **2013**, *32*, 4950–4959. [CrossRef]
95. Liu, G.; Asanoma, K.; Takao, T.; Tsukimori, K.; Uchi, H.; Furue, M.; Kato, K.; Wake, N. Aryl hydrocarbon receptor SNP -130 C/T associates with dioxins susceptibility through regulating its receptor activity and downstream effectors including interleukin. *Toxicol. Lett.* **2015**, *232*, 384–392. [CrossRef]
96. Hong, C.H.; Lee, C.H.; Yu, H.S.; Huang, S.K. Benzopyrene, a major polyaromatic hydrocarbon in smoke fume, mobilizes Langerhans cells and polarizes Th2/17 responses in epicutaneous protein sensitization through the aryl hydrocarbon receptor. *Int. Immunopharmacol.* **2016**, *36*, 111–117. [CrossRef]
97. Kim, H.O.; Kim, J.H.; Chung, B.Y.; Choi, M.G.; Park, C.W. Increased expression of the aryl hydrocarbon receptor in patients with chronic inflammatory skin diseases. *Exp. Dermatol.* **2014**, *23*, 278–281. [CrossRef] [PubMed]
98. Yu, J.; Luo, Y.; Zhu, Z.; Zhou, Y.; Sun, L.; Gao, J.; Sun, J.; Wang, G.; Yao, X.; Li, W. A tryptophan metabolite of the skin microbiota attenuates inflammation in patients with atopic dermatitis through the aryl hydrocarbon receptor. *J. Allergy Clin. Immunol.* **2019**, *143*, 2108–2119. [CrossRef] [PubMed]
99. Hidaka, T.; Ogawa, E.; Kobayashi, E.H.; Suzuki, T.; Funayama, R.; Nagashima, T.; Fujimura, T.; Aiba, S.; Nakayama, K.; Okuyama, R.; et al. The aryl hydrocarbon receptor AhR links atopic dermatitis and air pollution via induction of the neurotrophic factor artemin. *Nat. Immunol.* **2017**, *18*, 64–73. [CrossRef]

100. Bissonnette, R.; Poulin, Y.; Zhou, Y.; Tan, J.; Hong, H.C.; Webster, J.; Ip, W.; Tang, L.; Lyle, M. Efficacy and safety of topical WBI-1001 in patients with mild to severe atopic dermatitis: Results from a 12-week, multicentre, randomized, placebo-controlled double-blind trial. *Br. J. Dermatol.* **2012**, *166*, 853–860. [CrossRef]

101. Richardson, W.H.; Schmidt, T.M.; Nealson, K.H. Identification of an anthraquinone pigment and a hydroxystilbene antibiotic from Xenorhabdus luminescens. *Appl. Environ. Microbiol.* **1988**, *54*, 1602–16055.

102. Smith, S.H.; Jayawickreme, C.; Rickard, D.J.; Nicodeme, E.; Bui, T.; Simmons, C.; Coquery, C.M.; Neil, J.; Pryor, W.M.; Mayhew, D.; et al. Tapinarof is a natural AhR agonist that resolves skin inflammation in mice and humans. *J. Investig. Dermatol.* **2017**, *137*, 2110–2119. [CrossRef]

103. Zang, Y.N.; Jiang, D.L.; Cai, L.; Chen, X.; Wang, Q.; Xie, Z.W.; Liu, Y.; Zhang, C.Y.; Jing, S.; Chen, G.H.; et al. Use of a dose-response model to guide future clinical trial of Benvitimod cream to treat mild and moderate psoriasis. *Int. J. Clin. Pharmacol. Ther.* **2016**, *54*, 87–95. [CrossRef]

104. Bissonnette, R.; Vasist, L.S.; Bullman, J.N.; Collingwood, T.; Chen, G.; Maeda-Chubachi, T. Systemic pharmacokinetics, safety, and preliminary efficacy of topical AhR agonist Tapinarof: Results of a phase 1 study. *Clin. Pharmacol. Drug Dev.* **2018**, *7*, 524–531. [CrossRef]

105. Miake, S.; Tsuji, G.; Takemura, M.; Hashimoto-Hachiya, A.; Vu, Y.H.; Furue, M.; Nakahara, T. IL-4 augments IL-31/IL-31 receptor alpha interaction leading to enhanced Ccl17 and Ccl22 production in dendritic cells: Implications for atopic dermatitis. *Int. J. Mol. Sci.* **2019**, *20*, 4053. [CrossRef]

106. Koch, S.; Stroisch, T.J.; Vorac, J.; Herrmann, N.; Leib, N.; Schnautz, S.; Kirins, H.; Forster, I.; Weighardt, H.; Bieber, T. AhR mediates an anti-inflammatory feedback mechanism in human Langerhans cells involving FcεRI and IDO. *Allergy* **2017**, *72*, 1686–1693. [CrossRef]

107. Edamitsu, T.; Taguchi, K.; Kobayashi, E.H.; Okuyama, R.; Yamamoto, M. Aryl hydrocarbon receptor directly regulates artemin gene expression. *Mol. Cell Biol.* **2019**, *39*. [CrossRef]

108. Morita, A. Current developments in phototherapy for psoriasis. *J. Dermatol.* **2018**, *45*, 287–292. [CrossRef]

109. Ortiz-Salvador, J.M.; Pérez-Ferriols, A. Phototherapy in Atopic Dermatitis. *Adv. Exp. Med. Biol.* **2017**, *996*, 279–286.

110. Boehncke, W.H.; Schön, M.P. Psoriasis. *Lancet* **2015**, *386*, 983–994. [CrossRef]

111. Furue, M.; Kadono, T. The contribution of IL-17 to the development of autoimmunity in psoriasis. *Innate Immun.* **2019**, *25*, 337–343. [CrossRef]

112. Ogawa, E.; Okuyama, R.; Seki, T.; Kobayashi, A.; Oiso, N.; Muto, M.; Nakagawa, H.; Kawada, A. Epidemiological survey of patients with psoriasis in Matsumoto city, Nagano Prefecture, Japan. *J. Dermatol.* **2018**, *45*, 314–317. [CrossRef]

113. Ito, T.; Takahashi, H.; Kawada, A.; Iizuka, H.; Nakagawa, H. Epidemiological survey from 2009 to 2012 of psoriatic patients in Japanese Society for Psoriasis Research. *J. Dermatol.* **2018**, *45*, 293–301. [CrossRef]

114. Ichiyama, S.; Ito, M.; Funasaka, Y.; Abe, M.; Nishida, E.; Muramatsu, S.; Nishihara, H.; Kato, H.; Morita, A.; Imafuku, S.; et al. Assessment of medication adherence and treatment satisfaction in Japanese patients with psoriasis of various severities. *J. Dermatol.* **2018**, *45*, 727–731. [CrossRef]

115. Takahashi, H.; Satoh, K.; Takagi, A.; Iizuka, H. Cost-efficacy and pharmacoeconomics of psoriatic patients in Japan: Analysis from a single outpatient clinic. *J. Dermatol.* **2019**, *46*, 478–481. [CrossRef]

116. Komatsu-Fujii, T.; Honda, T.; Otsuka, A.; Kabashima, K. Improvement of nail lesions in a patient with psoriatic arthritis by switching the treatment from an anti-interleukin-17A antibody to an anti-tumor necrosis factor-α antibody. *J. Dermatol.* **2019**, *46*, e158–e160. [CrossRef]

117. Tsuruta, N.; Narisawa, Y.; Imafuku, S.; Ito, K.; Yamaguchi, K.; Miyagi, T.; Takahashi, K.; Fukamatsu, H.; Morizane, S.; Koketsu, H.; et al. Cross-sectional multicenter observational study of psoriatic arthritis in Japanese patients: Relationship between skin and joint symptoms and results of treatment with tumor necrosis factor-α inhibitors. *J. Dermatol.* **2019**, *46*, 193–198. [CrossRef]

118. Yamamoto, T.; Ohtsuki, M.; Sano, S.; Morita, A.; Igarashi, A.; Okuyama, R.; Kawada, A. Late-onset psoriatic arthritis in Japanese patients. *J. Dermatol.* **2019**, *46*, 169–170. [CrossRef]

119. Chujo, S.; Asahina, A.; Itoh, Y.; Kobayashi, K.; Sueki, H.; Ishiji, T.; Umezawa, Y.; Nakagawa, H. New onset of psoriasis during nivolumab treatment for lung cancer. *J. Dermatol.* **2018**, *45*, e55–e56. [CrossRef]

120. Furue, K.; Ito, T.; Tsuji, G.; Kadono, T.; Nakahara, T.; Furue, M. Autoimmunity and autoimmune co-morbidities in psoriasis. *Immunology* **2018**, *154*, 21–27. [CrossRef]

121. Ho, Y.H.; Hu, H.Y.; Chang, Y.T.; Li, C.P.; Wu, C.Y. Psoriasis is associated with increased risk of bullous pemphigoid: A nationwide population-based cohort study in Taiwan. *J. Dermatol.* **2019**, *46*, 604–609. [CrossRef]
122. Ichiyama, S.; Hoashi, T.; Kanda, N.; Hashimoto, H.; Matsushita, M.; Nozawa, K.; Ueno, T.; Saeki, H. Psoriasis vulgaris associated with systemic lupus erythematosus successfully treated with apremilast. *J. Dermatol.* **2019**, *46*, e219–e221. [CrossRef]
123. Kamata, M.; Asano, Y.; Shida, R.; Maeda, N.; Yoshizaki, A.; Miyagaki, T.; Kawashima, T.; Tada, Y.; Sato, S. Secukinumab decreased circulating anti-BP180-NC16a autoantibodies in a patient with coexisting psoriasis vulgaris and bullous pemphigoid. *J. Dermatol.* **2019**, *46*, e216–e217. [CrossRef]
124. Masaki, S.; Bayaraa, B.; Imafuku, S. Prevalence of inflammatory bowel disease in Japanese psoriatic patients. *J. Dermatol.* **2019**, *46*, 590–594. [CrossRef]
125. Chiu, H.Y.; Chang, W.L.; Shiu, M.N.; Huang, W.F.; Tsai, T.F. Psoriasis is associated with a greater risk for cardiovascular procedure and surgery in patients with hypertension: A nationwide cohort study. *J. Dermatol.* **2018**, *45*, 1381–1388. [CrossRef]
126. Momose, M.; Asahina, A.; Fukuda, T.; Sakuma, T.; Umezawa, Y.; Nakagawa, H. Evaluation of epicardial adipose tissue volume and coronary artery calcification in Japanese patients with psoriasis vulgaris. *J. Dermatol.* **2018**, *45*, 1349–1352. [CrossRef]
127. Takamura, S.; Takahashi, A.; Inoue, Y.; Teraki, Y. Effects of tumor necrosis factor-α, interleukin-23 and interleukin-17A inhibitors on bodyweight and body mass index in patients with psoriasis. *J. Dermatol.* **2018**, *45*, 1130–1134. [CrossRef]
128. Han, J.H.; Lee, J.H.; Han, K.D.; Kim, H.N.; Bang, C.H.; Park, Y.M.; Lee, J.Y.; Kim, T.Y. Increased risk of psoriasis in subjects with abdominal obesity: A nationwide population-based study. *J. Dermatol.* **2019**, *46*, 695–701. [CrossRef]
129. Yamazaki, F.; Takehana, K.; Tamashima, M.; Okamoto, H. Improvement in abnormal coronary arteries estimated by coronary computed tomography angiography after secukinumab treatment in a Japanese psoriatic patient. *J. Dermatol.* **2019**, *46*, e51–e52. [CrossRef]
130. Bayaraa, B.; Imafuku, S. Sustainability and switching of biologics for psoriasis and psoriatic arthritis at Fukuoka University Psoriasis Registry. *J. Dermatol.* **2019**, *46*, 389–398. [CrossRef]
131. Nakajima, K.; Sano, S. Mouse models of psoriasis and their relevance. *J. Dermatol.* **2018**, *45*, 252–263. [CrossRef]
132. Ogawa, E.; Sato, Y.; Minagawa, A.; Okuyama, R. Pathogenesis of psoriasis and development of treatment. *J. Dermatol.* **2018**, *45*, 264–272. [CrossRef]
133. Kamata, M.; Tada, Y. Safety of biologics in psoriasis. *J. Dermatol.* **2018**, *45*, 279–286. [CrossRef]
134. Tada, Y.; Ishii, K.; Kimura, J.; Hanada, K.; Kawaguchi, I. Patient preference for biologic treatments of psoriasis in Japan. *J. Dermatol.* **2019**, *46*, 466–477. [CrossRef]
135. Bayaraa, B.; Imafuku, S. Relationship between environmental factors, age of onset and familial history in Japanese patients with psoriasis. *J. Dermatol.* **2018**, *45*, 715–718. [CrossRef]
136. Elder, J.T. Expanded genome-wide association study meta-analysis of psoriasis expands the catalog of common psoriasis-associated variants. *J. Investig. Dermatol. Symp. Proc.* **2018**, *19*, S77–S78. [CrossRef]
137. Di Meglio, P.; Duarte, J.H.; Ahlfors, H.; Owens, N.D.; Li, Y.; Villanova, F.; Tosi, I.; Hirota, K.; Nestle, F.O.; Mrowietz, U.; et al. Activation of the aryl hydrocarbon receptor dampens the severity of inflammatory skin conditions. *Immunity* **2014**, *40*, 989–1001. [CrossRef]
138. Smith, S.H.; Peredo, C.E.; Takeda, Y.; Bui, T.; Neil, J.; Rickard, D.; Millerman, E.; Therrien, J.P.; Nicodeme, E.; Brusq, J.M.; et al. Development of a topical treatment for psoriasis targeting RORγ: From bench to skin. *PLoS ONE* **2016**, *11*, e0147979. [CrossRef]
139. Cochez, P.M.; Michiels, C.; Hendrickx, E.; Van Belle, A.B.; Lemaire, M.M.; Dauguet, N.; Warnier, G.; de Heusch, M.; Togbe, D.; Ryffel, B.; et al. AhR modulates the IL-22-producing cell proliferation/recruitment in imiquimod-induced psoriasis mouse model. *Eur. J. Immunol.* **2016**, *46*, 1449–1459. [CrossRef]
140. Mescher, M.; Tigges, J.; Rolfes, K.M.; Shen, A.L.; Yee, J.S.; Vogeley, C.; Krutmann, J.; Bradfield, C.A.; Lang, D.; Haarmann-Stemmann, T. The Toll-like receptor agonist imiquimod is metabolized by aryl hydrocarbon receptor-regulated cytochrome P450 enzymes in human keratinocytes and mouse liver. *Arch. Toxicol.* **2019**, *93*, 1917–1926. [CrossRef]

141. Beranek, M.; Fiala, Z.; Kremlacek, J.; Andrys, C.; Krejsek, J.; Hamakova, K.; Palicka, V.; Borska, L. Serum levels of aryl hydrocarbon receptor, cytochromes P450 1A1 and 1B1 in patients with exacerbated psoriasis vulgaris. *Folia Biol. (Praha)* **2018**, *64*, 97–102. [PubMed]
142. Bissonnette, R.; Bolduc, C.; Maari, C.; Nigen, S.; Webster, J.M.; Tang, L.; Lyle, M. Efficacy and safety of topical WBI-1001 in patients with mild to moderate psoriasis: Results from a randomized double-blind placebo-controlled, phase II trial. *J. Eur. Acad. Dermatol. Venereol.* **2012**, *26*, 1516–1521. [CrossRef] [PubMed]

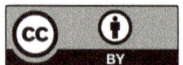

© 2019 by the authors. Licensee MDPI, Basel, Switzerland. This article is an open access article distributed under the terms and conditions of the Creative Commons Attribution (CC BY) license (http://creativecommons.org/licenses/by/4.0/).

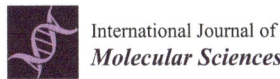

Article

Altered Lipid Metabolism in Blood Mononuclear Cells of Psoriatic Patients Indicates Differential Changes in Psoriasis Vulgaris and Psoriatic Arthritis

Piotr Wójcik [1], Michał Biernacki [1], Adam Wroński [2], Wojciech Łuczaj [1], Georg Waeg [3], Neven Žarković [4] and Elżbieta Skrzydlewska [1,*]

1. Department of Analytical Chemistry, Medical University of Bialystok, 15-089 Białystok, Poland
2. Dermatological Specialized Center "DERMAL" NZOZ in Bialystok, 15-453 Białystok, Poland
3. Institute of Molecular Biosciences, University of Graz, 8010 Graz, Austria
4. LabOS, Rudjer Boskovic Institute, Laboratory for Oxidative Stress, 10000 Zagreb, Croatia
* Correspondence: elzbieta.skrzydlewska@umb.edu.pl; Tel.: +48-857485882

Received: 26 July 2019; Accepted: 28 August 2019; Published: 30 August 2019

Abstract: The aim of this study was to investigate possible stress-associated disturbances in lipid metabolism in mononuclear cells, mainly lymphocytes of patients with psoriasis vulgaris (Ps, n = 32) or with psoriatic arthritis (PsA, n = 16) in respect to the healthy volunteers (n = 16). The results showed disturbances in lipid metabolism of psoriatic patients reflected by different phospholipid profiles. The levels of non-enzymatic lipid metabolites associated with oxidative stress 8-isoprostaglandin F2α (8-isoPGF2α) and free 4-hydroxynonenal (4-HNE) were higher in PsA, although levels of 4-HNE-His adducts were higher in Ps. In the case of the enzymatic metabolism of lipids, enhanced levels of endocannabinoids were observed in both forms of psoriasis, while higher expression of their receptors and activities of phospholipases were detected only in Ps. Moreover, cyclooxygenase-1 (COX-1) activity was enhanced only in Ps, but cyclooxygenase-2 (COX-2) was enhanced both in Ps and PsA, generating higher levels of eicosanoids: prostaglandin E1 (PGE1), leukotriene B4 (LTB4), 13-hydroxyoctadecadienoic acid (13HODE), thromboxane B2 (TXB2). Surprisingly, some of major eicosanoids 15-d-PGJ$_2$ (15-deoxy-Δ12,14-prostaglandin J$_2$), 15-hydroxyeicosatetraenoic acid (15-HETE) were elevated in Ps and reduced in PsA. The results of our study revealed changes in lipid metabolism with enhancement of immune system-modulating mediators in psoriatic mononuclear cells. Evaluating further differential stress responses in Ps and PsA affecting lipid metabolism and immunity might be useful to improve the prevention and therapeutic treatments of psoriasis.

Keywords: lipid mediators; psoriasis vulgaris; psoriatic arthritis; lipid peroxidation products; endocannabinoids; eicosanoids

---

1. Introduction

Psoriasis is a chronic autoimmune disease, the most common form of which is psoriasis vulgaris, characterized by pathological interactions between immune cells, especially lymphocytes, and skin cells, especially keratinocytes. In some patients, psoriasis is characterized by a more severe clinical course, leading to the development of psoriatic arthritis [1]. The cause of the disease remains unknown, although some genetic or environmental factors are associated with the development of psoriasis. Thus, it has been observed that lymphocytes and the cytokines they produce, especially interferon γ (IFNγ) and interleukin 17 (IL-17), affect other cells, leading to chronic inflammation and characteristic symptoms such as cutaneous plaques in psoriasis or arthrosis and loss of movement in psoriatic arthritis. Moreover, the pro-inflammatory phenotype of lymphocytes and other immune cells is observed not only locally in the skin or joints, but also in cells isolated from blood, which confirms that general inflammation is present in psoriasis [2]. However, that can only partially explain the course of the disease, still leaving many questions open in respect to the development of psoriasis or the transition of one form to another. Recent studies on immunological diseases have revealed that their development is often accompanied by oxidative stress and increased metabolism of phospholipids, suggesting that both ROS and lipid mediators play important roles in the pathophysiology of psoriasis [3]. In psoriasis, both systemic and local, oxidative stress and increased metabolism of phospholipids have been demonstrated. Among immune-competent, inflammatory cells of psoriatic patients were observed especially for granulocytes, which increasingly generate lipid peroxidation products, thus modulating their inflammatory activities [4]. Furthermore, it has been shown that activation of lymphocytes is also accompanied by the generation of large amounts of reactive oxygen species (ROS) that are important mediators of cytokine-mediated redox biology [5]. Biological activities of ROS are related to their ability to react with biomolecules, such as phospholipids, in particular polyunsaturated fatty acids (PUFA), which leads to lipid peroxidation and generation of reactive aldehydes, e.g., 4-hydroxynonenal (4-HNE), which is denoted also as a "second messenger of free radicals" [6].

In addition to lipid peroxidation, cellular phospholipids are also metabolized by enzymes, the activities of which are increased in various inflammatory processes. The most important enzymes involved in the generation of lipid mediators are phospholipases, cyclooxygenases (COXs), and lipoxygenases (LOXs) [7]. During this process phospholipases begin biosynthesis of endocannabinoids among which the best known are 2-acylglycerol (2-AG) and anandamide (AEA). Enhanced levels of them are observed in inflammatory diseases like osteoarthritis or systemic lupus erythematosus [8,9]. Endocannabinoids affect cells mostly by interactions with their receptors, cannabinoid receptors (CB1 and CB2). It is known that activation of CB2 receptor results in anti-inflammatory and anti-oxidative regulation, while activation of CB1 shows pro-inflammatory and pro-oxidative activity [10]. In addition, endocannabinoids have been found to be involved in the development of psoriatic comorbidities. Therefore, it can be assumed that disturbances of the endocannabinoid system may also play a significant role in the course of psoriasis.

Moreover, recent studies suggest, that effect of endocannabinoids action is also dependent on the action of their metabolites [11]. Anandamide is metabolized into arachidonic acid which together with arachidonic acid revealed from phospholipids is further metabolized into eicosanoids by (COXs) and LOX. Among cyclooxygenases COX-2 is believed to be the main enzyme responsible for generation of active lipid mediators during inflammation [12], while arachidonic acid is also a substrate to synthesis of thromboxanes, leukotrienes, and prostaglandins [13].

Since lipid mediators are commonly observed in autoimmune diseases, they are constantly gaining increased attention among researchers focused on autoimmune diseases. Lipid mediators might accordingly be important for studies on diseases with poorly understood pathophysiology and without effective therapy, like psoriasis. As such, the aim of this study was to investigate oxidative lipid modifications in mononuclear cells, mainly lymphocytes isolated from patients suffering from psoriasis vulgaris (Ps) or psoriatic arthritis (PsA).

2. Results

Phospholipids that could distinguish patients with psoriasis vulgaris and psoriatic arthritis were selected by use of multivariate statistics. Twenty phospholipid species with variable importance in projection (VIP ≥ 1) were selected, which were driving the separation of examined groups. Principal component analysis (PCA) model (Figure 1) was constructed to check classification of each group. The complete data set with the log transformed and auto-scaled phospholipid variables was used to carry out the analysis. The PCA model, on which each point represents an individual sample, showed that the group of healthy subjects was clearly separated from the patients groups, while the separation between both types of psoriasis almost did not occur. The model captured 78.1% of the total variance. The variation in the variables is represented by two principal components of PC1 (57.7%) versus PC2 (14.7%). It is highly probable that PC1 is associated with the age, while PC2 indicates a positive correlation with disease state. It was observed that the samples from both groups of psoriatic patients showed positive values for PC2, whereas those from healthy subjects presented negative values. Finally, we used partial least squares-discriminate analysis (PLS-DA) (Figure S1) and VIP for estimation of the importance of each phospholipid species which drove the separation of the examined groups (Table 1).

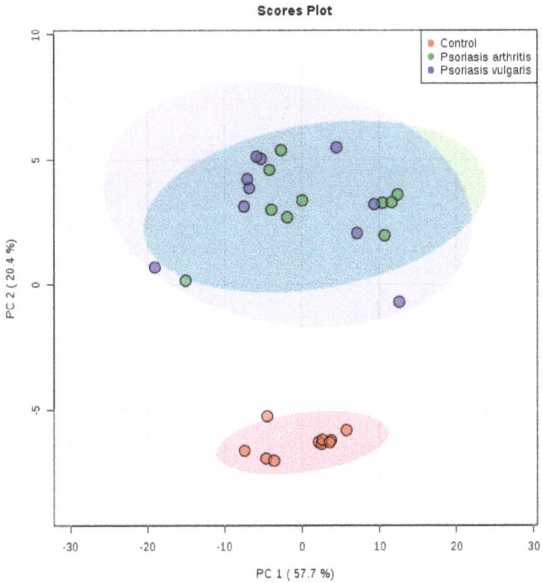

Figure 1. Principal component analysis (PCA) plot of the phospholipid species relative abundance determined by HILIC-LC-MS in lymphocytes of patient with psoriasis vulgaris (n = 10) and psoriatic arthritis (n = 10) as well as healthy subjects (n = 10); 95% confidential intervals are indicated by shaded area.

Table 1 shows the details of these species that belong to lysophosphatidylcholine (LPC), phosphatidylcholine (PC), phosphatidylinositol (PI), and sphingomyelin (SM) classes. Two phosphatidylcholines containing eicosatrienoic (20:3) and docosadienoic (22:2) acid, namely PC(20:0/22:2), and PC(20:3/24:0), had the highest VIP scores. In general, PC was down-regulated in patients of both types of psoriasis while two SM species, containing tetracosadienoic (24:2) and docosaenoic acid (22:1), respectively, were up-regulated. Other phospholipid species that were changed in the course of both forms of psoriasis belong to the PI class. PI species were down-regulated in both groups of patients with exception of PI(24:0/24:0), PI(24:0/24:1), and PI(18:0/22:0), which were highly up-regulated. Important to notice is that PI species containing arachidonic and linoleic acid, namely PI(16:0/20:4), PI(18:0/20:4), and PI(18:2/22:0) were significantly down-regulated in both groups of psoriatic patients in comparison to healthy subjects. Moreover, most of PI species were found to be more altered in PsA patients than those with Ps. LPC species with the score > 1, namely LPC(16:0) and LPC(18:0), were found to be highly up-regulated in psoriasis in comparison to healthy subjects. Hence, these two LPC species were mostly responsible for the differentiation of both types of psoriasis from healthy subjects (Table 1).

Table 1. Changes in mononuclear cells top 20 phospholipid species with VIP score greater than one comparing the healthy subjects (C; n = 10) to psoriasis vulgaris (n = 10) and psoriasis arthritis (n = 10) groups of patients; ns, not statistically significant.

m/z	RT	ID	Composition	VIP	Control vs. Psoriasis Vulgaris	p Value	Log2 (Fold-Change) Control vs. Psoriatic Arthritis	p Value	Psoriasis Vulgaris vs. Psoriatic Arthritis	p Value
928.6940	18.31	PC(42:2)	PC(20:0/22:2)	1.97	0.63	2.34×10^{-5}	0.34	1.17×10^{-3}	0.29	ns
954.7113	18.12	PC(44:3)	PC(20:3/24:0)	1.89	0.54	3.76×10^{-5}	0.26	2.84×10^{-3}	0.29	ns
917.6085	3.47	PI(40:2)	PI(18:2/22:0)	1.57	0.68	1.13×10^{-5}	0.90	1.81×10^{-8}	−0.21	ns
915.5954	3.47	PI(40:3)	PI(18:0/22:3)	1.57	0.75	1.13×10^{-5}	0.97	3.91×10^{-8}	−0.21	ns
1033.7629	3.90	PI(48:0)	PI(24:0/24:0)	1.52	−1.06	5.81×10^{-4}	−0.85	2.06×10^{-3}	−0.21	ns
857.6755	18.16	SM(d41:2)	SM(d17:0/24:2)	1.51	−0.50	5.81×10^{-4}	−0.26	3.36×10^{-2}	−0.23	ns
868.6052	16.49	PC(38:4)	PC(18:0/20:4)	1.47	−0.181	2.00×10^{-3}	0.31	1.66×10^{-2}	0.26	ns
1031.7489	3.90	PI(48:1)	PI(24:0/24:1)	1.44	−1.64	1.03×10^{-3}	−1.43	1.93×10^{-3}	−0.2109	ns
857.5159	3.85	PI(36:4)	PI(16:0/20:4)	1.39	0.68	5.81×10^{-4}	0.89	1.26×10^{-5}	−0.21	ns
840.5732	16.71	PC(36:4)	PC(16:0/20:4)	1.39	0.56	3.51×10^{-3}	0.31	3.00×10^{-2}	0.25	ns
896.6372	16.37	PC(40:4)	PC(18:0/22:4)	1.38	0.42	4.04×10^{-3}	0.14	ns	0.27	ns
909.5490	3.84	PI(40:6)	PI(18:2/22:4)	1.38	0.61	3.33×10^{-4}	0.82	2.76×10^{-6}	−0.21	ns
792.5746	17.39	PC(32:0)	PC(16:0/16:0)	1.37	0.54	4.04×10^{-3}	0.28	ns	0.25	ns
921.6399	3.99	PI(40:0)	PI(18:0/22:0)	1.36	−1.89	1.63×10^{-3}	−1.68	3.02×10^{-3}	−0.21	ns
885.5472	3.83	PI(38:4)	PI(18:0/20:4)	1.35	0.57	2.61×10^{-4}	−0.26	ns	−0.21	ns
554.3463	20.37	LPC(16:0)		1.33	−1.77	5.81×10^{-4}	−2.6	3.53×10^{-6}	0.83	ns
582.3771	20.10	LPC(18:0)		1.31	−1.50	3.32×10^{-5}	−2.3	7.98×10^{-8}	0.83	ns
894.6222	16.40	PC(40:5)	PC(18:1/22:4)	1.30	0.50	4.72×10^{-3}	0.80	ns	0.26	ns
843.6591	18.25	SM(d40:2)	SM(d18:1/22:1)	1.26	−0.50	4.70×10^{-3}	−0.20	ns	−0.29	ns
911.5644	3.84	PI(40:5)	PI(18:1/20:4)	1.26	0.59	1.63×10^{-3}	0.24	4.78×10^{-5}	−0.21	ns

It is often assumed that the reduced level of PUFAs is related to their ROS-dependent and enzyme-dependent metabolism. Consequently, the elevated levels of lipid peroxidation products belonging to compounds generated during PUFAs' oxidative fragmentation, such as 4-HNE, as well as to compounds generated during PUFAs oxidative cyclisation, such as 8-iso prostaglandin F2α (8-isoPGF2α), was observed, in particular in patients with PsA (Figure 2).

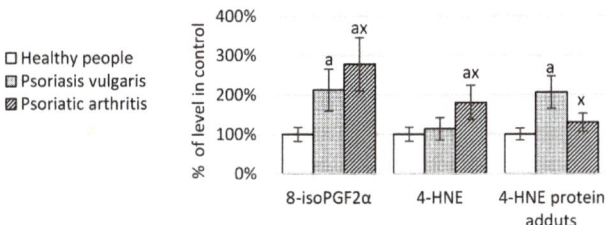

Figure 2. The level of phospholipid oxidative modifications products and of 4-HNE-protein adducts in mononuclear cells of healthy peoples (n = 16) and patients with psoriasis vulgaris (n = 32) and psoriatic arthritis (n = 16). 8-isoPGF2α, F2α-8-isoprostaglandin; 4-HNE, 4-hydroxynonenal. Data points represent the mean ± SD; a, significantly different from healthy subject, $p < 0.05$; x, significantly different from patients with psoriasis vulgaris, $p < 0.05$.

That might indeed be that case with psoriatic patients because their observed decrease of PUFAs was associated by enhanced activities of the enzymes metabolizing lipids including phospholipases (PLA2 and PAF-AH), as well as of cyclooxygenase 1 (COX1) and cyclooxygenase2 (COX2), especially in Ps (Figure 3).

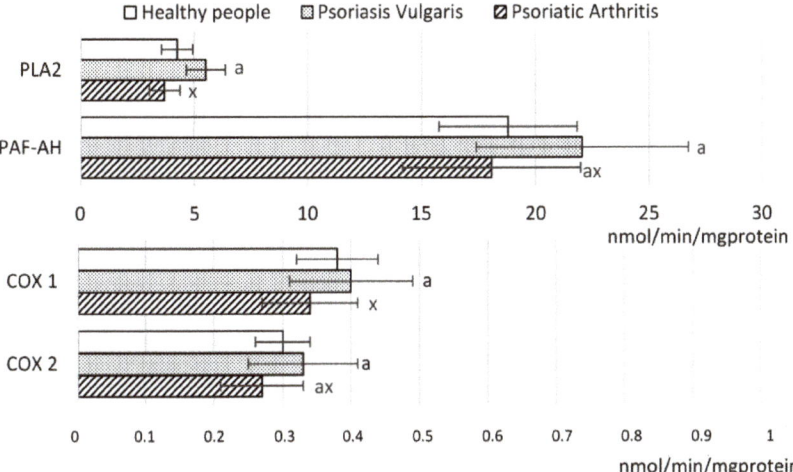

Figure 3. The activity of the enzymes involved in phospholipid metabolism in mononuclear cells of patients psoriasis vulgaris (n = 32) and psoriatic arthritis (n = 16) as well as healthy subjects (n = 16). PLA2, phosholipase A2; PAF-AF, platelet-activating factor acetylhydrolase; COX, cyclooxygenases. Data points represent the mean ± SD; a, significantly different from healthy subject, $p < 0.05$; x, significantly different from patients with psoriasis vulgaris, $p < 0.05$.

It is likely that increased activity of the above listed enzymes promoted generation of endocannabinoids. The levels of anandamide and LEA increased more in mononuclear cells of patients with PsA, while the concentration of 2-AG, 2-LG (2-linoleoylglycerol), and OEA (oleoylethanolamide) was higher in patients with Ps (Table 2). An elevated level of endocannabinoids was observed despite the increased activity of enzymes degrading them (FAAH—fatty acid amide hydrolase and MAGL—monoacylglycerol lipase), especially in mononuclear cells of patients with Ps (Table 2).

Table 2. The level of endocannabinoids and enzymes degrading them (FAAH and MAGL) in mononuclear cells of patients with psoriasis vulgaris (n = 32) and psoriatic arthritis (n = 16) Abbreviations: 2-AG, 2-arachidonoylglycerol; 2-LG, 2-linoleoylglycerol; AEA, anandamide; FAAH, fatty acid amide hydrolase; LEA, dihomo-γ-linolenoylethanolamine; MAGL, monoacylglycerol lipase; OEA, oleoylethanolamide. Data points represent the mean ± SD; a, significantly different from healthy subject, $p < 0.05$; x, significantly different from patients with Ps, $p < 0.05$.

Analyzed Parameters	Healthy Subjects	Psoriasis Vulgaris	Psoriatic Arthritis
AEA (pmol/mg protein)	0.17 ± 0.02	0.19 ± 0.03a	0.23 ± 0.04ax
2-AG (pmol/mg protein)	1.87 ± 0.18	3.24 ± 0.45a	2.78 ± 0.37ax
2-LG (pmol/mg protein)	5.59 ± 0.87	7.92 ± 0.99a	7.41 ± 0.93a
LEA (pmol/mg protein)	0.79 ± 0.08	0.94 ± 0.15a	1.17 ± 0.15ax
OEA (pmol/mg protein)	0.33 ± 0.05	0.47 ± 0.07a	0.36 ± 0.05a
FAAH (pmol/min/mg protein)	170 ± 16	219 ± 28a	242 ± 31ax
MAGL (pmol/min/mg protein)	55 ± 6	75 ± 10a	83 ± 14ax

Increased level of endocannabinoids resulted in enhanced expression of cannabinoids receptors (CB1 and CB2), as well as other receptors activated also by endocannabinoids (GPR55 and TRPV1) in Ps and decreased expression of these receptors in PsA (Figure 4). Products of phospholipid metabolism including endocannabinoids, but also fatty acids and eicosanoids, are ligands of nuclear peroxisome proliferator-activated receptors (PPARα, PPARγ, PPARδ). A significant increase in the expression of these receptors was observed in mononuclear cells obtained from patients with Ps, while it was only moderately raised in mononuclear cells of patients with PsA (Figure 4).

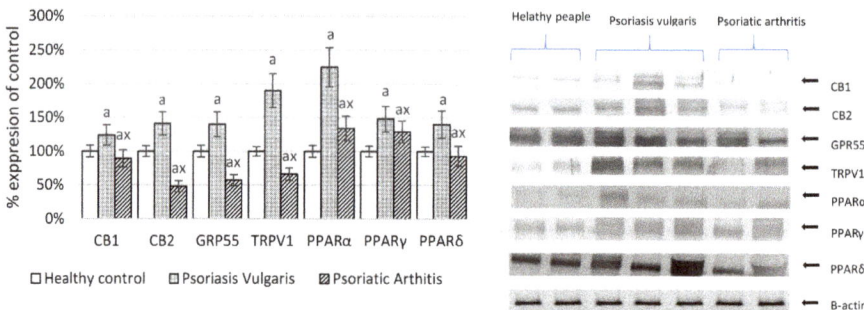

Figure 4. The expression of receptors involved in phospholipid metabolism in mononuclear cells of patients with psoriasis vulgaris (n = 16) and psoriatic arthritis (n = 8) and healthy peoples (n = 8). CB1, CB2, cannabinoid receptors; GRP55, G protein-coupled receptor 55; TRPV, the transient receptor potential cation channel subfamily V member 1; PPAR, peroxisome proliferator-activated receptor. Data points represent the mean ± SD; a, significantly different from healthy subjects, $p < 0.05$; x, significantly different from patients with psoriasis vulgaris, $p < 0.05$.

Increased activity of PLA2 lead to the enhanced release of arachidonic acid, which is further metabolized (mainly by cyclooxygenases and lipoxygenases) into another large group of active lipid mediators, notably eicosanoids (Figure 5) Among them, pro-inflammatory factors, such as 13-hydroxyoctadecadienoic acid (13-HODE) and leukotriene B$_4$ (LTB4) levels, were increased in both forms of the disease. In particular LTB4 level increased dramatically in psoriasis, especially in Ps. In addition, thromboxane B$_2$ (TxB2), (metabolite of pro-inflammatory thromboxane A$_2$ (TxA2) level was increased in Ps, which might be related to the activities of cyclooxygenases. The analysis of anti-inflammatory mediators revealed decreased levels of 15-deoxy-Δ12,14-prostaglandin J$_2$ (15-d-PGJ$_2$) in patients with Ps, while 15-hydroxyeicosatetraenoic acid (15-HETE) levels were slightly, but significantly, increased in Ps, and prostaglandin E1 (PGE$_1$) levels were increased both in Ps (four-fold) and in PsA (two-fold).

Since psoriasis is known to be associated with inflammation, basic pro-inflammatory and anti-inflammatory parameters were examined (Figure 6). The levels of pro-inflammatory cytokine IL-2 was increased above normal in mononuclear cells of both forms of psoriasis, while anti-inflammatory IL-10 levels were not changed in psoriatic patients.

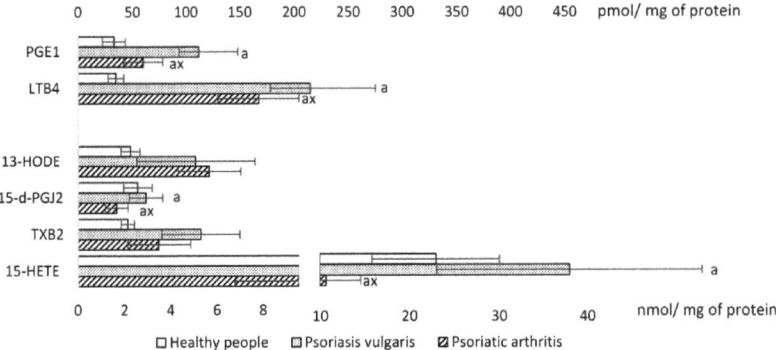

Figure 5. The level of the eicosanoids in mononuclear cells of patients with psoriasis (n = 32), psoriatic arthritis (n = 16), as well as healthy subjects (n = 16). Data points represent the mean ± SD; a, significantly different from healthy subject, $p < 0.05$; x, significantly different from patients with psoriasis vulgaris. Prostaglandin E1 (PGE1), leukotriene B4 (LTB4), 13-hydroxyoctadecadienoic acid (13HODE), thromboxane B2 (TXB2). Surprisingly, some of major eicosanoids 15-deoxy-Δ12,14-prostaglandin J$_2$ (15-d-PGJ$_2$), 15-hydroxyeicosatetraenoic acid (15-HETE). Data points represent the mean ± SD; a, significantly different from healthy subject, $p < 0.05$; x, significantly different from patients with Ps, $p < 0.05$.

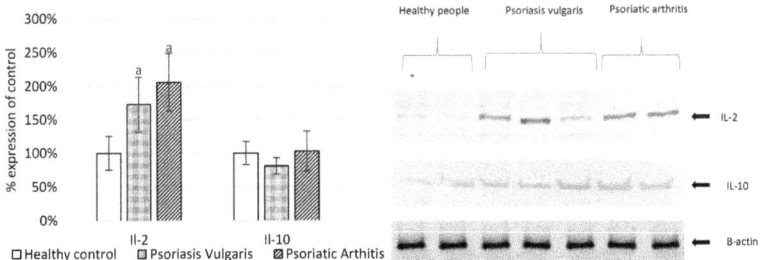

Figure 6. The expression of interleukins and pro-inflammatory mediators in mononuclear cells from patients with psoriasis vulgaris (n = 16), psoriatic arthritis (n = 8), and healthy subjects (n = 8). IL-interleukine. Data points represent the mean ± SD; a, significantly different from healthy subjects, $p < 0.05$.

3. Discussion

Psoriasis is a complex inflammatory disease associated with increased activation of lymphocytes [14], which leads to the generation of pro-inflammatory cytokines and to pro-oxidative processes causing oxidative stress [3]. The results of our study confirm the onset of oxidative stress in psoriasis, which is, in particular in PsA, manifested by changes in the metabolism of phospholipids in mononuclear cells, mainly containing lymphocytes, thus offering better understanding of the diseases, due to differentially expressed changes in lipid metabolism between Ps and PsA examined mononuclear cells.

The main source of ROS in cells are usually mitochondria whose respiratory chain may be disrupted by various factors, including phospholipids' metabolites, such as endocannabinoids, the levels of which were, in the current study, found to be increased in the mononuclear cells of psoriatic patients. It is known that the main endocannabinoids, AEA and 2-AG, may stimulate the function of mitochondria, including the production of hydrogen peroxide by enhanced entry of calcium ions into the cell [15]. In addition, activation of cannabinoid receptors (CB1), caused by endocannabinoids, which was, in our study, also found to be increased in mononuclear cells of psoriatic patients, may promote oxidative stress by enhanced inflammation, e.g., through NOS stimulation leading to increased generation of superoxide and nitric oxide [16]. In favor of this possibility are increased activities of cytosolic NADPH and xanthine oxidases in granulocytes and in plasma of patients with psoriasis, in particular if obtained from patients with PsA [4]. Such changes were accompanied by disturbances in the antioxidant system, which was spread in a stress-response manner lowering the level/activity of cellular antioxidants.

Similarly, redox imbalance and inflammation observed in psoriatic patients were, in the current study, associated with changes in ROS-dependent and enzyme-dependent phospholipid metabolism of mononuclear cells affecting especially PUFAs, which are lipid species the most sensitive to the ROS attack causing lipid peroxidation. Different phospholipid species, including phosphatidylcholines and phosphatidylinositols containing linoleic, arachidonic, eicosatetraenoic and docosadienoic acids, in particular, were down-regulated in mononuclear cells of psoriatic patients. Arachidonic acid and linoleic acid are the major PUFAs, which are oxidized in a ROS-dependent manner to biologically-active lipid mediators, including products of oxidative fragmentation (mainly α,β-unsaturated electrophilic aldehydes, with 4-HNE as the most important one) and products of oxidative cyclisation (mainly prostaglandin derivatives, such as 8-isoPGF2α) that further propagate oxidative damages altering functional activities of the immune-competent cells [17]. The mechanism of 8-isoPGF$_{2\alpha}$ action is based on TNFα activation [18]. So far, increased levels of 8-isoPGF$_{2\alpha}$ have been found in psoriatic patients' serum [19] as well as in the skin cells [20] being accompanied by elevated TNFα expression [21]. However, 4-HNE is a more potent biomarker of lipid peroxidation, which is involved in complex regulation of inflammatory and immunological responses [6]. The increased levels of the free 4-HNE were observed in our study especially in the mononuclear cells of PsA patients. Opposite to that, the levels of histidine-bound protein adducts of 4-HNE were higher in examined cells of patients with Ps indicating differential metabolic and scavenging pathways for this "second messenger of free radicals" in Ps and in PsA patients. It is known that unsaturated aldehydes, such as 4-HNE, have a strong affinity for covalently linking with nucleophilic amino and thiol groups of biomolecules, including proteins and glutathione (GSH) [17]. Since the thiol groups of protein cysteine residues act as redox switches controlling cell signaling and metabolism [22], versatile interactions of cysteine with signaling molecules, such as 4-HNE, can selectively modulate protein functions [23]. Complementary to that, modifications of protein residues, not only cysteine but also histidine or lysine, may lead to disturbances of biological functions of modified proteins and their translocation to the cell membrane and activation of protein G [24–26]. Our findings suggest that such protein adducts may participate in enhanced expression of protein G-coupled receptors (including cannabinoid receptors), as was observed in this study in mononuclear cells of psoriatic patients.

The cellular metabolism of phospholipids, independent of ROS, also includes enzymatic reactions leading to the generation of endocannabinoids dependent on the activity of phospholipases [27]. Despite the increased activity of endocannabinoid-metabolizing enzymes (FAAH and MAGL), endocannabinoid levels were elevated in our patients. The main endocannabinoids, anandamide and 2-arachidonoylglycerol (2-AG), participate in the modulation of inflammation and redox balance mainly through the activation of cannabinoid receptors [28]. Crosstalk between ROS and endocannabinoids has been proven in various diseases [27], but so far not in patients with psoriasis, as was done for the first time in the present study.

In addition, inflammation is associated with increased expression of lymphocyte receptors: GPR55 and TRPV1 [29,30]. According to in vitro studies endocannabinoids themselves may also act as anti-inflammatory agents by promoting the Th2 cell phenotype and further inhibit the production of pro-inflammatory cytokines by lymphocytes [31]. This may suggest that endocannabinoids are generated, among others, to alleviate the inflammatory aspects of psoriasis. In fact, in the case of Ps we observed a higher expression of endocannabinoid receptors but, surprisingly, in the case of PsA, the expression of these receptors has been reduced, suggesting no cellular response to the regulatory role of endocannabinoids. It is possible that the receptors or membrane protein G have been modified by 4-HNE, which can explain also less pronounced increase of the soluble 4-HNE-protein adducts in patients with PsA, who have otherwise higher levels of the free aldehyde than patients with Ps. In any case, the disrupted immunosuppressive effect of endocannabinoids in PsA may be an important factor differentiating the pathophysiology of both forms of psoriasis and may promote exacerbation of Ps into the form of PsA.

Enzymatic degradation of endocannabinoids, with COXs participation in particular, plays a critical role in the onset of the inflammatory cascade with the generation of different biologically-active compounds, including eicosanoids [32]. Among them are various bioactive agents, such as prostaglandins, thromboxanes, and leukotrienes, which can participate in the pathophysiology of psoriasis. Eicosanoids may have opposite inflammatory effects and, thus, modulate skin disorders. The results of this study revealed a significant increase in mononuclear cells of patients with psoriasis TxB2, a stable metabolite of TxA2, which plays a pro-inflammatory role in imiquimod-induced psoriatic dermatitis [33]. Additionally, elevated LTB4 levels may promote skin inflammation [34]. Inflammation may also be modified by 15d-PGJ$_2$, which is elevated in Ps, and which inhibits NFκB mediated metabolic pathways by inhibiting IκB kinase (IKK) activity [35].

Another mechanism of interactions redox biology-lipid metabolism in the mononuclear cells of psoriatic patients may be associated with the expression of nuclear receptors like peroxisome proliferator-activated receptors—PPARs [36], whose forms: PPARα, PPARγ, and PPARδ were enhanced in mononuclear cells of patients with psoriasis, particularly with Ps. Moreover, PUFAs, eicosanoids, and endocannabinoids may be ligands of PPARs, which in B and T lymphocytes serve as important regulators of the immune system as potential anti-inflammatory targets for PPAR ligands [37,38].

PPARα and PPARδ show antioxidant properties by suppressing enzymes involved in ROS/RNS generation [39], while enhanced activation of PPARα may also prevent NFκB–dependent inflammation [40]. The results obtained by the murine translation study indicated that PPARα activation may be one of the protective mechanisms against progression of skin inflammation [41]. Additionally, the PPARδ promotes synthesis of antioxidants, such as thioredoxin, superoxide dismutase, or heme oxygenase [42]. Thus, PPARδ enhanced expression seems to be an important antioxidative mechanism in patients with Ps. The significant decrease in their expression observed in PsA confirms that the lack of anti-stress protection against ROS leads to an increase the severity of this disease. In addition, increased PPARγ expression, as discovered in this study, may be involved in reduction of TNFα level, particularly in PsA [43].

4. Materials and Methods

4.1. Materials

Blood samples were collected from 32 patients with psoriasis vulgaris (Ps) (16 females, 16 men; mean age 38) and 16 patients with psoriatic arthritis (seven females, nine men; mean age 35).

Only patients with psoriasis vulgaris for at least six months and characterized by at least 10% of the total body surface affected by the disease were included in the study (the median of their psoriasis surface index and severity index (PASI) was 21, with a range of 15–25). Patients with psoriatic arthritis (PsA) were diagnosed on the basis of a questionnaire CASPAR (ClASsification criteria for Psoriatic Arthritis). All participants gave their informed consent for inclusion in the research. The research was carried out in accordance with the Helsinki Declaration, and the protocol was approved by the Local Bioethics Commission at the Medical University of Białystok (Poland), no. R-I-002/289/2017 (2017.09.28). People receiving topical or oral medications during the four weeks before the study and comorbidities/smoking or alcohol abuse were excluded from examinations.

Blood was collected into tubes with ethylenediaminetetraacetic acid as an anti-coagulant and butylhydroxytoluene as an antioxidant. Density gradient centrifugation (Gradisol L, 300 g, 25 min) was used to obtain mononuclear cells mainly containing lymphocytes fraction from blood. This fraction was washed in phosphate-buffered saline (PBS), then resuspended in PBS containing proteases inhibitors mix. Purity of the cells has been examined microscopically (Nikon Eclipse Ti, Nikon Instruments Inc., Melville, NY, USA). Isolated fractions were lysed by sonification on ice and stored at −80 °C before further analysis. All obtained parameters are expressed per mg of protein (protein levels were examined using Bradford method [44]).

4.2. Methods

4.2.1. Phospholipid Profile Estimation

Mononuclear cells from ten patients with Ps, ten patients with PsA (5f + 5m) and ten healthy subjects (5f + 5m) were used to estimate phospholipid profile of each group. Total lipids from all samples were extracted by the modified Bligh and Dyer method [45]. The total amount of phospholipids (PL) was calculated by using a phosphorus assay, performed according to Bartlett and Lewis [46]. Hydrophilic interaction chromatography liquid chromatography-mass spectrometry (HILIC-LC)-MS, performed on an Agilent 1290 ultra-performance liquid chromatography (UPLC) system coupled to an Agilent 6540 quadrupole time of flight mass spectrometer (Agilent Technologies, Palo Alto, CA, USA) was applied to obtain the phospholipid profile. An Ascentis Si HPLC Pore column (15 cm × 1.0 mm, 3 µm; Sigma Aldrich, St. Louis, MO, USA) was used for chromatographic separation in gradient mode. The method was described in details previously [47]. Internal standards PC 14:0/14:0, PI 16:0/16:0, and PE 14:0/14:0 (Avanti Polar Lipids, Alabaster, AL, USA) were used to confirm the ion variations observed in the MS spectra. Identification of each phospholipid species was performed according to the typical fragmentation pathways [48]. The area of each extracted ion chromatogram peak was normalized to the area of an internal standard to calculate relative abundance of each ion. Detailed description of the lipidomic methodology is provided in supplementary materials.

4.2.2. Determination of the Activity of Lipid Metabolizing Enzymes

Spectrophotometric method was used to assay phospholipase A2 (PLA2-EC.3.1.1.4) activity using PLA2 Assay Kit (no. 765021, Cayman Chemical Company, Ann Arbor, MI, USA) according to the kit instructions [49].

PAF acetylhydrolase (PAF-AH-EC.3.1.1.47) activity was measured spectrophotometrically using the Cayman's PAF Acetylhydrolase Assay Kit (no. 760901, Cayman Chemical Company, Ann Arbor, MI, USA) according to kit instructions [50].

Cyclooxygenase 1 and 2 (COX1/2-EC.1.14.99.1) activities were measured spectrophotometrically using a commercial assay kit (Cayman Chemical Company, Ann Arbor, MI, USA) [51]. For distinguishing COX1 activity from COX2 activity the specific COX1 inhibitor SC-560 was used [52].

4.2.3. 4-HNE Determination

Gas chromatography-mass spectrometry (GC/MS) using the selected ion monitoring (SIM) mode, as the O-PFB-oxime-TMS derivatives, using minor modifications of the method of Luo [53] was used to measure product of phospholipid fragmentation—4-HNE. Transitions of the precursor to the product ion were as follows: m/z 333.0 and 181.0 for 4-HNE-PFB-TMS and m/z 307 for IS (benzaldehyde-D_{6+}) derivative. (7890A GC-7000 quadrupole MS/MS, Agilent Technologies, Palo Alto, CA, USA).

4.2.4. 4-HNE-Protein Adducts Determination

The 4-HNE-protein adducts level was measured using ELISA method using anti-4-HNE-His murine monoclonal antibody (genuine anti-4-HNE-Hismurine monoclonal antibody, clone 4-HNE 1g4) and goat anti-mouse antibody (Dako, Carpinteria, CA, USA) as primary and secondary antibodies [54]. Results were shown as a percentage of the expression determined in control cells.

4.2.5. 8-isoPGF2α Determination

LC-MS/MS method of Coolen [55] was used to determination of phospholipid oxidative cyclisation product, 8-isoPGF2α, which was analyzed in negative-ion mode using MRM mode: m/z 353.2→193.1 (for 8-isoPGF2α) and 357.2→197.1 (for 8-isoPGF2α-d4 used as an internal standard) (LCMS 8060, Shimadzu, Kyoto, Japan).

4.2.6. Determination of Endocannabinoids and Enzymes Them Degradation

The LC-MS/MS method was used for the quantification of the endocannabinoids level [56]. Endocannabinoids were analyzed in positive-ion mode using MRM mode. Transitions of the precursors to the product ions were as follows: m/z 348.0→62.15 for AEA, m/z 379.0→269.35 for 2-AG, m/z 356.0→63.05 for AEA-d8, m/z 387.0→294.0 m/z for 2-AG-d8, m/z 430.0→66.0 for OEA-d4, m/z 324.0→62.0 for LEA, m/z 355.0→263.0 for 2-LG, 326.0→62.0 for OEA. (LCMS 8060, Shimadzu, Kyoto, Japan). Results were expressed as amount of cannabinoids per mg of protein. The Siegmund procedure [57] was used to determine FAAH (EC.3.5.1.99) activity, following the releasing of m-nitroaniline (m-NA) from decanoyl m-nitroaniline at 410 nm. Enzyme activity was expressed as the amount of enzyme metabolizing 1 pmol of substrat per minute per mg of protein. Releasing of 5′-thio-2-nitrobenzoic acid from arachidonoyl-1-thio-glycerol was used to spectrophotometric [340 nm] determination of MAGL (EC.3.1.1.23) activity [58]. Enzyme activity was expressed as the amount of enzyme metabolizing 1 pmol of substrate per minute per mg of protein.

4.2.7. Lipid Mediators Determination

Lipid mediators levels: TXB_2, PGE_1, 15d-PGJ_2, 13-HODE, LTB_4, and 15-HETE were estimated using ultra-performing liquid chromatography tandem mass spectrometry (LCMS 8060, Shimadzu, Kyoto, Japan) [59]. 15-HETE-d_8, LTB_4-d_4, PGF2α-d_4 and PGD_2-d_4 were used as internal standards for quantification. Lipid mediators were extracted using SPE and analyzed in negative-ion mode (MRM). The precursor to the product ion transition was as follows: m/z 369.3→169.1 for TXB_2, m/z 353.3→317.2 for PGE_1, 315.2→271.2 for 15-d-PGJ_2, m/z 295→277 for 13-HODE, and m/z 319→301.2 for 15-HETE.

4.2.8. Proteins Examination

Western blot analysis of protein expression was performed according to Eissa and Seada [60]. Samples were electrophoretically separated on 10% gels, transferred to 0.2 μm pore-sized nitrocellulose, and incubated overnight with primary antibodies against: GPR55, PPARα (host: rabbit) β-actin (host: mouse) that were purchased from Sigma-Aldrich, (St. Louis, MO, USA). Primary antibodies against: Il-10 (host mouse), CB1, CB2, TRPV1 (host rabbit) were purchased from Santa Cruz Biotechnology (Santa Cruz, CA, USA). Primary antibodies against PPARγ (host: rat) were purchased from Abcam (Cambridge, UK). Primary antibodies against PPARδ were purchased from Invitrogen (Carlsbad,

CA, USA). Primary antibodies against IL-2 (host: rat) were purchased from Thermo Fisher Scientific (Thermo Fisher Scientific, Waltham, MA, USA). Next membranes were incubated for 2 h with alkaline phosphatase secondary IgG antibody against corresponding primary antibody (Sigma-Aldrich, St. Louis, MO, USA). Protein bands were visualized using the BCIP/NBT Liquid substrate system (Sigma-Aldrich, St. Louis, MO, USA). To compare the proteins expression between samples, each band intensity was estimated using VersaDoc System and Quantity One software (Bio-Rad Laboratories Inc., Hercules, CA, USA). The results are expressed as a percentage of the expression determined in the control cells.

4.3. Statistical analysis

All data were expressed as mean ± SD. For data analysis program Statistica (Statistica 13.3, StatSoft Polska, Cracow, Poland) were used. These data were analyzed using one-way analysis of variance followed by a post hoc Tukey test. Values of $p < 0.05$ were considered significant.

5. Conclusions

In conclusion, the results of our research suggest that the development of both forms of psoriasis is strongly associated with oxidative stress resulting in altered lipid metabolism and cytokine production, leading to the development of pro-inflammatory preconditioning of the immune cells. In such a vicious circle, mononuclear cells additionally activate pro-inflammatory states and enhance pro-oxidative, stressful conditions. Thus, ROS and enzyme-dependent changes in mononuclear cell phospholipids can be considered as important processes associated with the pathophysiology of psoriasis. Moreover, the reduced expression of endocannabinoid receptors in PsA suggests the failure of the anti-inflammatory mechanism and may be an important factor leading to the transformation of Ps into a more severe form of PsA. Finally, we assume that monitoring the level of 4-HNE adducts can help predict the progression of Ps into PsA if done complementary to the other parameters of lipid metabolism and the levels of respective cytokines that should be analyzed in further studies.

Supplementary Materials: Supplementary materials can be found at http://www.mdpi.com/1422-0067/20/17/4249/s1

Author Contributions: Conceptualization: E.S. and N.Z.; methodology: P.W.; software: W.L.; validation: W.L., P.W.; formal analysis: W.L.; investigation: M.B.; G.W.; resources: P.W.; data curation: A.W.; writing—original draft preparation: P.W.; writing—review and editing: E.S.; visualization: P.W.; supervision: N.Z.; project administration: E.S.; funding acquisition: E.S.

Funding: This study was financed by the National Science Centre Poland (NCN), grant no. 2016/23/B/NZ7/02350. Cooperation between coauthors is financed by the Polish National Agency for Academic Exchange (NAWA) as part of the International Academic Partnerships (PPI/APM/2018/00015/U/001).

Conflicts of Interest: The authors declared no conflict of interest.

Abbreviations

2-AG	2-Arachidonylglycerol
2-LG	2-Linoleoylglycerol
4-HNE	4-Hydroxynonenal
4-ONE	4-Oxynonenal
8-isoPGF2α	8-iso prostaglandin F2α
13-HODE	13-hydroxyoctadecadienoic acid
15-HETE	15-Hydroxyeicosatetraenoic acid
15d-PGJ$_2$	15-deoxy-Δ12,14-prostaglandin J$_2$
AEA	Anandamide
AIDS	Acquired immunodeficiency syndrome
CB	Cannabinoid receptor
COX	Cyclooxygenase

EDTA	Ethylenediaminetetraacetic acid
ELISA	Enzyme-linked immunosorbent assay
ERK5	Extracellular-signal-regulated kinase 5
FAAH	Fatty acid amide hydrolase
GC	Gas chromatography
GPR55	G protein-coupled receptor 55
HILIC	Hydrophilic interaction chromatography
HPLC	High-performance liquid chromatography
IFNγ	Interferon γ
IKK	IκB kinase
IL	Interleukin
IMQ	Imiquimod
LC	Liquid chromatography
LEA	Dihomo-γ-linolenoylethanolamine
LOX	Lipoxygenases
LPC	Lysophosphatidylcholine
LTB$_4$	Leukotriene B4
MAGL	Monoacylglycerol lipase
MS	Mass spectrometry
NFκB	Nuclear factor kappa-light-chain-enhancer of activated B cells
NOX	NADPH oxidase
Ns	Not significant
OEA	Oleoylethanolamide
PAF-AH	Platelet-activating factor acetylhydrolase
PBS	Phosphate-buffered saline
PC	Phosphatidylcholine
PCA	Principal component analysis
PGE1	Prostaglandin E1
PI	Phosphatidylinositol
PLA2	Phospholipase A2
PLS-DA	partial least squares-discriminate analysis
PPAR	Peroxisome proliferator-activated receptor
Ps	Psoriasis vulgaris
PsA	Psoriatic arthritis
PUFAs	Polyunsaturated fatty acids
ROS	Reactive oxygen species
RT	Retention time
SIM	Selected ion monitoring
SLE	Systemic lupus erythematosus
SM	Sphingomyelin
Th	T helper lymphocytes
TNFα	Tumor necrosis factor α
TNFR	Tumor necrosis factor receptor
TRPV1	The transient receptor potential cation channel subfamily V member 1
TxA2	Thromboxane A2
TxB2	Thromboxane B2
UPLC	Ultra-performance liquid chromatography
VIP	variable importance in projection

References

1. Mease, P.J.; Armstrong, A.W. Managing Patients with Psoriatic Disease: The Diagnosis and Pharmacologic Treatment of Psoriatic Arthritis in Patients with Psoriasis. *Drugs* **2014**, *74*, 423–441. [CrossRef] [PubMed]
2. Hawkes, J.E.; Chan, T.C.; Krueger, J.G. Psoriasis pathogenesis and the development of novel targeted immune therapies. *J. Allergy Clin. Immunol.* **2017**, *140*, 645–653. [CrossRef] [PubMed]
3. Huang, N.; Perl, A. Metabolism as a Target for Modulation in Autoimmune Diseases. *Trends Immunol.* **2018**, *39*, 562–576. [CrossRef] [PubMed]
4. Ambrożewicz, E.; Wójcik, P.; Wroński, A.; Łuczaj, W.; Jastrząb, A.; Žarković, N.; Skrzydlewska, E. Pathophysiological Alterations of Redox Signaling and Endocannabinoid System in Granulocytes and Plasma of Psoriatic Patients. *Cells* **2018**, *7*, 159. [CrossRef] [PubMed]
5. Belikov, A.V.; Schraven, B.; Simeoni, L. T cells and reactive oxygen species. *J. Biomed. Sci.* **2015**, *22*. [CrossRef] [PubMed]
6. Łuczaj, W.; Gęgotek, A.; Skrzydlewska, E. Antioxidants and HNE in redox homeostasis. *Free Radic. Biol. Med.* **2017**, *111*, 87–101. [CrossRef] [PubMed]
7. Phillis, J.W.; O'Regan, M.H. The role of phospholipases, cyclooxygenases, and lipoxygenases in cerebral ischemic/traumatic injuries. *Crit. Rev. Neurobiol.* **2003**, *15*, 61–90. [CrossRef]
8. Barrie, N.; Manolios, N. The endocannabinoid system in pain and inflammation: Its relevance to rheumatic disease. *Eur. J. Rheumatol.* **2017**, *4*, 210–218. [CrossRef]
9. Navarini, L.; Bisogno, T.; Mozetic, P.; Piscitelli, F.; Margiotta, D.P.E.; Basta, F.; Afeltra, A.; Maccarrone, M. Endocannabinoid system in systemic lupus erythematosus: First evidence for a deranged 2-arachidonoylglycerol metabolism. *Int. J. Biochem. Cell Biol.* **2018**, *99*, 161–168. [CrossRef]
10. Mukhopadhyay, P.; Rajesh, M.; Bátkai, S.; Pan, H.; Mukhopadhyay, B.; Haskó, G.; Mackie, K.; Pacher, P. Opposing effects of cb1 and cb2 receptors on inflammation, oxidative stress, and cell death in nepropathy. *Faseb. J.* **2011**, *25*, 1087.
11. Siegmund, S.V.; Wojtalla, A.; Schlosser, M.; Schildberg, F.A.; Knolle, P.A.; Nüsing, R.M.; Zimmer, A.; Strassburg, C.P.; Singer, M.V. Cyclooxygenase-2 contributes to the selective induction of cell death by the endocannabinoid 2-arachidonoyl glycerin in hepatic stellate cells. *Biochem. Biophys. Res. Commun.* **2016**, *470*, 678–684. [CrossRef] [PubMed]
12. Meirer, K.; Steinhilber, D.; Proschak, E. Inhibitors of the Arachidonic Acid Cascade: Interfering with Multiple Pathways. *Basic Clin. Pharmacol. Toxicol.* **2014**, *114*, 83–91. [CrossRef] [PubMed]
13. Gachet, M.S.; Rhyn, P.; Bosch, O.G.; Quednow, B.B.; Gertsch, J. A quantitiative LC-MS/MS method for the measurement of arachidonic acid, prostanoids, endocannabinoids, N-acylethanolamines and steroids in human plasma. *J. Chromatogr. B Anal. Technol. Biomed. Life Sci.* **2015**, *976–977*, 6–18. [CrossRef] [PubMed]
14. Diani, M.; Altomare, G.; Reali, E. T cell responses in psoriasis and psoriatic arthritis. *Autoimmun. Rev.* **2015**, *14*, 286–292. [CrossRef] [PubMed]
15. Nunn, A.; Guy, G.; Bell, J.D. Endocannabinoids in neuroendopsychology: Multiphasic control of mitochondrial function. *Philos Trans. R Soc Lond B Biol Sci* **2012**, *367*, 3342–3352. [CrossRef] [PubMed]
16. Carney, S.T.; Lloyd, M.L.; MacKinnon, S.E.; Newton, D.C.; Jones, J.D.; Howlett, A.C.; Norford, D.C. Cannabinoid Regulation of Nitric Oxide Synthase I (nNOS) in Neuronal Cells. *J. Neuroimmune Pharm.* **2009**, *4*, 338–349. [CrossRef] [PubMed]
17. Csala, M.; Kardon, T.; Legeza, B.; Lizák, B.; Mandl, J.; Margittai, É.; Puskás, F.; Száraz, P.; Szelényi, P.; Bánhegyi, G. On the role of 4-hydroxynonenal in health and disease. *Biochim. Et Biophys. Acta (Bba)-Mol. Basis Dis.* **2015**, *1852*, 826–838. [CrossRef]
18. Timmermann, M.; Högger, P. Oxidative stress and 8-iso-prostaglandin F(2alpha) induce ectodomain shedding of CD163 and release of tumor necrosis factor-alpha from human monocytes. *Free Radic. Biol. Med.* **2005**, *39*, 98–107. [CrossRef]
19. Jiao, X.; Guo, Z.; Chen, T.; Zhang, Y.; Li, M. Determination of antioxidant capacity and 8-iso-prostaglandin F2α levels in patients with psoriasis and their significance. *Chin. J. Dermatol.* **2012**, *45*, 388–391.
20. Basu, S.; Whiteman, M.; Mattey, D.; Halliwell, B. Raised levels of F2-isoprostanes and prostaglandin F2α in different rheumatic diseases. *Ann. Rheum. Dis.* **2001**, *60*, 627–631. [CrossRef]
21. Man, X.-Y.; Zheng, M. Role of Angiogenic and Inflammatory Signal Pathways in Psoriasis. *J. Investig. Derm. Symp. Proc.* **2015**, *17*, 43–45. [CrossRef]

22. Miki, H.; Funato, Y. Regulation of intracellular signalling through cysteine oxidation by reactive oxygen species. *J. Biochem.* **2012**, *151*, 255–261. [CrossRef] [PubMed]
23. Castro, J.P.; Jung, T.; Grune, T.; Siems, W. 4-Hydroxynonenal (HNE) modified proteins in metabolic diseases. *Free Radic. Biol. Med.* **2017**, *111*, 309–315. [CrossRef] [PubMed]
24. Grabarczyk, D.B.; Chappell, P.E.; Eisel, B.; Johnson, S.; Lea, S.M.; Berks, B.C. Mechanism of Thiosulfate Oxidation in the SoxA Family of Cysteine-ligated Cytochromes. *J. Biol. Chem.* **2015**, *290*, 9209–9221. [CrossRef] [PubMed]
25. Agarwal, R.; MacMillan-Crow, L.A.; Rafferty, T.M.; Saba, H.; Roberts, D.W.; Fifer, E.K.; James, L.P.; Hinson, J.A. Acetaminophen-Induced Hepatotoxicity in Mice Occurs with Inhibition of Activity and Nitration of Mitochondrial Manganese Superoxide Dismutase. *J. Pharm. Exp.* **2011**, *337*, 110–118. [CrossRef] [PubMed]
26. Westcott, P.M.K.; To, M.D. The genetics and biology of KRAS in lung cancer. *Chin. J. Cancer* **2013**, *32*, 63–70. [CrossRef] [PubMed]
27. Turcotte, C.; Chouinard, F.; Lefebvre, J.S.; Flamand, N. Regulation of inflammation by cannabinoids, the endocannabinoids 2-arachidonoyl-glycerol and arachidonoyl-ethanolamide, and their metabolites. *J. Leukoc. Biol.* **2015**, *97*, 1049–1070. [CrossRef] [PubMed]
28. Jean-Gilles, L.; Braitch, M.; Latif, M.L.; Aram, J.; Fahey, A.J.; Edwards, L.J.; Robins, R.A.; Tanasescu, R.; Tighe, P.J.; Gran, B.; et al. Effects of pro-inflammatory cytokines on cannabinoid CB1 and CB2 receptors in immune cells. *Acta Physiol. (Oxf)* **2015**, *214*, 63–74. [CrossRef] [PubMed]
29. Włodarczyk, M.; Sobolewska-Włodarczyk, A.; Cygankiewicz, A.I.; Jacenik, D.; Krajewska, W.M.; Stec-Michalska, K.; Piechota-Polańczyk, A.; Wiśniewska-Jarosińska, M.; Fichna, J. G protein-coupled receptor 55 (GPR55) expresses differently in patients with Crohn's disease and ulcerative colitis. *Scand. J. Gastroenterol.* **2017**, *52*, 711–715. [CrossRef] [PubMed]
30. Gouin, O.; L'Herondelle, K.; Lebonvallet, N.; Le Gall-Ianotto, C.; Sakka, M.; Buhé, V.; Plée-Gautier, E.; Carré, J.-L.; Lefeuvre, L.; Misery, L.; et al. TRPV1 and TRPA1 in cutaneous neurogenic and chronic inflammation: Pro-inflammatory response induced by their activation and their sensitization. *Protein Cell* **2017**, *8*, 644–661. [CrossRef] [PubMed]
31. Klein, T.W.; Newton, C.; Larsen, K.; Chou, J.; Perkins, I.; Lu, L.; Nong, L.; Friedman, H. Cannabinoid receptors and T helper cells. *J. Neuroimmunol.* **2004**, *147*, 91–94. [CrossRef] [PubMed]
32. Camara-Lemarroy, C.R.; Gonzalez-Moreno, E.I.; Guzman-de la Garza, F.J.; Fernandez-Garza, N.E. Arachidonic Acid Derivatives and Their Role in Peripheral Nerve Degeneration and Regeneration. *Sci. World J.* **2012**, *2012*, 7. [CrossRef] [PubMed]
33. Tanada-Ueharaguchi, Y.; Honda, T.; Murata, T.; Arita, M.; Miyachi, Y.; Kabashima, K. Thromboxane A2 promotes the development of imiquimod-induced mouse psoriasis model via TP receptor. *J. Dermatol. Sci.* **2016**, *84*, e5. [CrossRef]
34. Del Prete, A.; Shao, W.-H.; Mitola, S.; Santoro, G.; Sozzani, S.; Haribabu, B. Regulation of dendritic cell migration and adaptive immune response by leukotriene B4 receptors: A role for LTB4 in up-regulation of CCR7 expression and function. *Blood* **2007**, *109*, 626–631. [CrossRef] [PubMed]
35. Paul, S.; Traver, M.K.; Kashyap, A.K.; Washington, M.A.; Latoche, J.R.; Schaefer, B.C. T cell receptor signals to NF-κB are transmitted by a cytosolic p62-Bcl10-Malt1-IKK signalosome. *Sci. Signal.* **2014**, *7*, ra45. [CrossRef] [PubMed]
36. Ament, Z.; Masoodi, M.; Griffin, J.L. Applications of metabolomics for understanding the action of peroxisome proliferator-activated receptors (PPARs) in diabetes, obesity and cancer. *Genome Med.* **2012**, *4*, 32. [CrossRef] [PubMed]
37. O'Sullivan, S.E. Cannabinoids go nuclear: Evidence for activation of peroxisome proliferator-activated receptors. *Br. J. Pharm.* **2007**, *152*, 576–582. [CrossRef] [PubMed]
38. Xu, Z.; Wang, G.; Zhu, Y.; Liu, R.; Song, J.; Ni, Y.; Sun, H.; Yang, B.; Hou, M.; Chen, L.; et al. PPAR-γ agonist ameliorates liver pathology accompanied by increasing regulatory B and T cells in high-fat-diet mice. *Obesity* **2017**, *25*, 581–590. [CrossRef]
39. Aleshin, S.; Reiser, G. Role of the peroxisome proliferator-activated receptors (PPAR)-α, β/δ and γ triad in regulation of reactive oxygen species signaling in brain. *Biol. Chem.* **2013**, *394*, 1553–1570. [CrossRef]
40. Contreras, A.V.; Torres, N.; Tovar, A.R. PPAR-α as a Key Nutritional and Environmental Sensor for Metabolic Adaptation. *Adv. Nutr.* **2013**, *4*, 439–452. [CrossRef]

41. Kim, M.-S.; Pyun, H.-B.; Hwang, J.-K. Panduratin A, an activator of PPAR-α/δ, suppresses the development of oxazolone-induced atopic dermatitis-like symptoms in hairless mice. *Life Sci.* **2014**, *100*, 45–54. [CrossRef] [PubMed]
42. Kim, H.J.; Ham, S.A.; Paek, K.S.; Hwang, J.S.; Jung, S.Y.; Kim, M.Y.; Jin, H.; Kang, E.S.; Woo, I.S.; Kim, H.J.; et al. Transcriptional up-regulation of antioxidant genes by PPARδ inhibits angiotensin II-induced premature senescence in vascular smooth muscle cells. *Biochem. Biophys. Res. Commun.* **2011**, *406*, 564–569. [CrossRef] [PubMed]
43. Marx, N.; Kehrle, B.; Kohlhammer, K.; Grüb, M.; Koenig, W.; Hombach, V.; Libby, P.; Plutzky, J. PPAR Activators as Antiinflammatory Mediators in Human T Lymphocytes. *Circ. Res.* **2002**, *90*, 703–710. [CrossRef] [PubMed]
44. Bradford, M.M. A rapid and sensitive method for the quantitation of microgram quantities of protein utilizing the principle of protein-dye binding. *Anal. Biochem.* **1976**, *72*, 248–254. [CrossRef]
45. Bligh, E.G.; Dyer, W.J. A Rapid Method of Total Lipid Extraction and Purification. *Can. J. Biochem. Physiol.* **1959**, *37*, 911–917. [CrossRef] [PubMed]
46. Bartlett, E.M.; Lewis, D.H. Spectrophotometric determination of phosphate esters in the presence and absence of orthophosphate. *Anal. Biochem.* **1970**, *36*, 159–167. [CrossRef]
47. Łuczaj, W.; Domingues, P.; Domingues, M.R.; Pancewicz, S.; Skrzydlewska, E. Phospholipidomic Analysis Reveals Changes in Sphingomyelin and Lysophosphatidylcholine Profiles in Plasma from Patients with Neuroborreliosis. *Lipids* **2017**, *52*, 93–98. [CrossRef] [PubMed]
48. Pulfer, M.; Murphy, R.C. Electrospray mass spectrometry of phospholipids. *Mass Spectrom. Rev.* **2003**, *22*, 332–364. [CrossRef] [PubMed]
49. Reynolds, L.J.; Hughes, L.L.; Yu, L.; Dennis, E.A. 1-Hexadecyl-2-arachidonoylthio-2-deoxy-sn-glycero-3-phosphorylcholine as a substrate for the microtiterplate assay of human cytosolic phospholipase A2. *Anal. Biochem.* **1994**, *217*, 25–32. [CrossRef] [PubMed]
50. Aarsman, A.J.; Neys, F.W.; Van den Bosch, H. Catabolism of platelet-activating factor and its acyl analog. Differentiation of the activities of lysophospholipase and platelet-activating-factor acetylhydrolase. *Eur. J. Biochem.* **1991**, *200*, 187–193. [CrossRef]
51. Kulmacz, R.J.; Lands, W.E. Requirements for hydroperoxide by the cyclooxygenase and peroxidase activities of prostaglandin H synthase. *Prostaglandins* **1983**, *25*, 531–540. [CrossRef]
52. Smith, C.J.; Zhang, Y.; Koboldt, C.M.; Muhammad, J.; Zweifel, B.S.; Shaffer, A.; Talley, J.J.; Masferrer, J.L.; Seibert, K.; Isakson, P.C. Pharmacological analysis of cyclooxygenase-1 in inflammation. *PNAS* **1998**, *95*, 13313–13318. [CrossRef] [PubMed]
53. Luo, X.P.; Yazdanpanah, M.; Bhooi, N.; Lehotay, D.C. Determination of aldehydes and other lipid peroxidation products in biological samples by gas chromatography-mass spectrometry. *Anal. Biochem.* **1995**, *228*, 294–298. [CrossRef]
54. Weber, D.; Milkovic, L.; Bennett, S.J.; Griffiths, H.R.; Zarkovic, N.; Grune, T. Measurement of HNE-protein adducts in human plasma and serum by ELISA—Comparison of two primary antibodies. *Redox Biol.* **2013**, *1*, 226–233. [CrossRef] [PubMed]
55. Coolen, S.A.J.; van Buuren, B.; Duchateau, G.; Upritchard, J.; Verhagen, H. Kinetics of biomarkers: Biological and technical validity of isoprostanes in plasma. *Amino Acids* **2005**, *29*, 429–436. [CrossRef] [PubMed]
56. Gouveia-Figueira, S.; Nording, M.L. Development and validation of a sensitive UPLC-ESI-MS/MS method for the simultaneous quantification of 15 endocannabinoids and related compounds in milk and other biofluids. *Anal. Chem.* **2014**, *86*, 1186–1195. [CrossRef] [PubMed]
57. Siegmund, S.V.; Seki, E.; Osawa, Y.; Uchinami, H.; Cravatt, B.F.; Schwabe, R.F. Fatty acid amide hydrolase determines anandamide-induced cell death in the liver. *J. Biol. Chem.* **2006**, *281*, 10431–10438. [CrossRef]
58. Ulloa, N.M.; Deutsch, D.G. Assessment of a Spectrophotometric Assay for Monoacylglycerol Lipase Activity. *AAPS J.* **2010**, *12*, 197–201. [CrossRef]

59. Watkins, B.A.; Kim, J.; Kenny, A.; Pedersen, T.L.; Pappan, K.L.; Newman, J.W. Circulating levels of endocannabinoids and oxylipins altered by dietary lipids in older women are likely associated with previously identified gene targets. *Biochim. et Biophys. Acta (BBA)-Mol. Cell Biol. Lipids* **2016**, *1861*, 1693–1704. [CrossRef]
60. Eissa, S.; Seada, L.S. Quantitation of bcl-2 protein in bladder cancer tissue by enzyme immunoassay: Comparison with Western blot and immunohistochemistry. *Clin. Chem.* **1998**, *44*, 1423–1429.

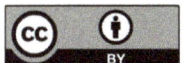

© 2019 by the authors. Licensee MDPI, Basel, Switzerland. This article is an open access article distributed under the terms and conditions of the Creative Commons Attribution (CC BY) license (http://creativecommons.org/licenses/by/4.0/).

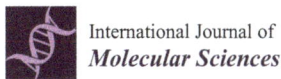

Review
Risk Factors for the Development of Psoriasis

Koji Kamiya *, Megumi Kishimoto, Junichi Sugai, Mayumi Komine and Mamitaro Ohtsuki

Department of Dermatology, Jichi Medical University, 3311-1 Yakushiji, Shimotsuke, Tochigi 329-0498, Japan
* Correspondence: m01023kk@jichi.ac.jp; Tel.: +81-285-58-7360

Received: 24 July 2019; Accepted: 3 September 2019; Published: 5 September 2019

Abstract: Psoriasis is an immune-mediated genetic skin disease. The underlying pathomechanisms involve complex interaction between the innate and adaptive immune system. T cells interact with dendritic cells, macrophages, and keratinocytes, which can be mediated by their secreted cytokines. In the past decade, biologics targeting tumor necrosis factor-α, interleukin (IL)-23, and IL-17 have been developed and approved for the treatment of psoriasis. These biologics have dramatically changed the treatment and management of psoriasis. In contrast, various triggering factors can elicit the disease in genetically predisposed individuals. Recent studies suggest that the exacerbation of psoriasis can lead to systemic inflammation and cardiovascular comorbidity. In addition, psoriasis may be associated with other auto-inflammatory and auto-immune diseases. In this review, we summarize the risk factors, which can be divided into two groups (namely, extrinsic and intrinsic risk factors), responsible for the onset and exacerbation of psoriasis in order to facilitate its prevention.

Keywords: psoriasis; risk factor; extrinsic risk factor; intrinsic risk factor; onset; exacerbation

1. Introduction

Psoriasis is a chronic inflammatory skin disease characterized by sharply demarcated erythematous plaques with whitish scale [1,2]. Psoriasis is one of the most frequent chronic inflammatory skin diseases. The prevalence of psoriasis varies with the country, and psoriasis can appear at any age [3,4], suggesting that ethnicity, genetic background, and environmental factors affect the onset of psoriasis. Genetic factors play a significant role in the pathogenesis of psoriasis. Psoriasis susceptibility 1 (PSORS1), which lies within an approximately 220 kb segment of the major histocompatibility complex on chromosome 6p21, is a major susceptibility locus for psoriasis [5–7]. HLA-Cw6 is the susceptibility allele within PSORS1 [8]; it is associated with early onset and severe and unstable disease [8,9]. In genetically predisposed individuals, various triggering factors can elicit the disease. In past surveys from 1982 to 2012, the exacerbating factors for the Japanese population were observed to be stress (6.4% to 16.6%), seasonal factors (9.7% to 13.3%), infection (3.5% to 8.3%), sun exposure (1.3% to 3.5%), and β-blockers (0.9% to 2.3%) [10–12]. The comorbidities included hypertension (1.1% to 27.8%), diabetes mellitus (DM) (7.0% to 13.9%), cardiovascular diseases (4.2% to 8.1%), and tonsillitis (3.5% to 5.4%) [10–12]. The risk factors for psoriasis can be divided into two groups, namely, extrinsic and intrinsic risk factors (Figure 1). In this review, we focus on each component of these groups and discuss their effects on the development of psoriasis.

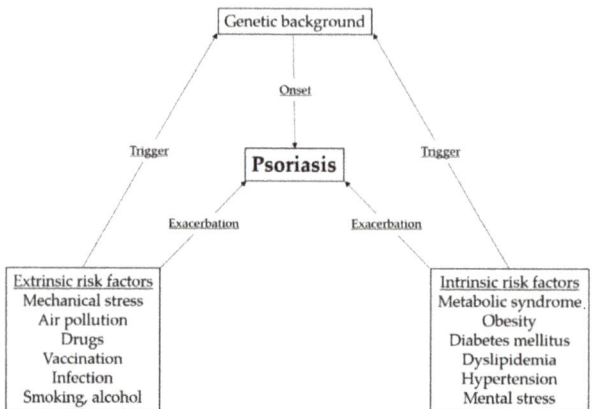

Figure 1. Risk factors for the onset and exacerbation of psoriasis. As shown in this figure, extrinsic and intrinsic factors are associated with the onset and exacerbation of psoriasis.

2. Extrinsic Risk Factors

2.1. Mechanical Stress

In patients with psoriasis, skin lesions appear in uninvolved areas after various injuries [13–16]; this is known as the Koebner phenomenon. Radiotherapy, ultraviolet (UV) B, and even a slight skin irritation have been reported to trigger new lesions of psoriasis [17–19]. However, psoriatic lesions are not always observed in the uninvolved skin after injuries [20,21]. Type, site, depth, and degree of trauma may affect the pathogenesis of the Koebner phenomenon [20]. Under appropriate conditions, the Koebner phenomenon may occur, especially when there is dermal trauma with epidermal involvement. It is speculated that increased papillary dermis blood flow helps bring mediators that play a part in the pathogenesis of psoriasis [20]. However, the mechanisms underlying the Koebner phenomenon remain to be completely elucidated [20,21]. Nerve growth factor (NGF) is a neurotrophic factor that is expressed in both the nervous system and peripheral organs. NGF is thought to be associated with the Koebner phenomenon [22]. After a cutaneous trauma, in a developing psoriasis lesion, keratinocyte proliferation and up-regulation of NGF in basal keratinocytes are early events and precede epidermotropism of T lymphocytes [22]. In addition, NGF secreted by the psoriatic keratinocytes is functionally active. Notably, the keratinocytes of patients with psoriasis produce higher levels of NGF. This study suggests that NGF plays a critical role in the pathogenesis of psoriasis and that the regulatory role of NGF and its receptor system is functionally active in the early stage of developing lesions of psoriasis. Resident memory T cells (T_{RM}) have been described as a non-circulating memory T cell subset that persists long-term in peripheral tissues; psoriasis is one of the T_{RM}-mediated autoimmune inflammatory skin diseases [23]. Interestingly, psoriasis lesions could be triggered and sustained by skin-resident pathogenic T cells in the non-lesioned skin of psoriasis patients [24,25]. Activation of resident T cells is necessary and sufficient for the development of lesions in psoriasis [24]. A subpopulation of T cells infiltrating the epidermis during active disease turn into T_{RM} cells, and T_{RM} cells are retained in resolved psoriasis [26]. These cells establish a site-specific disease memory and are capable of producing cytokines that play a critical role in the pathogenesis of psoriasis [26]. These observations suggest that T_{RM} cells are key players not only in the recurrent lesions of psoriasis but also in the lesions of the Koebner phenomenon. Type 1 interferons (IFNs), such as IFN-α and IFN-β, have been suggested to play an indispensable role in initiating psoriasis during skin injury [27]. Skin injury rapidly induces IFN-β from keratinocytes and IFN-α from dermal plasmacytoid dendritic cells through distinct mechanisms [27]. Host antimicrobial peptide LL37 potentiates double-stranded RNA immune pathways and single-stranded RNA or DNA pathways in plasmacytoid dendritic cells. Production of type 1 IFNs induced by skin injury may explain the Koebner phenomenon.

2.2. Air Pollutants and Sun Exposure

The increase in air pollution over the years has had major effects on the human skin, and various air pollutants such as polycyclic aromatic hydrocarbons, volatile organic compounds, oxides, particulate matter, ozone, heavy metals, and UV damage the skin by inducing oxidative stress [28]. Cadmium is one of the air pollutants which affect the pathogenesis of psoriasis. Patients with severe psoriasis had higher blood cadmium when compared with the general population [29]. This study suggests that environmental exposure to cadmium may compromise immunity, and microenvironmental perturbation can predispose one to the worsening of psoriasis. The UV radiation that reaches the Earth's surface is divided into two subtypes: more than 95% UVA (315–400 nm) and 1%–5% UVB (280–315 nm). In the past several decades, phototherapy has been widely used to treat psoriasis [30]. Both narrowband UVB (311 nm) and excimer laser (308 nm) are currently used as the first-line therapy for psoriasis, and psoralen UVA (PUVA) is also used as the second-line therapy with preference to refractory psoriatic plaques [30]. There is a subset of patients with severely photosensitive psoriasis in whom the condition is predominantly photodistributed and is severe in the summer months [31]. In this study, patients with photosensitive psoriasis showed striking female predominance, very low mean age of psoriasis onset, family history of psoriasis, a strong HLA-Cw*0602 association, and a rapid abnormal clinical response to broadband UVA, comprising erythema and/or scaling plaques [31]. A phenotypically distinct subset of psoriasis was characterized by histopathological analysis. In a certain group, psoriasis can develop after UV exposure.

2.3. Drugs

Drug-related psoriasis is recognized as the onset and exacerbation of psoriasis which is associated with certain drugs. It is often difficult to identify drug-related causes of psoriasis in clinical situations. This is because the latency period between the start of the medication and the onset of psoriatic skin lesions can vary considerably between drugs [32]. In some cases, the psoriasis flare can persist even after the suspected drug has been discontinued. Moreover, there may be little difference between psoriasis and drug-related psoriasis in terms of the clinical and histopathological findings [32]. Drug-related psoriasis would manifest as plaque psoriasis, palmoplantar psoriasis, nail psoriasis, scalp psoriasis, pustular psoriasis, and erythrodermic psoriasis [33]. In most cases, histopathological findings of drug-related psoriasis are virtually indistinguishable from those of conventional psoriasis [32]. Histopathological findings of eosinophilic infiltrates in the dermis and lichenoid reaction might help in the diagnosis of drug-related psoriasis [34]. While in psoriasis plaques unrelated to drugs, the capillaries in the upper dermis are convoluted and tortuous, that alteration is sometimes missing in drug-related psoriasis [34]. Moreover, there might also be differences regarding the formation of micro-abscesses of neutrophils in the upper layer of the epidermis [34]. However, these are just a few and not the most important clues that might orientate to a drug-related cause of psoriasis. Drug ingestion may result in the exacerbation of pre-existing psoriasis, induction of psoriatic lesions on clinically uninvolved skin in patients with psoriasis, or precipitation of the disease in patients without family history of psoriasis as well as in predisposed individuals [35]. The most widely accepted drugs are β-blockers, lithium, anti-malarial drugs, interferons, imiquimod, angiotensin-converting enzyme inhibitors, terbinafine, tetracycline, nonsteroidal anti-inflammatory drugs, and fibrate drugs [32,33,36,37]. The mechanisms of drug-related psoriasis still remain to be fully elucidated and the molecular mechanisms are complicated. However, some drugs have been known to affect keratinocyte hyperproliferation and the IL-23/IL-17 axis. Cyclic adenosine monophosphate (cAMP) is an intracellular messenger that is responsible for the stimulation of proteins for cellular differentiation and inhibition of proliferation, and β-blockers lead to a decrease in intraepidermal cAMP, causing keratinocyte hyperproliferation [32,33,38]. Imiquimod-induced skin inflammation is the most widely accepted psoriasis animal model [39]. Imiquimod, which activates the toll-like receptor-7/8, can induce and exacerbate psoriasis, critically dependent on the IL-23/IL-17 axis [39]. Recently, immune check point inhibitors and molecular inhibitors have been used for the treatment of malignancies and autoimmune diseases, and these drugs may affect the immune system, leading to the development of psoriasis [40–42]. The symptoms of psoriasis are rarely exacerbated during biologic therapy. However, psoriasis can also be triggered by biologics [43,44], and this is recognized as paradoxical reactions. Although most of the paradoxical reactions reported have been associated with the use of tumor necrosis factor (TNF)-α inhibitors, other biologics targeting interleukin (IL)-23 and IL-17 are increasingly common [45]. Biologics targeting TNF-α, IL-23, and IL-17 block immune signaling pathways, which can lead to cytokine imbalances [45]. Paradoxical reactions are thought to be due to an imbalance in cytokine production with an overproduction of IFN-α and altered lymphocyte recruitment and migration [45,46]. Suspected drugs should be discontinued and switched to an alternative drug in patients with drug-related psoriasis.

2.4. Vaccination

Patients with psoriasis are at increased risk of infection, mostly because of treatment with immunomodulatory or immunosuppressive drugs [47]. Thus, vaccination is recommended to prevent specific infections [47–49]. However, vaccination can often trigger and exacerbate psoriasis. Several studies support the association between influenza vaccination and the exacerbation of psoriasis [50,51]. Influenza vaccination may also trigger the onset of psoriasis [52]. Bacillus Calmette–Guerin (BCG) vaccine, which is a live attenuated strain of *Mycobacterium bovis*, is primarily used for the prevention of tuberculosis [53]. Psoriasis can be triggered post BCG vaccination [54,55]. BCG has also been used as local immunotherapy for bladder cancer, and a case of erythrodermic pustular psoriasis induced by BCG immunotherapy has been reported [56]. In a retrospective study, psoriasis was found to more frequently occur after adenovirus vaccination [57]. Psoriasis may also be triggered by other vaccines such as tetanus–diphtheria vaccination and pneumococcal polysaccharide vaccination [58,59]. These vaccinations are thought to generate T helper 1 (Th1) and Th17 immune responses which lead to the onset and exacerbation of psoriasis, although the precise pathomechanisms of psoriasis induced by vaccination remain to be elucidated. The incidence of psoriasis induced by vaccination is very low; rather, vaccination is therapeutically effective in patients with psoriasis.

2.5. Infection

The association between psoriasis and streptococcal infection is well established [60]. Psoriasis occurs after streptococcal infection, and the most common type is guttate psoriasis. Although the symptoms are self-limited, they can recur with the recurrence of streptococcal infection. Thus, tonsillectomy may be a potential treatment option for patients with recalcitrant psoriasis associated with episodes of tonsillitis [61]. Although prior infection with *Streptococcus pyogenes* is associated with guttate psoriasis, the ability to trigger guttate psoriasis is not serotype specific [60]. *Staphylococcus (S.) aureus* is also associated with the development of psoriasis [38]. Dysregulated skin microbiomes have been found to be associated with psoriasis [62]. Colonization of *S. aureus* in the lesions has been demonstrated in approximately 60% of patients with psoriasis, compared with 5% to 30% of normal healthy skin [38]. Moreover, the severity of psoriasis significantly correlates with enterotoxin production by the isolated *S. aureus* strains [63]. *Candida* species are a part of the normal human microbiota, and they were highly detected in either the skin or the mucosal membranes of patients with psoriasis [64]. A statistically significantly higher *Candida* species detection rate was also observed for mucosal membranes [64]. The detection rates of *Candida* species are significantly higher in patients with psoriasis as compared with those in healthy controls, especially in the oral mucosa milieux [64]. However, patients with psoriasis and healthy controls do not significantly differ in the rate of *Candida* species isolated from the skin [64]. *Candida albicans* is the most common disease-causing *Candida* species and its colonization promotes antifungal immunity, which may be associated with the pathogenesis of psoriasis [65]. *Malassezia* is a lipophilic yeast found on skin and body surfaces; it may contribute to the exacerbation of psoriasis [38]. It still remains to be established whether the species of *Malassezia* can initiate the development of psoriasis lesions. Human immunodeficiency virus (HIV) is also a well-known risk factor associated with psoriasis [66]. It is paradoxical that, while drugs that target T lymphocytes are effective in psoriasis, the condition should be exacerbated by HIV infection [66]. Although HIV infection causes the onset and exacerbation of psoriasis, the precise pathomechanisms still remain to be fully elucidated. Other viruses such as papilloma viruses, retroviruses, and endogenous retroviruses have also been implicated in psoriasis [67].

2.6. Lifestyle

Smoking and alcohol consumption have been associated with psoriasis. A systematic review and meta-analysis revealed that patients with psoriasis are more likely to be current or former smokers [68]. Smoking is associated with an increased risk of developing psoriasis [69]. In addition, smoking is strongly associated with pustular lesions of psoriasis [70]. A trend was found toward an increased risk of psoriasis with increasing pack-years or duration of smoking. Another study also showed that there was a positive correlation between the amount and/or duration of smoking and the occurrence of psoriasis [71]. Alcohol consumption appears to be a risk factor for psoriasis. However, a past systematic review concluded that there was not enough evidence to establish whether the alcohol consumption was indeed a risk factor [72]. Nonetheless, alcohol consumption was observed to be greater in patients with psoriasis than in the general population. Although the relationship between psoriasis and alcohol consumption is complex and multifactorial, alcohol abuse positively correlates with psoriasis severity and reduced treatment efficacy [73]. In addition, alcohol abuse is associated with significantly increased mortality rates [74]. Qualitative changes to the diet may play a significant role in maintaining the intestinal microbiome, and diet-induced dysbiosis may induce the cytokine imbalances associated with the pathogenesis of psoriasis [75–77]. Dietary modifications such as supplementation with polyunsaturated fatty acids, folic acid, vitamin D, and antioxidants can also be considered as adjuncts in the management of psoriasis [73]. To date, randomized controlled trials have produced conflicting results. Diet is a complex combination of foods from various groups; nutrients and the rich diversity of such foods may contribute to its protective effects against psoriasis [78].

3. Intrinsic Risk Factors

3.1. Obesity

Metabolic syndrome is common in patients with psoriasis [79–83] and obesity is strongly associated with the onset and exacerbation of psoriasis [78,84,85]. Patients with psoriasis have a significantly higher prevalence of obesity [70,86–88] as well as a higher risk of obesity [89–91]. In a previous meta-analysis, obesity was associated with severe psoriasis [92]. A large prospective cohort study also showed a positive association between body mass index (BMI) and psoriasis [93]. However, BMI has high specificity but low sensitivity to identify adiposity, as it fails to identify half of the people with excess body fat [94,95]. In contrast, waist circumference is more reliable measure of body fat, and many studies have shown a strong association between waist circumference and psoriasis [93,96,97]. Obesity can be defined as the expansion of white adipose tissue [85], and various mediators secreted by adipose tissue lead to a low-grade inflammatory state, contributing to the pathogenesis of psoriasis [98–101]. Pro-inflammatory adipokines such as TNF-α, IL-6, leptin, and adiponectin are produced in adipose tissue [98]. Blocking the TNF-α signaling pathway improves the inflammatory cycle of psoriasis, while it does not improve insulin sensitivity in patients with type 2 DM [102]. Leptin is an adipose tissue hormone that functions as an afferent signal in a negative feedback loop that maintains homeostatic control of adipose tissue mass [103]. Leptin is an important regulator of metabolic status and influences inflammatory and immune responses [104]. Leptin can enhance immune functions, including inflammatory cytokine production in macrophages, granulocyte chemotaxis, and increased Th17 proliferation [105,106]. The presence of elevated leptin inhibits the differentiation of regulatory

T cells, which maintain tolerance and prevent psoriasis, in adipose tissue [106]. In fact, serum or plasma levels of leptin are higher in patients with psoriasis as compared to the healthy controls [107]. In addition, tissue levels of leptin are increased in the skin of patients with psoriasis [108]. Adiponectin is an adipocyte-specific factor which contributes to a beneficial metabolic action in whole-body energy homeostasis [109]. In contrast to leptin, adiponectin protects cells from apoptosis and reduces inflammation in various cell types [109]. Although adiponectin may act as an anti-inflammatory adipokine in patients with psoriasis, the association still remains unclear [110]. Weight loss itself appears to improve psoriasis symptoms [111,112] and is likely to improve decreased response to oral systemic therapies and biologics [113–117]. Moreover, weight loss may decrease the risk of drug toxicity of systemic therapies [118–121].

3.2. Diabetes Mellitus

The prevalence of DM is generally influenced by ethnic origin and lifestyle factors. However, the prevalence of DM might be similar among diverse patient populations, ethnic backgrounds, and baseline therapy [122]. A meta-analysis revealed that psoriasis was associated with DM [122]. Other meta-analyses have also demonstrated the association between psoriasis and the risk of DM [81,123]. DM is divided into two groups, namely, type 2 and type 1 DM. Patients with psoriasis have a significantly higher risk of type 2 DM. However, the prevalence of type 2 DM does not correlate with patient age or severity of psoriasis [124]. Psoriasis is a marker for increased risk of type 2 DM independent of its severity. It is unclear which disease comes first, psoriasis or type 2 DM [124]. As mentioned above, obesity is a risk factor for psoriasis. Obesity contributes to the onset and exacerbation of type 2 DM directly. Thus, obesity is associated with psoriasis as well as type 2 DM, and type 2 DM may not contribute to the pathogenesis of psoriasis directly. In contrast to type 2 DM, type 1 DM is a chronic disease characterized by insulin deficiency due to autoimmune destruction of insulin-producing pancreatic β-cells, leading to hyperglycemia [125]. Proinflammatory cytokines, including TNF-α, are involved in the pathogenesis of type 1 DM [126,127]. Interestingly, both Th1 and Th17 cells may contribute to the onset of type 1 DM [128,129]. Although type 1 DM may not contribute to the pathogenesis of psoriasis directly, the TNF-α/IL-23/IL-17 axis plays a crucial role in the pathogenesis of psoriasis and type 1 DM.

3.3. Dyslipidemia

Psoriasis is associated with obesity [70,86–88], and excess adipose tissue may contribute to dyslipidemia. Patients with psoriasis have a higher prevalence of dyslipidemia, which is likely to increase with the severity of psoriasis [130–133]. A past study including 70 patients with psoriasis revealed that dyslipidemia was observed in 62.85% of the patients [133]. Most often it was hypertriglyceridemia (39%) and hypertriglyceridemia with a lowered value of high-density lipoprotein (HDL). Dyslipidemia can also appear during oral systemic therapies for psoriasis [134]. Retinoids have the most potent activity leading to dyslipidemia, such as increased levels of triglycerides, total cholesterol, low-density lipoprotein cholesterol, and very-low-density lipoprotein cholesterol and simultaneously decreased levels of HDL cholesterol [135–137]. Cyclosporin can also lead to dyslipidemia [138]. It is possible that cyclosporine unmasks a latent tendency for mild to moderate hypertriglyceridemia [138], and this study concluded that fasting triglyceride levels should be monitored during cyclosporine therapy, especially after 1 to 2 months of use, and in patients with preexisting increased triglycerides and/or a history of etretinate use. Although dyslipidemia is associated with immunological abnormalities [134], it still remains unknown whether dyslipidemia affects the onset and exacerbation of psoriasis.

3.4. Hypertension

In a meta-analysis, patients with psoriasis showed greater prevalence and incidence of hypertension [139]. This meta-analysis also revealed that severe psoriasis was associated with greater incidence of hypertension [139]. Patients with psoriasis appear to have more severe hypertension [140,141]. A multicenter noninterventional observational study including 2210 patients with psoriasis revealed that 26% of patients with psoriasis had hypertension, and the incidence of hypertension was higher when compared with the general population [142]. Conversely, hypertension may be associated with the incidence of psoriasis [143]. Although psoriasis and hypertension have shared risk factors such as obesity and smoking, most studies have shown an independent association of psoriasis with hypertension after adjusting for these risk factors [139]. The mechanisms underlying this association remain unknown.

3.5. Mental Stress

Mental stress is a feeling of strain and pressure caused by internal perceptions which lead to anxiety or other negative emotions. Mental stress occurs when individuals think the demands exceed their ability to cope. Mental stress is commonly regarded as a well-established trigger of psoriasis and many patients with psoriasis and physicians believe that mental stress exacerbates psoriasis. Although psoriasis leads to higher degree of distress as proved by measurements on Dermatology Life Quality Index scales, the relation between mental stress and psoriasis is complex. In a past systematic review including 39 studies (32,537 patients), 46% of patients believed their disease was stress reactive and 54% recalled preceding stressful events [144]. However, there was no high-quality evidence to support the notion that the preceding stress was strongly associated with the onset and exacerbation of psoriasis. The association was based primarily on retrospective studies with many limitations. It seems unclear whether mental stress affects the clinical course of psoriasis. In contrast, a prospective study concluded that cognitive and behavioral patterns of worrying and scratching were both independently related to an increase four weeks later in disease severity and itch, at moments when patients experienced a high level of daily stressors [145]. At these moments, stressors also interacted with vulnerability factors, suggesting that patients with more daily stress and high worrying and scratching had particularly worsened disease severity and itch. Scratching in response to itch subsequently leads to an itch–scratch–itch cycle causing the exacerbation of psoriasis. Further studies are necessary to elucidate the association between mental stress and psoriasis.

4. Conclusions

In this review, both extrinsic and intrinsic risk factors for the development of psoriasis were discussed in detail. Biologics have dramatically changed the treatment of psoriasis. In contrast, elimination of the risk factors is also important for controlling the disease. From the clinicians' perspective, the exacerbation of psoriasis induced by the Koebner phenomenon and drugs can be avoided by proper knowledge. From the patients' perspective, lifestyle could be modified by proper education, although the extent varies among patients. However, various factors interact with each other and can affect the pathogenesis of psoriasis directly and/or indirectly. For example, obesity, dyslipidemia, and hypertension are associated with the course of psoriasis and are also dependent on the patient's age, lifestyle, and concomitant diseases. Moreover, the impacts of the patient's age, lifestyle, and concomitant diseases vary among individuals. The risk factors of psoriasis are not fully understood, and future studies need to successfully establish preventive approaches for psoriasis.

Author Contributions: K.K., M.Ki., J.S., M.K., and M.O. collected information. K.K., M.K., and M.O. wrote the manuscript. All authors approved the final version of the manuscript for submission.

Funding: This research received no external funding.

Conflicts of Interest: The authors declare no conflict of interest.

Abbreviations

PSORS1	Psoriasis susceptibility 1
DM	Diabetes mellitus
UV	Ultraviolet
NGF	Nerve growth factor
T_{RM}	Resident memory T cells
IFN	Interferon
PUVA	Psoralen ultraviolet A
cAMP	Cyclic adenosine monophosphate
TNF	Tumor necrosis factor
IL	Interleukin
BCG	Bacillus Calmette–Guerin
Th	T helper
S.	Staphylococcus
HIV	Human immunodeficiency virus
BMI	Body mass index
HDL	High-density lipoprotein

References

1. Boehncke, W.H.; Schon, M.P. Psoriasis. *Lancet* **2015**, *386*, 983–994. [CrossRef]
2. Nestle, F.O.; Kaplan, D.H.; Barker, J. Psoriasis. *N. Engl. J. Med.* **2009**, *361*, 496–509. [CrossRef] [PubMed]
3. Parisi, R.; Symmons, D.P.; Griffiths, C.E.; Ashcroft, D.M.; IMPACT project team. Global epidemiology of psoriasis: A systematic review of incidence and prevalence. *J. Invest. Dermatol.* **2013**, *133*, 377–385. [CrossRef] [PubMed]
4. Michalek, I.M.; Loring, B.; John, S.M. A systematic review of worldwide epidemiology of psoriasis. *J. Eur. Acad. Dermatol. Venereol.* **2017**, *31*, 205–212. [CrossRef] [PubMed]
5. Trembath, R.C.; Clough, R.L.; Rosbotham, J.L.; Jones, A.B.; Camp, R.D.; Frodsham, A.; Browne, J.; Barber, R.; Terwilliger, J.; Lathrop, G.M.; et al. Identification of a major susceptibility locus on chromosome 6p and evidence for further disease loci revealed by a two stage genome-wide search in psoriasis. *Hum. Mol. Genet.* **1997**, *6*, 813–820. [CrossRef]
6. Burden, A.D.; Javed, S.; Bailey, M.; Hodgins, M.; Connor, M.; Tillman, D. Genetics of psoriasis: Paternal inheritance and a locus on chromosome 6p. *J. Invest. Dermatol.* **1998**, *110*, 958–960. [CrossRef] [PubMed]
7. Sagoo, G.S.; Tazi-Ahnini, R.; Barker, J.W.; Elder, J.T.; Nair, R.P.; Samuelsson, L.; Traupe, H.; Trembath, R.C.; Robinson, D.A.; Iles, M.M. Meta-analysis of genome-wide studies of psoriasis susceptibility reveals linkage to chromosomes 6p21 and 4q28-q31 in Caucasian and Chinese Hans population. *J. Invest. Dermatol.* **2004**, *122*, 1401–1405. [CrossRef]
8. Nair, R.P.; Stuart, P.E.; Nistor, I.; Hiremagalore, R.; Chia, N.V.C.; Jenisch, S.; Weichenthal, M.; Abecasis, G.R.; Lim, H.W.; Christophers, E. Sequence and haplotype analysis supports HLA-C as the psoriasis susceptibility 1 gene. *Am. J. Hum. Genet.* **2006**, *78*, 827–851. [CrossRef]
9. Chen, L.; Tsai, T.F. HLA-Cw6 and psoriasis. *Br. J. Dermatol.* **2018**, *178*, 854–862. [CrossRef]
10. Kawada, A.; Tezuka, T.; Nakamizo, Y.; Kimura, H.; Nakagawa, H.; Ohkido, M.; Ozawa, A.; Ohkawara, A.; Kobayashi, H.; Harada, S.; et al. A survey of psoriasis patients in Japan from 1982 to 2001. *J. Dermatol. Sci.* **2003**, *31*, 59–64. [CrossRef]
11. Takahashi, H.; Nakamura, K.; Kaneko, F.; Nakagawa, H.; Iizuka, H.; Japanese Society for Psoriasis Research. Analysis of psoriasis patients registered with the Japanese Society for Psoriasis Research from 2002–2008. *J. Dermatol.* **2011**, *38*, 1125–1129. [CrossRef] [PubMed]
12. Ito, T.; Takahashi, H.; Kawada, A.; Iizuka, H.; Nakagawa, H.; Japanese Society for Psoriasis Research. Epidemiological survey from 2009 to 2012 of psoriatic patients in Japanese Society for Psoriasis Research. *J. Dermatol.* **2018**, *45*, 293–301. [CrossRef]
13. Alolabi, N.; White, CP.; Cin, A.D. The Koebner phenomenon and breast reconstruction: Psoriasis eruption along the surgical incision. *Can. J. Plast. Surg.* **2011**, *19*, 143–144. [CrossRef] [PubMed]

14. Arias-Santiago, S.; Espineira-Carmona, M.J.; Aneiros-Fernandez, J. The Koebner phenomenon: Psoriasis in tattoos. *CMAJ* **2013**, *185*, 585. [CrossRef]
15. Binitha, M.P.; Betsy, A.; Lekha, T. Psoriasis occurring as a koebner phenomenon over keloids. *Indian J. Dermatol.* **2013**, *58*, 329. [CrossRef]
16. Morais, P.; Oliveira, M.; Matos, J. Striae: A potential precipitating factor for Koebner phenomenon in psoriasis? *Dermatol. Online J.* **2013**, *19*, 18186. [PubMed]
17. Charalambous, H.; Bloomfield, D. Psoriasis and radiotherapy: Exacerbation of psoriasis following radiotherapy for carcinoma of the breast (the Koebner phenomenon). *Clin. Oncol.* **2000**, *12*, 192–193.
18. Muller, H.; Fah, J.; Dummer, R. Unusual Koebner phenomenon in psoriasis caused by varicella and UVB. *Hautarzt* **1997**, *48*, 130–132.
19. Streit, E.; Vogelgsang, L.E. ECG-induced Koebner phenomenon. *N. Engl. J. Med.* **2017**, *377*, 2180. [CrossRef]
20. Weiss, G.; Shemer, A.; Trau, H. The Koebner phenomenon: Review of the literature. *J. Eur. Acad. Dermatol. Venereol.* **2002**, *16*, 241–248. [CrossRef]
21. Camargo, C.M.; Brotas, A.M.; Ramos-e-Silva, M.; Carneiro, S. Isomorphic phenomenon of Koebner: Facts and controversies. *Clin. Dermatol.* **2013**, *31*, 741–749. [CrossRef] [PubMed]
22. Raychaudhuri, S.P.; Jiang, W.Y.; Raychaudhuri, S.K. Revisiting the Koebner phenomenon: Role of NGF and its receptor system in the pathogenesis of psoriasis. *Am. J. Pathol.* **2008**, *172*, 961–971. [CrossRef] [PubMed]
23. Clark, L.; Lebwohl, M. The effect of weight on the efficacy of biologic therapy in patients with psoriasis. *J. Am. Acad. Dermatol.* **2008**, *58*, 443–446. [CrossRef]
24. Boyman, O.; Hefti, H.P.; Conrad, C.; Nickoloff, B.J.; Suter, M.; Nestle, F.O. Spontaneous development of psoriasis in a new animal model shows an essential role for resident T cells and tumor necrosis factor-alpha. *J. Exp. Med.* **2004**, *199*, 731–736. [CrossRef] [PubMed]
25. Boyman, O.; Conrad, C.; Tonel, G.; Gilliet, M.; Nestle, F.O. The pathogenic role of tissue-resident immune cells in psoriasis. *Trends. Immunol.* **2007**, *28*, 51–57. [CrossRef] [PubMed]
26. Cheuk, S.; Wiken, M.; Blomqvist, L.; Nylen, S.; Talme, T.; Stahle, M.; Eidsmo, L. Epidermal Th22 and Tc17 cells form a localized disease memory in clinically healed psoriasis. *J. Immunol.* **2014**, *192*, 3111–3120. [CrossRef]
27. Zhang, L.J. Type1 interferons potential initiating factors linking skin wounds with psoriasis pathogenesis. *Front. Immunol.* **2019**, *10*, 1440. [CrossRef]
28. Puri, P.; Nandar, S.K.; Kathuria, S.; Ramesh, V. Effects of air pollution on the skin: A review. *Indian J. Dermatol. Venereol. Leprol.* **2017**, *83*, 415–423.
29. Liaw, F.Y.; Chen, W.L.; Kao, T.W.; Chang, Y.W.; Huang, C.F. Exploring the link between cadmium and psoriasis in a nationally representative sample. *Sci. Rep.* **2017**, *7*, 1723. [CrossRef]
30. Zhang, P.; Wu, M.X. A clinical review of phototherapy for psoriasis. *Lasers Med. Sci.* **2018**, *33*, 173–180. [CrossRef]
31. Rutter, K.J.; Watson, R.E.; Cotterell, L.F.; Brenn, T.; Griffiths, C.E.; Rhodes, L.E. Severely photosensitive psoriasis: A phenotypically defined patient subset. *J. Invest. Dermatol.* **2009**, *129*, 2861–2867. [CrossRef] [PubMed]
32. Balak, D.M.; Hajdarbegovic, E. Drug-induced psoriasis: Clinical perspectives. *Psoriasis* **2017**, *7*, 87–94. [CrossRef] [PubMed]
33. Kim, G.K.; Del Rosso, J.Q. Drug-provoked psoriasis: Is it drug induced or drug aggravated?: Understanding pathophysiology and clinical relevance. *J. Clin. Aesthet. Dermatol.* **2010**, *3*, 32–38.
34. Justiniano, H.; Berlingeri-Ramos, A.C.; Sanchez, J.L. Pattern analysis of drug-induced skin diseases. *Am. J. Dermatopathol.* **2008**, *30*, 352–369. [CrossRef] [PubMed]
35. Tsankov, N.; Angelova, I.; Kazandjieva, J. Drug-induced psoriasis. Recognition and management. *Am. J. Clin. Dermatol.* **2000**, *1*, 159–165. [CrossRef] [PubMed]
36. Jacobi, T.C.; Highet, A. A clinical dilemma while treating hypercholesterolaemia in psoriasis. *Br. J. Dermatol.* **2003**, *149*, 1305–1306. [CrossRef] [PubMed]
37. Fisher, D.A.; Elias, P.M.; LeBoit, P.L. Exacerbation of psoriasis by the hypolipidemic agent, gemfibrozil. *Arch. Dermatol.* **1988**, *124*, 854–855. [CrossRef] [PubMed]
38. Fry, L.; Baker, B.S. Triggering psoriasis: The role of infections and medications. *Clin. Dermatol.* **2007**, *25*, 606–615. [CrossRef]

39. van der Fits, L.; Mourits, S.; Voerman, J.S.; Kant, M.; Boon, L.; Laman, J.D.; Cornelissen, F.; Mus, A.M.; Florencia, E.; Prens, E.P.; et al. Imiquimod-induced psoriasis-like skin inflammation in mice is mediated via the IL-23/IL-17 axis. *J. Immunol.* **2009**, *182*, 5836–45. [CrossRef]
40. Bonigen, J.; Raynaud-Donzel, C.; Hureaux, J.; Kramkimel, N.; Blom, A.; Jeudy, G.; Berton, A.L.; Hubiche, T.; Bedane, C.; Legoupil, D.; et al. Anti-PD1-induced psoriasis: A study of 21 patients. *J. Eur. Acad. Dermatol. Venereol.* **2017**, *31*, e254–e257. [CrossRef]
41. Kim, D.W.; Park, S.K.; Woo, S.H.; Yun, S.K.; Kim, H.U.; Park, J. New-onset psoriasis induced by rituximab therapy for non-Hodgkin lymphoma in a child. *Eur. J. Dermatol.* **2016**, *26*, 190–191. [CrossRef] [PubMed]
42. Guidelli, G.M.; Fioravanti, A.; Rubegni, P.; Feci, L. Induced psoriasis after rituximab therapy for rheumatoid arthritis: A case report and review of the literature. *Rheumatol. Int.* **2013**, *33*, 2927–2930. [CrossRef] [PubMed]
43. Brown, G.; Wang, E.; Leon, A.; Huynh, M.; Wehner, M.; Matro, R.; Lions, E.; Liao, W.; Haemel, A. Tumor necrosis factor-alpha inhibitor-induced psoriasis: Systematic review of clinical features, histopathological findings, and management experience. *J. Am. Acad. Dermatol.* **2017**, *76*, 334–341. [CrossRef]
44. Collamer, A.N.; Guerrero, K.T.; Henning, J.S.; Battafarano, D.F. Psoriatic skin lesions induced by tumor necrosis factor antagonist therapy: A literature review and potential mechanisms of action. *Arthritis Rheum.* **2008**, *59*, 996–1001. [CrossRef] [PubMed]
45. Munera-Campos, M.; Ballesca, F.; Carrascosa, J.M. Paradoxical reactions to biologic therapy in psoriasis: A review of the literature. *Actas Dermosifiliogr.* **2018**, *109*, 791–800. [CrossRef]
46. Collamer, A.N.; Battafarano, D.F. Psoriatic skin lesions induced by tumor necrosis factor antagonist therapy: Clinical features and possible immunopathogenesis. *Semin. Arthritis. Rheum.* **2010**, *40*, 233–240. [CrossRef]
47. Rahier, J.F.; Moutschen, M.; Van Gompel, A.; Van Ranst, M.; Louis, E.; Segaert, S.; Masson, P.; Keyser, D.F. Vaccinations in patients with immune-mediated inflammatory diseases. *Rheumatology* **2010**, *49*, 1815–1827. [CrossRef]
48. Lopez, A.; Mariette, X.; Bachelez, H.; Belot, A.; Bonnotte, B.; Hachulla, E.; Lahfa, M.; Lortholary, O.; Loulergue, P.; Paul, S.; et al. Vaccination recommendations for the adult immunosuppressed patient: A systematic review and comprehensive field synopsis. *J. Autoimmun.* **2017**, *80*, 10–27. [CrossRef]
49. Wine-Lee, L.; Keller, S.C.; Wilck, M.B.; Gluckman, S.J.; Van Voorhees, A.S. From the Medical Board of the National Psoriasis Foundation: Vaccination in adult patients on systemic therapy for psoriasis. *J. Am. Acad. Dermatol.* **2013**, *69*, 1003–1013. [CrossRef]
50. Gunes, A.T.; Fetil, E.; Akarsu, S.; Ozbagcivan, O.; Babayeva, L. Possible triggering effect of influenza vaccination on psoriasis. *J. Immunol. Res.* **2015**, *2015*, 258430. [CrossRef]
51. Sbidian, E.; Eftekahri, P.; Viguier, M.; Laroche, L.; Chosidow, O.; Gosselin, P.; Trouche, F.; Bonnet, N.; Arfi, C.; Tubach, F.; et al. National survey of psoriasis flares after 2009 monovalent H1N1/seasonal vaccines. *Dermatology* **2014**, *229*, 130–135. [CrossRef] [PubMed]
52. Shin, M.S.; Kim, S.J.; Kim, S.H.; Kwak, Y.G.; Park, H.J. New onset guttate psoriasis following pandemic H1N1 influenza vaccination. *Ann. Dermatol.* **2013**, *25*, 489–492. [CrossRef] [PubMed]
53. Luca, S.; Mihaescu, T. History of BCG vaccine. *Maedica* **2013**, *8*, 53–58. [PubMed]
54. Koca, R.; Altinyazar, H.C.; Numanoglu, G.; Unalacak, M. Guttate psoriasis-like lesions following BCG vaccination. *J. Trop. Pediatr.* **2004**, *50*, 178–179. [CrossRef] [PubMed]
55. Takayama, K.; Satoh, T.; Hayashi, M.; Yokozeki, H. Psoriatic skin lesions induced by BCG vaccination. *Acta. Derm. Venereol.* **2008**, *88*, 621–622.
56. Wee, J.S.; Natkunarajah, J.; Moosa, Y.; Marsden, R.A. Erythrodermic pustular psoriasis triggered by intravesical bacillus Calmette-Guerin immunotherapy. *Clin. Exp. Dermatol.* **2012**, *37*, 455–457. [CrossRef] [PubMed]
57. Choudhry, A.; Mathena, J.; Albano, J.D.; Yacovone, M.; Collins, L. Safety evaluation of adenovirus type 4 and type 7 vaccine live, oral in military recruits. *Vaccine* **2016**, *34*, 4558–4564. [CrossRef] [PubMed]
58. Macias, V.C.; Cunha, D. Psoriasis triggered by tetanus-diphtheria vaccination. *Cutan. Ocul. Toxicol.* **2013**, *32*, 164–165. [CrossRef]
59. Yoneyama, S.; Kamiya, K.; Kishimoto, M.; Komine, M.; Ohtsuki, M. Generalized exacerbation of psoriasis vulgaris induced by pneumococcal polysaccharide vaccine. *J. Dermatol.* **2019**, (in press). [CrossRef]
60. Telfer, N.R.; Chalmers, R.J.; Whale, K.; Colman, G. The role of streptococcal infection in the initiation of guttate psoriasis. *Arch. Dermatol.* **1992**, *128*, 39–42. [CrossRef]

61. Rachakonda, T.D.; Dhillon, J.S.; Florek, A.G.; Armstrong, A.W. Effect of tonsillectomy on psoriasis: A systematic review. *J. Am. Acad. Dermatol.* **2015**, *72*, 261–275. [CrossRef] [PubMed]
62. Visser, M.J.E.; Kell, D.B.; Pretorius, E. Bacterial dysbiosis and translocation in psoriasis vulgaris. *Front. Cell. Infect. Microbiol.* **2019**, *9*, 7. [CrossRef] [PubMed]
63. Tomi, N.S.; Kranke, B.; Aberer, E. Staphylococcal toxins in patients with psoriasis, atopic dermatitis, and erythroderma, and in healthy control subjects. *J. Am. Acad. Dermatol.* **2005**, *53*, 67–72. [CrossRef] [PubMed]
64. Pietrzak, A.; Grywalska, E.; Socha, M.; Rolinski, J.; Franciszkiewicz-Pietrzak, K.; Rudnicka, L.; Rudzki, M.; Krasowska, D. Prevalence and possible role of candida species in patients with psoriasis: A systematic review and meta-analysis. *Mediat. Inflamm.* **2018**, *2018*, 9602362. [CrossRef] [PubMed]
65. Kashem, S.W.; Kaplan, D.H. Skin immunity to candida albicans. *Trends Immunol.* **2016**, *37*, 440–450. [CrossRef] [PubMed]
66. Mallon, E.; Bunker, C.B. HIV-associated psoriasis. *AIDS Patient Care STDS* **2000**, *14*, 239–246. [CrossRef] [PubMed]
67. Lee, E.B.; Wu, K.K.; Lee, M.P.; Bhutani, T.; Wu, J.J. Psoriasis risk factors and triggers. *Cutis.* **2018**, *102*, 18–20. [PubMed]
68. Armstrong, A.W.; Harskamp, C.T.; Dhillon, J.S.; Armstrong, E.J. Psoriasis and smoking: A systematic review and meta-analysis. *Br. J. Dermatol.* **2014**, *170*, 304–314. [CrossRef] [PubMed]
69. Li, W.; Han, J.; Choi, H.K.; Qureshi, A.A. Smoking and risk of incident psoriasis among women and men in the United States: A combined analysis. *Am. J. Epidemiol.* **2012**, *175*, 402–413. [CrossRef]
70. Naldi, L.; Chatenoud, L.; Linder, D.; Belloni, F.A.; Peserico, A.; Virgili, A.R.; Bruni, P.L.; Ingordo, V.; Scocco, G.L.; Solaroli, C.; et al. Cigarette smoking, body mass index, and stressful life events as risk factors for psoriasis: Results from an Italian case-control study. *J. Dermatol.* **2005**, *125*, 61–67. [CrossRef]
71. Lee, E.J.; Han, K.D.; Han, J.H.; Lee, J.H. Smoking and risk of psoriasis: A nationwide cohort study. *J. Am. Acad. Dermatol.* **2017**, *77*, 573–575. [CrossRef] [PubMed]
72. Brenaut, E.; Horreau, C.; Pouplard, C.; Barnetche, T.; Paul, C.; Richard, M.A.; Joly, P.; Matire, M.L.; Aractingi, S.; Aubin, F.; et al. Alcohol consumption and psoriasis: A systematic literature review. *J. Eur. Acad. Dermatol. Venereol.* **2013**, *27*, 30–35. [CrossRef] [PubMed]
73. Murzaku, E.C.; Bronsnick, T.; Rao, B.K. Diet in dermatology: Part II. Melanoma, chronic urticaria, and psoriasis. *J. Am. Acad. Dermatol.* **2014**, *71*, 1053-e1. [CrossRef] [PubMed]
74. Poikolainen, K.; Karvonen, J.; Pukkala, E. Excess mortality related to alcohol and smoking among hospital-treated patients with psoriasis. *Arch. Dermatol.* **1999**, *135*, 1490–1493. [CrossRef] [PubMed]
75. Brown, K.; DeCoffe, D.; Molcan, E.; Gibson, D.L. Diet-induced dysbiosis of the intestinal microbiota and the effects on immunity and disease. *Nutrients* **2012**, *4*, 1095–1119. [CrossRef] [PubMed]
76. Van der Meer, J.W.; Netea, M.G. A salty taste to autoimmunity. *N. Engl. J. Med.* **2013**, *368*, 2520–2521. [CrossRef] [PubMed]
77. Manzel, A.; Muller, D.N.; Hafler, D.A.; Erdman, S.E.; Linker, R.A.; Kleinewietfeld, M. Role of "Western diet" in inflammatory autoimmune diseases. *Curr. Allergy Asthma Rep.* **2014**, *14*, 404. [CrossRef]
78. Barrea, L.; Nappi, F.; Di Somma, C.; Savanelli, M.C.; Falco, A.; Balato, A.; Balato, N.; Savastano, S. Environmental risk factors in psoriasis: The point of view of the nutritionist. *Int. J. Environ. Res. Public Health* **2016**, *13*, 743. [CrossRef]
79. Love, T.J.; Qureshi, A.A.; Karlson, E.W.; Gelfand, J.M.; Choi, H.K. Prevalence of the metabolic syndrome in psoriasis: Results from the national health and nutrition examination survey, 2003–2006. *Arch. Dermatol.* **2011**, *147*, 419–424. [CrossRef]
80. Langan, S.M.; Seminara, N.M.; Shin, D.B.; Troxel, A.B.; Kimmel, S.E.; Mehta, N.N.; Margolis, D.J.; Gelfand, J.M. Prevalence of metabolic syndrome in patients with psoriasis: A population-based study in the United Kingdom. *J. Invest. Dermatol.* **2012**, *132*, 556–562. [CrossRef]
81. Coto-Segura, P.; Eiris-Salvado, N.; Gonzalez-Lara, L.; Queiro-Silva, R.; Martinez-Camblor, P.; Maldonado-Seral, C.; Garcia-Garcia, B.; Palacios-Garcia, L.; Gomez-Bernal, S.; Santos-Juanes, J.; et al. Psoriasis, psoriatic arthritis and type 2 diabetes mellitus: A systematic review and meta-analysis. *Br. J. Dermatol.* **2013**, *169*, 783–793. [CrossRef] [PubMed]
82. Takahashi, H.; Takahashi, I.; Honma, M.; Ishida-Yamamoto, A.; Iizuka, H. Prevalence of metabolic syndrome in Japanese psoriasis patients. *J. Dermatol. Sci.* **2010**, *57*, 143–144. [CrossRef] [PubMed]

83. Takahashi, H.; Iizuka, H. Psoriasis and metabolic syndrome. *J. Dermatol.* **2012**, *39*, 212–218. [CrossRef] [PubMed]
84. Bremmer, S.; Van Voorhees, A.S.; Hsu, S.; Korman, N.J.; Lebwohl, M.G.; Young, M.; Bebo Jr, B.F.; Blauvelt, A. Obesity and psoriasis: From the medical board of the national psoriasis foundation. *J. Am. Cad. Dermatol.* **2010**, *63*, 1058–1069. [CrossRef] [PubMed]
85. Jensen, P.; Skov, L. Psoriasis and obesity. *Dermatology* **2016**, *232*, 633–639. [CrossRef] [PubMed]
86. Lindegard, B. Diseases associated with psoriasis in a general population of 159,200 middle-aged, urban, native Swedes. *Dermatologica* **1986**, *172*, 298–304. [CrossRef] [PubMed]
87. Henseler, T.; Christophers, E. Disease concomitance in psoriasis. *J. Am. Acad. Dermatol.* **1995**, *32*, 982–986. [CrossRef]
88. Debbaneh, M.; Millsop, J.W.; Bhatia, B.K.; Koo, J.; Liao, W. Diet and psoriasis, part I: Impact of weight loss interventions. *J. Am. Acad. Dermatol.* **2014**, *71*, 133–140. [CrossRef] [PubMed]
89. Neimann, A.L.; Shin, D.B.; Wang, X.; Margolis, D.J.; Troxel, A.B.; Gelfand, J.M. Prevalence of cardiovascular risk factors in patients with psoriasis. *J. Am. Acad. Dermatol.* **2006**, *55*, 829–835. [CrossRef]
90. Herron, M.D.; Hinckley, M.; Hoffman, M.S.; Papenfuss, J.; Hansen, C.B.; Callis, K.P.; Krueger, G.G. Impact of obesity and smoking on psoriasis presentation and management. *Arch. Dermatol.* **2005**, *141*, 1527–1534. [CrossRef]
91. Mallbris, L.; Granath, F.; Hamsten, A.; Stahle, M. Psoriasis is associated with lipid abnormalities at the onset of skin disease. *J. Am. Acad. Dermatol.* **2006**, *54*, 614–621. [CrossRef] [PubMed]
92. Armstrong, A.W.; Harskamp, C.T.; Armstrong, E.J. The association between psoriasis and obesity: A systematic review and meta-analysis of observational studies. *Nutr. Diabetes* **2012**, *2*, e54. [CrossRef] [PubMed]
93. Setty, A.R.; Curhan, G.; Choi, H.K. Obesity, waist circumference, weight change, and the risk of psoriasis in women: Nurses' Health Study II. *Arch. Intern. Med.* **2007**, *167*, 1670–1675. [CrossRef] [PubMed]
94. Okorodudu, D.O.; Jumean, M.F.; Montori, V.M.; Romero-Corral, A.; Somers, V.K.; Erwin, P.J.; Jimenez, F.L. Diagnostic performance of body mass index to identify obesity as defined by body adiposity: A systematic review and meta-analysis. *Int. J. Obes.* **2010**, *34*, 791–799. [CrossRef] [PubMed]
95. De Lorenzo, A.; Bianchi, A.; Maroni, P.; Iannarelli, A.; Di Daniele, N.; Iacopino, L.; Renzo, L.D. Adiposity rather than BMI determines metabolic risk. *Int. J. Cardiol.* **2013**, *166*, 111–117. [CrossRef] [PubMed]
96. Tobin, A.M.; Hackett, C.B.; Rogers, S.; Collins, P.; Richards, H.L.; O'Shea, D.; Kirby, B. Body mass index, waist circumference and HOMA-IR correlate with the psoriasis area and severity index in patients with psoriasis receiving phototherapy. *Br. J. Dermatol.* **2014**, *171*, 436–438. [CrossRef]
97. Kumar, S.; Han, J.; Li, T.; Qureshi, A.A. Obesity, waist circumference, weight change and the risk of psoriasis in US women. *J. Eur. Acad. Dermatol. Venereol.* **2013**, *27*, 1293–1298. [CrossRef] [PubMed]
98. Cao, H. Adipocytokines in obesity and metabolic disease. *J. Endocrinol.* **2014**, *220*, T47–T59. [CrossRef]
99. Versini, M.; Jeandel, P.Y.; Rosenthal, E.; Shoenfeld, Y. Obesity in autoimmune diseases: Not a passive bystander. *Autoimmun. Rev.* **2014**, *13*, 981–1000. [CrossRef]
100. Brembilla, N.C.; Boehncke, W.H. Dermal adipocytes' claim for fame in psoriasis. *Exp. Dermatol.* **2017**, *26*, 392–393. [CrossRef]
101. Wellen, K.E.; Hotamisligil, G.S. Inflammation, stress, and diabetes. *J. Clin. Invest.* **2005**, *115*, 1111–1119. [CrossRef] [PubMed]
102. Yamauchi, P.S.; Bissonnette, R.; Teixeira, H.D.; Valdecantos, W.C. Systematic review of efficacy of anti-tumor necrosis factor (TNF) therapy in patients with psoriasis previously treated with a different anti-TNF agent. *J. Am. Acad. Dermatol.* **2016**, *75*, 612–618. [CrossRef] [PubMed]
103. Friedman, J. The long road to leptin. *J. Clin. Invest.* **2016**, *126*, 4727–4734. [CrossRef] [PubMed]
104. Francisco, V.; Pino, J.; Campos-Cabaleiro, V.; Ruiz-Fernandez, C.; Mera, A.; Gonzalez-Gay, M.A.; Gómez, R.; Gualillo, O. Obesity, Fat mass and immune system: Role for leptin. *Front. Physiol.* **2018**, *9*, 640. [CrossRef] [PubMed]
105. Shen, J.; Sakaida, I.; Uchida, K.; Terai, S.; Okita, K. Leptin enhances TNF-alpha production via p38 and JNK MAPK in LPS-stimulated Kupffer cells. *Life Sci.* **2005**, *77*, 1502–1515. [CrossRef] [PubMed]
106. Naylor, C.; Petri, W.A., Jr. Leptin regulation of immune responses. *Trends Mol. Med.* **2016**, *22*, 88–98. [CrossRef] [PubMed]

107. Zhu, K.J.; Zhang, C.; Li, M.; Zhu, C.Y.; Shi, G.; Fan, Y.M. Leptin levels in patients with psoriasis: A meta-analysis. *Clin. Exp. Dermatol.* **2013**, *38*, 478–483. [CrossRef] [PubMed]
108. Cerman, A.A.; Bozkurt, S.; Sav, A.; Tulunay, A.; Elbasi, M.O.; Ergun, T. Serum leptin levels, skin leptin and leptin receptor expression in psoriasis. *Br. J. Dermatol.* **2008**, *159*, 820–826. [CrossRef] [PubMed]
109. Wang, Z.V.; Scherer, P.E. Adiponectin, the past two decades. *J. Mol. Cell Biol.* **2016**, *8*, 93–100. [CrossRef]
110. Zhu, K.J.; Shi, G.; Zhang, C.; Li, M.; Zhu, C.Y.; Fan, Y.M. Adiponectin levels in patients with psoriasis: A meta-analysis. *J. Dermatol.* **2013**, *40*, 438–442. [CrossRef]
111. Jensen, P.; Zachariae, C.; Christensen, R.; Geiker, N.R.; Schaadt, B.K.; Stender, S.; Hansen, P.R.; Astrup, A.; Skov, L. Effect of weight loss on the severity of psoriasis: A randomized clinical study. *JAMA Dermatol.* **2013**, *149*, 795–801. [CrossRef] [PubMed]
112. Roongpisuthipong, W.; Pongpudpunth, M.; Roongpisuthipong, C.; Rajatanavin, N. The effect of weight loss in obese patients with chronic stable plaque-type psoriasis. *Dermatol. Res. Pract.* **2013**, *2013*, 795932. [CrossRef] [PubMed]
113. Murray, M.L.; Bergstresser, P.R.; Adams-Huet, B.; Cohen, J.B. Relationship of psoriasis severity to obesity using same-gender siblings as controls for obesity. *Clin. Exp. Dermatol.* **2009**, *34*, 140–144. [CrossRef] [PubMed]
114. Gisondi, P.; Del Giglio, M.; Di Francesco, V.; Zamboni, M.; Girolomoni, G. Weight loss improves the response of obese patients with moderate-to-severe chronic plaque psoriasis to low-dose cyclosporine therapy: A randomized, controlled, investigator-blinded clinical trial. *Am. J. Clin. Nutr.* **2008**, *88*, 1242–1247. [PubMed]
115. Gelfand, J.M.; Abuabara, K. Diet and weight loss as a treatment for psoriasis. *Arch. Dermatol.* **2010**, *146*, 544–546. [CrossRef] [PubMed]
116. Bardazzi, F.; Balestri, R.; Baldi, E.; Antonucci, A.; De Tommaso, S.; Patrizi, A. Correlation between BMI and PASI in patients affected by moderate to severe psoriasis undergoing biological therapy. *Dermatol. Ther.* **2010**, *23*, S14–S19. [CrossRef] [PubMed]
117. Al-Mutairi, N.; Nour, T. The effect of weight reduction on treatment outcomes in obese patients with psoriasis on biologic therapy: A randomized controlled prospective trial. *Expert Opin. Biol. Ther.* **2014**, *14*, 749–756. [CrossRef]
118. Berends, M.A.; Snoek, J.; de Jong, E.M.; van de Kerkhof, P.C.; van Oijen, M.G.; van Krieken, J.H.; Drenth, J.P.H. Liver injury in long-term methotrexate treatment in psoriasis is relatively infrequent. *Aliment. Pharmacol. Ther.* **2006**, *24*, 805–811. [CrossRef]
119. Malatjalian, D.A.; Ross, J.B.; Williams, C.N.; Colwell, S.J.; Eastwood, B.J. Methotrexate hepatotoxicity in psoriatics: Report of 104 patients from Nova Scotia, with analysis of risks from obesity, diabetes and alcohol consumption during long term follow-up. *Can. J. Gastroenterol.* **1996**, *10*, 369–375. [CrossRef]
120. Montaudie, H.; Sbidian, E.; Paul, C.; Maza, A.; Gallini, A.; Aractingi, S.; Aubin, F.; Bachelez, H.; Cribier, B.; Joly, P.; et al. Methotrexate in psoriasis: A systematic review of treatment modalities, incidence, risk factors and monitoring of liver toxicity. *J. Eur. Acad. Dermatol. Venereol.* **2011**, *25*, 12–18. [CrossRef]
121. Shibata, N.; Hayakawa, T.; Hoshino, N.; Minouchi, T.; Yamaji, A.; Uehara, M. Effect of obesity on cyclosporine trough concentrations in psoriasis patients. *Am. J. Health. Syst. Pharm.* **1998**, *55*, 1598–1602. [CrossRef] [PubMed]
122. Armstrong, A.W.; Harskamp, C.T.; Armstrong, E.J. Psoriasis and the risk of diabetes mellitus: A systematic review and meta-analysis. *JAMA Dermatol.* **2013**, *149*, 84–91. [CrossRef] [PubMed]
123. Cheng, J.; Kuai, D.; Zhang, L.; Yang, X.; Qiu, B. Psoriasis increased the risk of diabetes: A meta-analysis. *Arch. Dermatol. Res.* **2012**, *304*, 119–125. [CrossRef] [PubMed]
124. Holm, J.G.; Thomsen, S.F. Type 2 diabetes and psoriasis: Links and risks. *Psoriasis* **2019**, *9*, 1–6. [CrossRef] [PubMed]
125. Granata, M.; Skarmoutsou, E.; Trovato, C.; Rossi, G.A.; Mazzarino, M.C.; D'Amico, F. Obesity, type 1 diabetes, and psoriasis: an autoimmune triple flip. *Pathobiology* **2017**, *84*, 71–79. [CrossRef] [PubMed]
126. Wang, C.; Guan, Y.; Yang, J. Cytokines in the progression of pancreatic beta-cell dysfunction. *Int. J. Endocrinol.* **2010**, *2010*, 515136. [CrossRef] [PubMed]
127. Wilcox, N.S.; Rui, J.; Hebrok, M.; Herold, K.C. Life and death of beta cells in Type 1 diabetes: A comprehensive review. *J. Autoimmun.* **2016**, *71*, 51–58. [CrossRef] [PubMed]

128. Alnek, K.; Kisand, K.; Heilman, K.; Peet, A.; Varik, K.; Uibo, R. Increased blood levels of growth factors, proinflammatory cytokines, and Th17 cytokines in patients with newly diagnosed type 1 diabetes. *PLoS ONE* **2015**, *10*, e0142976. [CrossRef] [PubMed]
129. Honkanen, J.; Nieminen, J.K.; Gao, R.; Luopajarvi, K.; Salo, H.M.; Ilonen, J.; Knip, M.; Otonkoski, T.; Vaarala, O. IL-17 immunity in human type 1 diabetes. *J. Immunol.* **2010**, *185*, 1959–1967. [CrossRef]
130. Rocha-Pereira, P.; Santos-Silva, A.; Rebelo, I.; Figueiredo, A.; Quintanilha, A.; Teixeira, F. Dislipidemia and oxidative stress in mild and in severe psoriasis as a risk for cardiovascular disease. *Clin. Chim. Acta.* **2001**, *303*, 33–39. [CrossRef]
131. Uyanik, B.S.; Ari, Z.; Onur, E.; Gunduz, K.; Tanulku, S.; Durkan, K. Serum lipids and apolipoproteins in patients with psoriasis. *Clin. Chem. Lab. Med.* **2002**, *40*, 65–68. [CrossRef] [PubMed]
132. Pietrzak, A.; Lecewicz-Torun, B. Activity of serum lipase and the diversity of serum lipid profile in psoriasis. *Med. Sci. Monit.* **2002**, *8*, CR9–CR13. [PubMed]
133. Salihbegovic, E.M.; Hadzigrahic, N.; Suljagic, E.; Kurtalic, N.; Hadzic, J.; Zejcirovic, A.; Bijedic, M.; Handanagic, A. Psoriasis and dyslipidemia. *Mater Sociomed* **2015**, *27*, 15–17. [CrossRef] [PubMed]
134. Pietrzak, A.; Michalak-Stoma, A.; Chodorowska, G.; Szepietowski, J.C. Lipid disturbances in psoriasis: An update. *Mediators Inflamm.* **2010**. [CrossRef] [PubMed]
135. Corbetta, S.; Angioni, R.; Cattaneo, A.; Beck-Peccoz, P.; Spada, A. Effects of retinoid therapy on insulin sensitivity, lipid profile and circulating adipocytokines. *Eur. J. Endocrinol.* **2006**, *154*, 83–86. [CrossRef] [PubMed]
136. Gupta, A.K.; Goldfarb, M.T.; Ellis, C.N.; Voorhees, J.J. Side-effect profile of acitretin therapy in psoriasis. *J. Am. Acad. Dermatol.* **1989**, *20*, 1088–1093. [CrossRef]
137. Ellis, C.N.; Kang, S.; Vinik, A.I.; Grekin, R.C.; Cunningham, W.J.; Voorhees, J.J. Glucose and insulin responses are improved in patients with psoriasis during therapy with etretinate. *Arch. Dermatol.* **1987**, *123*, 471–475. [CrossRef]
138. Grossman, R.M.; Delaney, R.J.; Brinton, E.A.; Carter, D.M.; Gottlieb, A.B. Hypertriglyceridemia in patients with psoriasis treated with cyclosporine. *J. Am. Acad. Dermatol.* **1991**, *25*, 648–651. [CrossRef]
139. Armstrong, A.W.; Harskamp, C.T.; Armstrong, E.J. The association between psoriasis and hypertension: A systematic review and meta-analysis of observational studies. *J. Hypertens.* **2013**, *31*, 433–442. [CrossRef]
140. Armstrong, A.W.; Lin, S.W.; Chambers, C.J.; Sockolov, M.E.; Chin, D.L. Psoriasis and hypertension severity: Results from a case-control study. *PLoS ONE* **2011**, *6*, e18227. [CrossRef]
141. Salihbegovic, E.M.; Hadzigrahic, N.; Suljagic, E.; Kurtalic, N.; Sadic, S.; Zejcirovic, A.; Mujacic, A. Psoriasis and high blood pressure. *Med. Arch.* **2015**, *69*, 13–15. [CrossRef]
142. Phan, C.; Sigal, M.L.; Lhafa, M.; Barthelemy, H.; Maccari, F.; Esteve, E.; Reguiai, Z.; Perrot, J.L.; Chaby, G.; Maillard, H.; et al. Metabolic comorbidities and hypertension in psoriasis patients in France. Comparisons with French national databases. *Ann. Dermatol. Venereol.* **2016**, *143*, 264–274. [CrossRef] [PubMed]
143. Kim, H.N.; Han, K.; Song, S.W.; Lee, J.H. Hypertension and risk of psoriasis incidence: An 11-year nationwide population-based cohort study. *PLoS ONE* **2018**, *13*, e0202854. [CrossRef] [PubMed]
144. Snast, I.; Reiter, O.; Atzmony, L.; Leshem, Y.A.; Hodak, E.; Mimouni, D. Psychological stress and psoriasis: A systematic review and meta-analysis. *Br. J. Dermatol.* **2018**, *178*, 1044–1055. [CrossRef] [PubMed]
145. Verhoeven, E.W.; Kraaimaat, F.W.; de Jong, E.M.; Schalkwijk, J.; van de Kerkhof, P.C.; Evers, A.W. Individual differences in the effect of daily stressors on psoriasis: A prospective study. *Br. J. Dermatol.* **2009**, *161*, 295–299. [CrossRef] [PubMed]

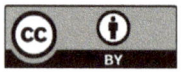

© 2019 by the authors. Licensee MDPI, Basel, Switzerland. This article is an open access article distributed under the terms and conditions of the Creative Commons Attribution (CC BY) license (http://creativecommons.org/licenses/by/4.0/).

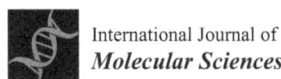

Article

Differences in Osteoimmunological Biomarkers Predictive of Psoriatic Arthritis among a Large Italian Cohort of Psoriatic Patients

Marco Diani [1,†], Silvia Perego [2,†], Veronica Sansoni [2,†], Lucrezia Bertino [3], Marta Gomarasca [2], Martina Faraldi [2], Paolo Daniele Maria Pigatto [1,4], Giovanni Damiani [1,4,5,6,*], Giuseppe Banfi [2,7], Gianfranco Altomare [1] and Giovanni Lombardi [2,8]

1. Department of Dermatology and Venereology, IRCCS Istituto Ortopedico Galeazzi, 20161 Milan, Italy; marco.diani@unimi.it (M.D.); paolo.pigatto@unimi.it (P.D.M.P.); gianfranco.altomare@unimi.it (G.A.)
2. Laboratory of Experimental Biochemistry and Molecular Biology, IRCCS Istituto Ortopedico Galeazzi, 20161 Milan, Italy; silvia.perego@grupposandonato.it (S.P.); veronica.sansoni@grupposandonato.it (V.S.); marta.gomarasca@grupposandonato.it (M.G.); martina.faraldi@grupposandonato.it (M.F.); banfi.giuseppe@fondazionesanraffaele.it (G.B.); giovanni.lombardi@grupposandonato.it (G.L.)
3. Department of Clinical and Experimental Medicine, section of Dermatology, University of Messina, 98122 Messina, Italy; bertino.lucrezia@gmail.com
4. Department of Biomedical, Surgical and Dental Sciences, University of Milan, 20122 Milano, Italy
5. Department of Dermatology, Case Western Reserve University, Cleveland, OH 44106, USA
6. Young Dermatologists Italian Network, Centro Studi GISED, 24121 Bergamo, Italy
7. Vita-Salute San Raffaele University, 20132 Milan, Italy
8. Department of Physiology and Pharmacology, Gdańsk University of Physical Education and Sport, 80336 Gdańsk, Poland
* Correspondence: dr.giovanni.damiani@gmail.com; Tel.: +39-0266214068
† These authors contributed equally to this work.

Received: 16 September 2019; Accepted: 7 November 2019; Published: 10 November 2019

Abstract: (1) Background: In literature it is reported that 20–30% of psoriatic patients evolve to psoriatic arthritis over time. Currently, no specific biochemical markers can either predict progression to psoriatic arthritis or response to therapies. This study aimed to identify osteoimmunological markers applicable to clinical practice, giving a quantitative tool for evaluating pathological status and, eventually, to provide prognostic support in diagnosis. (2) Methods: Soluble (serum) bone and cartilage markers were quantified in 50 patients with only psoriasis, 50 psoriatic patients with psoriatic arthritis, and 20 healthy controls by means of multiplex and enzyme-linked immunoassays. (3) Results: Differences in the concentrations of matrix metalloproteases (MMPs), tissue inhibitors of metalloproteinases (TIMPs), receptor activator of nuclear factor kappa-B- ligand (RANK-L), procollagen type I N propeptide (PINP), C-terminal telopeptide of type I collagen (CTx-I), dickkopf-related protein 1 (DKK1), and sclerostin (SOST) distinguished healthy controls from psoriasis and psoriatic arthritis patients. We found that MMP2, MMP12, MMP13, TIMP2, and TIMP4 distinguished psoriasis from psoriatic arthritis patients undergoing a systemic treatment, with a good diagnostic accuracy (Area under the ROC Curve (AUC) > 0.7). Then, chitinase-3-like protein 1 (CHI3L1) and MMP10 distinguished psoriasis from psoriatic arthritis not undergoing systemic therapy and, in the presence of onychopathy, MMP8 levels were higher in psoriasis than in psoriatic arthritis. However, in these latter cases, the diagnostic accuracy of the identified biomarkers was low (0.5 < AUC < 0.7). (4) Conclusions: By highlighting never exploited differences, the wide osteoimmunological biomarkers panel provides a novel clue to the development of diagnostic paths in psoriasis and psoriasis-associated arthropathic disease.

Keywords: psoriasis; psoriatic arthritis; osteoimmunological markers; bone resorption

1. Introduction

Adult psoriatic disease depicts a continuum encompassing disease progression from psoriasis (Ps) to psoriatic arthritis (PsA) [1]. In contrast to children, in adults, PsA manifests mainly after Ps and its musculoskeletal damages may be prevented with an early diagnosis and treatment [1,2]. Remarkably, 20–30% of Ps patients develop PsA but the non-clinically oriented instrumental screening of psoriatic patients is neither routinely adopted nor recommended due to the connected costs [1]. Thus, both clinical signs, such as psoriatic onychopathy and non-specific inflammatory parameters, are considered to identify Ps patients with a putative higher risk of developing PsA [3]. This is also accompanied by other proposed tools, such as the psoriasis epidemiology screening tool (PEST) questionnaire, evaluating the risk of developing PsA [4]. However, epidemiological studies based on clinical health records comparing Ps and PsA cohorts displayed contrasting results about the possible risk factors implicated in the evolution from Ps to PsA [5].

A biochemical marker that clearly predicts PsA in a cohort of Ps patients is still elusive. A biomarker is defined as a measurable characteristic indicating a biological or pathophysiological process and can be used to identify the risk to develop a certain disease [6]. Several studies investigated the association of different biomarkers with PsA. This condition has been associated with higher levels of cartilage oligomeric matrix protein (COMP), osteoprotegerin (OPG), matrix metalloproteinase 3 (MMP3), and the ratio between C-propeptide of type II collagen (CIIP) and collagen fragment neoepitope Col2–3/4 (C2C) [7]. Other studies found higher levels of CXCL10 in PsA patients compared to Ps patients [8], interleukin (IL)-6 [9], Dikkopf-1 (DKK-1), and macrophage-colony stimulating factor (M-CSF) [10]. However, the clinical significance of these studies is somehow limited due to the restricted panel of biomarkers considered and, more importantly, the lack of consideration of the therapeutic regimens and comorbidities/clinical signs (e.g., nail involvement).

Based on this background, this study aimed to investigate the possible association between a wide panel of osteoimmunological biomarkers with Ps and PsA, and in the relative sub-cohorts in order to identify a possible laboratory tool that could support PsA diagnosis and early prediction.

2. Results

2.1. Clinical Features of the Study Cohorts

Table 1 summarizes the study population demographics and clinical features.

Table 1. Clinical features of patients at the time of recruitment.

Variables	Total Cases ($n = 100$)	Ps Group ($n = 50$)	PsA Group ($n = 50$)	CTRL Group ($n = 20$)
Age median (IQR), years	49 (19–82)	48 (19–82)	48 (28–79)	48 (29–67)
Female, n (%)	28 (28)	17 (34)	11 (22)	10 (50)
Male, n (%)	72 (72)	33 (66)	39 (78)	10 (50)
BMI median (IQR), kg/m^2	25 (23–28)	25 (23–29)	26 (23–28)	24 (22–25)
Ps duration median (IQR), months	195 (83–319)	200 (67–347)	195 (110–317)	-
Eruptive/stable Ps, (n)	-	39/11	-	-
PsA duration median (IQR), months	-	-	25 (4–110)	-
PASI median (IQR)	5 (2–8)	6 (5–12)	4 (1–7)	-
Onychopathy (n)	43	19	24	-
Non systemic therapy (n)	64	31	33	-
Systemic therapy (n)	36	19	17	-
Acitretin (n) (dose)	1 (20 mg/die)	1 (20 mg/die)	0	-
CsA (n) (dose)	6 (237.5 (221.3–257.5) mg/die)	5 (250 (220–260) mg/die)	1 (225 mg/die)	-
MTX (n) (dose)	28 (15 (15–17.5) mg/week)	13 (15 (15–17.5) mg/die)	15 (15 (15–16.25) mg/die)	-
Systemic prednisone (n) (dose)	1 (10 mg/die)	-	1 (10 mg/die)	-

BMI: Body mass index, CsA: Cyclosporin, CTRL: Controls, IQR: Interquartile range, MTX: Methotrexate, n: number, Ps: Psoriasis, PsA: Psoriatic arthritis.

In both Ps and PsA groups, a prevalence of male subjects, 66% and 78%, respectively, was observed despite no gender prevalence being reported. Median ages were 48 (19–82) years in Ps, 51(28–79) years in PsA, and 48 (29–67) years in controls. The body mass index (BMI), in the three groups, was 25 (23–29), 26 (23–28), and 24 (22–25) kg/m^2, respectively.

The Psoriasis Area Severity Score (PASI) was higher in Ps (6 (5–12)) than in PsA (4 (1–7)).

Onychopathic signs were present in 38% of Ps subjects and 48% of PsA subjects, according to the literature [11,12], PsA occurred after the diagnosis of Ps in 88% of patients. At recruitment, patients undergoing systemic therapy (ST) were 38% Ps and 34% PsA patients, respectively. Among these, 28 patients were treated with methotrexate (MTX, 13 Ps and 15 PsA), 6 with cyclosporine (CsA, 5 Ps and 1 PsA), 1 with acitretin (Ps), and 1 with cortisone (PsA).

2.2. Biochemical Characterization of the Study Cohorts

When considered in their entirety, without any subgrouping for treatment status, no significant differences were observed for any of the tested markers between Ps and PsA. Conversely, compared to the control group (CTRL), both Ps and PsA groups differed for most of the analyzed molecules, except for MMP3, MMP7, MMP12, tissue inhibitors of metalloproteinase (TIMP)-1, TIMP-2, OPG, C-telopeptide of type II collagen (CTx-II), and chitinase-3-like protein 1 (CHI3L1) (Table 2).

Table 2. Concentration of serum osteoimmunological markers measured in the study cohorts.

Markers	CTRL Group (n = 20)	Ps Group (n = 50)	PsA Group (n = 50)	CTRL vs. Ps p-Value	CTRL vs. PsA p-Value
MMP1 (pg/mL)	35.00 (35.00–35.00)	471.20 (159.10–1033.00)	608.00 (35.00–1266.00)	$p < 0.001$ ⇑	$p = 0.001$ ⇑
MMP2 (ng/mL)	91.70 (74.58–102.26)	21.18 (7.8–76.60)	16.52 (4.75–78.11)	$p < 0.001$ ⇓	$p < 0.001$ ⇓
MMP3 (ng/mL)	6.27 (3.10–11.67)	2.39 (1.14–4.93)	2.29 (0.74–4.44)	n.s	n.s
MMP7 (ng/mL)	0.86 (0.47–1.16)	0.42 (0.22–1.08)	0.38 (0.19–1.31)	n.s	n.s
MMP8 (ng/mL)	0.61 (0.51–0.71)	1.35 (0.83–3.01)	1.32 (0.71–3.15)	$p = 0.001$ ⇑	$p = 0.009$ ⇑
MMP9 (ng/mL)	0.83 (0.61–1.25)	8.22 (3.31–11.72)	6.59 (3.35–11.63)	$p < 0.001$ ⇑	$p < 0.001$ ⇑
MMP10 (pg/mL)	1.60 (1.60–1.60)	317 (1.60–824.30)	257.47 (1.60–541.60)	$p < 0.001$ ⇑	$p < 0.001$ ⇑
MMP12 (pg/mL)	1.00 (1.00–444.20)	86.63 (11.76–165.40)	76.99 (7.65–144.10)	n.s	n.s
MMP13 (pg/mL)	4.90 (4.90–4.90)	24.85 (4.90–63.21)	4.90 (4.90–49.19)	$p = 0.004$ ⇑	n.s
TIMP1 (ng/mL)	78.74 (66.65–109.45)	101.19 (17.17–114.69)	85.53 (17.71–113.35)	n.s	n.s
TIMP2 (ng/mL)	90.71 (72.38–105.16)	70.77 (10.09–83.73)	59.83 (8.91–76.81)	$p = 0.011$ ⇓	$p < 0.001$ ⇓
TIMP3 (ng/mL)	0.09 (0.09–1.66)	8.79 (0.76–10.73)	6.98 (0.61–9.17)	$p < 0.001$ ⇑	$p < 0.001$ ⇑
TIMP4 (pg/mL)	1072.75 (701.90–1934.00)	27.11 (1.70–320.90)	1.70 (1.70–175.20)	$p < 0.001$ ⇓	$p < 0.001$ ⇓
OPG (pmol/L)	6.46 (3.83–8.51)	5.58 (4.23–6.99)	5.67 (4.51–6.95)	n.s	n.s
RANKL (pmol/L)	393.95 (295.50–943.00)	148.20 (81.75–293.20)	165.40 (86.79–235.20)	$p < 0.001$ ⇓	$p < 0.001$ ⇓
PINP (ng/mL)	46.17 (33.55–62.88)	5.94 (5.01–7.40)	7.08 (4.87–8.22)	$p < 0.001$ ⇓	$p < 0.001$ ⇓
CTx-I (ng/mL)	1.70 (1.38–2.14)	0.55 (0.44–0.61)	0.51 (0.40–0.62)	$p < 0.001$ ⇓	$p < 0.001$ ⇓
CTx-II (ng/mL)	0.25 (0.19–0.29)	0.26 (0.20–0.31)	0.26 (0.20–0.30)	n.s	n.s
DKK1 (ng/mL)	0.27 (0.23–0.37)	2.79 (2.30–3.74)	2.80 (2.02–3.53)	$p < 0.001$ ⇑	$p < 0.001$ ⇑
SOST (pg/mL)	55.17 (35.37–97.10)	147.95 (111.20–186.70)	154.20 (126.90–196.60)	$p < 0.001$ ⇑	$p < 0.001$ ⇑
CHI3L1 (pg/mL)	70.19 (31.87–118.80)	65.98 (47.81–107.00)	83.11 (47.33–114.90)	n.s	n.s

Measures are expressed as median (IQR). CHI3L1: chitinase-3-like protein 1, CTRL: controls, CTx-I: C-terminal cross-linked telopetide of type I collagen, CTx-II: C-terminal cross-linked telopeptides of type II collagen, DKK1: Dickkopf-related protein 1, IQR: Interquartile range, MMP: Matrix metalloproteinases, n.s.: Not significant, PINP: procollagen type I N-terminal propeptide, Ps: Psoriasis, PsA: Psoriatic arthritis, RANKL: receptor activator of NF-κB ligand, TIMP: tissue inhibitor of metalloproteinases, SOST: sclerostin.

Furthermore, statistically significant correlations were found between markers' concentration and duration of both Ps and PsA: MMP2, MMP12, MMP13, TIMP1, TIMP2, TIMP3, sclerostin (SOST), and CHI3L1 in Ps (positive correlation) and with MMP10 and TIMP2 in PsA (negative correlation). Moreover, in Ps group, MMP8, MMP10, and CTx-I positively correlated with PASI score, while TIMP4 was negatively correlated (Table 3).

Table 3. Correlation analysis between osteoimmunological biomarker concentrations and duration of disease or PASI score. Correlations reaching statistical significance are given in bold.

Markers	Ps Duration		PsA Duration		Ps PASI		PsA PASI	
	p	r	p	r	p	r	p	r
MMP1	0.486	−0.10	0.790	−0.04	0.216	0.18	0.647	0.07
MMP2	**0.001**	**0.46**	0.929	0.01	0.322	−0.14	0.205	−0.18
MMP3	0.549	0.09	0.458	0.11	0.459	−0.11	0.829	−0.03
MMP7	0.651	0.07	0.120	−0.23	0.316	0.14	0.746	−0.05
MMP8	0.177	0.19	0.098	−0.24	**0.040**	**0.29**	0.054	0.27
MMP9	0.630	0.07	0.306	−0.15	0.257	0.16	0.226	0.17
MMP10	0.876	0.02	**0.025**	**−0.32**	**0.004**	**0.40**	0.057	0.27
MMP12	**0.001**	**0.45**	0.418	−0.12	0.372	−0.13	0.313	−0.15
MMP13	**0.010**	**0.36**	0.392	−0.13	0.667	−0.06	0.781	−0.04
TIMP1	**0.016**	**0.34**	**0.049**	**−0.29**	0.935	0.01	0.361	−0.13
TIMP2	**0.037**	**0.30**	0.203	−0.19	0.871	0.02	0.372	−0.13
TIMP3	**0.042**	**0.29**	0.087	−0.25	0.946	0.01	0.709	−0.05
TIMP4	0.065	0.26	0.052	0.28	**0.041**	**−0.29**	0.497	−0.10
OPG	0.341	0.14	0.176	0.20	0.067	−0.26	0.448	−0.11
RANKL	0.335	−0.14	0.616	−0.07	0.450	−0.11	0.680	0.06
PINP	0.571	−0.08	0.638	−0.07	0.999	0.00	0.480	0.10
CTX-I	0.215	−0.18	0.341	0.14	**0.048**	**0.28**	0.440	0.11
CTX-II	0.398	0.12	0.956	−0.01	0.124	−0.22	0.161	−0.20
DKK1	0.233	0.17	0.684	−0.06	0.474	−0.10	0.985	0.00
SOST	**0.015**	**0.34**	0.343	−0.14	0.286	−0.15	0.421	−0.12
CHI3L1	**0.010**	**0.36**	0.384	0.13	0.284	−0.15	0.596	0.08

CHI3L1: Chitinase-3-like protein 1, CTx-I: C-terminal cross-linked telopetide of type I collagen, CTx-II: C-terminal cross-linked telopeptides of type II collagen, DKK1: Dickkopf-related protein 1, MMP: Matrix metalloproteinases, PASI: Psoriasis area severity index, p: p value, PINP: Procollagen type I N-terminal propeptide, Ps: Psoriasis, PsA: Psoriatic arthritis, RANKL: Receptor activator of NF-κB ligand, r: Pearson coefficient, TIMP: Tissue inhibitor of metalloproteinases, SOST: Sclerostin.

2.3. Effect of Systemic Treatments

The Ps and PsA cohorts were further divided based on the therapy regimen (subjects undergone to systemic treatments (ST) and not systemically treated (NST)).

When Ps and PsA subjects ST ($n = 19$ and $n = 17$, respectively) were compared, MMP2 (57.47 vs. 11.50 ng/mL, $p = 0.006$), MMP12 (124.10 vs. 76.43 pg/mL, $p = 0.013$), MMP13 (62.48 vs. 4.90 pg/mL, $p = 0.029$), TIMP2 (80.00 vs. 50.34 ng/mL, $p = 0.001$), and TIMP4 (177.7 vs. 1.7 pg/mL, $p = 0.012$) were higher in Ps to PsA (Figure 1A). As expected, PASI score was higher in Ps than in PsA patients (5.5 vs. 1.8, $p = 0.004$).

The Relative Operating Characteristic (ROC) analysis shows that the area under the ROC curve (AUC) for both the single markers (MMP2: 0.768, MMP12: 0.743, TIMP2: 0.811, TIMP4: 0.724) and their combination (0.755 to 0.845) display a moderately accurate diagnostic potential in discriminating Ps from PsA ST patients. Noteworthy, the combination of all these markers gave the highest diagnostic accuracy (AUC = 0.845) (Figure S1).

By focusing on the NST group, Ps NST ($n = 31$) and PsA NST ($n = 33$) significantly differed for MMP10 (340.9 vs. 224.9 pg/mL, $p = 0.031$), and CHI3L1 (65.21 vs. 91.54 pg/mL, $p = 0.042$) (Figure 1B), with the PASI score being always higher in Ps than in PsA (7 vs. 4, $p = 0.002$).

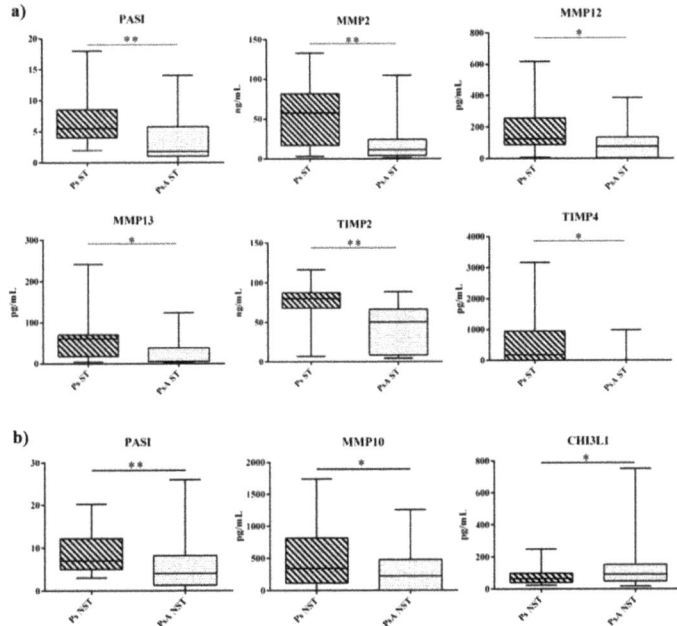

Figure 1. (a) Changes in PASI and serum profile of osteoimmunological markers in Ps ST group (hashed box) and PsA ST group (gray box). (b) Changes in PASI and serum profile of osteoimmunological markers in Ps NST group (hashed box) and PsA NST group (gray box). The box and whiskers plot identify, respectively, the value of the median (intermediate line), the 25th and 75th percentile (box), and the minimum and maximum value (whiskers). Asterisks indicate significant intergroup differences (* $p < 0.05$, ** $p < 0.01$). CHI3L1: Chitinase-3-like protein 1, MMP: Matrix metalloproteinases, NST: not systemically treated, PASI: Psoriasis area severity index, Ps: Psoriasis, PsA: Psoriatic arthritis, ST: systemically treated, TIMP: Tissue inhibitor of metalloproteinases.

In Ps NST, MMP10 positively correlated with CHI3L1 ($r = 0.446$, $p = 0.011$), and negatively with PsA duration ($r = -0.32$, $p = 0.024$).

From the ROC analysis emerges the AUC for these markers and their combinations are below 0.700 (Figure S2). Compared to Ps NST ($n = 31$), Ps ST ($n = 19$) had significantly increased serum levels of MMP2 (57.47 vs. 10.37 ng/mL, $p = 0.007$), MMP3 (3.52 vs. 1.65 ng/mL, $p = 0.026$), MMP12 (124.1 vs. 31.84 pg/mL, $p = 0.002$), MMP13 (62.48 vs. 12.21 pg/mL, $p = 0.013$), TIMP2 (80.00 vs. 14.34 ng/mL, $p = 0.003$), TIMP3 (9.83 vs. 1.33 ng/mL, $p = 0.022$), and CTx-I (265.2 vs. 246.8 pg/mL, $p = 0.01$) (Figure 2).

Interestingly, no osteoimmunological biomarkers were statistically different in the comparison PsA ST ($n = 17$) vs. PsA NST ($n = 33$).

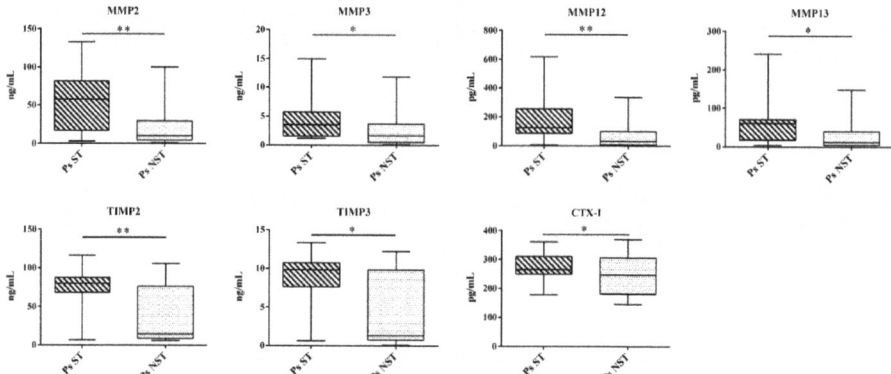

Figure 2. Changes in the serum profile of osteoimmunological markers in Ps ST group (hashed box) and Ps NST group (grey box). The box and whiskers plot identifies, respectively, the value of the median (intermediate line), the 25th and 75th percentile (box), and the minimum and maximum value (whiskers). Asterisks indicate significant intergroup differences (* $p < 0.05$, ** $p < 0.01$). CTx-I: C-terminal cross-linked telopetide of type I collagen, MMP: Matrix metalloproteinases, NST: not systemically treated, Ps: Psoriasis, PsA: Psoriatic arthritis, ST: systemically treated, TIMP: Tissue inhibitor of metalloproteinases.

2.4. Onychopathy Biochemical Signature

Ps patients with onychopathy (Ps O) had higher PASI (6.5 vs. 3.7 $p = 0.009$) and higher circulating MMP8 (1.96 vs. 1.26 ng/mL, $p = 0.028$) compared to onychopathic PsA patients (PsA O) (Figure 3). ROC analysis gave an AUC below 0.700, for MMP8 (Figure S3).

Non-onychopathic Ps compared to PsA counterparts achieved significance only for PASI (6.6 vs. 1.7 $p = 0.002$).

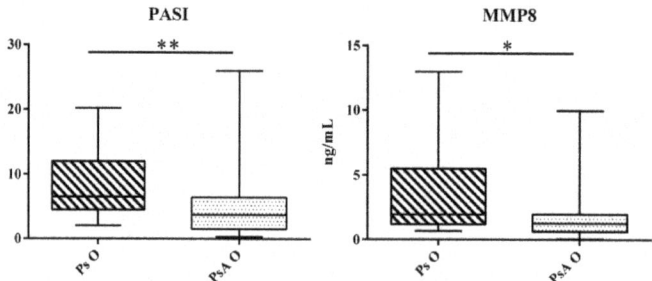

Figure 3. Changes in PASI and serum profile of MMP8 in Ps O group (hashed box) and PsA O group (dotted box). The box and whiskers plot identifies, respectively, the value of the median (intermediate line), the 25th and 75th percentile (box), and the minimum and maximum value (whiskers). Asterisks indicate significant intergroup differences (* $p < 0.05$, ** $p < 0.01$). MMP: Matrix metalloproteinasis, PASI: Psoriasis area severity index, Ps O: Psoriatic onychopathy, PsA O: Psoriatic arthritis with onychopathy.

3. Discussion

The present study investigated two different possible sets of osteoimmunological biomarkers to screen for PsA among Ps. This is of particular interest because Ps patients, especially those with a mild cutaneous involvement, having a subclinical PsA are hardly identifiable using standard measures. The consequent delayed diagnosis of PsA results in a more severe impact on the joint status. Imaging techniques have a high diagnostic potential, but they are intrinsically limited in terms of predictability.

Contrarily, since biochemical markers expression anticipates the micro/macro-structural changes, they have a predictive potential. However, markers discriminating between Ps and PsA have not been identified, although advances have been gained in the biochemical differential characterization between RA and seronegative arthropathies [13].

Previous findings gave controversy results, eventually due to the high within-cohort heterogeneity. Indeed, in our study, when the entire cohorts are considered, the main differences were between Ps and PsA and healthy controls. Similarly, previous studies failed in determining any difference between Ps and PsA in sRANKL, COMP, and OPG concentrations. A possible explanation of differences found comparing Ps and PsA patients with their healthy counterparts is that, actually, some Ps patients that are asymptomatic for PsA are, instead, suffering from subclinical cartilage and bone changing [14]. In particular, the pathological changes in cartilage and bone can be associated with enthesitis, dactylitis, nail dystrophy, and new bone apposition. Importantly, aberrant bone formation characterizes and clearly differentiates PsA from rheumatoid arthritis (RA) and other inflammatory arthritis where resorptive phenomena prevail [15,16]. On the other hand, the inclusion of patients under different treatment regimens and/or with different clinical features within the same cohorts makes the comparison less fine.

A first set of biomarkers, composed matrix metalloproteinases, and their tissue inhibitors comprises of MMP2, MMP12, MMP13, TIMP2, and TIMP4 whose circulating levels are higher in Ps undergoing systemic therapy compared to the parallel PsA cohort. Moreover, the ROC analysis of both single and differently combined markers (even more, the combination of all five) gave a good diagnostic accuracy. Consequently, this panel is particularly promising because of the wide use of MTX in both Ps and PsA. The effects of systemic treatments on the osteoimmune function is clearly depicted, in our study, by the decrease in the circulating levels of most of the markers here considered.

A second set of biomarkers seems to be useful in differentiating between Ps and PsA that have never undergone systemic treatments (NST). Given their naïve condition, the comparison of Ps NST and PsA NST patients could be considered as the most useful. This set comprises of MMP10 and CHI3L1 whose levels are, moreover, reciprocally correlated. CHI3L1 is an inactive chitinase due to the lack of the catalytic domain whose physiological functions have not been fully clarified, although it may play a role in inflammation [17–19]. Biological activities of CHI3L1 include regulation of cell proliferation, adhesion, migration, and activation. Furthermore, CHI3L1 is produced by a variety of inflammatory cells, including neutrophils, monocytes/macrophages, and osteoclasts [20], and its induction has been reported in patients suffering from many diseases, including several autoimmune disorders [21]. In addition, elevated plasma levels of CHI3L1 have also been found in RA [22]. According to previous findings, Ps patients experience higher CHI3L1 circulating levels than healthy subjects [23]. Our result seems to indicate that this protein could be a new inflammatory biomarker associated with PsA.

Nail psoriasis is, among others, a risk factor for the development of PsA, especially within the distal interphalangeal joints, as suggested by McGonagle and colleagues [24,25]. Remarkably, the enthesitis of the extensor tendon of the finger in the distal interphalangeal joint of the hand may clinically manifest with psoriatic onychopathy [26]. Although it is reported in literature that psoriatic onychopathy appears in 50% of Ps and in 93% of PsA patients [27], PsA is diagnosed after Ps development in 88% of adult patients. Several epidemiological studies associated psoriatic onychopathy with Ps duration, Ps early onset, high PASI, and concurrent PsA [28]. Systemic therapies, both biologics and non-biological, are regarded as effective and as a possible secondary treatment step in case of lack/loss of response to topical therapies in patients with high PASI or high DLQI (the dermatology life quality index) or PsA [29]. MTX and CsA can improve the nail lesions, with MTX being more effective in treating nail matrix changes, while CsA is more effective in improving nail bed scores [30].

In those subjects presenting onychopathy signs, MMP8 concentrations were higher in Ps than in PsA. Being a collagenase, MMP8 preferentially cleaves the interstitial type I collagen and is the first collagenase that appears during dermal wound-healing [31,32]. MMP8 is expressed by keratinocytes, fibroblasts, and granulocytes, at the level of the cutaneous lesions, and by synovial cells. In this latter case it was hypothesized that MMP8 solves a function in osteo-articular remodeling [33]. It is known that MMP-expressing cells are found in high amounts in the flogotic joint [34]. Therefore, it could be hypothesized that the circulating levels of MMP8 in PsA patients with onychopathy, compared to their Ps counterparts, were low because of its release into the close joint structures rather than into the blood stream. In fact, in PsA patients, as in those with RA, the levels of MMPs are elevated within the joint, which is a closed environment [35]. On the contrary, in Ps subjects without any joint involvement, MMP8 is released directly into the bloodstream, since expressed at the skin level which is, instead, an open system. Although possible, this speculation needs to be demonstrated.

The cross-sectional nature of this study and the somehow limited sample size (pilot study) represent the main limitations, although this is compensated by the great homogeneity of the selected cohorts that limits the number of variables potentially affecting the circulating levels of the analyzed biomarkers. Remarkably, due to the exiguity of the sample, it was not possible to evaluate the influences of drugs and severity on the biomarker's levels. Future studies are mandatory to assess the osteoimmunological biomarker specificity for PsA and further compare the present findings with other autoimmune diseases involving joints, such as RA or gout.

4. Methods

4.1. Ethical Committee

The clinical trial was approved by the ethical committee (BioArp, Ospedale San Raffaele, Milano, Italia), and registered at clinicaltrials.gov (NCT03455166). The study was carried out following the rules of the Declaration of Helsinki of 1975, revised in 2008 (https://www.wma.net/what-we-do/medical-ethics/declaration-of-helsinki/).

A written consent to the use of clinical data was obtained from all patients after being informed about the study procedures, their benefits, and eventual risks.

4.2. Patients Selection and Study Design

Patients with a diagnosis of plaque psoriasis (Ps, $n = 50$) and patients with Ps and PsA (PsA, $n = 50$) were enrolled at the department of dermatology and venereology of the IRCCS Istituto Ortopedico Galeazzi (Milan, Italy), starting from June 2015 until April 2017, during routine clinical activities. Inclusion criteria for Ps patients were plaque psoriasis (no erythrodermic, inverse, or guttate forms) for more than six months, neither current nor previous treatment with biological drugs, and no joint involvement.

Inclusion criteria for PsA patients fulfilling classification for psoriatic arthritis (CASPAR) criteria [36] were active peripheral (disease activity index for psoriatic arthritis (DAPSA) [37] ≥5 points) and axial arthropathy (Bath ankylosing spondylitis disease activity index (BASDAI) [38] ≥4 points), as well as enthesitis (Leeds enthesitis index (LEI) [39] >0 points), and dactylitis (dactylitis severity score (DSS) [40] >2 points) with cutaneous involvement (PASI >3), neither current treatment with biological drugs nor biological treatment. For PsA, we included a new diagnosis of PsA in order, but also of patients without an experience with biologics or patients unresponsive to biological treatments willing to start a new systemic treatment, or, if they experienced biologics, they stopped them in favor of a systemic conventional treatment for a minimum of 4 months before entering in this study. Remarkably, patients should have suspended topical therapy for at least 4 weeks.

Psoriatic onychopathy was included only if nail psoriasis severity index (NAPSI) [41] ≥ 3 points.

Exclusion criteria, common to the two groups, included pregnancy, current or previous malignancies, other acute or chronic inflammatory diseases, infectious diseases (human immunodeficiency virus (HIV), hepatitis B and C [42], tuberculosis), other rheumatologic diseases, primary bone metabolic diseases, recent bone fractures (within 6 months), anxiety, psychosis, or depressive disorders, supplementations, or particular diets (included fasting) [43–45].

4.3. Dermatology and Rheumatology Assessment of Patients

During the outpatient visit, Ps history, disease onset and evolution were evaluated. The most prevalent type of Ps was determined, along with the body sites involved and the presence of the onychopathic trait. A psoriasis area and severity index (PASI) score was assigned by two independent board-certified dermatologists.

PsA diagnosis was formulated by two independent board certified rheumatologists prior to the dermatological examination, based on anamnestic and clinical evaluations of the patient's inflammatory and imaging indexes. In particular, based on CASPAR criteria [36] and ultrasound (US) or nuclear magnetic resonance imaging (NMRI), the specialist evaluated the presence of Ps, signs and symptoms of joint inflammation (i.e., dactylitis, enthesitis), and reduced joint mobility.

Finally, laboratory analyses completed the diagnostic path by investigating markers useful in the differential diagnosis with other forms of inflammatory arthritis (e.g., rheumatoid factor, anti-CCP, inflammatory indices).

4.4. Blood Sampling and Biochemical Determinations

Blood samples were collected by standard venipuncture of the antecubital vein in SST II Advance Vacutainer® (Becton, Dickinson and Co., Franklin Lakes, NJ, USA). Blood was immediately centrifuged at 1300× g (10 min, 15 °C) and serum was aliquoted and stored at −80 °C until assayed. Serum samples from 20 healthy Caucasian age- and sex-matched subjects (10 males and 10 females, Cliniscience, Nanterre, FR, EU) were used as a control (CTRL).

Serum matrix metalloproteinases (MMP1, MMP2, MMP3, MMP7, MMP8, MMP9, MMP10, MMP12, MMP13) and their tissue inhibitors (TIMP1, TIMP2, TIMP3, TIMP4) were quantified using a multiplex assay on a Bio-Plex® Multiplex System (Bio-Rad Laboratories Inc., Hercules, CA, USA).

Osteoimmune markers, OPG, and RANKL, concentrations were measured in serum using monoclonal antibody-based immunoassays (ELISA) (BioVendor-Laboratorni Medicina A.S., Brno, CZ, EU). A marker of bone resorption, CTx-I, and a marker of bone formation, PINP, were measured in serum by monoclonal antibody-based immunoassays (Cloud-Clone Corp©, Houston, TX, USA). Serum markers of cartilage degradation and inflammation, CTx-II and CHI3L1, also known as YKL-40, were measured by a competitive enzyme immunoassay (Cloud-Clone Corp©) and a sandwich enzyme immunoassay (BioVendor-Laboratorni Medicina A.S.), respectively. Inhibitors of the Wnt signaling pathway, DKK1, and SOST, were assayed in serum by a solid-phase ELISA (Quantikine® R&D Systems Inc., Minneapolis, MN, USA).

The lower limits of detection (LOD) were 0.03 pmol/L for OPG, 0.4 pmol/L for RANKL, 44.3 pg/mL for CTx-I, 12.4 pg/mL for PINP, 52.3 pg/mL for CTx-II, 5.0 pg/mL for CHI3L1, 4.20 pg/mL for DKK1, and 1.78 pg/mL for SOST. Intra-assay (CV_w) and inter-assay (CV_b) variations were: 2.5–4.9% and 1.7–9.0% for OPG, 7.25–11.51% and 11.21–12.77% for RANKL, <10% and <12% for CTx-I, PINP, CTx-II, CHI3L1, 4.2% and 7.6% for DKK1, 2.1% and 10.8% for SOST.

Strict warnings were applied during the pre-analytical phase (i.e., collection, handling, and storage) in order to limit variability in the final analytical output [12,13].

4.5. Statistical Analysis

Shapiro–Wilk's normality test was performed on data from the entire cohort. Since the non-parametrical distribution of the values, quantitative parameters are expressed as the median and the interquartile range in the descriptive analysis. The within-group comparisons were performed using Mann–Whitney U-test. Kruskall–Wallis test was used for multiple comparison. Spearman's rank correlation test was applied to evaluate correlations that were considered significant when $r \geq 0.25$.

Diagnostic accuracy of those markers displaying a statistically significant difference in the subgroup's comparison was determined by the ROC (receiver operating characteristic) curves analysis. The AUC (area under curve)-based accuracy was classified according to Swets JA [14].

The significance was set at $p < 0.05$. Analyses were performed using SPSS software (IBM, Armonk, NY, USA).

5. Conclusions

This study, comparing a large panel of osteoimmunological biomarkers, highlighted profound differences between Ps, PsA, and healthy controls. These phenotypic differences, which are attenuated in the comparison between Ps and PsA, reinforces the thesis according to which these two diseases belong to the same pathological spectrum. However, we also identified important differences in the expression of specific tissue-remodeling associated enzymatic activities in selected sub-cohorts of Ps and PsA subjects that seem to be dependent upon the treatment (systemic vs. topic) and the presence nail involvement (onychopathy).

Supplementary Materials: Supplementary Materials can be found at http://www.mdpi.com/1422-0067/20/22/5617/s1.

Author Contributions: Conceptualization, G.A. and G.L.; methodology, M.D., S.P., V.S., L.B., M.G., M.F.; validation, G.B., G.A., G.L., and G.D.; formal analysis, S.P., V.S., and G.D.; investigation, M.D., S.P., V.S., and L.B.; data curation, S.P., V.S., G.A., and G.L.; writing—original draft preparation, M.D., S.P., V.S., and G.D.; writing—review and editing, P.D.M.P., G.B., G.A., and G.L.; supervision, P.D.M.P., G.B., and G.L.; project administration, G.A. and G.L.; funding acquisition, P.D.M.P., G.B., G.A., and G.L.

Funding: This study was partially supported by the Italian Ministry of Health and by an unrestricted grant from Pfizer Italy (granted to G.A.). G.D. is supported by the P50 AR 070590 01A1 National Institute of Arthritis and Musculoskeletal and Skin Diseases. The funding sources had no role in the conception and design of the study.

Conflicts of Interest: The authors declare no conflict of interest.

References

1. Ritchlin, C.T.; Colbert, R.A.; Gladman, D.D. Psoriatic Arthritis. *N. Eng. J. Med.* **2017**, *376*, 957–970. [CrossRef] [PubMed]
2. Kane, D.; Stafford, L.; Bresnihan, B.; FitzGerald, O. A prospective, clinical and radiological study of early psoriatic arthritis: An early synovitis clinic experience. *Rheumatology* **2003**, *42*, 1460–1468. [CrossRef] [PubMed]
3. Haneke, E. Nail psoriasis: Clinical features, pathogenesis, differential diagnoses, and management. *Psoriasis* **2017**, *7*, 51–63. [CrossRef]
4. Ibrahim, G.H.; Buch, M.H.; Lawson, C.; Waxman, R.; Helliwell, P.S. Evaluation of an existing screening tool for psoriatic arthritis in people with psoriasis and the development of a new instrument: The Psoriasis Epidemiology Screening Tool (PEST) questionnaire. *Clin. Exp. Rheumatol.* **2009**, *27*, 469–474. [PubMed]
5. Ogdie, A. The preclinical phase of PsA: A challenge for the epidemiologist. *Ann. Rheum. Dis.* **2017**, *76*, 1481–1483. [CrossRef] [PubMed]
6. Biomarkers Definitions Working Group. Biomarkers and surrogate endpoints: Preferred definitions and conceptual framework. *Clin. Pharmacol. Ther.* **2001**, *69*, 89–95. [CrossRef]
7. Chandran, V.; Cook, R.J.; Edwin, J.; Shen, H.; Pellett, F.J.; Shanmugarajah, S.; Rosen, C.F.; Gladman, D.D. Soluble biomarkers differentiate patients with psoriatic arthritis from those with psoriasis without arthritis. *Rheumatology* **2010**, *49*, 1399–1405. [CrossRef]
8. Abji, F.; Pollock, R.A.; Liang, K.; Chandran, V.; Gladman, D.D. CXCL10 Is a Possible Biomarker for the Development of Psoriatic Arthritis among Patients with Psoriasis. *Arthritis Rheumatol.* **2016**, *68*, 2911–2916. [CrossRef]
9. Alenius, G.M.; Eriksson, C.; Rantapaa Dahlqvist, S. Interleukin-6 and soluble interleukin-2 receptor alpha-markers of inflammation in patients with psoriatic arthritis? *Clin. Exp. Rheumatol.* **2009**, *27*, 120–123.
10. Dalbeth, N.; Pool, B.; Smith, T.; Callon, K.E.; Lobo, M.; Taylor, W.J.; Cornish, J.; McQueen, F.M. Circulating mediators of bone remodeling in psoriatic arthritis: Implications for disordered osteoclastogenesis and bone erosion. *Arthritis Res. Ther.* **2010**, *12*, R164. [CrossRef]

11. Armesto, S.; Esteve, A.; Coto-Segura, P.; Drake, M.; Galache, C.; Martinez-Borra, J.; Santos-Juanes, J. [Nail psoriasis in individuals with psoriasis vulgaris: A study of 661 patients]. *Actas Dermo-Sifiliogr.* **2011**, *102*, 365–372. [CrossRef] [PubMed]
12. Augustin, M.; Reich, K.; Blome, C.; Schafer, I.; Laass, A.; Radtke, M.A. Nail psoriasis in Germany: Epidemiology and burden of disease. *Br. J. Dermatol.* **2010**, *163*, 580–585. [CrossRef] [PubMed]
13. Sakellariou, G.; Lombardi, G.; Vitolo, B.; Gomarasca, M.; Faraldi, M.; Caporali, R.; Banfi, G.; Montecucco, C. Serum calprotectin as a marker of ultrasound-detected synovitis in early psoriatic and rheumatoid arthritis: Results from a cross-sectional retrospective study. *Clin. Exp. Rheumatol.* **2019**, *37*, 429–436. [PubMed]
14. Bartosinska, J.; Michalak-Stoma, A.; Juszkiewicz-Borowiec, M.; Kowal, M.; Chodorowska, G. The Assessment of Selected Bone and Cartilage Biomarkers in Psoriatic Patients from Poland. *Mediat. Inflamm.* **2015**, *2015*, 194535. [CrossRef]
15. Merola, J.F.; Espinoza, L.R.; Fleischmann, R. Distinguishing rheumatoid arthritis from psoriatic arthritis. *RMD Open* **2018**, *4*, e000656. [CrossRef]
16. Mc Ardle, A.; Flatley, B.; Pennington, S.R.; FitzGerald, O. Early biomarkers of joint damage in rheumatoid and psoriatic arthritis. *Arthritis Res. Ther.* **2015**, *17*, 141. [CrossRef]
17. Lee, C.G.; Hartl, D.; Lee, G.R.; Koller, B.; Matsuura, H.; Da Silva, C.A.; Sohn, M.H.; Cohn, L.; Homer, R.J.; Kozhich, A.A.; et al. Role of breast regression protein 39 (BRP-39)/chitinase 3-like-1 in Th2 and IL-13-induced tissue responses and apoptosis. *J. Exp. Med.* **2009**, *206*, 1149–1166. [CrossRef]
18. Di Rosa, M.; Distefano, G.; Zorena, K.; Malaguarnera, L. Chitinases and immunity: Ancestral molecules with new functions. *Immunobiology* **2016**, *221*, 399–411. [CrossRef]
19. Rathcke, C.N.; Johansen, J.S.; Vestergaard, H. YKL-40, a biomarker of inflammation, is elevated in patients with type 2 diabetes and is related to insulin resistance. *Inflamm. Res.* **2006**, *55*, 53–59. [CrossRef]
20. Di Rosa, M.; Tibullo, D.; Vecchio, M.; Nunnari, G.; Saccone, S.; Di Raimondo, F.; Malaguarnera, L. Determination of chitinases family during osteoclastogenesis. *Bone* **2014**, *61*, 55–63. [CrossRef]
21. Coffman, F.D. Chitinase 3-Like-1 (CHI3L1): A putative disease marker at the interface of proteomics and glycomics. *Crit. Rev. Clin. Lab. Sci.* **2008**, *45*, 531–562. [CrossRef] [PubMed]
22. Andersen, O.A.; Dixon, M.J.; Eggleston, I.M.; van Aalten, D.M. Natural product family 18 chitinase inhibitors. *Nat. Prod. Rep.* **2005**, *22*, 563–579. [CrossRef] [PubMed]
23. Imai, Y.; Tsuda, T.; Aochi, S.; Futatsugi-Yumikura, S.; Sakaguchi, Y.; Nakagawa, N.; Iwatsuki, K.; Yamanishi, K. YKL-40 (chitinase 3-like-1) as a biomarker for psoriasis vulgaris and pustular psoriasis. *J. Dermatol. Sci.* **2011**, *64*, 75–77. [CrossRef] [PubMed]
24. Tan, A.L.; Benjamin, M.; Toumi, H.; Grainger, A.J.; Tanner, S.F.; Emery, P.; McGonagle, D. The relationship between the extensor tendon enthesis and the nail in distal interphalangeal joint disease in psoriatic arthritis–a high-resolution MRI and histological study. *Rheumatology* **2007**, *46*, 253–256. [CrossRef] [PubMed]
25. Aydin, S.Z.; Castillo-Gallego, C.; Ash, Z.R.; Marzo-Ortega, H.; Emery, P.; Wakefield, R.J.; Wittmann, M.; McGonagle, D. Ultrasonographic assessment of nail in psoriatic disease shows a link between onychopathy and distal interphalangeal joint extensor tendon enthesopathy. *Dermatology* **2012**, *225*, 231–235. [CrossRef] [PubMed]
26. Sandre, M.K.; Rohekar, S. Psoriatic arthritis and nail changes: Exploring the relationship. *Semin. Arthritis Rheum.* **2014**, *44*, 162–169. [CrossRef] [PubMed]
27. Skroza, N.; Proietti, I.; Pampena, R.; La Viola, G.; Bernardini, N.; Nicolucci, F.; Tolino, E.; Zuber, S.; Soccodato, V.; Potenza, C. Correlations between psoriasis and inflammatory bowel diseases. *BioMed Res. Int.* **2013**, *2013*, 983902. [CrossRef]
28. Schons, K.R.; Beber, A.A.; Beck Mde, O.; Monticielo, O.A. Nail involvement in adult patients with plaque-type psoriasis: Prevalence and clinical features. *An. Bras. Dermatol.* **2015**, *90*, 314–319. [CrossRef]
29. Lombardi, G.; Perego, S.; Sansoni, V.; Diani, M.; Banfi, G.; Altomare, G. Anti-adalimumab antibodies in psoriasis: Lack of clinical utility and laboratory evidence. *BMJ Open* **2016**, *6*, e011941. [CrossRef]
30. Sobolewski, P.; Walecka, I.; Dopytalska, K. Nail involvement in psoriatic arthritis. *Reumatologia* **2017**, *55*, 131–135. [CrossRef]
31. Nwomeh, B.C.; Liang, H.X.; Diegelmann, R.F.; Cohen, I.K.; Yager, D.R. Dynamics of the matrix metalloproteinases MMP-1 and MMP-8 in acute open human dermal wounds. *Wound Repair Regen.* **1998**, *6*, 127–134. [CrossRef] [PubMed]

32. Mezentsev, A.; Nikolaev, A.; Bruskin, S. Matrix metalloproteinases and their role in psoriasis. *Gene* **2014**, *540*, 1–10. [CrossRef] [PubMed]
33. Hitchon, C.A.; Danning, C.L.; Illei, G.G.; El-Gabalawy, H.S.; Boumpas, D.T. Gelatinase expression and activity in the synovium and skin of patients with erosive psoriatic arthritis. *J. Rheumatol.* **2002**, *29*, 107–117.
34. Ritchlin, C. Psoriatic disease-from skin to bone. *Nat. Clin. Pract. Rheumatol.* **2007**, *3*, 698–706. [CrossRef] [PubMed]
35. Alenius, G.M.; Jonsson, S.; Wallberg Jonsson, S.; Ny, A.; Rantapaa Dahlqvist, S. Matrix metalloproteinase 9 (MMP-9) in patients with psoriatic arthritis and rheumatoid arthritis. *Clin. Exp. Rheumatol.* **2001**, *19*, 760. [PubMed]
36. Palazzi, C.; Lubrano, E.; D'Angelo, S.; Olivieri, I. Beyond early diagnosis: Occult psoriatic arthritis. *J. Rheumatol.* **2010**, *37*, 1556–1558. [CrossRef] [PubMed]
37. Schoels, M.M.; Aletaha, D.; Alasti, F.; Smolen, J.S. Disease activity in psoriatic arthritis (PsA): Defining remission and treatment success using the DAPSA score. *Ann. Rheum. Dis.* **2016**, *75*, 811–818. [CrossRef]
38. Garrett, S.; Jenkinson, T.; Kennedy, L.G.; Whitelock, H.; Gaisford, P.; Calin, A. A new approach to defining disease status in ankylosing spondylitis: The Bath Ankylosing Spondylitis Disease Activity Index. *J. Rheumatol.* **1994**, *21*, 2286–2291.
39. Healy, P.J.; Helliwell, P.S. Measuring clinical enthesitis in psoriatic arthritis: Assessment of existing measures and development of an instrument specific to psoriatic arthritis. *Arthritis Rheum.* **2008**, *59*, 686–691. [CrossRef]
40. Helliwell, P.S.; Firth, J.; Ibrahim, G.H.; Melsom, R.D.; Shah, I.; Turner, D.E. Development of an assessment tool for dactylitis in patients with psoriatic arthritis. *J. Rheumatol.* **2005**, *32*, 1745–1750.
41. Rich, P.; Scher, R.K. Nail Psoriasis Severity Index: A useful tool for evaluation of nail psoriasis. *J. Am. Acad. Dermatol.* **2003**, *49*, 206–212. [CrossRef]
42. Damiani, G.; Franchi, C.; Pigatto, P.; Altomare, A.; Pacifico, A.; Petrou, S.; Leone, S.; Pace, M.C.; Fiore, M. Outcomes assessment of hepatitis C virus-positive psoriatic patients treated using pegylated interferon in combination with ribavirin compared to new Direct-Acting Antiviral agents. *World J. Hepatol.* **2018**, *10*, 329–336. [CrossRef] [PubMed]
43. Adawi, M.; Damiani, G.; Bragazzi, N.L.; Bridgewood, C.; Pacifico, A.; Conic, R.R.Z.; Morrone, A.; Malagoli, P.; Pigatto, P.D.M.; Amital, H.; et al. The Impact of Intermittent Fasting (Ramadan Fasting) on Psoriatic Arthritis Disease Activity, Enthesitis, and Dactylitis: A Multicentre Study. *Nutrients* **2019**, *11*, 601. [CrossRef] [PubMed]
44. Damiani, G.; Watad, A.; Bridgewood, C.; Pigatto, P.D.M.; Pacifico, A.; Malagoli, P.; Bragazzi, N.L.; Adawi, M. The Impact of Ramadan Fasting on the Reduction of PASI Score, in Moderate-To-Severe Psoriatic Patients: A Real-Life Multicenter Study. *Nutrients* **2019**, *11*, 277. [CrossRef] [PubMed]
45. Kocic, H.; Damiani, G.; Stamenkovic, B.; Tirant, M.; Jovic, A.; Tiodorovic, D.; Peris, K. Dietary compounds as potential modulators of microRNA expression in psoriasis. *Ther. Adv. Chronic Dis.* **2019**, *10*. [CrossRef]

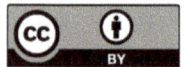

© 2019 by the authors. Licensee MDPI, Basel, Switzerland. This article is an open access article distributed under the terms and conditions of the Creative Commons Attribution (CC BY) license (http://creativecommons.org/licenses/by/4.0/).

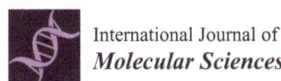

Article

The EGFR-ERK/JNK-CCL20 Pathway in Scratched Keratinocytes May Underpin Koebnerization in Psoriasis Patients

Kazuhisa Furue [1], Takamichi Ito [1], Yuka Tanaka [1], Akiko Hashimoto-Hachiya [2], Masaki Takemura [1], Maho Murata [1], Makiko Kido-Nakahara [1], Gaku Tsuji [2], Takeshi Nakahara [3] and Masutaka Furue [1,2,3,*]

1. Department of Dermatology, Faculty of Medical Sciences, Kyushu University, Maidashi 3-1-1, Fukuoka 812-8582, Japan; ffff5113@gmail.com (K.F.); takamiti@dermatol.med.kyushu-u.ac.jp (T.I.); yukat53@med.kyushu-u.ac.jp (Y.T.); take0917@dermatol.med.kyushu-u.ac.jp (M.T.); muratama@dermatol.med.kyushu-u.ac.jp (M.M.); macky@dermatol.med.kyushu-u.ac.jp (M.K.-N.)
2. Research and Clinical Center for Yusho and Dioxin, Kyushu University Hospital, Maidashi 3-1-1, Fukuoka 812-8582, Japan; ahachi@dermatol.med.kyushu-u.ac.jp (A.H.-H.); gakku@dermatol.med.kyushu-u.ac.jp (G.T.)
3. Division of Skin Surface Sensing, Department of Dermatology, Faculty of Medical Sciences, Kyushu University, Maidashi 3-1-1, Fukuoka 812-8582, Japan; nakahara@dermatol.med.kyushu-u.ac.jp
* Correspondence: furue@dermatol.med.kyushu-u.ac.jp; Tel.: +81-92-642-5581; Fax: +81-92-642-5600

Received: 23 December 2019; Accepted: 8 January 2020; Published: 9 January 2020

Abstract: Epidermal keratinocytes represent a rich source of C-C motif chemokine 20 (CCL20) and recruit CCR6[+] interleukin (IL)-17A–producing T cells that are known to be pathogenic for psoriasis. A previous study revealed that scratch injury on keratinocytes upregulates CCL20 production, which is implicated in the Koebner phenomenon characteristically seen in psoriasis patients. However, the molecular mechanisms leading to scratch-induced CCL20 production remain elusive. In this study, we demonstrate that scratch injury upregulates the phosphorylation of epidermal growth factor receptor (EGFR) and that the specific EGFR inhibitor PD153035 attenuates scratch-induced CCL20 upregulation in an extracellular signal-related kinase (ERK)-dependent, and to a lesser extent, a c-Jun N-terminal kinase (JNK)-dependent but p38 mitogen-activated protein kinase (MAPK)–independent manner. Immunoreactive CCL20 was visualized in the keratinocytes that lined the scratched wound. IL-17A also induced the phosphorylation of EGFR and further augmented scratch-induced CCL20 upregulation. The EGFR-ERK/JNK-CCL20 pathway in scratched keratinocytes may explain why Koebnerization is frequently seen in psoriasis patients.

Keywords: CCL20; IL-17A; psoriasis; scratch injury; epidermal growth factor receptor; Koebner phenomenon; ERK; JNK; p38 MAPK; keratinocyte

---

1. Introduction

Psoriasis is an immune-mediated skin disease characterized by epidermal hyperproliferation and dermal inflammatory cell infiltrates such as dendritic cells and T cells [1]. Psoriasis has shown a diverse prevalence across populations worldwide: 2.5% in Europeans, 0.05–3% in Africans, and 0.1–0.5% in Asians [1,2]. Psoriasis markedly diminishes the quality of life, treatment adherence/satisfaction, and socioeconomic stability of afflicted patients [3,4]. Skin injury triggers or exacerbates psoriatic lesions in a condition named the Koebner phenomenon [5,6]. Although the Koebner phenomenon is observed in other skin diseases such as lichen planus and vitiligo, it is particularly associated with psoriasis [5,6]. However, the pathogenetic mechanism of Koebnerization is not clear [5,6].

A number of biologic therapies are currently approved for the management of moderate to severe psoriasis. These biologics target specific molecules in the immune system, and they have a favorable safety and efficacy profiles than the traditional systemic agents such as methotrexate and cyclosporine [7]. Therapeutic success by specific biologics points to the pathogenic role of the tumor necrosis factor-α (TNF-α) axis and the interleukin (IL)-23/IL-17A axis in psoriasis [8–13]. The gene expression of *TNF*, *IL23*, and *IL17A* is upregulated in the skin lesions of psoriasis patients [13–15]. Infiltration of IL-17A–producing T helper (Th17) cells is detected in the lesional skin of psoriatic patients, and certain Th17 cells are reactive to selective autoantigens [16–18].

The recruitment of Th17 cells into the lesion is governed by CCL20-CCR6 engagement [19,20]. The expression of CCR6 has been confirmed in other IL-17A–producing cytotoxic T cells (Tc17) [21,22], innate lymphoid cell group3 (ILC3) [23,24], and γδT cells [25,26]. CCL20 is a potent chemoattractant for CCR6$^+$ T cells as well as dendritic cells [20,27–29]. Psoriatic lesions are associated with abundant epidermal CCL20 expression and dermal skin–homing CCR6$^+$ Th17 cells [17,30,31]. Epidermal keratinocytes represent a rich source of CCL20 secretion [32]. In addition, mechanical suctioning or scratching upregulates the mRNA and protein expression of CCL20 [27,32], and keratinocytes release large amounts of CCL20 in a time- and scratch line number-dependent manner [32]. In a murine psoriasis model generated by intradermal IL-23 injection, treatment with an anti–CCL20 antibody significantly reduced the recruitment of CCR6$^+$ cells and attenuated IL-23–induced psoriasiform dermatitis [33]. Getschman et al. designed a CCL20 variant, CCL20S64C, that acts as a partial agonist of CCR6 [34]. After administration, CCL20S64C competes with CCL20 and significantly attenuates IL-23–induced psoriasiform inflammation in mice [34]. These preclinical studies reinforce the crucial role of the CCL20-CCR6 axis in the pathogenesis of psoriasis.

We have previously demonstrated an upregulated production of CCL20 following scratch injury in keratinocytes and proposed a potential link to the Koebner phenomenon in psoriasis [32]. However, the subcellular mechanisms of scratch-induced CCL20 production in keratinocytes remain elusive. One of the prominent biological alterations following scratch wounding is the activation of epidermal growth factor receptor (EGFR) in epithelial cells, including keratinocytes and corneal cells [35,36]. Therefore, we hypothesized that EGFR activation induces upstream signal transduction for CCL20 production. In this study, we demonstrated that scratch-induced CCL20 production was mediated by EGFR-extracellular signal-related kinase (ERK), and to a lesser extent, by the EGFR–c-Jun N-terminal kinase (JNK) pathway in keratinocytes. IL-17A also upregulated CCL20 production via EGFR activation and further potentiated scratch-induced CCL20 production, suggesting that epidermal CCL20 production is an integral part in the pathogenesis of psoriasis and Koebnerization.

2. Results

2.1. Scratch-Induced CCL20 Expression Is Ameliorated by EGFR Inhibition

Consistent with our previous report [32], scratch injury augmented the protein production of CCL20 compared with non-scratched control human keratinocytes (Figure 1). Significant amounts of CCL20 were released from scratched keratinocytes as early as 3 h after scratch injury (Figure 1). Notably, the EGFR inhibitor PD153035 significantly inhibited scratch-induced CCL20 upregulation (Figure 2A). Moreover, PD153035 significantly decreased the baseline production of CCL20 even in non-scratched controls (Figure 2A). We next examined whether or not scratch injury phosphorylates EGFR. In accordance with previous reports [35,36], scratch injury upregulated the phosphorylation of EGFR (P-EGFR) compared with non-scratched controls, and scratch-induced P-EGFR upregulation was attenuated in the presence of PD153035 (Figure 2B). These results suggest a pivotal regulatory role of EGFR signaling in scratch-induced CCL20 production in keratinocytes.

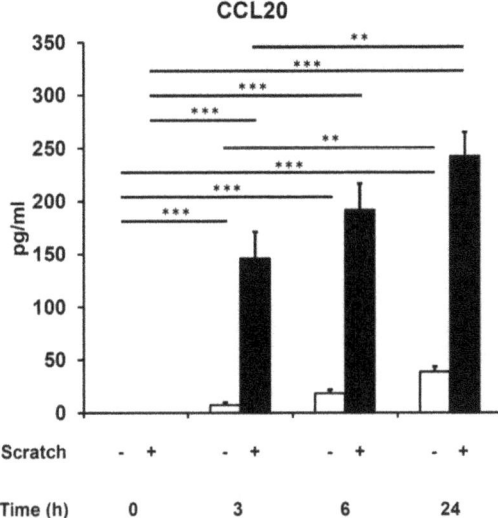

Figure 1. Scratch injury–induced CCL20 production. The production of CCL20 was measured at 3, 6, and 24 h after the initiation of culture in non-scratched control and scratched keratinocyte cultures. Representative data of three independent experiments are shown. ** $p < 0.01$. *** $p < 0.001$.

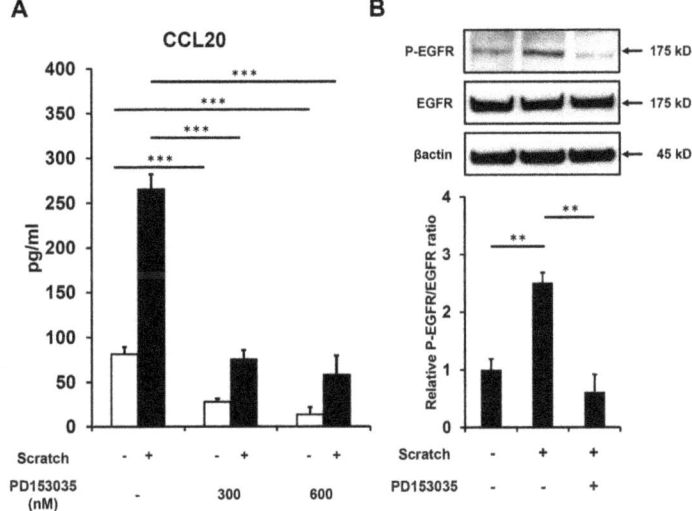

Figure 2. Scratch injury-induced CCL20 production depends on activation of epidermal growth factor receptor (EGFR). (**A**) Scratch injury-induced CCL20 production was measured in the presence or absence of PD153035 (EGFR inhibitor, 300 or 600 nM) at 24 h after scratching. (**B**) The phosphorylation of EGFR (P-EGFR) was measured by western blot analysis at 1 h after scratching. Representative enzyme-linked immunosorbent assay (ELISA) data and Western blot images of three independent experiments are shown. ** $p < 0.01$. *** $p < 0.001$.

2.2. Spatial Distribution of CCL20 Expression in Keratinocytes

Subsequently, we attempted to visualize the CCL20 expression using an immunofluorescence technique. Compared with IgG staining in negative controls (Figure 3A), the immunoreactive CCL20 was positively but faintly and diffusely stained in the non-scratched control keratinocytes (Figure 3B). Compared with staining in negative controls (Figure 3C), CCL20 expression was clearly enhanced in the keratinocytes residing along the scratch-edge area (Figure 3D, arrows). These findings strongly suggest that the scratch injury triggers CCL20 production in keratinocytes adjacent to the wound.

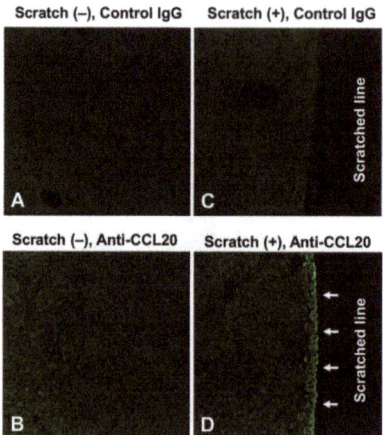

Figure 3. Immunofluorescent visualization of CCL20 at 6 h after scratching. (**A**) Non-scratched control keratinocytes stained with control IgG. (**B**) Non-scratched control keratinocytes stained with anti–CCL20 antibody. (**C**) Scratched keratinocytes stained with control IgG. (**D**) Scratched keratinocytes stained with anti–CCL20 antibody. Original magnification 100×. Representative data of three independent experiments are shown.

2.3. Scratch-Induced CCL20 Production Depends on ERK and, to a Lesser Extent, JNK, but Not the p38 Mitogen-Activated Protein Kinase (MAPK) Pathway

The variable involvement of MAPKs (ERK, JNK, and p38 MAPK) in CCL20 expression has been reported in stimuli-specific and cell type–specific manners [37–41]. Therefore, we examined whether scratch injury activates MAPKs in our system. As shown in Figure 4, scratch injury phosphorylated ERK, JNK, and p38 MAPK molecules compared with nonscratched controls. We then investigated whether scratch-induced CCL20 expression is affected by the ERK inhibitor U0126, the JNK inhibitor SP600125, and the p38 MAPK inhibitor SB203580 (Figure 5). Of note, the scratch-induced CCL20 expression was strongly and significantly inhibited by U0126 and partially by SP600125 (Figure 5). U0126 and SP600125 also inhibited the baseline production of CCL20 in nonscratched keratinocytes (Figure 5). SB203580 did not inhibit baseline and scratch-induced CCL20 production (Figure 5). These results indicate that scratch-induced CCL20 expression is regulated by ERK and partially by JNK activation in keratinocytes.

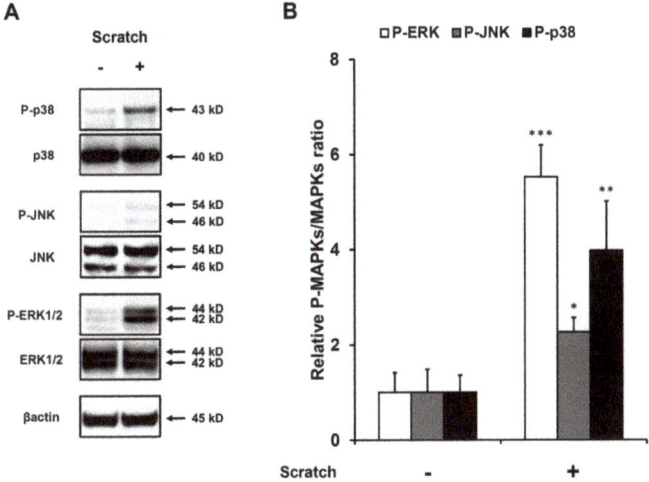

Figure 4. Scratch injury induces phosphorylation of ERK1/2, JNK, and p38 MAPK at 1 h after scratching. Phosphorylation of ERK1/2, JNK, and p38 MAPK was examined by western blotting in non-scratched control and scratched keratinocytes. Representative blot images of three independent experiments (**A**) and the relative expressions of phosphorylated proteins (**B**) are shown. * $p < 0.05$. ** $p < 0.01$. *** $p < 0.001$.

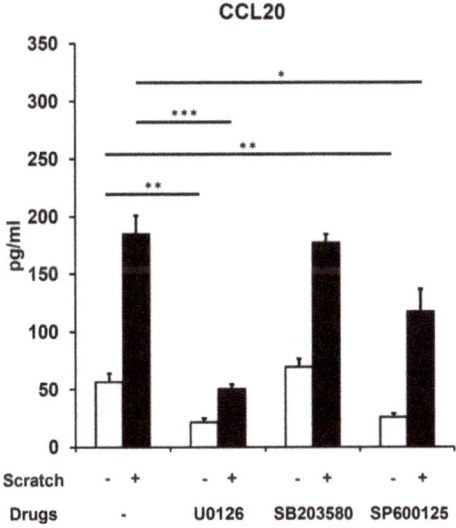

Figure 5. Scratch-induced CCL20 (24 h after scratching) upregulation depends on ERK1/2 and JNK activation. The CCL20 production was measured in nonscratched control and scratched keratinocytes in the presence or absence of U0126 (ERK1/2 inhibitor, 10 μM), SB203580 (p38 MAPK inhibitor, 10 μM), and SP600125 (JNK inhibitor, 10 μM). Representative data of three independent experiments are shown. * $p < 0.05$. ** $p < 0.01$. *** $p < 0.001$.

2.4. IL-17A Synergistically Enhances Scratch-Induced CCL20 Production

Because IL-17A feasibly upregulates CCL20 production in keratinocytes [42], we next checked whether IL-17A augments scratch-induced CCL20 expression. IL-17A alone upregulated CCL20 production in non-scratched control keratinocytes in a dose-dependent fashion (Figure 6A).

When combined with scratch injury, IL-17A additively or synergistically enhanced scratch-induced CCL20 production (Figure 6A). Interestingly, the IL-17A–induced CCL20 production was also attenuated by the EGFR inhibitor PD153035 (Figure 6B). In accordance with this result, IL-17A alone induced the phosphorylation of EGFR and was attenuated by PD153035 in non-scratched control keratinocytes (Figure 7). IL-17A induced similar levels of EGFR activation as did scratch injury. Significant enhancement of phosphorylated EGFR (P-EGFR) was not observed in combined treatment with scratch and IL-17A compared with IL-17A monotreatment (Figure 7). These results stress the crucial role of EGFR activation in IL-17A–induced, as well as in scratch-induced CCL20 production.

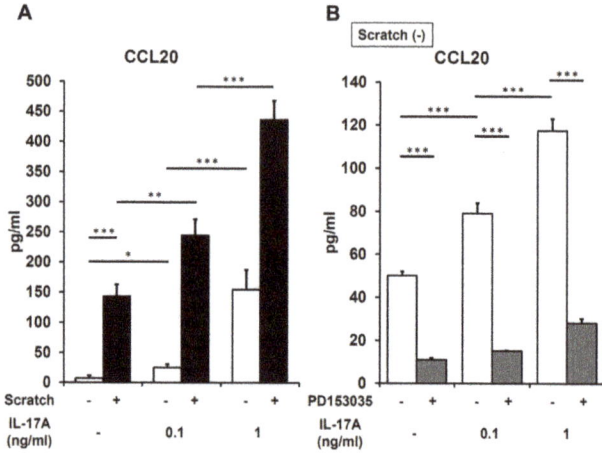

Figure 6. IL-17A augments scratch-induced CCL20 upregulation at 3 h after scratching. (**A**) CCL20 production was measured in non-scratched control and scratched keratinocytes in the presence or absence of IL-17A (0.1 or 1 ng/mL). (**B**) Non-scratched keratinocytes were stimulated with IL-17A (0.1 or 1 ng/mL) with or without PD153035 (EGFR inhibitor, 300 nM). Representative data of three independent experiments are shown. * $p < 0.05$. ** $p < 0.01$. *** $p < 0.001$.

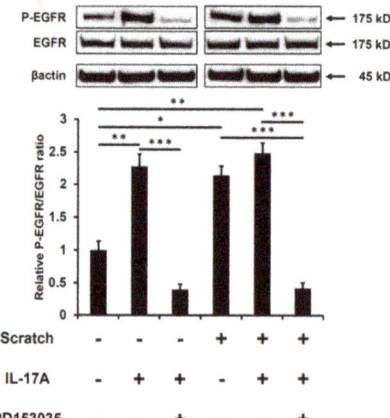

Figure 7. IL-17A upregulates the phosphorylation of EGFR at 3 h after scratching. The phosphorylation of EGFR was measured by western blot in non-scratched control keratinocytes and scratched-keratinocytes in the presence or absence of IL-17A (1 ng/mL) or PD153035 (EGFR inhibitor, 300 nM). Representative blot images of three independent experiments and the relative expressions of phosphorylated proteins are shown. * $p < 0.05$. ** $p < 0.01$. *** $p < 0.001$.

3. Discussion

CCR6 is a representative surface marker for IL-17A–producing immune cells [19–21,23,28,43]. CCL20 and CCR6 engagement is critical for the recruitment of CCR6+ Th17 cells [27,29,44]. Although immune cells can feasibly produce CCL20 [45–48], the expression of CCL20 seems to be confined to peripheral tissues, including skin [32,42,44]. Epidermal keratinocytes constitutively produce CCL20 in culture conditions [32,42]. The lesional epidermal keratinocytes express abundant CCL20 in patients with psoriasis [30,31]. Following stimulation with IL-17A, keratinocyte production of CCL20 is markedly enhanced [42].

We have previously shown that mechanical scratching also upregulates CCL20 production in keratinocytes [32]. However, the underlying mechanisms remain elusive. In this study, we demonstrated that scratch-induced CCL20 expression is mediated by the EGFR-ERK (and, to a lesser extent, by the EGFR-JNK) pathway. The scratch injury induced the phosphorylation of EGFR in keratinocytes. The scratch-induced activation of EGFR is consistent with previous reports [35,36]. The production of CCL20 was detected as early as 3 h after scratch injury, and the blockade of EGFR activation by its specific inhibitor, PD153035, significantly reduced scratch-induced CCL20 upregulation. PD153035 also significantly decreased the baseline production of CCL20 in non-scratched control keratinocytes. These results indicate that CCL20 production is highly dependent on EGFR signaling. Notably, the immunofluorescence study revealed that CCL20 expression was markedly augmented in keratinocytes lining the scratched edge, suggesting a clear relationship between scratch injury and CCL20 upregulation.

Scratch injury activated and induced the phosphorylation of ERK1/2, JNK, and p38 MAPK in keratinocytes. However, in the present study, scratch-induced CCL20 protein upregulation was strongly blocked by an ERK inhibitor and partially by a JNK inhibitor but not by a p38 MAPK inhibitor. In hepatocellular carcinoma cells and murine colonic epithelial cells, CCL20 expression is known to depend on the ERK pathway [37,38]. TNF-α–induced CCL20 upregulation depends on ERK and p38 MAPK in bronchial epithelial cells [39]. Prolactin upregulated CCL20 expression in keratinocytes and was dependent on ERK and JNK [40]. Evidence from our own and previous studies suggests that the ERK (partially JNK) pathway plays a pivotal role in scratch/EGFR-mediated CCL20 production. Although p38 MAPK is not directly involved in scratch-induced CCL20 production, a recent study suggests that p38 MAPK may regulate the recycling of EGFR by accelerating the latter's endocytosis [49].

Positive therapeutic responses to biologics and lesional transcriptomic analysis have highlighted the critical pathogenic role of IL-17A in psoriasis [15,32,50]. Scratch injury triggers the development of psoriatic lesions (Koebner phenomenon) in patients with psoriasis [6]. Therefore, we next examined the effects of IL-17A on scratch-induced CCL20 production. IL-17A dose-dependently increased CCL20 production in non-scratched control keratinocytes, as reported previously [42]. When they were combined with the scratch injury, we observed an additive or synergistic augmentation of CCL20 production by scratch and IL-17A. In line with a previous study that elucidated EGFR activation by IL-17A [51,52], we also demonstrated that IL-17A upregulated the phosphorylation of EGFR and that the EGFR inhibitor PD153035 attenuated IL-17A–mediated CCL20 production. These results suggest that, in patients with psoriasis, the scratch injury stimulates keratinocytes to produce CCL20, which attracts circulating Th17 cells into the scratched skin. IL-17A produced from recruited Th17 cells may further accelerate CCL20 production from the scratched epidermis and further recruit circulating Th17 cells to the injured skin, leading to a feed-forward positive loop that develops into the Koebnerized psoriatic eruption. Both scratch-induced and IL-17A–induced CCL20 expression depend on EGFR activation. Consistent with the present results, it has been demonstrated that the inhibition of EGFR by erlotinib or cetuximab successfully improves severe psoriasis [53–56].

A first-in-human study using a humanized anti–CCL20 antibody, GSK3050002, has already been reported for the treatment of psoriasis [27]. Intravenous GSK305002 inhibits the infiltration of Th17 cells, but not Th1 or Th2 cells, into the suction blisters (rich in CCL20) in treated individuals, suggesting the active and selective involvement of the CCL20/CCR6 axis in Th17 cell homing into the skin [27]. In addition, preclinical studies reveal that a humanized anti–CCR6 antibody or a small-molecule CCR6 antagonist efficiently inhibits the infiltration of immune cells and inflammatory symptoms in a murine psoriatic model [29,43]. These studies stress the significance of CCL20 as a potential therapeutic target for psoriasis. In parallel, the increased expression of CCL20 and CCR6 has been demonstrated in lichen planus which also manifests Koebnerization [57]. There are several limitations in this study. We only examined the effects of scratch injury on the monolayer keratinocyte culture system. Further studies are warranted using three-dimensional skin equivalent, ex vivo human skin, or in vivo mouse models. Fibroblasts may affect the scratch-induced, keratinocyte-derived CCL20 expression in coculture models. More extensive studies may be necessary to draw a concrete conclusion.

In conclusion, scratch-induced CCL20 production depends on the EGFR-ERK (and partially on the JNK) pathway. As has been proposed previously [58], EGFR signaling may be a significant and integral component in the pathogenesis of Koebnerization and psoriasis. Our study underscores the potential role of new therapies such as anti-CCL20 antibody and EGFR/ERK inhibitors in the management of psoriasis.

4. Materials and Methods

4.1. Reagents and Antibodies

Dimethyl sulfoxide (DMSO) was purchased from Sigma-Aldrich (St. Louis, MO, USA). $CaCl_2$ (Fujifilm Wako Pure Chemical Corporation, Osaka, Japan) was dissolved in UltraPure distilled water (Invitrogen, Carlsbad, CA, USA) and added to culture medium at a final concentration of 1.6 mM. In the same way, recombinant human IL-17A (PeproTech, Rocky Hill, NJ, USA) was used at final concentrations of 0.1 and 1.0 ng/mL. An EGFR–tyrosine kinase inhibitor, PD153035 (ChemScene LLC, Monmouth Junction, NJ, USA), was dissolved in DMSO and added to culture medium at final concentrations of 300 and 600 nM. Control cultures contained comparable amounts of DMSO (0.01%) and UltraPure distilled water (1.6%). Signal-transduction inhibitors U0126 (ERK1/2 inhibitor) and SB203580 (p38 inhibitor) were purchased from Tocris Bioscience (Bristol, UK), and SP600125 (JNK inhibitor) was obtained from Abcam (Cambridge, UK). The antibodies used for immunofluorescence staining were as follows: rabbit anti–human macrophage inflammatory protein 3 alpha (MIP-3α, CCL20) polyclonal antibody, and normal rabbit polyclonal IgG (all from Abcam); and goat anti–rabbit IgG (H + L) cross-adsorbed secondary antibody with Alexa Fluor 488 dye (Thermo Fisher Scientific, Waltham, MA, USA). The antibodies (catalog numbers) used for western blotting were as follows: rabbit anti–human ERK1/2 (9102S), JNK (9252S), p38 MAPK (8690S), phospho-ERK1/2 (4370S, Thr202/Tyr204), phospho-JNK (4668S, Thr183/Tyr185), phospho-p38 MAPK (4511S, Thr180/Tyr182), EGFR (4267S), phosphor-EGFR (3777S, Tyr1068), and β-actin (4970S) monoclonal antibodies (all from Cell Signaling Technology, Danvers, MA, USA) as primary antibodies, and goat anti-rabbit IgG HRP-linked antibody (7074S) (Cell Signaling Technology) as a secondary antibody.

4.2. Cell Culture

Normal human epidermal keratinocytes (NHEKs) from neonatal foreskin were cultured in KBM-GOLD Keratinocyte Basal Medium supplemented with KGM-GOLD SingleQuots (all from Lonza, Basel, Switzerland) containing bovine pituitary extract, recombinant epidermal growth factor, insulin, hydrocortisone, transferrin, gentamicin sulfate–amphotericin (GA-1000) (Lonza), and epinephrine and were maintained at 37 °C in 5% CO_2. The culture medium was replaced every day, and the cells were serially passaged at 70–80% confluence. In all experiments, cells were used at the third passage. Cells (3.5×10^5 cells/well) were seeded in 6-well culture plates (Corning Inc., Corning, NY, USA), and the culture medium was replaced every day. At 100% confluence, cells were treated with a high level of $CaCl_2$ (1.6 mM, high-Ca^{2+} conditions), which converted the cells from the proliferative state to the differentiating state.

4.3. CCL20 Secretion in an In Vitro Scratched Keratinocyte Model

The in vitro scratched keratinocyte model was performed as previously described [32]. Briefly, NHEKs at 100% confluence were incubated for 24 h under high-Ca^{2+} conditions at 37 °C in 5% CO_2. Then, the cell sheets were scratched (10 lines) with a 250-µL Long Tip (Watson Bio Lab, Tokyo, Japan). In several assays, the scratched cell sheets were also treated with IL-17A (0.1 or 1.0 ng/mL) [42,59], PD153035 (300 or 600 nM) [60], U0126 (10 µM), SB203580 (10 µM), or SP600125 (10 µM).

4.4. Enzyme-Linked Immunosorbent Assay (ELISA)

Culture supernatants were collected, and the concentrations of CCL20 were measured using Quantikine Human CCL20 ELISA Kits (R&D Systems, Minneapolis, MN, USA) in accordance with the manufacturer's instructions. Absorbance at 450 nM was measured with an iMark microplate reader (Bio-Rad Laboratories Inc., Hercules, CA, USA), and the concentrations of CCL20 were determined in each sample by comparison with a standard curve.

4.5. Western Blotting

Protein lysates of NHEKs were isolated from cells with 100 µL/well of lysis buffer (25 mM HEPES, 10 mM $Na_4P_2O_7$/10 H_2O, 100 mM NaF, 5 mM EDTA, 2 mM Na_3VO_4, and 1% Triton X-100), supplemented with 10 µL/well of proteinase inhibitor cocktail (Sigma-Aldrich). The lysates were then centrifuged at 14,000 rpm for 20 min, and the supernatants were used for analysis. The protein concentration of each lysate was measured with a BCA protein assay kit (Thermo Fisher Scientific). Equal amounts of protein (30 µg for EGFR, phosphor-EGFR; 20 µg for the other proteins) were mixed with 2× sample buffer (Nacalai Tesque, Inc., Kyoto, Japan), boiled at 95 °C for 5 min, loaded onto Bolt 4–12% Bis-Tris Plus Gels (Invitrogen), and electrophoresed at 200 V and 160 mA for 22 min. The proteins were then transferred to a polyvinylidene fluoride (PVDF) membrane (Invitrogen) using the Power Blotter XL System (Invitrogen). Membranes were blocked with 2% bovine serum albumin (BSA; Sigma-Aldrich) in 0.1% tris buffered saline with tween (TBS-T). Membranes were probed with primary antibodies overnight at 4 °C. After incubation with anti–rabbit IgG HRP-linked secondary antibody at room temperature for 1 h, protein bands were visualized with SuperSignal West Pico Chemiluminescent Substrate (Thermo Fisher Scientific) using the ChemiDoc Touch Imaging System (Bio-Rad Laboratories Inc.).

4.6. Immunofluorescence Analysis

Immunofluorescence analysis was performed as reported previously [61]. The cells were cultured in 4-well slide chambers (1.5×10^5 cells/well) (Lab-Tek, Rochester, NY, USA) in accordance with the culture methods described herein. Then, the cell sheets were scratched and incubated for 6 h at 37 °C in 5% CO_2. The cell sheets were washed with PBS 3 times for 5 min each and fixed in cold acetone for 10 min at room temperature. The cell sheets were blocked with 10% BSA (Roche Diagnostics, Basel, Switzerland) and incubated with rabbit anti-human CCL20 polyclonal antibody or control normal rabbit polyclonal IgG. Goat anti-rabbit IgG (H + L) cross-adsorbed secondary antibody with Alexa Fluor 488 dye was used as the secondary antibody. The nucleus was stained with 4′,6-diamino-2-phenylindole (DAPI). Slides were then mounted with Ultra Cruz mounting medium (Santa Cruz Biotechnology, Dallas, TX, USA) and were observed using a D-Eclipse confocal laser scanning microscope (Nikon, Tokyo, Japan).

4.7. Statistical Analysis

All data are presented as mean ± standard deviation (SD). The significance of differences between groups was assessed using unpaired 2-tailed student's *t*-test (2 groups) or 1-way analysis of variance (ANOVA), followed by Tukey's multiple comparison test (multiple groups) using GraphPad

PRISM 7.0 software (GraphPad Software, La Jolla, CA, USA). A p-value of < 0.05 was considered statistically significant.

Author Contributions: K.F. performed all the experiments with the help and advice of T.I., Y.T., A.H.-H., M.T., M.M., M.K.-N., G.T. and T.N. K.F. wrote the first draft of the article. M.F. designed the experimental protocol finalized the article. All authors approved the finalized article. All authors have read and agreed to the published version of the manuscript.

Funding: This work was partly supported by a grant from The Ministry of Health, Labour, and Welfare in Japan (H30-Shokuhin-Shitei-005).

Conflicts of Interest: The authors declare no conflict of interest.

References

1. Boehncke, W.H.; Schön, M.P. Psoriasis. *Lancet* **2015**, *386*, 983–994. [CrossRef]
2. Furue, K.; Yamamura, K.; Tsuji, G.; Mitoma, C.; Uchi, H.; Nakahara, T.; Kido-Nakahara, M.; Kadono, T.; Furue, M. Highlighting interleukin-36 signalling in plaque psoriasis and pustular psoriasis. *Acta Derm. Venereol.* **2018**, *98*, 5–13. [CrossRef]
3. Ichiyama, S.; Ito, M.; Funasaka, Y.; Abe, M.; Nishida, E.; Muramatsu, S.; Nishihara, H.; Kato, H.; Morita, A.; Imafuku, S.; et al. Assessment of medication adherence and treatment satisfaction in Japanese patients with psoriasis of various severities. *J. Dermatol.* **2018**, *45*, 727–731. [CrossRef]
4. Takahashi, H.; Satoh, K.; Takagi, A.; Iizuka, H. Cost-efficacy and pharmacoeconomics of psoriatic patients in Japan: Analysis from a single outpatient clinic. *J. Dermatol.* **2019**, *46*, 478–481. [CrossRef]
5. Miller, R.A. The Koebner phenomenon. *Int. J. Dermatol.* **1982**, *21*, 192–197. [CrossRef]
6. Weiss, G.; Shemer, A.; Trau, H. The Koebner phenomenon: Review of the literature. *J. Eur. Acad. Dermatol. Venereol.* **2002**, *16*, 241–248. [CrossRef]
7. Kaushik, S.B.; Lebwohl, M.G. Review of safety and efficacy of approved systemic psoriasis therapies. *Int. J. Dermatol.* **2019**, *58*, 649–658. [CrossRef]
8. Nakajima, K.; Sano, S. Mouse models of psoriasis and their relevance. *J. Dermatol.* **2018**, *45*, 252–263. [CrossRef]
9. Ogawa, E.; Sato, Y.; Minagawa, A.; Okuyama, R. Pathogenesis of psoriasis and development of treatment. *J. Dermatol.* **2018**, *45*, 264–272. [CrossRef]
10. Furue, K.; Ito, T.; Furue, M. Differential efficacy of biologic treatments targeting the TNF-α/IL-23/IL-17 axis in psoriasis and psoriatic arthritis. *Cytokine* **2018**, *111*, 182–188. [CrossRef]
11. Furue, K.; Ito, T.; Tsuji, G.; Kadono, T.; Furue, M. Psoriasis and the TNF/IL23/IL17 axis. *G. Ital. Dermatol. Venereol.* **2019**, *154*, 418–424. [CrossRef]
12. Sano, S.; Kubo, H.; Morishima, H.; Goto, R.; Zheng, R.; Nakagawa, H. Guselkumab, a human interleukin-23 monoclonal antibody in Japanese patients with generalized pustular psoriasis and erythrodermic psoriasis: Efficacy and safety analyses of a 52-week, phase 3, multicenter, open-label study. *J. Dermatol.* **2018**, *45*, 529–539. [CrossRef]
13. Krueger, J.G.; Brunner, P.M. Interleukin-17 alters the biology of many cell types involved in the genesis of psoriasis, systemic inflammation and associated comorbidities. *Exp. Dermatol.* **2018**, *27*, 115–123. [CrossRef]
14. Lowes, M.A.; Russell, C.B.; Martin, D.A.; Towne, J.E.; Krueger, J.G. The IL-23/T17 pathogenic axis in psoriasis is amplified by keratinocyte responses. *Trends Immunol.* **2013**, *34*, 174–181. [CrossRef]
15. Tsoi, L.C.; Rodriguez, E.; Degenhardt, F.; Baurecht, H.; Wehkamp, U.; Volks, N.; Szymczak, S.; Swindell, W.R.; Sarkar, M.K.; Raja, K.; et al. Atopic dermatitis is an IL-13-dominant disease with greater molecular heterogeneity compared to psoriasis. *J. Investig. Dermatol.* **2019**, *139*, 1480–1489. [CrossRef]
16. Furue, M.; Kadono, T. The contribution of IL-17 to the development of autoimmunity in psoriasis. *Innate Immun.* **2019**, *25*, 337–343. [CrossRef]
17. Pène, J.; Chevalier, S.; Preisser, L.; Vénéreau, E.; Guilleux, M.H.; Ghannam, S.; Molès, J.P.; Danger, Y.; Ravon, E.; Lesaux, S.; et al. Chronically inflamed human tissues are infiltrated by highly differentiated Th17 lymphocytes. *J. Immunol.* **2008**, *180*, 7423–7430. [CrossRef]
18. Villanova, F.; Flutter, B.; Tosi, I.; Grys, K.; Sreeneebus, H.; Perera, G.K.; Chapman, A.; Smith, C.H.; Di Meglio, P.; Nestle, F.O. Characterization of innate lymphoid cells in human skin and blood demonstrates increase of NKp44+ ILC3 in psoriasis. *J. Investig. Dermatol.* **2014**, *134*, 984–991. [CrossRef]

19. Singh, S.P.; Zhang, H.H.; Foley, J.F.; Hedrick, M.N.; Farber, J.M. Human T cells that are able to produce IL-17 express the chemokine receptor CCR6. *J. Immunol.* **2008**, *180*, 214–221. [CrossRef]
20. Sallusto, F.; Impellizzieri, D.; Basso, C.; Laroni, A.; Uccelli, A.; Lanzavecchia, A.; Engelhardt, B. T-cell trafficking in the central nervous system. *Immunol. Rev.* **2012**, *248*, 216–227. [CrossRef]
21. Diani, M.; Casciano, F.; Marongiu, L.; Longhi, M.; Altomare, A.; Pigatto, P.D.; Secchiero, P.; Gambari, R.; Banfi, G.; Manfredi, A.A.; et al. Increased frequency of activated CD8+ T cell effectors in patients with psoriatic arthritis. *Sci. Rep.* **2019**, *9*, 10870. [CrossRef]
22. Steel, K.J.A.; Srenathan, U.; Ridley, M.; Durham, L.E.; Wu, S.Y.; Ryan, S.E.; Hughes, C.D.; Chan, E.; Kirkham, B.W.; Taams, L.S. Synovial IL-17A+ CD8+ T cells display a polyfunctional, pro-inflammatory and tissue-resident memory phenotype and function in psoriatic arthritis. *Arthritis Rheumatol.* **2019**. [CrossRef]
23. Bando, J.K.; Gilfillan, S.; Song, C.; McDonald, K.G.; Huang, S.C.; Newberry, R.D.; Kobayashi, Y.; Allan, D.S.J.; Carlyle, J.R.; Cella, M.; et al. The tumor necrosis f actor superfamily member RANKL suppresses effector cytokine production in group 3 innate lymphoid cells. *Immunity* **2018**, *48*, 1208–1219. [CrossRef]
24. Talayero, P.; Mancebo, E.; Calvo-Pulido, J.; Rodríguez-Muñoz, S.; Bernardo, I.; Laguna-Goya, R.; Cano-Romero, F.L.; García-Sesma, A.; Loinaz, C.; Jiménez, C.; et al. Innate lymphoid cells groups 1 and 3 in the epithelial compartment of functional human intestinal allografts. *Am. J. Transplant.* **2016**, *16*, 72–82. [CrossRef]
25. Campbell, J.J.; Ebsworth, K.; Ertl, L.S.; McMahon, J.P.; Newland, D.; Wang, Y.; Liu, S.; Miao, Z.; Dang, T.; Zhang, P.; et al. IL-17-secreting γδ T cells are completely dependent upon CCR6 for homing to inflamed skin. *J. Immunol.* **2017**, *199*, 3129–3136. [CrossRef]
26. Mabuchi, T.; Takekoshi, T.; Hwang, S.T. Epidermal CCR6+ γδ T cells are major producers of IL-22 and IL-17 in a murine model of psoriasiform dermatitis. *J. Immunol.* **2011**, *187*, 5026–5031. [CrossRef]
27. Bouma, G.; Zamuner, S.; Hicks, K.; Want, A.; Oliveira, J.; Choudhury, A.; Brett, S.; Robertson, D.; Felton, L.; Norris, V.; et al. CCL20 neutralization by a monoclonal antibody in healthy subjects selectively inhibits recruitment of CCR6+ cells in an experimental suction blister. *Br. J. Clin. Pharmacol.* **2017**, *83*, 1976–1990. [CrossRef]
28. Maecker, H.T.; McCoy, J.P.; Nussenblatt, R. Standarizing immunophenotyping for the Human Immunology Project. *Nat. Rev. Immunol.* **2012**, *12*, 191–200. [CrossRef]
29. Robert, R.; Ang, C.; Sun, G.; Juglair, L.; Lim, E.X.; Mason, L.J.; Payne, N.L.; Bernard, C.C.; Mackay, C.R. Essential role for CCR6 in certain inflammatory diseases demonstrated using specific antagonist and knockin mice. *JCI Insight* **2017**, *2*, e94821. [CrossRef]
30. Homey, B.; Dieu-Nosjean, M.C.; Wiesenborn, A.; Massacrier, C.; Pin, J.J.; Oldham, E.; Catron, D.; Buchanan, M.E.; Müller, A.; de Waal Malefyt, R.; et al. Up-regulation of macrophage inflammatory protein-3 alpha/CCL20 and CC chemokine receptor 6 in psoriasis. *J. Immunol.* **2000**, *164*, 6621–6632. [CrossRef]
31. Kim, T.G.; Jee, H.; Fuentes-Duculan, J.; Wu, W.H.; Byamba, D.; Kim, D.S.; Kim, D.Y.; Lew, D.H.; Yang, W.I.; Krueger, J.G.; et al. Dermal clusters of mature dendritic cells and T cells are associated with the CCL20/CCR6 chemokine system in chronic psoriasis. *J. Investig. Dermatol.* **2014**, *134*, 1462–1465. [CrossRef]
32. Furue, K.; Ito, T.; Tanaka, Y.; Yumine, A.; Hashimoto-Hachiya, A.; Takemura, M.; Murata, M.; Yamamura, K.; Tsuji, G.; Furue, M. Cyto/chemokine profile of in vitro scratched keratinocyte model: Implications of significant upregulation of CCL20, CXCL8 and IL36G in Koebner phenomenon. *J. Dermatol. Sci.* **2019**, *94*, 244–251. [CrossRef]
33. Mabuchi, T.; Singh, T.P.; Takekoshi, T.; Jia, G.F.; Wu, X.; Kao, M.C.; Weiss, I.; Farber, J.M.; Hwang, S.T. CCR6 is required for epidermal trafficking of γδ-T cells in an IL-23-induced model of psoriasiform dermatitis. *J. Investig. Dermatol.* **2013**, *133*, 164–171. [CrossRef]
34. Getschman, A.E.; Imai, Y.; Larsen, O.; Peterson, F.C.; Wu, X.; Rosenkilde, M.M.; Hwang, S.T.; Volkman, B.F. Protein engineering of the chemokine CCL20 prevents psoriasiform dermatitis in an IL-23-dependent murine model. *Proc. Natl. Acad. Sci. USA* **2017**, *114*, 12460–12465. [CrossRef]
35. Tokumaru, S.; Higashiyama, S.; Endo, T.; Nakagawa, T.; Miyagawa, J.I.; Yamamori, K.; Hanakawa, Y.; Ohmoto, H.; Yoshino, K.; Shirakata, Y.; et al. Ectodomain shedding of epidermal growth factor receptor ligands is required for keratinocyte migration in cutaneous wound healing. *J. Cell Biol.* **2000**, *151*, 209–220. [CrossRef]

36. Xu, K.P.; Ding, Y.; Ling, J.; Dong, Z.; Yu, F.S. Wound-induced HB-EGF ectodomain shedding and EGFR activation in corneal epithelial cells. *Invest. Ophthalmol. Vis. Sci.* **2004**, *45*, 813–820. [CrossRef]
37. Benkheil, M.; Paeshuyse, J.; Neyts, J.; van Haele, M.; Roskams, T.; Liekens, S. HCV-induced EGFR-ERK signaling promotes a pro-inflammatory and pro-angiogenic signature contributing to liver cancer pathogenesis. *Biochem. Pharmacol.* **2018**, *155*, 305–315. [CrossRef]
38. Dutta, P.; Ta, A.; Thakur, B.K.; Dasgupta, N.; Das, S. Biphasic Ccl20 regulation by toll-like receptor 9 through the activation of ERK-AP-1 and non-canonical NF-κB signaling pathways. *Biochim. Biophys. Acta Gen. Subj.* **2017**, *1861*, 3365–3377. [CrossRef]
39. Zijlstra, G.J.; Fattahi, F.; Rozeveld, D.; Jonker, M.R.; Kliphuis, N.M.; van den Berge, M.; Hylkema, M.N.; ten Hacken, N.H.; van Oosterhout, A.J.; Heijink, I.H. Glucocorticoids induce the production of the chemoattractant CCL20 in airway epithelium. *Eur. Respir. J.* **2014**, *44*, 361–370. [CrossRef]
40. Kanda, N.; Shibata, S.; Tada, Y.; Nashiro, K.; Tamaki, K.; Watanabe, S. Prolactin enhances basal and IL-17-induced CCL20 production by human keratinocytes. *Eur. J. Immunol.* **2009**, *39*, 996–1006. [CrossRef]
41. Liu, Y.; Lagowski, J.P.; Gao, S.; Raymond, J.H.; White, C.R.; Kulesz-Martin, M.F. Regulation of the psoriatic chemokine CCL20 by E3 ligases Trim32 and Piasy in keratinocytes. *J. Investig. Dermatol.* **2010**, *130*, 1384–1390. [CrossRef]
42. Harper, E.G.; Guo, C.; Rizzo, H.; Lillis, J.V.; Kurtz, S.E.; Skorcheva, I.; Purdy, D.; Fitch, E.; Iordanov, M.; Blauvelt, A. Th17 cytokines stimulate CCL20 expression in keratinocytes in vitro and in vivo: Implications for psoriasis pathogenesis. *J. Investig. Dermatol.* **2009**, *129*, 2175–2183. [CrossRef]
43. Campbell, J.J.; Ebsworth, K.; Ertl, L.S.; McMahon, J.P.; Wang, Y.; Yau, S.; Mali, V.R.; Chhina, V.; Kumamoto, A.; Liu, S.; et al. Efficacy of Chemokine Receptor Inhibition in Treating IL-36α-Induced Psoriasiform Inflammation. *J. Immunol.* **2019**, *202*, 1687–1692. [CrossRef]
44. Schutyser, E.; Struyf, S.; Van Damme, J. The CC chemokine CCL20 and its receptor CCR6. *Cytokine Growth Factor Rev.* **2003**, *14*, 409–426. [CrossRef]
45. Bridgewood, C.; Watad, A.; Russell, T.; Palmer, T.M.; Marzo-Ortega, H.; Khan, A.; Millner, P.A.; Dunsmuir, R.; Rao, A.; Loughenbury, P.; et al. Identification of myeloid cells in the human enthesis as the main source of local IL-23 production. *Ann. Rheum. Dis.* **2019**, *78*, 929–933. [CrossRef]
46. Hedrick, M.N.; Lonsdorf, A.S.; Shirakawa, A.K.; Lee, C.C.R.; Liao, F.; Singh, S.P.; Zhang, H.H.; Grinberg, A.; Love, P.E.; Hwang, S.T.; et al. CCR6 is required for IL-23-induced psoriasis-like inflammation in mice. *J. Clin. Investig.* **2009**, *119*, 2317–2329. [CrossRef]
47. Komatsu, N.; Okamoto, K.; Sawa, S.; Nakashima, T.; Oh-hora, M.; Kodama, T.; Tanaka, S.; Bluestone, J.A.; Takayanagi, H. Pathogenic conversion of Foxp3+ T cells into TH17 cells in autoimmune arthritis. *Nat. Med.* **2014**, *20*, 62–68. [CrossRef]
48. Yamazaki, T.; Yang, X.O.; Chung, Y.; Fukunaga, A.; Nurieva, R.; Pappu, B.; Martin-Orozco, N.; Kang, H.S.; Ma, L.; Panopoulos, A.D.; et al. CCR6 regulates the migration of inflammatory and regulatory T cells. *J. Immunol.* **2008**, *181*, 8391–8401. [CrossRef]
49. Tanaka, T.; Zhou, Y.; Ozawa, T.; Okizono, R.; Banba, A.; Yamamura, T.; Oga, E.; Muraguchi, A.; Sakurai, H. Ligand-activated epidermal growth factor receptor (EGFR) signaling governs endocytic trafficking of unliganded receptor monomers by non-canonical phosphorylation. *J. Biol. Chem.* **2018**, *293*, 2288–2301. [CrossRef]
50. Momose, M.; Asahina, A.; Umezawa, Y.; Nakagawa, H. Long-term clinical efficacy and safety of secukinumab for Japanese patients with psoriasis: A single-center experience. *J. Dermatol.* **2018**, *45*, 318–321. [CrossRef]
51. Acciani, T.H.; Suzuki, T.; Trapnell, B.C.; Le Cras, T.D. Epidermal growth factor receptor signalling regulates granulocyte-macrophage colony-stimulating factor production by airway epithelial cells and established allergic airway disease. *Clin. Exp. Allergy* **2016**, *46*, 317–328. [CrossRef]
52. Chen, X.; Cai, G.; Liu, C.; Zhao, J.; Gu, C.; Wu, L.; Hamilton, T.A.; Zhang, C.J.; Ko, J.; Zhu, L.; et al. IL-17R-EGFR axis links wound healing to tumorigenesis in Lrig1$^+$ stem cells. *J. Exp. Med.* **2019**, *216*, 195–214. [CrossRef]
53. Goepel, L.; Jacobi, A.; Augustin, M.; Radtke, M.A. Rapid improvement of psoriasis in a patient with lung cancer after treatment with erlotinib. *J. Eur. Acad. Dermatol. Venereol.* **2018**, *32*, e311–e313. [CrossRef]
54. Overbeck, T.R.; Griesinger, F. Two cases of psoriasis responding to erlotinib: Time to revisiting inhibition of epidermal growth factor receptor in psoriasis therapy? *Dermatology* **2012**, *225*, 179–182. [CrossRef]

55. Trivin, F.; Boucher, E.; Raoul, J.L. Complete sustained regression of extensive psoriasis with cetuximab combination chemotherapy. *Acta Oncol.* **2004**, *43*, 592–593. [CrossRef]
56. Neyns, B.; Meert, V.; Vandenbroucke, F. Cetuximab treatment in a patient with metastatic colorectal cancer and psoriasis. *Curr. Oncol.* **2008**, *15*, 196–197. [CrossRef]
57. Ichimura, M.; Hiratsuka, K.; Ogura, N.; Utsunomiya, T.; Sakamaki, H.; Kondoh, T.; Abiko, Y.; Otake, S.; Yamamoto, M. Expression profile of chemokines and chemokine receptors in epithelial cell layers of oral lichen planus. *J. Oral Pathol. Med.* **2006**, *35*, 167–174. [CrossRef]
58. Johnston, A.; Gudjonsson, J.E.; Aphale, A.; Guzman, A.M.; Stoll, S.W.; Elder, J.T. EGFR and IL-1 signaling synergistically promote keratinocyte antimicrobial defenses in a differentiation-dependent manner. *J. Investig. Dermatol.* **2011**, *131*, 329–337. [CrossRef]
59. Tohyama, M.; Hanakawa, Y.; Shirakata, Y.; Dai, X.; Yang, L.; Hirakawa, S.; Tokumaru, S.; Okazaki, H.; Sayama, K.; Hashimoto, K. IL-17 and IL-22 mediate IL-20 subfamily cytokine production in cultured keratinocytes via increased IL-22 receptor expression. *Eur. J. Immunol.* **2009**, *39*, 2779–2788. [CrossRef]
60. Sutter, C.H.; Yin, H.; Li, Y.; Mammen, J.S.; Bodreddigari, S.; Stevens, G.; Cole, J.A.; Sutter, T.R. EGF receptor signaling blocks aryl hydrocarbon receptor-mediated transcription and cell differentiation in human epidermal keratinocytes. *Proc. Natl. Acad. Sci. USA* **2009**, *106*, 4266–4271. [CrossRef]
61. Ulzii, D.; Kido-Nakahara, M.; Nakahara, T.; Tsuji, G.; Furue, K.; Hashimoto-Hachiya, A.; Furue, M. Scratching counteracts IL-13 signaling by upregulating the decoy receptor IL-13Rα2 in deratinocytes. *Int. J. Mol. Sci.* **2019**, *20*, 3324. [CrossRef] [PubMed]

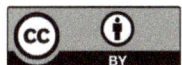

© 2020 by the authors. Licensee MDPI, Basel, Switzerland. This article is an open access article distributed under the terms and conditions of the Creative Commons Attribution (CC BY) license (http://creativecommons.org/licenses/by/4.0/).

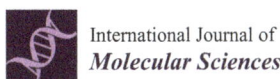

Review

Immunological Memory of Psoriatic Lesions

Agnieszka Owczarczyk-Saczonek [1,*], Magdalena Krajewska-Włodarczyk [2,3], Marta Kasprowicz-Furmańczyk [1] and Waldemar Placek [1]

1. Department of Dermatology, Sexually Transmitted Diseases and Clinical Immunology, The University of Warmia and Mazury, Al. Wojska Polskiego 30, 10-229 Olsztyn, Poland; martak03@wp.pl (M.K.-F.); w.placek@wp.pl (W.P.)
2. Department of Rheumatology, Municipal Hospital in Olsztyn, 10-229 Olsztyn, Poland; magdalenakw@op.pl
3. Department of Internal Medicine, School of Medicine, Collegium Medicum, University of Warmia and Mazury, 10-900 Olsztyn, Poland
* Correspondence: aganek@wp.pl; Tel.: +48-89-678-6670; Fax: +48-89-678-6675

Received: 16 December 2019; Accepted: 15 January 2020; Published: 17 January 2020

Abstract: The natural course of psoriasis is the appearance of new lesions in the place of previous ones, which disappeared after a successful therapy. Recent studies of psoriasis etiopathogenesis showed that after psoriatic plaques have disappeared, in healthy skin we can still find a trace of inflammation in the form of tissue resident memory cells (TRM). They are originally responsible for protection against viral and bacterial infections in non-lymphatic tissues. In psoriatic inflammation, they are characterized by heterogeneity depending on their origin. CD8+ T cells TRM are abundantly present in psoriatic epidermis, while CD4+ TRM preferentially populate the dermis. In psoriasis, epidermal CD8+ TRM cells express CLA, CCR6, CD103 and IL-23R antigen and produce IL-17A during ex vivo stimulation. However, CD4+ CD103+ TRM can also colonize the epidermis and produce IL-22 during stimulation. Besides T cells, Th22 and epidermal DCs proved that epidermal cells in healed skin were still present and functioning after several years of disease remission. It explains the clinical phenomenon of the tendency of psoriatic lesions to relapse in the same location and it allows to develop new therapeutic strategies in the future.

Keywords: psoriasis; tissue resident memory cells; IL-17

1. Introduction

The natural course of psoriasis is the long-term persistence of lesions in the same anatomical regions and the appearance of new ones in places where they have resolved after successful therapy. The appearance of new lesions in the place of previous ones, which disappeared after a successful therapy, evokes feelings of depression, hopelessness and depression in patients and induces conviction in the lack of effective therapies. Recent studies of psoriasis etiopathogenesis showed that after psoriatic plaques have disappeared, in healthy skin we can still find a trace of inflammation in the form of tissue resident memory cells (TRM). They are able to initiate an inflammatory cascade and cause a relapse in the same location. In psoriasis, even during remission, they become a source of important inflammatory cytokines IL-17A and IL-22 [1–4]. T cell-associated gene (*LCK* and *TRCB1*) and inflammatory gene (*IL17*, *IL22* and *IFN-γ*) activity remains increased in the skin after psoriasis lesions, at least three months after the onset of the treatment with TNF-α inhibitors [5,6]. However, not only TRMs are responsible for clinical relapses at the same location (Figure 1) (Table 1). This article is a review of current knowledge about the "immune memory" of psoriatic lesions.

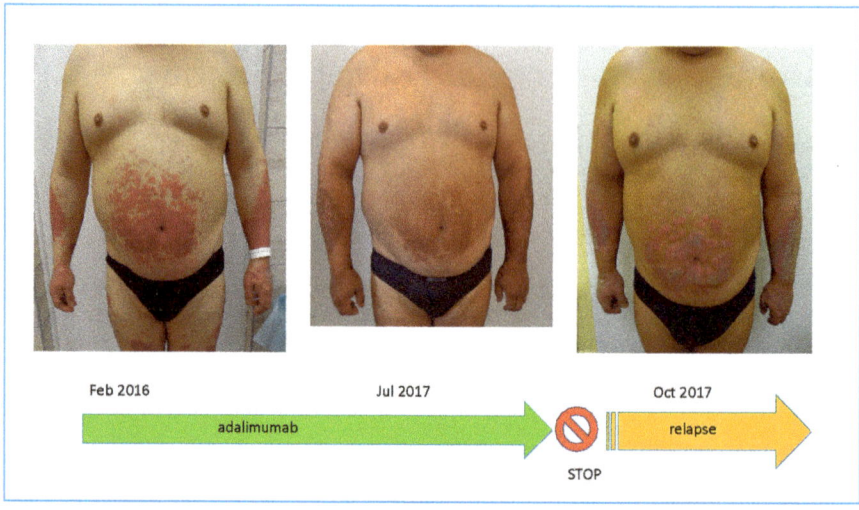

Figure 1. The relapse of psoriatic lesions in the same localization despite efficient treatment.

Table 1. The Cells Responsible for the "memory" of Psoriatic Lesions.

Type of Cells			Psoriasis Lesions	Resolved Psoriasis Skin
TRM	CD4+		A few in dermis CD103- and a low number in epidermis CD103+	A few
	CD8+		A lot of in epidermis CD103+: CD8+CD49a+ producing perforin, IFN-γ CD8+CD49a- producing IL-17 IL-22, IFN-γ, a few in dermis CD103- and a low number CD103+	A few in epidermis
Dendritic Cells	LC		In epidermis producing a lot of IL-23	In epidermis producing IL-23
	eDC		In epidermis producing of IL-1β, IL-23, TNFα	Absent

2. Tissue Resident Memory Cells (TRM)

TRM cells are transcriptionally, phenotypically and functionally different from traditional central memory cells (TCM) and effector memory T cells (TEM). They recirculate among blood, T cell zones of secondary lymphoid organs, lymph and non-lymphoid tissues, such as the skin, where they act as alarm sensors or cytotoxic killers. They are characterized by heterogeneity depending on their origin [5,7–11].

They are originally responsible for protection against viral and bacterial infections in non-lymphatic tissues. The protective activity of TRM has been confirmed in HSV infection, vaccinia pox, lymphocytic choriomeningitis virus (LCMV), influenza, listeriosis, malaria, as well as in some types of cancer. The vaccination task is, among others, the education of TRM to react very quickly against an infection [9]. TRM cells are locally found in many tissues providing a rapid in situ response to infectious agents more effectively than T cells of effector memory. They also secrete granzyme B, which helps to reduce the spread of pathogens at the site of infection. They can activate the innate and adaptive mechanisms of the immune response [2,10,12–15]. TRM acts as a bridge between the adaptive and innate immune systems. Because many viruses have tissue tropism, TRM also provides protective immune responses for tissue that it has previously encountered. Since, HSV-specific TRMs have been found in the skin, rotavirus-specific TRMs in the intestines and flu-specific TRMs in the lungs [16,17]. However, in addition to their protective functions, there is more and more evidence of their involvement in the pathogenesis of autoimmune disorders such as psoriasis, vitiligo, autoimmune hepatitis, rheumatoid arthritis and lymphomas [11].

The main surface markers of human TRM cells are CD49a, CD69 and CD103. The CD103 marker (integrin αE subunit) is only expressed on CD8+ TRM cells, not CD4+ TRM. Its expression is most prominent on epidermal CD4+ and CD8+ TRM cells because it enables TRM binding to E-cadherin, which is widely expressed by epithelial cells [8,13,18]. The CD69 marker plays a key role in distinguishing T cells in tissues from those in circulation and it is responsible for the colonization of these cells in tissues, preventing them from recirculating. CD69 binds and inhibits the expression of the cell surface of sphingosine-1-phosphate receptor (S1PR1). The transcription factor KLF2 promotes the expression of S1PR1, thereby CD69 and may allow recirculation of TRM in unusual situations [19]. S1PR1 reacts to the S1P ligand, which is released by endothelial cells in the blood and lymph, allowing TRM cells to leave the tissues for circulation. This situation is observed, among others, after exposure to an allergen resulting in formation of secondary TRM cells [19]. However, the latest findings indicate that the importance of CD69 for TRM residence may depend on the tissue in which they are located (essential for TRM in the kidneys, no relevance in the gut) [18]. However, expression levels may vary between T cells in different tissues. Another marker that can be used to differentiate two subsets of TRM cells is CD49a—the α-subunit of the α1β1 integrin receptor (also known as very late antigen VLA-1). It determines a subset of CD8+ TRM cells that are localized in the epidermis. These cells produce IFN-γ and acquire high cytotoxic capacity upon IL-15 stimulation [20]. CD8+ CD49a+ TRM cells produce perforin and IFN-γ, which is a key cytokine in fighting viral infections. CD8+ CD49-TRM cells produce IL-17 [20,21]. TRM also expresses the Program Cell Death Protein-1 (PD-1) and T-cell immunoglobulin mucin receptor 3 (TIM3), which are the surface proteins that suppress T cell activity. Their expression occurs in inflamed tissues. In such situations, TRMs have an anti-inflammatory effect, which indicates the ambiguous nature of these cells [22,23].

In healthy individuals, CD8$^+$CD103$^+$CD49a$^-$TRM cells were present in both dermis and epidermis, whereas CD8$^+$CD103$^+$CD49a$^+$TRM cells were localized in the epidermis. Epidermal CD8$^+$CD103$^+$CD49a$^-$TRM cells were predominant IL-17 producers, whereas CD8$^+$CD103$^+$CD49a$^+$TRM cells excelled at IFN-γ production and rapidly gained a cytotoxic capacity following IL-15 stimulation [21].

TRM cells develop from circulating effector T cell precursors in response to an antigen. CD103 plays a major role in their formation, and the expression of this integrin depends on the TGF-β cytokine. CD8+ T effector cells, which do not produce TGF-β, have no expression of CD103 and they do not differentiate into TRM cells. The homeostatic IL-15 cytokine, pro-inflammatory cytokines (IL-12 and IL-18) and barrier cytokines, such as IL-33, which support TRM cell formation and survival, play an important role in the development of TRM cells [7,8].

The second type of TRM are CD4+ cells, which are less-known ones, and are located near the vessels in the dermis; they do not express CD103 and have a high proliferative capacity. They are responsible for defense against *Leishmania* and *Candida albicans* in the gut, lungs and reproductive system [24].

3. Tissue Resident Memory Cells in Psoriasis

CD4+ T cells with the Th1 and Th17 phenotype have long been considered the main pathogenic subpopulations of T cells. LL37 (antimicrobial peptide derived from keratinocytes) and ADAMTSL5 (protein produced by melanocytes) in the pathogenesis of the disease has been more appreciated. The abovementioned proteins are considered as autoantigens in psoriasis. Similarly, CD4 T-cells recognize LL37 as an autoantigen and they correlate with PASI [25,26]. CD8+ T cells with resident memory tissue phenotype (TRM) are abundantly present in psoriatic epidermis, while CD4+ TRM preferentially populate the dermis. The differences in colonization result from the expression of CD69, which blocks the sphingosine-1-phosphate receptor (S1P1), a receptor normally allowing lymph entry. In addition, a significant proportion of skin TRM expresses CD103, the αEβ7 integrin chain, which interacts with E-cadherin expressed by keratinocytes (Figure 2). The signal required for their residence is TGF-β via TGF-βRII [9]. Hair follicles through IL-15 and IL-7 production are also important in their recruitment [27]. In addition to cytokines, lipids available in the skin are essential to maintain TRM [10,17]

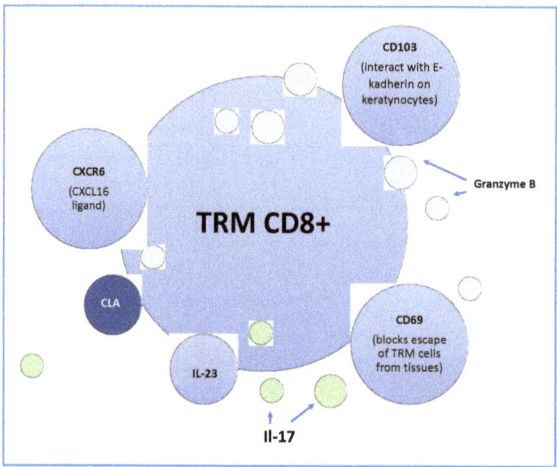

Figure 2. The receptors and secretory activity of tissue resident memory (TRM) CD8+ [5,22]

TRMs have been described in unchanged, healed skin in places of recurrent psoriasis, which indicates their role in the disease's local memory [28]. Recirculation of memory T cells between the skin and circulation is a newly recognized immunological mechanism that plays an important role in the initiation of psoriasiform response [3,29,30] (Figure 3). Their particular pathogenicity is determined by the fact that they have the ability to produce IL-17 and IL-22, pro-inflammatory, key cytokines involved in this process [23,29].

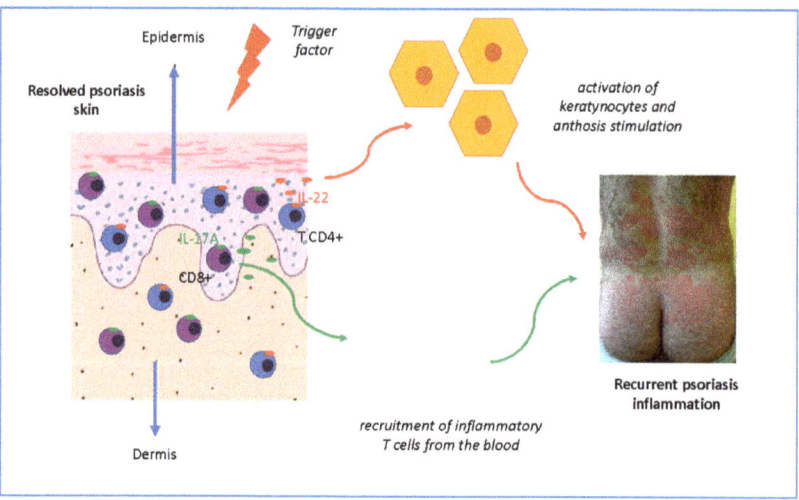

Figure 3. The role of TRM in psoriatic inflammation.

The first study that highlighted the role of resident skin T cells in psoriasis was the experiment of Boyman et al. [31]. They implanted unchanged human psoriatic skin to immunodeficient mice (AGR129 mice, deficient in type I and II interferon receptors and the recombination activating gene 2). The reproduction of resident human T cells and the formation of psoriatic lesions were observed within eight weeks. They showed the CD8+ phenotype with TNF-α susceptibility and were located mainly in the epidermis and the dermal–epidermal junction [31].

Diani et al. [1] analyzed the phenotype of circulating T cells in patients with psoriasis with the assessment of gene expression in psoriatic skin. It was found that circulating CCR6+ CD4+ TEM (effector memory cells) and T effector cells significantly correlated with the severity of skin lesions and inflammation (CRP) while the percentage of CXCR3+ CD4+ TEM cells correlated negatively. In addition, CLA+ CD4+ TCM cells expressing CCR6+ or CCR4+ CXCR3+ negatively correlated with the severity of psoriasis. CLA expression is associated with the recruitment of CD4+ T cells into the skin, mainly when expressed on TCM cells, in particular on CD4+ TCM with the CCR4+ and CCR6+ phenotype [1,26]. In an earlier study, Bose et al. [32] proved that inhibition of the CCR7/CCL19 axis was critical for remission of psoriasis induced by TNF inhibitors [3]. In psoriasis, circulating CCR4 + CD4+ T cells significantly correlate with disease severity (PASI), and a strong negative correlation has been found for CCR5+ CD4+ T cells [32]. A subset of T effector CCR4+ CD8+ CD103+ cells also positively correlates with both systemic inflammation (CRP) and the severity of skin lesions [4,33]. It was also found that the fraction of IL-17 secreting CD4+ T-lymphocytes and probably γδ T-lymphocytes may play a role in the formation of a self-sustaining inflammatory loop [1].

Lymphocytes CD4+ Th producing pro-inflammatory cytokines, such as IL-17A, IL-22 and IFN-γ, are considered to be the main pathogenic T cell subpopulation, whereas CD8+, present in healthy skin as memory T cells, have a similar pro-inflammatory cytokine profile. They are in large quantities in the psoriatic epidermis and can recognize peptide antigens presented on MHC class I molecules like HLA-Cw6 [29]. Blockade of β1-integrin hinders entry of T cells into the epidermis, which prevents the development of disease eruptions on the murine AGR model of psoriasis [34]. Di Meglio et al. [29] showed that the accumulation of epidermal CD8+ cells induces both hyperproliferation of keratinocytes and papillomatosis (increase in CD8 + a parallel to the intensity of Ki67 staining in keratinocytes) [29]. CD8+ T cells isolated from psoriasis patients produce psoriasis-related cytokines. After treatment they remain in the skin as TRM and LL-37-specific CD8 + T cells, expressing integrin α1β1 [29].

In the study of Kurihara et al. [13], biopsies from psoriatic lesions were examined. The number of CD8+CD103+ TRM cells in the epidermis correlated with the thickness of the epidermis ($p = 0.016$), suggesting their role in the formation of psoriatic lesions [13]. They were mostly CD8+ CD69+ T cells, expressing skin colonization antigens, and the count of CD4+ CD103+ TRM was low. Some CD8+ CD103+ T cells produced IFN-γ, IL-17A or IL-22. In addition, CD8+ CD103+ TRM cells more frequently produced IL-17A than CD8+ CD103- and effector cells CD8+ CD103 or CD4+ CD103+. Interestingly, the number of CD8+ CD103+ IL-17A + TRM cells in patients treated with biological or systemic therapy was higher [13]. In contrast, in the dermis of the psoriatic plaques, TRM cells show lower expression of CD103, as demonstrated by Cheuk et al. [5]. In the first stage of psoriatic inflammation, in the skin without lesions yet, epidermal TRM cells expressing CCR6 cooperate with CCL20 expressing keratinocytes [35,36].

In turn, Vo et al. [36] evaluated the phenotypic features of TRM in non-lesional, lesional psoriasis and healthy skin. Immunofluorescence study showed that CD103+ CD8 TRM, both in non-lesional and lesional were dominant in the epidermis compared to the skin of healthy volunteers. In addition, IL-17A production was higher in patients with longer disease duration [36].

The optimal treatment time needed to completely silence TRM, which could ensure that there is no recurrence of lesions at the location is unknown [37]. Therefore, psoriatic lesions preferentially recur in previously affected areas of the skin, and pathogenic TRM cells exposed to IL-17A and IL-22 accumulate in resolved lesions [5,35]. In the study of Gallais Serezal et al. [38], tissue responses after T cell stimulation in healthy and psoriatic lesions were analyzed. An increase in the number of epidermal IL-17 and IL-22—producing skin-resident T CCR6 + cells—may be a genetically predisposed reaction to microbial stimulation in never-lesional skin in patients with psoriasis. The consequence is an increase in IFN-g production and stimulation of keratinocytes that release INF-a, which stimulates psoriatic inflammation.

At the same time psoriasis plaques showed IL-17-induced response patterns, indicating a relapse. The proportional amount of induced IFN-γ, IL-10e and IL-17A correlated with relapse time in patients after discontinuation of the treatment [38].

For the complete remission of the disease, full TRM suppression is required. Unfortunately, TRM cells are long-lived, and resistant to damaging factors and apoptosis. This explains the frequent relapses at the same location for psoriasis. Even after the clinical lesions have resolved, they are capable of producing IL-17A, and effective therapy only suppresses their activity [3,37]. Furthermore, CD8+ TRM cells accumulate in untreated psoriasis localizations, probably in correlation with disease duration [4,11]. An interesting issue is the explanation of the longevity of memory cells. One of the reasons is its resistance to apoptosis. The heterodimeric marker molecule CD8+ (αEβ7) consists of CD103 and β7 subunits and plays a key role in the stability of CD8+ TRM cells by increasing the level of the Bcl-2 molecule with anti-apoptotic activity [8,13]. In contrast, TRM can produce granzyme B (serine protease), which can induce cellular apoptosis [23]. Moreover, IL-15 probably plays an important role in TRM cell survival [24].

What is surprising, the effector T cells use glycolysis energy, which is less efficient in generating ATP, but faster. TCM, on the other hand, use endogenously synthesized fatty acids, glucose catabolism and oxidative phosphorylation to support their long-term survival and function [17,39]. TCMs use extracellular glucose from the blood to synthesize fatty acids in the endoplasmic reticulum, using lysosomal acid lipase, which is important in the hydrolysis of cholesteryl esters and triglycerides in LDL molecules to cholesterol and free fatty acids (FFA). Thanks to such mechanisms, they can be long-lived and able to react quickly to antigen [17]. Cui et al. additionally showed that IL-7, a cytokine critical for TCM differentiation and survival, induced glycerol transport and triacylglycerol synthesis via enhanced gene expression of glycerol channel aquaporin 9, thus providing substrates for mitochondria via fatty acid oxidation (FAO) [17,40].

Unfortunately, there is currently no detailed data on the metabolic properties of TRM. However, it is known that CD8+ TRM develop a transcriptional program with overexpression of FABP4 (adipocyte-FABP), FABP5 (epidermal-FABP), CD36 (a lipid scavenger receptor) and lipoprotein lipase (cleaves triglycerides to yield FFA and diacylglycerol). Such activity of genes responsible for the activity of these molecules is not found in naive T cells, TCM or effector memory cells [17].

The study by Pan et al. [17] showed that mouse CD8 + TRM cells generated by skin viral infection show different expression level of genes of proteins mediating the intracellular uptake and transport of lipids, including fatty acid-binding protein—FABP4 (adipocyte-FABP) and FABP5 (epidermal-FABP). These are molecules facilitating exogenous FFAs acquisition and metabolism [17]. CD8 + TRM upregulated the gene expression of FABP4/FABP5 in a peroxisome proliferator-activated receptor gamma (PPAR-γ)—dependent manner [17,41]. T-specific deficiency of these molecules has been shown to impair the uptake of exogenous FFA by CD8+ TRM cells, which significantly reduces their long-term survival in vivo, but does not affect the survival of TCM in lymph nodes. In addition, CD8+ TRM skin cells lacking FABP4/FABP5 were less effective in protecting mice against cutaneous viral infection [41]. It is interesting whether in patients with psoriasis the described situation will be similar to the one in healthy individuals. No studies have been published on this subject yet.

In vitro, CD8+ TRM cells showed increased oxidative metabolism of mitochondria in the presence of exogenous FFA in normal and psoriatic skin. These results suggest that FABP4 and FABP5 play a key role in the maintenance, longevity and function of CD8+ TRM cells, and suggest that CD8+ TRM cells use exogenous FFA and their oxidative metabolism to survive in tissue. It has been shown that the lack of FABP4 and FABP5 does not affect CD8+ T cell proliferation or skin recruitment, but they are necessary for their long-term survival in the skin [41]. Perhaps the blockade of PPAR-γ functions will allow the development of strategies for the treatment of psoriatic lesions.

Oxidative stress plays an important role in psoriatic inflammation. In the study of Esmaeili et al. [42], the redox status of TRM CD4+ and its correlation with IL-17 response were assessed. The increased intracellular ROS production in memory CD4+ T cells in psoriasis patients decreased catalase gene expression compared to healthy ones, but no differences in intracellular glutathione levels and plasma total antioxidant capacity were revealed. However, the above disorders did not affect the IL-17 response in memory T cells [42].

4. Tissue Resident Memory Cells in Psoriatic Arthritis (PsA)

Recently, data has shown that TRM cells are responsible for the development of synovitis in PsA. However, they were not observed in rheumatoid arthritis [23].

The latest study on psoriatic arthritis (PsA) and other spondyloarthritides (SpA) assessed the molecular profile, phenotype and function of synovial Tc17 cells (IL-17A + CD8 + T cells) to clarify their role in pathogenesis. It turned out that, as in psoriasis, they were mainly TCRαβ +, and their number was increased in synovial fluid vs. peripheral blood in patients with PsA or other SpA. In addition, synovial TA17 PsA cells had the characteristics of Th17 (RORC/IL23R/CCR6/CD161) and Tc1 cells (A/B granzyme). The synovial marker Tc17 was CXCR6, and elevated levels of CXCR6 CXCL16 ligand in PsA were found in synovial fluid, which could contribute to their retention in the joints [43]. However, there are many doubts if TRMs are responsible for the initiation of inflammation and whether it is the same phenotype that persists after the treatment [23].

A new theory has emerged that TRMs involved in synovitis migrate from the skin and gut. Although TRMs do not circulate in the blood, they can sometimes be activated so that they travel within the lymphatic system [23,44,45]. A study by Guggino et al. [45], assessing TRM cells in peripheral blood, gut and synovium in patients with SpA, showed that the expression of α4β7 may support the recirculation of these cells from the gut and peripheral blood to foci of inflammation in the joints. Although this study applies to the entire group of patients with ankylosing spondylitis, probably patients with PSA were also included. Unfortunately, PSA patients were not analyzed separately and there is no research on these patients.

5. The Role of Memory γδ T Cells

Matos et al. found that TRM in psoriasis patients had specific properties that TRM did not have in healthy skin. These pathogenic clones preferentially had Vβ and Vα in the TCR region. Researchers identified 15 TCRβ and 4 TCRα antigen receptor sequences in patients with psoriasis that were not seen in the skin of healthy patients or atopic dermatitis patients. In addition, they observed a reduced amount of γδ T cells in psoriasis compared to αβ T cells. It has been proven that IL-17- and IL-22-producing T-cell clones with IL-17- and IL-22-specific antigen receptors still exist in the skin after the active psoriatic lesions have resolved. Therefore, for full disease remission, suppression of these resident T lymphocyte populations is required [3].

However, in psoriasis a reduced amount of γδ T cells was observed compared to αβ T cells [3]. In contrast, γδ T lymphocytes, considered innate immune cells that can also give rise to TRM populations, are far less known. Recently it has been shown in a mouse model that they can produce IL-17A and IL-17F in the skin in response to imiquimod. Each subsequent test with imiquimod resulted in an ever stronger proliferation of γδ T cells compared to the skin of mice after the first provocation [46].

6. Th22 and Tc17 Lymphocytes

In active psoriasis, we observe increased expression of IL17A, IL22 and IFN-γ in the effector T CD4+ and CD8+ cells of the epidermis in the immediate vicinity of keratinocytes, whereas cutaneous T cells show less activity of these genes. Cheuk et al. [5] proved that Th22 epidermal cells in healed skin were still present and functioning after several years of disease remission. After their stimulation, an increase in local IL-22, IL-17A and IFN-γ production by CD4+ T cells was observed. The percentage of IL-22-producing CD4+ epidermal cells did not correlate with the number of years of treatment, which indicates a preserved effector function even after 6 years of the treatment [5]. It has been shown that CD4+ epidermal T cells produced mainly IL-22, which activates keratinocytes leading to acanthosis. In contrast, epidermal CD8+ T cells mainly produced IL-17A, which drives the production of pro-inflammatory cytokines and chemokines by keratinocytes and is involved in the recruitment of neutrophils [5].

Studies have also shown that there are T-cells producing both IL-22 and IL-17 in the epidermis, which are present in lesions and healed skin in patients receiving nb-UVB therapy, and are practically absent in patients treated with biological drugs. Perhaps this type of T cell is more pathogenic [5]. It is known that effective nb-UVB therapy induces T cell apoptosis in the skin, but highly active effector lymphocytes can be constantly recruited from circulation [5].

Of note, active effector T cells involved in the inflammatory process may develop into long-lived epidermal TRM cells as the disease subsides [5,7,8].

7. Epidermal Langerhans Cells (LCs)

Psoriatic lesions' "memory" may also be affected by Langerhans cells dysfunction. In normal skin, epidermal Langerhans cells (eLC) are located in the epidermis and separated from dendritic skin cells (DC) by the basal membrane. Compared with cutaneous DC, LCs express fewer Toll-like receptors (TLRs), indicating an impaired ability to respond to TLR signaling, probably to maintain a state of tolerance to commensal [47]. In active psoriasis, under the influence of IL-23 and IL-17, inflammatory DCs penetrate both to the epidermis and dermis. In inflammatory DC epidermal expression of CCR2+ (eDC) occurs only in psoriasis and is phenotypically different from normal DCs'. Their number is higher than eLC and they show high expression of genes involved in the recruitment of neutrophils, keratinocytes and T lymphocytes. On the other hand, colonization of epidermis by eLC, under the influence of TLR-4 and TLR-7/8 activation, produce large amounts of IL-23, and eDCs secrete IL-1β together with IL-23 and TNF-α. After the psoriasis eruption, eDCs are absent in unchanged skin, while eLC retain high IL-23A expression and continue to respond to TLR stimulation, producing IL-23 [47,48]. Although eDCs are 3–10 times more numerous than eLC and drive the psoriatic condition, they also have the ability to produce anti-inflammatory IL-10 [48].

In individuals with early type of psoriasis (under 40 years of age) LCs do not show the ability to migrate under the influence of stimuli (chemical allergens, IL-1b and TNF-α). It is probably a phenomenon caused by the influence of the psoriatic environment rather than their defect [49,50]. Their ability to migrate is restored under the influence of treatment (among others anti-TNF, anti-IL-12/23, fumaric acid esters and UVB), except for therapies directed mainly towards T cells (ciclosporin A, MTX) [50–52]. Therefore, the observed rapid relapses after discontinuation of ciclosporin A may be explained by the role of LC in the rapid initiation of the inflammation in the same location (effect on TRM expressing IL-23R), which thus affects the memory of psoriatic eruptions [48].

8. Clinical Significance of the Memory of Psoriasis Lesions

Psoriatic lesions are characterized by the presence of massive inflammatory infiltrates (lymphocytes, neutrophils), proliferation and disturbance of epidermal differentiation (parakeratosis) as well as the formation of new blood vessels. Despite being such large structures, their resolution leaves no scars. This is quite unusual, especially comparing to other conditions in which neutrophils (pyoderma gangrenosum) are involved, where scars are present [12]. However, after discontinuation of treatment, a rapid recurrence of lesions is usually observed (90% in the same location) [24]. The understanding of the psoriasis context and the role of TRM can explain the key issues associated with this disease:

- the role in resistance to treatment and reactivation of changes in the same location [24];
- the role in the Koebner isomorphic symptom [24];

- the decision about adequate treatment time to limit lesions relapse and withdraw and reduce the amount of TRM.

The clinical characteristics of recurrence of psoriatic lesions mirrors the biology of TRMs. Since TRM does not work, inflammatory lesions induced by TRM are usually well demarcated with clear margins. The relapse of lesions can be fast because they occur in TRM skin and cooperate with local dendritic cells [12,52]. In understanding the abovementioned mechanisms, one stands a chance to provide more effective treatment and thus long-lasting remissions in psoriasis patients.

9. Conclusions

The discovery of TRM cells in psoriasis allows a better understanding of the complicated relationships between mediators and cells of the innate and adaptive immune system, keratinocytes and endothelial cells. It explains the clinical phenomenon of the tendency of psoriatic lesions to relapse in the same location and it allows to develop new therapeutic strategies in the future.

Author Contributions: A.O.-S. and W.P. conceived and designed manuscript; A.O.-S., M.K.-W., M.K.-F. analyzed the data; A.O.-S., M.K.-W., M.K.-F. contributed materials; A.O.-S. wrote the paper. All authors have read and agreed to the published version of the manuscript.

Funding: This research received no external funding.

Conflicts of Interest: The authors declare no conflict of interest.

References

1. Diani, M.; Altomare, G.; Reali, E. T helper cell subsets in clinical manifestations of psoriasis. *J. Immunol. Res.* **2016**, *2016*, 1–7. [CrossRef]
2. Eberle, F.C.; Brück, J.; Holstein, J.; Hirahara, K.; Ghoreshi, K. Recent advances in understanding psoriasis. *F1000 Res.* **2016**, *5*, 770. [CrossRef]
3. Matos, T.; O'Malley, J.T.; Lowry, E.L.; Hamm, D.; Kirsch, I.R.; Robins, H.S.; Kupper, T.S.; Krueger, J.G.; Clark, R.A. Clinically resolved psoriatic lesions contain psoriasis-specific IL-17–producing αβ T cell clones. *J. Clin. Invest.* **2017**, *127*, 4031–4041. [CrossRef]
4. Watanabe, R. Protective and pathogenic roles of resident memory T cells in human skin disorders. *J. Dermatol. Sci.* **2019**, *95*, 2–7. [CrossRef]
5. Cheuk, S.; Wikén, M.; Blomqvist, L.; Nylén, S.; Talme, T.; Ståhle, M.; Eidsmo, L. Epidermal Th22 and Tc17 cells form a localized disease memory in clinically healed psoriasis. *J. Immunol.* **2014**, *192*, 3111–3120. [CrossRef]
6. Suarez-Farinas, M.; Fuentes-Duculan, J.; Lowes, M.A.; Krueger, J.G. Resolved psoriasis lesions retain expression of a subset of disease-related genes. *J. Investig. Dermatol.* **2011**, *131*, 391–400. [CrossRef]
7. Casey, K.A.; Fraser, K.A.; Schenkelm, J.M.; Moran, A.; Abt, M.C.; Beura, L.K.; Lucas, P.J.; Artis, D.; Wherry, E.J.; Hogquist, K.; et al. Antigen-independent differentiation and maintenance of effector-like resident memory T cells in tissues. *J. Immunol.* **2012**, *188*, 4866–4875. [CrossRef]
8. Mackay, L.K.; Rahimpour, A.; Ma, J.Z.; Collins, N.; Stock, A.T.; Hafon, M.L.; Vega-Ramos, J.; Lauzurica, P.; Mueller, S.N.; Stefanovic, T.; et al. The developmental pathway for CD103(+)CD8+ tissue-resident memory T cells of skin. *Nat. Immunol.* **2013**, *14*, 1294–1301. [CrossRef]
9. Milner, J.J.; Goldrath, A.W. Transcriptional programming of tissue-resident memory CD8$^+$ T cells. *Curr. Opin. Immunol.* **2018**, *51*, 162–169. [CrossRef]
10. Patra, V.; Laoubi, L.; Nicolas, J.F.; Vocanson, M.; Wolf, P. A perspective on the interplay of ultraviolet-radiation, skin microbiome and skin resident memory TCRαβ+ cells. *Front. Med. (Lausanne)* **2018**, *5*, 166. [CrossRef]
11. Wu, H.; Liao, W.; Li, Q.; Long, H.; Yin, H.; Zhao, M.; Chan, V.; Lau, C.S.; Lu, Q. Pathogenic role of tissue-resident memory T cells in autoimmune diseases. *Autoimmun. Rev.* **2018**, *17*, 906–911. [CrossRef]
12. Clark, R.A. Resident memory T cells in human health and diseases. *Sci. Transl. Med.* **2015**, *7*, 269rv1. [CrossRef]
13. Kurihara, K.; Fujiyama, T.; Phadungsaksawasdi, P.; Ito, T.; Tokura, Y. Significance of IL-17A-producing CD8$^+$CD103$^+$ skin resident memory T cells in psoriasis lesion and their possible relationship to clinical course. *J. Dermatol. Sci.* **2019**, *95*, 21–27. [CrossRef]

14. Rosato, P.C.; Beura, L.K.; Masopust, D. Tissue resident memory T cells and viral immunity. *Curr. Opin. Virol.* **2017**, *22*, 44–50. [CrossRef]
15. Shin, H.; Iwasaki, A. Tissue-resident memory T cells. *Immunol. Rev.* **2013**, *255*, 165–181. [CrossRef]
16. Khan, A.A.; Srivastava, R.; Chentoufi, A.A.; Kritzer, E.; Chilukuri, S.; Garg, S.; Yu, D.C; Vahed, H.; Huang, L.; Syed, S.A.; et al. Bolstering the number and function of HSV-1-specific CD8(+) effector memory T cells and tissue-resident memory T cells in latently infected trigeminal ganglia reduces recurrent ocular herpes infection and disease. *J. Immunol.* **2017**, *199*, 186–203. [CrossRef]
17. Pan, Y.; Kupper, T.S. Metabolic reprogramming and longevity of tissue-resident memory T cells. *Front. Immunol.* **2018**, *9*, 1347. [CrossRef]
18. Walsh, D.A.; Borges da Silva, H.; Beura, L.K.; Peng, C.; Hamilton, S.E.; Masopust, D.; Jameson, S.C. The functional requirement for CD69 in establishment of resident memory $CD8^+$ T cells varies with tissue location. *J. Immunol.* **2019**, *203*, 946–955. [CrossRef]
19. Behr, F.M.; Chuwonpad, A.; Stark, R.; van Gisbergen, K. Armed and ready: Transcriptional regulation of Tissue-Resident Memory CD8 T cells. *Front. Immunol.* **2018**, *9*, 1770. [CrossRef]
20. Schenkel, J.M.; Masopust, D. Tissue-resident memory T cells. *Immunity* **2014**, *41*, 886–897. [CrossRef]
21. Cheuk, S.; Schlums, H.; Gallais Sérézal, I.; Martini, E.; Chiang, S.C.; Marquardt, N.; Gibbs, A.; Detlofsson, E.; Introini, A.; Forkel, M.; et al. CD49a expression defines tissue-resident $CD8^+$ T cells poised for cytotoxic function in human skin. *Immunity* **2017**, *46*, 287–300. [CrossRef] [PubMed]
22. Petrelli, A.; van Wijk, F. CD8(+) T cells in human autoimmune arthritis: The unusual suspects. *Nat. Rev. Rheumatol.* **2016**, *12*, 421–428. [CrossRef] [PubMed]
23. Ritchlin, C. Tissue-resident T cells: Sequestered immune sensors and effectors of inflammation in spondyloarthritis. *Arthritis Rheumatol.* **2019**, *17*. [CrossRef]
24. Chen, L.; Shen, Z. Tissue-resident memory T cells and their biological characteristics in the recurrence of inflammatory skin disorders. *Cell. Mol. Immunol.* **2019**, *8*. [CrossRef]
25. Lande, R.; Botti, E.; Jandus, C.; Dojcinovic, D.; Fanelli, G.; Conrad, C.; Chamilos, G.; Feldmeyer, L.; Marinari, B.; Chon, S.; et al. The antimicrobial peptide LL37 is a T-cell autoantigen in psoriasis. *Nat. Commun.* **2014**, *5*, 5621. [CrossRef]
26. Arakawa, A.; Siewert, K.; Stöhr, J.; Besgen, P.; Kim, S.M.; Rühl, G.; Nickel, J.; Vollmer, S.; Thomas, P.; Krebs, S.; et al. Melanocyte antigen triggers autoimmunity in human psoriasis. *J. Exp. Med.* **2015**, *212*, 2203–2212. [CrossRef]
27. Adachi, T.; Kobayashi, T.; Sugihara, E.; Yamada, T.; Ikuta, K.; Pittaluga, S.; Saya, H.; Amagai, M.; Nagao, K. Hair follicle-derived IL-7 and IL-15 mediate skin-resident memory T cell homeostasis and lymphoma. *Nat. Med.* **2015**, *21*, 1272–1279. [CrossRef]
28. Diani, M.; Galasso, M.; Cozzi, C.; Sgambelluri, F.; Altomare, A.; Cigni, C.; Frigerio, E.; Drago, L.; Volinia, S.; Granucci, F.; et al. Blood to skin recirculation of CD4+ memory T cells associates with cutaneous and systemic manifestations of psoriatic disease. *Clin. Immunol.* **2017**, *180*, 84–94. [CrossRef]
29. Di Meglio, P.; Villanova, F.; Navarini, A.A.; Mylonas, A.; Tosi, I.; Nestle, F.O.; Conrad, C. Targeting CD8(+) T cells prevents psoriasis development. *J. Allergy Clin. Immunol.* **2016**, *138*, 274–276. [CrossRef]
30. Farber, D.L.; Yudanin, N.A.; Restifo, N.P. Human memory T cells: Generation, compartmentalization and homeostasis. *Nat. Rev. Immunol.* **2014**, *14*, 24–35. [CrossRef]
31. Boyman, O.; Hefti, H.P.; Conrad, C.; Nickoloff, B.J.; Suter, M.; Nestle, F.O. Spontaneous development of psoriasis in a new animal model shows an essential role for resident T cells and tumor necrosis factor-alpha. *J. Exp. Med.* **2004**, *199*, 731–736. [CrossRef] [PubMed]
32. Bosè, F.; Petti, L.; Diani, M.; Moscheni, C.; Molteni, S.; Altomare, A.; Rossi, R.L.; Talarico, D.; Fontana, R.; Russo, V.; et al. Inhibition of CCR7/CCL19 axis in lesional skin is a critical event for clinical remission induced by TNF blockade in patients with psoriasis. *Am. J. Pathol.* **2013**, *183*, 413–421. [CrossRef] [PubMed]
33. Sgambelluri, F.; Diani, M.; Altomare, A.; Frigerio, E.; Drago, L.; Granucci, F.; Banfi, G.; Altomare, G.; Reali, E. A role for CCR5(+)CD4 T cells in cutaneous psoriasis and for CD103(+) CCR4(+) CD8 Teff cells in the associated systemic inflammation. *J. Autoimmun.* **2016**, *70*, 80–90. [CrossRef] [PubMed]
34. Conrad, C.; Boyman, O.; Tonel, G.; Tun-Kyi, A.; Laggner, U.; de Fougerolles, A.; Kotelianski, V.; Gardner, H.; Nestle, F.O. Alpha1beta1 integrin is crucial for accumulation of epidermal T cells and the development of psoriasis. *Nat. Med.* **2007**, *13*, 836–842. [CrossRef] [PubMed]

35. Gallais Sérézal, I.; Classon, C.; Cheuk, S.; Barrientos-Somarribas, M.; Wadman, E.; Martini, E.; Chang, D.; Xu Landén, N.; Ehrström, M.; Nylén, S.; et al. Resident T cells in resolved psoriasis steer tissue responses that stratify clinical outcome. *J. Invest. Dermatol.* **2018**, *138*, 1754–1763. [CrossRef] [PubMed]
36. Vo, S.; Watanabe, R.; Koguchi-Yoshioka, H.; Matsumura, Y.; Ishitsuka, Y.; Nakamura, Y.; Okiyama, N.; Fujisawa, Y.; Fujimoto, M. CD8 resident memory T cells with interleukin 17A producing potential are accumulated in disease-naïve nonlesional sites of psoriasis possibly in correlation with disease duration. *Br. J. Dermatol.* **2019**, *181*, 410–412. [CrossRef]
37. Campbell, J.J.; Clark, R.A.; Watanabe, R.; Kupper, T.S. Sezary syndrome and mycosis fungoides arise from distinct T-cell subsets: A biologic rationale for their distinct clinical behaviors. *Blood* **2010**, *116*, 767–771. [CrossRef]
38. Gallais Sérézal, I.; Hoffer, E.; Ignatov, B.; Martini, E.; Zitti, B.; Ehrström, M.; Eidsmo, L. A skewed pool of resident T cells triggers psoriasis-associated tissue responses in never-lesional skin from patients with psoriasis. *J. Allergy Clin. Immunol.* **2019**, *143*, 1444–1454. [CrossRef]
39. Pearce, E.L.; Walsh, M.C.; Cejas, P.J.; Harms, G.M.; Shen, H.; Wang, L.S.; Jones, R.G.; Choi, Y. Enhancing CD8 T-cell memory by modulating fatty acid metabolism. *Nature* **2009**, *460*, 103–107. [CrossRef]
40. Cui, G.; Staron, M.M.; Gray, S.M.; Ho, P.C.; Amezquita, R.A.; Wu, J.; Kaech, S.M. IL-7-induced glycerol transport and TAG synthesis promotes memory CD8+ T cell longevity. *Cell* **2015**, *161*, 750–761. [CrossRef]
41. Pan, Y.; Tian, T.; Park, C.O.; Lofftus, S.Y.; Mei, S.; Liu, X.; Luo, C.; O'Malley, J.T.; Gehad, A.; Teague, J.E.; et al. Survival of tissue-resident memory T cells requires exogenous lipid uptake and metabolism. *Nature* **2017**, *9*, 252–256. [CrossRef] [PubMed]
42. Esmaeili, B.; Mansouri, P.; Doustimotlagh, A.H.; Izad, M. Redox imbalance and IL-17 responses in memory CD4+ T cells from patients with psoriasis. *Scand. J. Immunol.* **2019**, *89*, e12730. [CrossRef] [PubMed]
43. Steel, K.J.A.; Srenathan, U.; Ridley, M.; Durham, L.E.; Wu, S.Y.; Ryan, S.E.; Hughes, C.D.; Chan, E.; Kirkham, B.W.; Taams, L.S. Synovial IL-17A+ CD8+ T cells display a polyfunctional, pro-inflammatory and tissue-resident memory phenotype and function in psoriatic arthritis. *Arthritis Rheumatol.* **2019**, *2*. [CrossRef] [PubMed]
44. Beura, L.K.; Wijeyesinghe, S.; Thompson, E.A.; Macchietto, M.G.; Rosato, P.C.; Pierson, M.J.; Schenkel, J.M.; Mitchell, J.S.; Vezys, V.; Fife, B.T.; et al. T cells in nonlymphoid tissues give rise to lymph-node-resident memory T Cells. *Immunity* **2018**, *48*, 327–338e5. [CrossRef] [PubMed]
45. Guggino, G.; Rizzo, A.; Mauro, D.; Macaluso, F.; Ciccia, F. Gut-derived CD8+ tissue-resident memory T cells are expanded in the peripheral blood and synovia of SpA patients. *Ann. Rheum. Dis.* **2019**, *18*. [CrossRef]
46. Lalor, S.J.; McLoughlin, R.M. Memory γδ T cells-newly appreciated protagonists in infection and immunity. *Trends Immunol.* **2016**, *37*, 690–702. [CrossRef] [PubMed]
47. Eidsmo, L.; Martini, E. Human langerhans cells with pro-inflammatory features relocate within psoriasis lesions. *Front. Immunol.* **2018**, *22*, 300. [CrossRef]
48. Martini, E.; Wikén, M.; Cheuk, S.; Gallais Sérézal, I.; Baharom, F.; Ståhle, M.; Smed Sörensen, A.; Eidsmo, L. Dynamic changes in resident and infiltrating epidermal dendritic cells in active and resolved psoriasis. *J. Invest. Dermatol.* **2017**, *137*, 865–873. [CrossRef]
49. Cumberbatch, M.; Singh, M.; Dearman, R.J.; Young, H.S.; Kimber, I.; Griffiths, C.E. Impaired Langerhans cell migration in psoriasis. *J. Exp. Med.* **2006**, *203*, 953–960. [CrossRef]
50. Shaw, F.L.; Mellody, K.T.; Ogden, S.; Dearman, R.J.; Kimber, I.; Griffiths, C. Treatment-related restoration of Langerhans cell migration in psoriasis. *J. Investig. Dermatol.* **2014**, *134*, 268–271. [CrossRef]
51. Mohammed, J.; Beura, L.K.; Bobr, A.; Astry, B.; Chicoine, B.; Kashem, S.W.; Welty, N.E.; Igyártó, B.Z.; Wijeyesinghe, S.; Thompson, E.A.; et al. Stromal cells control the epithelial residence of DCs and memory T cells by regulated activation of TGF-beta. *Nat. Immunol.* **2016**, *17*, 414–421. [CrossRef] [PubMed]
52. Clark, R.A. Gone but not forgotten: Lesional memory in psoriatic skin. *J. Invest. Dermatol.* **2011**, *131*, 283–285. [CrossRef] [PubMed]

 © 2020 by the authors. Licensee MDPI, Basel, Switzerland. This article is an open access article distributed under the terms and conditions of the Creative Commons Attribution (CC BY) license (http://creativecommons.org/licenses/by/4.0/).

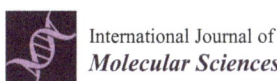

Review

The Roles of Lipoprotein in Psoriasis

Chun-Ming Shih [1,2,3,†], Chang-Cyuan Chen [4,†], Chen-Kuo Chu [5,†], Kuo-Hsien Wang [6], Chun-Yao Huang [1,2,3] and Ai-Wei Lee [2,3,4,*]

1. Department of Internal Medicine, School of Medicine, College of Medicine, Taipei Medical University, Taipei 11031, Taiwan; cmshih53@tmu.edu.tw (C.-M.S.); cyhuang@tmu.edu.tw (C.-Y.H.)
2. Cardiovascular Research Center, Taipei Medical University Hospital, Taipei 11031, Taiwan
3. Taipei Heart Institute, Taipei Medical University, Taipei 11031, Taiwan
4. Department of Anatomy and Cell Biology, School of Medicine, College of Medicine, Taipei Medical University, Taipei 11031, Taiwan; chance03070307@gmail.com
5. Department of Emergency Medicine, Taichung Veterans General Hospital, Taichung 40705, Taiwan; drckchu@gmail.com
6. Department of Dermatology, Taipei Medical University Hospital, Taipei 11031, Taiwan; khwang40@gmail.com
* Correspondence: ammielee@tmu.edu.tw; Tel.: +(886-2)-2736-1661 (ext. 3255)
† These authors contributed equally to this work.

Received: 30 November 2019; Accepted: 26 January 2020; Published: 29 January 2020

Abstract: The association between psoriasis and cardiovascular disease risk has been supported by recent epidemiological data. Patients with psoriasis have an increased adjusted relative risk for myocardial infarction. As such, the cardiovascular risk conferred by severe psoriasis may be comparable to what is seen with other well-established risk factors, such as diabetes mellitus. Previous studies demonstrated that low-density lipoprotein (LDL) plays critical roles during atherogenesis. It may be caused by the accumulation of macrophages and lipoprotein in the vessel wall. Oxidized LDL (ox-LDL) stimulates the expression of adhesion molecules, such as ICAM-1 and VCAM-1, on endothelial cells and increases the attachment of mononuclear cells and the endothelium. Even though previous evidence demonstrated that psoriasis patients have tortuous and dilated blood vessels in the dermis, which results in the leakage of ox-LDL, the leaked ox-LDL may increase the expression of adhesion molecules and cytokines, and disturb the static balance of osmosis. Therefore, exploration of the relationship between hyperlipidemia and psoriasis may be another novel treatment option for psoriasis and may represent the most promising strategy.

Keywords: lipid; psoriasis; inflammation

1. Introduction

Psoriasis is a chronic inflammatory disease related to many diseases, especially cardiovascular disease. Among these diseases, atherosclerosis plays the most important role [1]. Atherosclerosis is caused by inflammation and an imbalance of the lipid metabolism. Psoriasis and atherosclerosis not only share the same cytokines involved in the immunological mechanism, such as interleukin (IL)-17, but also have common angiogenic factors and oxidative pathways [2]. In addition, both of them have similar lipid profiles, including decreased high-density lipoprotein (HDL) levels and/or increased low-density lipoprotein (LDL) levels [3]. In the pathological process of atherosclerosis, the accumulation of cholesterol triggers the production of pro-inflammatory cytokines, such as tumor necrosis factor alpha (TNFα), and also leads to the aggregation of monocytes and differentiation into foam cells [4]. TNFα eventually induces an inflammatory cascade in blood vessels [5]. In chronic inflammation, TNFα may also influence the lipid profile, such as LDL-C levels, via a decreased concentration of apolipoproteins. Moreover, TNFα lowers the quality of lipoprotein by inducing the production of

LDL and oxLDL and reducing the level of HDL-C at the same time [6]. Oxidized LDL (oxLDL) not only exacerbates inflammation but also promotes cholesterol accumulation in lysosomes, which eventually leads to cell death [7]. On the other hand, HDL has a reverse cholesterol transport (RCT) function, anti-oxidative capacity, and anti-inflammatory properties by regulating dendritic cells' (DCs) differentiation [8], and reducing T cell activation and IL-12 production [9]. However, these properties are reduced during chronic inflammation, such as psoriasis [10]. Previous studies have clarified the immunological pathway of psoriasis; however, the mechanism between psoriasis and an abnormal lipid profile remains unknown. Thus, identification of the relationship between hyperlipidemia and psoriasis is of paramount importance to develop a new therapeutic prospect for psoriasis.

2. Psoriasis

2.1. The Etiology of Psoriasis

Psoriasis is a chronic inflammatory skin disease related to immune inheritance. However, to date, the true cause of the disease remains unclear. According to epidemiological statistics, approximately 1%–3% of people worldwide develop psoriasis every year [11]. Psoriasis has long been considered a skin disease. However, according to recent research findings, psoriasis is actually a multisystem disease. It may be related to the occurrence and course of other diseases, including rheumatological (psoriatic arthritis (PsA)), cardiovascular and psychiatric complications [12,13], as well as cardiometabolic diseases, such as obesity, hypertension, and dyslipidemia [14]. At present, comorbid cardiovascular diseases are the main cause of death in patients with psoriasis [15]. The risk of suffering myocardial infarction in patients with severe psoriasis is seven times that in individuals with corresponding age, sex, body mass index (BMI), and cardiovascular risk factors, and the risk of cardiovascular mortality increases by 57% in patients with severe psoriasis [16]. In addition, patients with psoriasis are at a higher risk for cardiovascular diseases. Psoriasis is also related to accelerated atherosclerosis. It has been found that all T cells involved in the pathogenesis of psoriasis are also involved in atherosclerosis [17]. Clinically, psoriasis is divided into many categories, and psoriasis vulgaris (PV) accounts for approximately 90%. Psoriasis often causes symptoms, such as desquamation, skin redness, and itching. In addition to affecting appearance, psoriasis causes great psychological pressure and social distress to patients, thus reducing quality of life [18].

2.2. The Molecular Mechanism of Psoriasis

Previous studies have shown that CD4+ helper T cells may differentiate into regulatory T cells and effector T cells (including T-helper cell type 1 (Th1) cells, T-helper cell type 2 (Th2) cells, T-helper cell type 17 (Th17) cells, follicular helper T (Tfh) cells, and regulatory T cells (Tregs)), which are subsequently activated. Before the discovery of other cell lineages, Th1 and Th2 cells were considered to be the only T cells that differentiated from progenitor CD4+ helper T cells [19]. However, a new CD4+ helper T cell subset was discovered, named Th17 cells [20]. Th17 cells produce interleukin 17 (IL-17). Among all Th cell subsets, IL-17-producing T cells play an important role in autoimmune diseases, including multiple sclerosis, psoriasis, inflammatory bowel diseases, and steroid-resistant asthma [21]. At present, psoriasis is generally considered to be derived from the chronic activation of the IL-23/Th17 cell signaling axis, in which dominant T cell subsets are Th1 and Th17 cells. The cytokines released by Th1 and Th17 cells facilitate immune cell aggregation, promote keratinocyte proliferation, and increase the inflammatory response [22]. More precisely, CD4+ and CD8+ T cells with an IL-17-secretory phenotype are most important because they produce pro-inflammatory cytokines IL-17, IL-22, and tumor necrosis factor alpha (TNFα) [23]. The pathogenic mechanism of psoriasis is divided into the primary initiation phase and the chronic inflammatory phase. In the primary initiation phase, the pathogenic inflammatory response is initiated. The subsequent chronic inflammatory phase is continued by feedback loops and amplification signals. During the development of psoriasis, T cell predominance shifts from Th1 predominance in the initiation phase to Th17 predominance in the chronic inflammatory phase [24]. External stimuli, such as trauma, infection, or drug administration, cause the release of self-nucleotides. Self-nucleotides then bind to antimicrobial peptides (AMPs) released by keratinocytes, forming complexes [19]. AMPs are positively charged proteins and members of the innate immune system and include cathelicidin antimicrobial peptide (CAMP), pro-inflammatory cytokines and chemokines (for example, TNF, IL-17, IL-22, and CC-chemokine ligand 20 (CCL20), among numerous others), and angiogenic factors [24]. Among the AMPs, CAMP is not produced when keratinocytes are healthy. However, CAMP is upregulated when epidermal cells are destroyed. In psoriasis lesions, the increase in CAMP production initiates pathogenic interferon (IFN) signaling cascades and the activation of DCs, resulting in uncontrolled inflammatory reactions [25]. The complexes of self-nucleotides and AMPs then bind to the receptors on antigen-presenting cells, such as toll-like receptor 7 (TLR7) and TLR9 on the surface of plasmacytoid dendritic cells (pDCs). pDCs are a member of the innate immune system circulating in the blood. After antigen presentation, pDCs promote the activation and clonal expansion of antigen-specific CD8+ T cells, and such processes occur in the dermis (activation of memory resident T cells) and local lymph nodes (activation of naive T cells). In addition, in the initiation phase of psoriasis, pDCs release the inflammatory mediators IFNα and IFNβ, thereby stimulating the secretion of pro-inflammatory mediators (such as IL-12, IL-23, and TNF) by myeloid DCs. Subsequently, the activated CD8+ T cells migrate to the epidermal layer and encounter class I major histocompatibility complex (MHC) receptors on the surface of keratinocytes (or melanocytes), triggering the local release of soluble factors, including cytokines, chemokines, and innate immune mediators, to increase local inflammation and stimulate keratinocyte proliferation [24]. In addition to being a skin barrier, keratinocytes release inflammatory cytokines, such as TNF; express IL-17 receptors; and participate in the initiation and amplification of psoriasis [26]. The IL-17 family consists of 6 members, IL-17A to IL-17F, among which IL-17A is the most studied member while IL-17E (also known as IL-25) is an inhibitor of IL-17 [27]. In addition to IL-17A, Th17 cells also release various inflammatory cytokines, including IL-17F, IL-21, IL-22, and granulocyte macrophage colony-stimulating factor (GM-CSF). Therefore, targeting the Th17 cell subset is more therapeutically effective than targeting a single cytokine [21]. Innate immunity mediators stimulate the activation of T cell populations, such as Th1, Th17, and Th22 cells, and then release additional cytokines and chemokines. In particular, IL-1 allows Th17 cells to respond to IL-23 [24]. Th17 cells then release IL-17, IL-22, TNF-α, and other cytokines [28], and participate in the macrophage-dependent and -independent stimulation of DCs, thereby enhancing the immune response [29]. They may participate in the production of angiogenic inflammatory mediators, including monocyte chemoattractant protein (MCP-1), nitric oxide, and vascular endothelial growth factor [30]. The expression of vascular endothelial growth factor receptors on epidermal cells induces cardiovascular endothelial hyperplasia and the expression of adhesion molecules in the vascular endothelium, thereby aggregating immune cells. Angiogenic factors induce tortuous characteristics in papillary dermal vessels at the sites of psoriasis lesions, manifesting as the Auspitz sign. In addition, IL-17 acts on the IL-17 receptor on keratinocytes to stimulate the production of TNF and CCL20 (a chemotactic for T cells and DCs208) by keratinocytes [24]. IL-17 and TNF and/or other pro-inflammatory cytokines stimulate the activation of defensins and chemokines to promote host defense and the accumulation of other immune cells [31]. IL-22 is related to the pathological characteristics of psoriasis, including epidermal hyperplasia, acanthosis, and parakeratosis. Important transcription factors in psoriasis include cyclic AMP, the Janus kinase (JAK) signal transducer and activator of transcription (STAT) family, and nuclear factor-κB (NF-κB). Activation of these transcription factors results in the production of other factors, such as TNF and IL-17, as well as downstream amplification loops. Notably, although IL-17 is a signature cytokine of TH17 cells, other innate and acquired immune cells also produce IL-17, including CD8+ T cells, γδ T cells, innate lymphoid cells, and natural killer (NK) T cells [32]. Compared with a healthy control group, patients with psoriasis display higher serum concentrations of IL-17. However, the paradigm of Th17 cells as the main cellular source of IL-17 is no longer fully valid [33].

Recent studies have noted that the innate immune system, including neutrophils, mast cells, γδ T cells, and innate lymphoid cells, is the most important source of IL-17 in patients with psoriasis [34].

3. The Relationships among Psoriasis, Cardiovascular Diseases, and Dyslipidemia

3.1. Normal Function of Fat and Cholesterol in Skin Cells

The stratum corneum is the outermost layer of the epidermis, and is a barrier protecting humans from the external environment. In addition to protecting humans against external harm, the stratum corneum prevents water loss from the body [35]. The structure of the stratum corneum is often described as bricks and mortar [36]. The bricks are fully differentiated keratinocytes, mostly consisting of keratin filaments and filaggrin [37]. The mortar refers to intracellular lipids, which consist of ceramides (CERs), free fatty acids (FFAs), and cholesterol. These lipids are arranged into a lamellar structure, and CERs account for 50%. CERs are the main polar lipids in the stratum corneum, and their basic composition is a sphingoid base connected to fatty acids by amide bonds. However, the composition of CERs varies appreciably in the human body. CERs are divided into 12 categories according to the head group composition or fatty acid esterification [38]. CERs play an important role in skin barriers, cell adhesion, and epidermal differentiation. In addition, CERs act as second messengers in stress-induced apoptosis [39]. CERs induce the apoptosis of tumor cells and reduce the resistance of tumor cells to chemotherapy drugs [40]. In psoriasis, the barrier function of the skin and water loss by the epidermis are mainly related to an abnormal composition ratio of CERs [41]. However, the total amount of CERs does not differ significantly between patients with psoriasis and healthy individuals [42]. Studies have shown that prosaposin, a precursor of saposin, and its mRNA were decreased in patients with psoriasis [43]. Saposins are a class of nonenzymatic proteins involved in the hydrolysis of sphingolipids, including the postsecretory glucosyl-CERs in the stratum corneum [44]. Sphingomyelinase is also significantly downregulated in the stratum corneum of patients with psoriasis. The reduction in the enzymes involved in CER production and metabolism may lead to decreases in ceramide 1 and other CERs at the sites of psoriasis lesions [41] as well as decreases in long-chain CERs containing ester-linked fatty acids and CERs containing phytosphingosine, thereby altering CER composition and increasing transepidermal water loss. In addition, the proportion of the three major intracellular lipids varies in the stratum corneum. At the sites of psoriasis lesions, the FFA content is significantly reduced while the cholesterol content is slightly increased [42]. Cholesterol constitutes approximately 25% of animal cell membranes and maintains cell integrity and fluidity. Moreover, the dynamic arrangement of cholesterol enhances the coating ability of the cell membrane, allowing the cell membrane to increase fluidity at low temperatures and increase stability at high temperatures [45]. For circulating low-density lipoprotein (LDL), cholesterol is transported via LDL receptor (LDL-R)-mediated endocytosis of holo-particles. Cholesteryl esters (CEs) delivered by the endocytosed LDL are hydrolyzed by lysosomal acid lipase in the lysosomes. The released unesterified (free) cholesterol is transported to the endoplasmic reticulum (ER), in which the cholesterol is re-esterified to form CEs. The CEs are stored in cytoplasmic lipid droplets (LDs) or are transported to the cell membrane or mitochondria. HDL binds to scavenger receptor class B type 1 (SR-B1) on the cell surface, and CEs are selectively transported into the cells without the internalization of the whole lipoprotein molecule. Subsequently, the CEs are hydrolyzed into free cholesterol by hormone-sensitive lipase (HSL). This mechanism is used by steroidogenic cells that rely on cholesterol as a precursor. Large amounts of CE-rich LDs are found in steroidogenic cells, in which the CEs are hydrolyzed into cholesterol by HSL to supply the steroidogenic cells [46]. Each has a unique receptor specificity and mechanism of transporting cholesterol. SR-B1 is a lipoprotein receptor [47] and plays an important role in cholesterol efflux and steroid hormone production [48]. In addition, SR-B1 has an RCT function and determines HDL-C levels through selectively transporting HDL-CEs to the liver, where the HDL-CEs are converted to bile acids, or through biliary cholesterol secretion [49]. Various mouse model studies have shown that SR-B1-null mice exhibit an increase in the amount and size of HDL-CE, which is accompanied by a reduced level of cholesterol in secreted bile and accelerated atherosclerosis. In contrast, SR-B1-overexpressing mice exhibit decreased levels of HDL-CE, a reduced degree of atherosclerosis, and a reduced extent of atherosclerosis in the liver [49]. Binding of HDL to SR-B1 increases anti-inflammatory cytokines, such as IL-10 and transforming growth factor-beta (TGF-β), by initiating Akt and reducing NF-κB activation, thereby regulating the inflammatory response of macrophages. SR-B1 in macrophages also regulates efferocytosis or the removal of apoptotic cells through the Src/phosphoinositide 3-kinase (PI3K)/Akt/Rac1 signaling pathway, thereby enhancing survival and the anti-inflammatory response of phagocytes. In endothelial cells, SR-B1 participates in the translocation of HDL from the apical to basolateral side, which further promotes the removal of cholesterol from intimal macrophages and lymphatic vessels [50].

3.2. The Correlation Between Psoriasis and Atherosclerosis

Patients with psoriasis are at a high risk for the incidence of cardiovascular disease and myocardial infarction [51]. Compared with the general population, the risk factors for cardiovascular diseases in patients with psoriasis have a high incidence, such as diabetes, hypertension, obesity, and hyperlipidemia [51]. Psoriasis is highly correlated with cardiovascular diseases, and hyperlipidemia-induced atherosclerosis is the predominant disease [1]. A large amount of evidence indicates that psoriasis is related to severe atherosclerosis and cardiovascular diseases while inflammation plays an important role in psoriasis and atherosclerosis [1]. Atherosclerosis and psoriasis have very similar immune response profiles. In addition, atherosclerosis and psoriasis share the same immunological pathways (including DCs, Th1 cells, Th17 cells, and Tregs) as well as angiogenic factors and oxidative mechanisms [2]. A number of studies show that patients with psoriasis exhibit decreased HDL levels and/or increased low-density lipoprotein (LDL), very-low-density lipoprotein (VLDL), and triglyceride (TG) levels [3].

3.3. The Relationship Between Psoriasis and Blood Lipids

Obesity is related to many immune diseases, including cardiovascular diseases, arteriosclerosis, and psoriasis [52]. However, in mouse models, both obese and lean mice develop severe psoriasiform skin inflammation after being fed a high-fat diet (HFD). Such a phenomenon is related to FFAs but is not related to the fat mass extension, blood glucose levels, and adipose tissue-derived mediators. The increase in FFAs leads to an immune response and insulin resistance, which alters the homeostasis and function of immune cells. HFD also increases the level of saturated fatty acids (SFAs). SFAs stimulate myeloid cells to produce TLR-like stimuli, which induce a pro-immune response, thus resulting in keratinocyte activation. Therefore, decreasing the SFA content in food reduces psoriasiform inflammation. HFD-induced obesity does not directly alter the proinflammatory status of skin and immune cells. However, it renders the skin and immune cells more susceptible to proinflammatory stimuli, such as imiquimod (IMQ), thereby enhancing the immune response [53]. Certain studies failed to establish a correlation between psoriasis and lipid serum levels [54], including a large population-based cross-sectional study conducted in the UK [55].

3.4. The Relationships among Oxidized LDL (oxLDL), the Inflammatory Response, and Psoriasis

The accumulation of excessive cholesterol in blood vessel walls could promote the dysfunction and activation of epidermal cells, which induces an inflammatory response and eventually leads to the production of pro-inflammatory cytokines and reactive oxygen species, the overexpression of adhesion molecules and chemokines, and a reduction in nitric oxide levels [4]. The above processes lead to the aggregation and invasion of monocytes and the differentiation of monocytes into macrophages. After receiving modified LDL via scavenger receptors, macrophages are converted to foam cells. In addition, TNFα triggers endothelial dysfunction and induces an inflammatory cascade in the blood vessel wall, ultimately resulting in vascular sclerosis [5]. Although elevated TNFα exerts a protective effect during acute immunity, the maintenance of a high concentration of TNFα during chronic inflammation may alter lipid and carbohydrate metabolism. In fact, TNFα decreases the concentration of LDL-C through diminishing the secretion of apolipoproteins and reducing cholesterol catabolism and excretion, thereby interfering with cholesterol metabolism. In addition, TNFα promotes the production of pro-atherogenic small dense LDL and oxLDL to alter the quality of lipoproteins. TNFα also reduces HDL-C levels and changes HDL composition [6]. Patients with chronic inflammatory responses experience qualitative and quantitative changes in lipid and lipoprotein profiles, including decreases in cholesterol, HDL-C, and apolipoprotein A-1, and increases in small dense LDL, lipoprotein(a) [Lp(a)], and TG. In addition to TNFα, IL-6 and IL-1ß also alter lipid metabolism, including increasing VLDL and reducing TG-rich lipoprotein clearance. An increase in serum TG levels enhances the expression of cholesteryl ester transfer protein (CETP), which transfers TG from VLDL/LDL to LDL/HDL. These TG-enriched particles become the substrate for hepatic lipase and lipoprotein lipase, resulting in the production of small dense LDL and HDL as the final products. Small dense LDL more readily enters into the arteries [9] and is more susceptible to oxidation. As a result, the antioxidant and anti-inflammatory activities of small dense HDL become limited [56]. LDL levels and composition are also altered due to inflammation. First, the increase in LDLR expression reduces LDL-C levels and thus promotes the intracellular accumulation of cholesterol. Second, circulating LDL is more prone to oxidation. Therefore, patients with chronic inflammatory diseases have high plasma levels of oxLDL. oxLDL is more atherogenic and can enhance the inflammatory response. Moreover, oxLDL promotes the accumulation of cholesterol and the formation of cholesterol crystals in lysosomes, which causes lysosomal disruption and leads to increased cellular toxicity [7].

3.5. The Relationships among HDL, the Inflammatory Response, and Psoriasis

HDL has RCT, anti-inflammatory, and antioxidant functions, which are related to the prevention of cardiovascular diseases [57]. In addition, HDL has anti-apoptotic and anti-thrombotic activities. The protective effect of HDL is mostly due to its role in RCT. RCT refers to the process of cholesterol transport from the peripheral tissues to the liver, where the cholesterol is secreted, converted into bile acid, or synthesized into sterol hormones [58]. The first step in RCT is the removal of excess cholesterol from macrophage foam cells at sclerotic sites via HDL or macrophage-derived apolipoproteins [59]. Cholesterol efflux can be achieved through a number of ways, including (a) unidirectional efflux to lipid-free apolipoproteins, particularly apoA-1, mediated by ATP-binding cassette A1 (ABCA1); (b) unidirectional efflux to mature HDL particles mediated by ABCG1; and (c) efflux to mature HDL particles via passive diffusion facilitated by SR-B1 [60]. Once cholesterol is transferred to the cytoplasm, SR-B1 delivers the macrophage-derived (HDL) cholesterol to the liver for bile acid production. The next step is biliary secretion or transport to steroidogenic tissues, especially the adrenal gland and ovary, for steroid production and storage. HDL terminates lipid peroxidation chain reactions via apolipoproteins (such as apoA) and enzymes (paraoxonase (PON1), lecithin-cholesterol acyltransferase (LCAT), and platelet activating factor-acetyl hydrolase), thereby exhibiting an antioxidant function [61]. HDL not only inhibits monocyte transmigration and the expression of adhesion molecules in endothelial cells but also plays an immunomodulating role in the innate and acquired immune systems. HDL regulates DCs, monocytes, macrophages, T cells, and B cells mainly through modification of the cholesterol content of lipid rafts [62]. The anti-inflammatory properties of HDL are achieved through apoA-1, a major HDL-associated protein. apoA-1 stimulates the production of IL-10 and prostaglandin E2 (PGE2), thereby inhibiting the differentiation and functions of DCs [63], and reducing T cell activation and IL-12 production [8]. During a chronic inflammatory response, the antioxidative and anti-inflammatory properties of HDL are reduced. In addition, RCT and the ability to resist LDL oxidation are affected. The decrease in the antioxidative property is due to proteome alterations, including decreased activity of HDL-associated enzymes and the accumulation of complement (C3), ceruloplasmin, and serum amyloid A (SAA) [58]. The reduced anti-inflammatory property may be related to decreased apoA-1 and apoM levels. In addition, enhancement of the pro-inflammatory mechanism is due to the impaired cellular efflux of lipids to HDL, which initiates intracellular STAT3 signaling and induces vascular inflammation. In addition to low plasma levels of HDL [9], HDL proteomic and lipid composition are altered in psoriasis [15,16], which leads to a decrease in the cholesterol efflux capacity [12,15] and a reduction in the anti-inflammatory and antioxidant capacities of HDL. Moreover, other properties of HDL are also altered, such as the anti-LDL oxidation capability, inhibition of TNF-α-induced monocyte adhesion to epidermal cells, prevention of the ox-LDL-induced monocyte migration, and protection of epidermal cells from TNF-α-induced apoptosis [14]. Patients with psoriasis exhibit low PON-1 activity, which is negatively correlated with psoriasis area and severity index (PASI) scores [58]. Conversely, anti-psoriatic therapy restores the composition and function of HDL [64]. HDL-associated proteins also undergo changes, among which apoA-1 and apoM are significantly reduced. In contrast, the levels of acute-phase proteins, such as SAA, prothrombin, α-1-antitrypsin, and α-1-acid glycoprotein 1, are significantly increased. The cholesterol efflux capacity is related to decreased apoA-1, phosphatidylcholine, and sphingomyelin in HDL. Under chronic inflammatory conditions, such as psoriasis, the changes in protein structure and the appearance of neo-epitopes may lead to autoantibody production and HDL dysfunction and are even related to cardiovascular diseases [10]. Therefore, these antibodies may serve as new biomarkers for autoimmune diseases in cardiovascular diseases. High titers of autoantibodies against HDL (aHDL) and apoA-I are present in chronic inflammatory diseases, which is related to high cardiovascular risk. aHDL and aapoA-I are also found in patients with psoriasis. These antibodies are correlated with the severity of diseases and may be related to the development of vascular sclerosis.

4. Conclusions

Psoriasis affects at least 125 million people across the world. Additional development and evaluation of the relationship between the lipid profile and psoriasis to explore treatment efficacy is required. In chronic inflammation, TNFα may influence the lipid profile, such as LDL-C levels, via decreased concentrations of apolipoproteins. Moreover, TNFα lowers the quality of lipoprotein by inducing the production of LDL and oxLDL but reducing the level of HDL-C at the same time. Oxidized LDL (oxLDL) not only exacerbates inflammation but also promotes cholesterol accumulation in lysosomes, which eventually leads to cell death. On the other hand, HDL has a reverse cholesterol transport (RCT) function, anti-oxidative capacity, and anti-inflammatory properties by regulating dendritic cells' (DCs) differentiation and reducing T cell activation and cytokine production. However, these properties are reduced during chronic inflammation, such as psoriasis. Thus, identification of the relationship between hyperlipidemia and psoriasis is of paramount importance to develop a new therapeutic prospect for psoriasis (Figure 1).

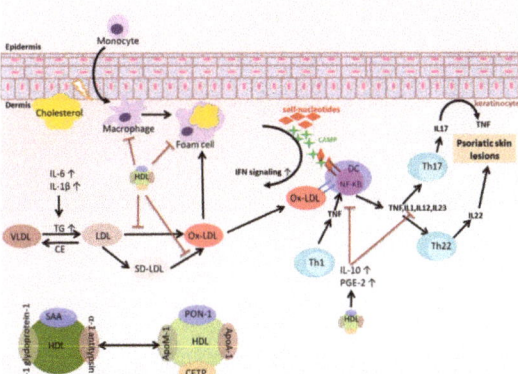

Figure 1. Immune cells and lipoprotein-associated cytokines implicated in psoriasis pathogenesis. Characteristic markers and cytokines related to the interleukin (IL)-17/IL-23 immune signature of T cells, lipoprotein, dendritic cells (DCs), and associated immune cells in psoriatic skin inflammation.

Author Contributions: Conceptualization, methodology, A.-W.L. and K.-H.W.; writing—original draft preparation, C.-C.C.; writing—review and editing, C.-M.S., C.-Y.H. and C.-K.C. All authors have read and agreed to the published version of the manuscript.

Acknowledgments: This work was supported by grants from National Science Council (MOST 108-2320-B-038-046) in Taiwan.

Conflicts of Interest: The authors declare no conflict of interest.

Abbreviations

apoA-I	Apolipoprotein A1
ABCA1	ATP-binding cassette A1
aHDL	autoantibodies against HDL
AMP	Antimicrobial peptide
apo	apolipoprotein
BMI	Body mass index
C3	Complement 3
CAMP	Cathelicidin antimicrobial peptide
CCL20	C-C motif chemokine ligand 20
CD	Cluster of differentiation
CE	Cholesteryl ester
CER	Ceramide
CETP	Cholesteryl ester transfer protein
DC	Dendritic cell
ER	Endoplasmic reticulum
FFA	Free fatty acid
GM-CSF	Granulocyte macrophage colony stimulating factor
HDL	High density lipoprotein
HDL-C	High-density lipoprotein cholesterol
HDL-CE	High density lipoprotein cholesteryl ester
HFD	High fat diet
HSL	Hormone-sensitive lipase
ICAM-1	Intercellular Adhesion Molecule 1
IFN	Interferon
IL	Interleukin
IMQ	Imiquimod
JAK	Janus kinase
LCAT	Lecithin-cholesterol acyltransferase
LD	Lipid droplet
LDL	Low density lipoprotein
LDL-R	Low density lipoprotein receptor
Lp(a)	Lipoprotein(a)
MCP-1	Monocyte chemoattractant protein 1
MHC	Major histocompatibility complex
NF-κB	Nuclear factor-κB
NK	Natural killer
ox-LDL	Oxidized LDL
pDC	Plasmacytoid dendritic cell
PI3K	Phosphoinositide 3 kinase
PON	Paraoxonase
PsA	Psoriatic arthritis
PV	Psoriasis vulgaris
RCT	Reverse cholesterol transport
SAA	Serum amyloid A
SFA	Saturated fatty acid
SR-B1	Scavenger receptor class B type 1

STAT	Signal transducer and activator of transcription
Th	T helper cell
Tfh	T follicular helper cells
TG	Triglyceride
TGF-β	Transforming growth factor beta
TLR	Toll-like receptor
TNF	Tumor necrosis factor
Treg	Regulatory T cell
VCAM-1	Vascular cell adhesion molecule 1
VLDL	Very-low-density lipoprotein

References

1. Ghazizadeh, R.; Tosa, M.; Ghazizadeh, M. Clinical improvement in psoriasis with treatment of associated hyperlipidemia. *Am. J. Med. Sci.* **2011**, *341*, 394–398. [CrossRef]
2. Harrington, C.L.; Dey, A.K.; Yunus, R.; Joshi, A.A.; Mehta, N.N. Psoriasis as a human model of disease to study inflammatory atherogenesis. *Am. J. Physiol. Heart Circ. Physiol.* **2017**, *312*, H867–H873. [CrossRef]
3. Kimball, A.B.; Szapary, P.; Mrowietz, U.; Reich, K.; Langley, R.G.; You, Y.; Hsu, M.C.; Yeilding, N.; Rader, D.J.; Mehta, N.N. Underdiagnosis and undertreatment of cardiovascular risk factors in patients with moderate to severe psoriasis. *J. Am. Acad Derm.* **2012**, *67*, 76–85. [CrossRef]
4. Gimbrone, M.A., Jr.; Garcia-Cardena, G. Endothelial Cell Dysfunction and the Pathobiology of Atherosclerosis. *Circ. Res.* **2016**, *118*, 620–636. [CrossRef] [PubMed]
5. Sorci-Thomas, M.G.; Thomas, M.J. Microdomains, Inflammation, and Atherosclerosis. *Circ. Res.* **2016**, *118*, 679–691. [CrossRef] [PubMed]
6. Amezaga Urruela, M.; Suarez-Almazor, M.E. Lipid paradox in rheumatoid arthritis: Changes with rheumatoid arthritis therapies. *Curr. Rheumatol. Rep.* **2012**, *14*, 428–437. [CrossRef] [PubMed]
7. Favari, E.; Thomas, M.J.; Sorci-Thomas, M.G. High-Density Lipoprotein Functionality as a New Pharmacological Target on Cardiovascular Disease: Unifying Mechanism That Explains High-Density Lipoprotein Protection Toward the Progression of Atherosclerosis. *J. Cardiovasc. Pharm.* **2018**, *71*, 325–331. [CrossRef]
8. Wang, S.H.; Yuan, S.G.; Peng, D.Q.; Zhao, S.P. HDL and ApoA-I inhibit antigen presentation-mediated T cell activation by disrupting lipid rafts in antigen presenting cells. *Atherosclerosis* **2012**, *225*, 105–114. [CrossRef]
9. Whetzel, A.M.; Sturek, J.M.; Nagelin, M.H.; Bolick, D.T.; Gebre, A.K.; Parks, J.S.; Bruce, A.C.; Skaflen, M.D.; Hedrick, C.C. ABCG1 deficiency in mice promotes endothelial activation and monocyte-endothelial interactions. *Arter. Thromb Vasc. Biol.* **2010**, *30*, 809–817. [CrossRef]
10. Batuca, J.R.; Ames, P.R.; Amaral, M.; Favas, C.; Isenberg, D.A.; Delgado Alves, J. Anti-atherogenic and anti-inflammatory properties of high-density lipoprotein are affected by specific antibodies in systemic lupus erythematosus. *Rheumatol. (Oxf.)* **2009**, *48*, 26–31. [CrossRef]
11. Spah, F. Inflammation in atherosclerosis and psoriasis: Common pathogenic mechanisms and the potential for an integrated treatment approach. *Br. J. Derm.* **2008**, *159*, 10–17. [CrossRef] [PubMed]
12. Gelfand, J.M.; Feldman, S.R.; Stern, R.S.; Thomas, J.; Rolstad, T.; Margolis, D.J. Determinants of quality of life in patients with psoriasis: A study from the US population. *J. Am. Acad Derm.* **2004**, *51*, 704–708. [CrossRef] [PubMed]
13. Kim, N.; Thrash, B.; Menter, A. Comorbidities in psoriasis patients. *Semin Cutan Med. Surg.* **2010**, *29*, 10–15. [CrossRef] [PubMed]
14. Langan, S.M.; Seminara, N.M.; Shin, D.B.; Troxel, A.B.; Kimmel, S.E.; Mehta, N.N.; Margolis, D.J.; Gelfand, J.M. Prevalence of metabolic syndrome in patients with psoriasis: A population-based study in the United Kingdom. *J. Invest. Derm.* **2012**, *132*, 556–562. [CrossRef]
15. Yeung, H.; Takeshita, J.; Mehta, N.N.; Kimmel, S.E.; Ogdie, A.; Margolis, D.J.; Shin, D.B.; Attor, R.; Troxel, A.B.; Gelfand, J.M. Psoriasis severity and the prevalence of major medical comorbidity: A population-based study. *Jama Derm.* **2013**, *149*, 1173–1179. [CrossRef]
16. Gelfand, J.M.; Neimann, A.L.; Shin, D.B.; Wang, X.; Margolis, D.J.; Troxel, A.B. Risk of myocardial infarction in patients with psoriasis. *JAMA* **2006**, *296*, 1735–1741. [CrossRef]
17. Hansson, G.K.; Hermansson, A. The immune system in atherosclerosis. *Nat. Immunol.* **2011**, *12*, 204–212. [CrossRef]

18. Parisi, R.; Symmons, D.P.; Griffiths, C.E.; Ashcroft, D.M.; Identification and Management of Psoriasis and Associated ComorbidiTy (IMPACT) project team. Global epidemiology of psoriasis: A systematic review of incidence and prevalence. *J. Invest. Derm.* **2013**, *133*, 377–385. [CrossRef]
19. Zhu, J.; Yamane, H.; Paul, W.E. Differentiation of effector CD4 T cell populations (*). *Annu Rev. Immunol.* **2010**, *28*, 445–489. [CrossRef]
20. Harrington, L.E.; Hatton, R.D.; Mangan, P.R.; Turner, H.; Murphy, T.L.; Murphy, K.M.; Weaver, C.T. Interleukin 17-producing CD4+ effector T cells develop via a lineage distinct from the T helper type 1 and 2 lineages. *Nat. Immunol.* **2005**, *6*, 1123–1132. [CrossRef]
21. Yang, J.; Sundrud, M.S.; Skepner, J.; Yamagata, T. Targeting Th17 cells in autoimmune diseases. *Trends Pharm. Sci.* **2014**, *35*, 493–500. [CrossRef] [PubMed]
22. Furue, M.; Tsuji, G.; Chiba, T.; Kadono, T. Cardiovascular and Metabolic Diseases Comorbid with Psoriasis: Beyond the Skin. *Intern. Med.* **2017**, *56*, 1613–1619. [CrossRef] [PubMed]
23. Karczewski, J.; Dobrowolska, A.; Rychlewska-Hanczewska, A.; Adamski, Z. New insights into the role of T cells in pathogenesis of psoriasis and psoriatic arthritis. *Autoimmunity* **2016**, *49*, 435–450. [CrossRef]
24. Greb, J.E.; Goldminz, A.M.; Elder, J.T.; Lebwohl, M.G.; Gladman, D.D.; Wu, J.J.; Mehta, N.N.; Finlay, A.Y.; Gottlieb, A.B. Psoriasis. *Nat. Rev. Dis. Primers* **2016**, *2*, 16082. [CrossRef]
25. Lande, R.; Gregorio, J.; Facchinetti, V.; Chatterjee, B.; Wang, Y.H.; Homey, B.; Cao, W.; Wang, Y.H.; Su, B.; Nestle, F.O.; et al. Plasmacytoid dendritic cells sense self-DNA coupled with antimicrobial peptide. *Nature* **2007**, *449*, 564–569. [CrossRef] [PubMed]
26. Chiricozzi, A.; Nograles, K.E.; Johnson-Huang, L.M.; Fuentes-Duculan, J.; Cardinale, I.; Bonifacio, K.M.; Gulati, N.; Mitsui, H.; Guttman-Yassky, E.; Suarez-Farinas, M.; et al. IL-17 induces an expanded range of downstream genes in reconstituted human epidermis model. *PLoS ONE* **2014**, *9*, e90284. [CrossRef]
27. Lavocat, F.; Ndongo-Thiam, N.; Miossec, P. Interleukin-25 Produced by Synoviocytes Has Anti-inflammatory Effects by Acting As a Receptor Antagonist for Interleukin-17A Function. *Front. Immunol.* **2017**, *8*, 647. [CrossRef]
28. Chiricozzi, A.; Guttman-Yassky, E.; Suarez-Farinas, M.; Nograles, K.E.; Tian, S.; Cardinale, I.; Chimenti, S.; Krueger, J.G. Integrative responses to IL-17 and TNF-alpha in human keratinocytes account for key inflammatory pathogenic circuits in psoriasis. *J. Invest. Derm.* **2011**, *131*, 677–687. [CrossRef]
29. Nestle, F.O.; Kaplan, D.H.; Barker, J. Psoriasis. *N. Engl. J. Med.* **2009**, *361*, 496–509. [CrossRef]
30. Takahashi, H.; Numasaki, M.; Lotze, M.T.; Sasaki, H. Interleukin-17 enhances bFGF-, HGF- and VEGF-induced growth of vascular endothelial cells. *Immunol. Lett.* **2005**, *98*, 189–193. [CrossRef]
31. Leonardi, C.; Matheson, R.; Zachariae, C.; Cameron, G.; Li, L.; Edson-Heredia, E.; Braun, D.; Banerjee, S. Anti-interleukin-17 monoclonal antibody ixekizumab in chronic plaque psoriasis. *N. Engl. J. Med.* **2012**, *366*, 1190–1199. [CrossRef] [PubMed]
32. Gaffen, S.L.; Jain, R.; Garg, A.V.; Cua, D.J. The IL-23-IL-17 immune axis: From mechanisms to therapeutic testing. *Nat. Rev. Immunol.* **2014**, *14*, 585–600. [CrossRef] [PubMed]
33. Keijsers, R.R.; Joosten, I.; van Erp, P.E.; Koenen, H.J.; van de Kerkhof, P.C. Cellular sources of IL-17 in psoriasis: A paradigm shift? *Exp. Derm.* **2014**, *23*, 799–803. [CrossRef] [PubMed]
34. Zheng, Y.; Wang, Z.; Deng, L.; Zhang, G.; Yuan, X.; Huang, L.; Xu, W.; Shen, L. Modulation of STAT3 and STAT5 activity rectifies the imbalance of Th17 and Treg cells in patients with acute coronary syndrome. *Clin. Immunol.* **2015**, *157*, 65–77. [CrossRef]
35. Del Rosso, J.Q.; Levin, J. Clinical relevance of maintaining the structural and functional integrity of the stratum corneum: Why is it important to you? *J. Drugs Derm.* **2011**, *10*, s5–s12.
36. Harding, C.R. The stratum corneum: Structure and function in health and disease. *Dermatol. Ther.* **2004**, *17*, 6–15. [CrossRef]
37. Proksch, E.; Brandner, J.M.; Jensen, J.M. The skin: An indispensable barrier. *Exp. Derm.* **2008**, *17*, 1063–1072. [CrossRef]
38. van Smeden, J.; Hoppel, L.; van der Heijden, R.; Hankemeier, T.; Vreeken, R.J.; Bouwstra, J.A. LC/MS analysis of stratum corneum lipids: Ceramide profiling and discovery. *J. Lipid Res.* **2011**, *52*, 1211–1221. [CrossRef]
39. Komatsu, M.; Takahashi, T.; Abe, T.; Takahashi, I.; Ida, H.; Takada, G. Evidence for the association of ultraviolet-C and H(2)O(2)-induced apoptosis with acid sphingomyelinase activation. *Biochim. Biophys. Acta* **2001**, *1533*, 47–54. [CrossRef]
40. Charles, A.G.; Han, T.Y.; Liu, Y.Y.; Hansen, N.; Giuliano, A.E.; Cabot, M.C. Taxol-induced ceramide generation and apoptosis in human breast cancer cells. *Cancer Chemother Pharm.* **2001**, *47*, 444–450. [CrossRef]

41. Motta, S.; Monti, M.; Sesana, S.; Mellesi, L.; Ghidoni, R.; Caputo, R. Abnormality of water barrier function in psoriasis. Role of ceramide fractions. *Arch. Derm.* **1994**, *130*, 452–456. [CrossRef]
42. Motta, S.; Monti, M.; Sesana, S.; Caputo, R.; Carelli, S.; Ghidoni, R. Ceramide composition of the psoriatic scale. *Biochim. Biophys. Acta* **1993**, *1182*, 147–151. [CrossRef]
43. Alessandrini, F.; Stachowitz, S.; Ring, J.; Behrendt, H. The level of prosaposin is decreased in the skin of patients with psoriasis vulgaris. *J. Invest. Derm.* **2001**, *116*, 394–400. [CrossRef]
44. Nemes, Z.; Marekov, L.N.; Fesus, L.; Steinert, P.M. A novel function for transglutaminase 1: Attachment of long-chain omega-hydroxyceramides to involucrin by ester bond formation. *Proc. Natl. Acad. Sci. USA* **1999**, *96*, 8402–8407. [CrossRef]
45. Incardona, J.P.; Eaton, S. Cholesterol in signal transduction. *Curr. Opin. Cell Biol.* **2000**, *12*, 193–203. [CrossRef]
46. Kraemer, F.B.; Shen, W.J.; Harada, K.; Patel, S.; Osuga, J.; Ishibashi, S.; Azhar, S. Hormone-sensitive lipase is required for high-density lipoprotein cholesteryl ester-supported adrenal steroidogenesis. *Mol. Endocrinol.* **2004**, *18*, 549–557. [CrossRef]
47. Shen, W.J.; Azhar, S.; Kraemer, F.B. Lipid droplets and steroidogenic cells. *Exp. Cell Res.* **2016**, *340*, 209–214. [CrossRef]
48. Shen, W.J.; Hu, J.; Hu, Z.; Kraemer, F.B.; Azhar, S. Scavenger receptor class B type I (SR-BI): A versatile receptor with multiple functions and actions. *Metabolism* **2014**, *63*, 875–886. [CrossRef]
49. Ueda, Y.; Royer, L.; Gong, E.; Zhang, J.; Cooper, P.N.; Francone, O.; Rubin, E.M. Lower plasma levels and accelerated clearance of high density lipoprotein (HDL) and non-HDL cholesterol in scavenger receptor class B type I transgenic mice. *J. Biol. Chem.* **1999**, *274*, 7165–7171. [CrossRef]
50. Lim, H.Y.; Thiam, C.H.; Yeo, K.P.; Bisoendial, R.; Hii, C.S.; McGrath, K.C.; Tan, K.W.; Heather, A.; Alexander, J.S.; Angeli, V. Lymphatic vessels are essential for the removal of cholesterol from peripheral tissues by SR-BI-mediated transport of HDL. *Cell Metab.* **2013**, *17*, 671–684. [CrossRef]
51. Kaye, J.A.; Li, L.; Jick, S.S. Incidence of risk factors for myocardial infarction and other vascular diseases in patients with psoriasis. *Br. J. Derm.* **2008**, *159*, 895–902. [CrossRef] [PubMed]
52. Kanneganti, T.D.; Dixit, V.D. Immunological complications of obesity. *Nat. Immunol.* **2012**, *13*, 707–712. [CrossRef] [PubMed]
53. Herbert, D.; Franz, S.; Popkova, Y.; Anderegg, U.; Schiller, J.; Schwede, K.; Lorz, A.; Simon, J.C.; Saalbach, A. High-Fat Diet Exacerbates Early Psoriatic Skin Inflammation Independent of Obesity: Saturated Fatty Acids as Key Players. *J. Invest. Derm.* **2018**, *138*, 1999–2009. [CrossRef]
54. Farshchian, M.; Zamanian, A.; Farshchian, M.; Monsef, A.R.; Mahjub, H. Serum lipid level in Iranian patients with psoriasis. *J. Eur. Acad. Derm. Venereol.* **2007**, *21*, 802–805. [CrossRef] [PubMed]
55. Neimann, A.L.; Shin, D.B.; Wang, X.; Margolis, D.J.; Troxel, A.B.; Gelfand, J.M. Prevalence of cardiovascular risk factors in patients with psoriasis. *J. Am. Acad. Derm.* **2006**, *55*, 829–835. [CrossRef] [PubMed]
56. Catapano, A.L.; Pirillo, A.; Norata, G.D. Vascular inflammation and low-density lipoproteins: Is cholesterol the link? A lesson from the clinical trials. *Br. J. Pharm.* **2017**, *174*, 3973–3985. [CrossRef] [PubMed]
57. Paiva-Lopes, M.J.; Delgado Alves, J. Psoriasis-associated vascular disease: The role of HDL. *J. Biomed. Sci.* **2017**, *24*, 73. [CrossRef]
58. Goren, A.; Ozsolak, F.; Shoresh, N.; Ku, M.; Adli, M.; Hart, C.; Gymrek, M.; Zuk, O.; Regev, A.; Milos, P.M.; et al. Chromatin profiling by directly sequencing small quantities of immunoprecipitated DNA. *Nat. Methods* **2010**, *7*, 47–49. [CrossRef]
59. Ono, K. Current concept of reverse cholesterol transport and novel strategy for atheroprotection. *J. Cardiol.* **2012**, *60*, 339–343. [CrossRef]
60. Phillips, M.C. Molecular mechanisms of cellular cholesterol efflux. *J. Biol. Chem.* **2014**, *289*, 24020–24029. [CrossRef]
61. Rosenson, R.S.; Brewer, H.B., Jr.; Ansell, B.; Barter, P.; Chapman, M.J.; Heinecke, J.W.; Kontush, A.; Tall, A.R.; Webb, N.R. Translation of high-density lipoprotein function into clinical practice: Current prospects and future challenges. *Circulation* **2013**, *128*, 1256–1267. [CrossRef]
62. Barter, P.J.; Nicholls, S.; Rye, K.A.; Anantharamaiah, G.M.; Navab, M.; Fogelman, A.M. Antiinflammatory properties of HDL. *Circ. Res.* **2004**, *95*, 764–772. [CrossRef] [PubMed]

63. Kim, K.D.; Lim, H.Y.; Lee, H.G.; Yoon, D.Y.; Choe, Y.K.; Choi, I.; Paik, S.G.; Kim, Y.S.; Yang, Y.; Lim, J.S. Apolipoprotein A-I induces IL-10 and PGE2 production in human monocytes and inhibits dendritic cell differentiation and maturation. *Biochem. Biophys. Res. Commun.* **2005**, *338*, 1126–1136. [CrossRef] [PubMed]
64. Marsche, G.; Saemann, M.D.; Heinemann, A.; Holzer, M. Inflammation alters HDL composition and function: Implications for HDL-raising therapies. *Pharmacol. Ther.* **2013**, *137*, 341–351. [CrossRef] [PubMed]

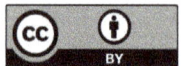

© 2020 by the authors. Licensee MDPI, Basel, Switzerland. This article is an open access article distributed under the terms and conditions of the Creative Commons Attribution (CC BY) license (http://creativecommons.org/licenses/by/4.0/).

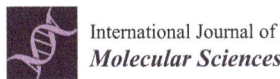

Review

Recent Advances in Psoriasis Research; the Clue to Mysterious Relation to Gut Microbiome

Mayumi Komine [1,2]

[1] Department of Dermatology, Jichi Medical University, 3311-1 Yakushiji, Shimotsuke, Tochigi 329-0498, Japan; mkomine12@jichi.ac.jp; Tel.: +81-285-58-7360
[2] Department of Biochemistry, Jichi Medical University, 3311-1 Yakushiji, Shimotsuke, Tochigi 329-0498, Japan

Received: 29 February 2020; Accepted: 1 April 2020; Published: 8 April 2020

Abstract: Psoriasis is a chronic inflammatory cutaneous disease, characterized by activated plasmacytoid dendritic cells, myeloid dendritic cells, Th17 cells, and hyperproliferating keratinocytes. Recent studies revealed skin-resident cells have pivotal roles in developing psoriatic skin lesions. The balance in effector T cells and regulatory T cells is disturbed, leading Foxp3-positive regulatory T cells to produce proinflammatory IL-17. Not only acquired but also innate immunity is important in psoriasis pathogenesis, especially in triggering the disease. Group 3 innate lymphoid cell are considered one of IL-17-producing cells in psoriasis. Short chain fatty acids produced by gut microbiota stabilize expression of Foxp3 in regulatory T cells, thereby stabilizing their function. The composition of gut microbiota influences the systemic inflammatory status, and associations been shown with diabetes mellitus, cardiovascular diseases, psychomotor diseases, and other systemic inflammatory disorders. Psoriasis has been shown to frequently comorbid with diabetes mellitus, cardiovascular diseases, psychomotor disease and obesity, and recent report suggested the similar abnormality in gut microbiota as the above comorbid diseases. However, the precise mechanism and relation between psoriasis pathogenesis and gut microbiota needs further investigation. This review introduces the recent advances in psoriasis research and tries to provide clues to solve the mysterious relation of psoriasis and gut microbiota.

Keywords: psoriasis; tissue resident cells; innate lymphoid cells; regulatory T cells; Foxp3; gut microbiome; systemic inflammation

1. Introduction

Psoriasis is a chronic inflammatory skin disease, with diverse disease severity and clinical phenotypes. Currently, no curative treatment exists, however, recent advances in therapeutics have made it possible to suppress the disease almost to disappearance. Progress in immunology and molecular biology has dramatically changed understanding of psoriasis pathogenesis, enabling development of novel treatment modalities.

In this review, several recent findings in psoriasis research are reviewed, to support further investigation.

2. Present Understanding of Psoriasis Pathogenesis

Plaque psoriasis is clinically defined as a cutaneous disease with multiple plaques of scaly erythematous lesions. The diagnosis is usually simple with macroscopic findings, but sometimes difficult to differentiate from eczematous, lichenoid, or other conditions. Microscopic investigation is sometimes helpful, but macroscopically difficult cases are also usually difficult to diagnose microscopically. The reason may be that there are heterogeneous clinical groups of psoriasis patients, suggesting that there are heterogenous pathogenetic groups in psoriasis patients. This is supported by the fact certain biologic drugs are efficient in some psoriasis patients but not in others. It has also been postulated that there is mixed pathogenesis of autoimmune and autoinflammatory conditions in psoriasis [1], and the balance of these conditions may differ among patients.

Krueger and Guttman [2] proposed a novel concept which positioned psoriasis and atopic dermatitis at the both ends of the same inflammatory disease spectrum: Psoriasis is located at pure Th17 inflammation, and atopic dermatitis is a combination of Th17, Th2, and Th1 inflammation.

Recent development of biologics for psoriasis treatment produced a novel skin condition, named "paradoxical psoriasis-like eruption" [3]. Paradoxical reactions have been noted for the first time in rheumatoid arthritis patients treated with anti-tumor necrosis factor (TNF) antibodies who developed psoriasis-like skin eruptions. Recently other immunological conditions provoked by targeted biological agents are included in paradoxical reactions, considered "class-effect of targeted biological agents". The interaction between genetically predisposed conditions and targeted biological agents may result in the development of paradoxical reaction development. This itself is of scientific interest, in the context of understanding mechanisms of inflammatory diseases.

The present understanding of psoriasis pathogenesis is summarized in Figure 1. Dendritic cells, T lymphocytes, and keratinocytes are the three major cellular players. Genetic background predisposes patients susceptible to psoriasis: epithelial cells exposed to various stimuli such as bacteria, virus, ultraviolet light, or mechanical stress, leads to apoptosis or necrosis of these cells resulting in exposure of self nucleic acids to tissues [4]. Self DNA bound to LL-37, a part of antimicrobial peptide cathelicidine produced by keratinocytes (KC), stimulating plasmacytoid dendritic cells (pDC) to produce large amount of type I interferons. Simultaneously, self RNA bound to LL-37 stimulate myeloid dendritic cells (mDC) produce tumor necrosis factor alpha (TNFα) and inducible nitric oxide synthase (iNOS). These cytokines produced by DCs stimulate immature T cells to develop into inflammatory T cells, especially Th17 cells, producing interleukin (IL)-17 and IL-22, which develop psoriatic phenotype in KC. KCs produce antimicrobial peptides such as cathelicidine, beta defensine (BD), psoriasin and S100 proteins, chemokines e.g., CXCL1, 2, 8, 10, 11, and CCL20 which attract neutrophils and Th17 cells; and proinflammatory cytokines, such as TNFα, IL-1, and IL-17. These inflammatory reactions cause an inflammatory loop sustaining chronic psoriasis [4].

Recent findings also imply psoriasis inflammation's systemic nature. Obesity's genetic background is distinct from that of psoriasis, however, psoriasis is highly associated with obesity. One explanation is adipose tissue in obese persons produce inflammatory adipocytokines, such as leptin, resistin, and TNFα, leading genetically predisposed patients to develop psoriasis. Increased amount of inflammatory adipocytokines and decreased regulatory adipocytokines have been reported in psoriasis patients, which also correlate with disease severity. This adipocytokine imbalance accelerates insulin resistance and endothelial dysfunction, leading to atherosclerosis and cardiovascular events [5].

3. Tissue Resident Cells

Tissue resident cells have been identified and have focused attention on the possibility of disclosing one of the unsolved mysteries: why systemic inflammation of psoriasis chooses skin and articular as the most involved inflammatory sites.

Clark R. et al. [6] proposed resident memory T cells as pathogenic cells of fixed and recurrent skin lesions of psoriasis. Resident memory T cells are a recently identified T cell subset residing in epithelial barrier tissues such as skin, gut, lung, and reproductive tracts. They are highly protective against pathogens frequently encountered in each tissue. Boyman O et al. [7] in 2004 disclosed that normal appearing, uninvolved skin of psoriasis patients transplanted on immune deficient mice developed psoriatic lesions, indicating that there existed pathogenic skin resident immune cells in non-lesional skin of psoriasis patients. Subsequent studies revealed almost 20 billion T cells reside in healthy human skin, twice as many T cells in the entire blood volume. These skin resident T cells express CD45RO, CLA, and CCR4, and strong effector functions with various T cell receptor (TCR) repertoires.

Large numbers of antigenically active tissue resident T cells have subsequently been disclosed in the gastrointestinal tract, lung, reproductive tract, peritoneum, and bone marrow [8–13].

Clinical trials of anti-E-selectin which completely block the migration of circulating T cells from blood to skin on psoriasis patients revealed its ineffectiveness, suggesting the clue to Tissue resident cell involvement in psoriasis [14]. Another study demonstrating transplanted normal-appearing uninvolved skin of psoriasis patients on immunodeficient mice developed psoriasis lesions suggested psoriasis patients' normal-appearing skin contains pathogenic cells which can develop psoriasis lesions without the circulating blood cells [7]. Subsequent studies revealed CD4-positive T cells with IL-22 and CD8-positive T cells producing IL-17 remained resident in previously involved psoriasis lesions after complete clinical resolution from a variety of treatments [15,16].

Gallais serezal I et al. [17] proposed a skewed pool of resident T cells in psoriasis patients trigger non-lesional skin of psoriasis patients to develop psoriasis lesion. They collected never lesional psoriasis (NLP) skin from mild psoriasis patients instead of from severe psoriasis, because in severe psoriasis, patients' uninvolved skin shows psoriatic gene expression profiles. These NLP with normal gene expression profiles exhibited IL-17- and IFN-γ-producing T cell accumulation after stimulation, which triggers keratinocytes to produce IFNα introducing an alternative source of Type I interferons in initiation of psoriasis. Their analysis revealed skewed T cell population in NLP with CD8-positive CD49a-negative T cells, and CCR6-positive T cells producing IL-22, IL-17, and IFNγ. NLP keratinocytes produce increased amounts of CCL20 upon stimulation with *Candida albicans* or mannan suggesting the role of KC, weakly stimulated by resident fungi, in accumulation of IL-17 and IL-22 producing CCR6-positive resident T cells in NLP skin of psoriasis patients. Resident T cells are insufficient to develop psoriasis lesions, but upon stimulation with various stimuli, such as mechanical stress, viral infection, and bacterial infection, these skewed population of resident memory T cells produce inflammatory cytokines, such as IL-17, IL-22, and IFNγ, which initiate psoriasis inflammation (Figure 2). Their study also demonstrated for the first time the role of KC in production of IFNα in psoriasis pathogenesis.

4. Innate Lymphoid Cells

Innate lymphoid cells (ILCs) are recently identified innate immune cells. They were found among lineage-negative cell populations not expressing any mature cell markers, such as Mac-1 for myeloid cells, CD4 and CD8 for T cells, CD19 for B cells, or Ter-119 for erythrocytes. They have a high potency for cytokine production without specific antigen stimulation [18]. Psoriasis has been considered an "autoimmune" disease; however, no specific antigens have been identified so far. The innate immune system is a relatively primitive immune system, directly activated by components of virus, bacteria, fungi, or self-DNAs and RNAs, without specific antigens. Many cell types were included in innate immune cells, such as neutrophils, mast cells, and natural killer cells as well as innate lymphoid cells. It is not surprising that these innate immune cells take part in psoriasis pathogenesis.

ILCs have been subdivided into three groups: ILC1, ILC2, and ILC3. ILC1 (group 1 ILC) characteristically produces IFN gamma, perforin, and granzyme, while ILC2 (group 2 ILC) produces IL-5, IL-13, and IL-4, with nuclear expression of GATA3. ILC3 (group 3 ILC) expresses IL-7Rα, matures with IL-7 and IL-23, and produces IL-17, IL-22, and lymphotoxin with nuclear expression of RORγt [18,19]. ILC3 in humans is further divided into three subsets on the basis of expression of natural cytotoxicity receptors: NKp44, NKp46, and NKp30. NKp44-positive ILC3 produces IL-22 and is dependent on aryl hydrocarbon receptor (AhR). NKp44-negative ILC3 produces IL-17A following stimulation, but NKp44-negative ILC3s have plasticity, and they are able to develop into NKp44-positive ILC3s or into ILC1s with IFNγ production [20]. In inflammatory bowel diseases, ILC3s have been shown to produce IL-17 in the gut [21]. Therefore, the world of ILCs looks as if it were the parallel world of helper T cells (Figure 3).

Soare A et al. [22] reported increased numbers of ILC3 exist in the circulating blood of psoriatic arthritis patients, and ILC3/ILC2 ratios correlated well with disease severity. ILC3 also increased in the lesional and non-lesional skin of psoriasis patients. Keren A et al. [23] revealed that injection of NKp44-positive ILC3 without T cells was able to develop psoriatic skin eruption in SCID mice with implantation of healthy human skin.

These results indicate that ILC3 may have a pathogenic role in psoriasis, which compensates the absence of specific self-antigen.

5. Regulatory T Cells

Regulatory T cells (Treg) have immune suppressive function to suppress excess immunity against a diverse range of antigens, such as self-antigens, commensal bacteria-derived antigens, and environmental allergens. Many autoimmune and inflammatory diseases, such as systemic erythematosus, inflammatory bowel diseases, and rheumatoid arthritis, show decreased Treg numbers and function. Foxp3 (Forkhead box P3) is a transcription factor playing a crucial role in development, maintenance and function of Tregs. Deficiency of Foxp3 results in lack of Tregs, and causes severe systemic inflammatory diseases characterized by autoimmunity, colitis, and allergies.

Tregs usually develop in the thymus from CD4−, CD8−, double negative thymocytes, called thymus-derived regulatory T cells (tTregs) or natural occurring Tregs (nTregs). Expression of Foxp3 are strongly induced through T cell receptor (TCR) signals after the recognition of self-antigen-MHC complex present on antigen presenting cells (APCs). tTregs are believed to comprise most of the systemic Treg population. A second subset of Tregs is induced in the peripheral tissues from CD4-positive naïve T cells by stimulation with cytokine combination, such as TGFβ and IL-2. This type of Tregs is called induced Tregs (iTregs) or peripherally induced Tregs (pTregs). iTregs usually represent Tregs induced in vitro, while pTregs indicates Tregs developed from naïve T cells in vivo.

tTregs matured in thymus have constitutive and stable expression of Foxp3, supported by the binding of several transcription factors to its corresponding promoter and enhancer regions. Several enhancer regions are identified, designated as conserved non-coding sequences (CNS) 1, 2, and 3, and CNS0 has recently been identified upstream of CNS1 [24].

Promoter region and each CNS binds specific transcription factors, which regulate the expression of Foxp3.

The most fundamental transcription factor for Foxp3 expression may be the recently identified Satb1, which binds to CNS0 inducing both transcriptional and epigenetic regulation. Satb1 binds to CNS0 at the beginning of Treg commitment and serves as a pioneering element involved in the transcriptional regulation sequence in Treg development. Nr4a is a transcription factor which binds to CNS2 and the promoter region of Foxp3, necessary for both pTerg and tTreg development. TCR activation induces Nr4a expression, which is essential for pTreg and tTreg development and maintenance after TCR activation. IL-2 and TGFβ are well-known inducers of Tregs, and IL-2 is essential in inducing both tTregs and pTregs, while TGFβ is needed in pTreg development. STAT5 is activated downstream of IL-2R, and STAT5 response elements exist in CNS2 and Foxp3 promoter region. CNS1 contains binding sites for Smads, NFAT, AP-1, and retinoic acid receptor (RAR). Smad2 and Smad3 are redundantly essential for development of iTregs/pTregs in the downstream of TGFβ. CNS2 region contains biding sites for multiple transcription factors, such as STAT5, NFAT, Runx1/Cbfβ, CREB, and Foxp3. This enhancer is very important in maintaining its own expression under inflammatory circumstances where Tregs are subjected to inflammatory cytokines and stronger TCR stimulation. CNS2 locus has multiple CpG sites making this region susceptible for methylation/demethylation status. In tTregs, CNS2 is fully demethylated: full sets of transcription factors bind to this locus enabling stable expression of Foxp3, and stable phenotype of tTregs. In pTregs, CNS2 locus is also demethylated, but with a slightly lower stability compared to tTregs. In iTregs, CNS2 locus is rarely demethylated, which makes this subset very unstable. This CNS2 locus is the major Treg-specific demethylated resion (TSDR) whose demethylated status confers the stability of Foxp3 expression, and the function of Tregs [25] (Figure 4).

The inducers and stabilizers of Foxp3 expression are summarized in Table 1.

Table 1. Factors which induce or stabilize Foxp3 expression.

Factors	Mechanism
Retinoic acids	Binding to *Foxp3* enhancer CNS1 through RAR
Progesterone	Suppression of mTOR
Vitamine D3	Binding to *Foxp3* enhancer CNS1 through VDR
Short chain fatty acids	Activation of GPR43
Butyrates	Inhibition of HDAC
Vitamine C	Activation of TET enzymes
Hydrogen sulfide	Induction of TET1 and TET2
Rapamycin	Inhibition of mTOR
JAK1 inhibitor	Suppression of Th17
AhR ligands	Suppression of Th17

Modified from Kanamori M. et al. Trends in Immunol 2016 [24].

Retinoic acids and vitamin D3 are ligands for their specific nuclear receptors, retinoic acid receptor (RAR), retinoid X receptor (RXR), and vitamin D receptor (VDR). Retinoids binds to RARs and/or RXRs, which make homo or heterodimers to bind to their binding sequences in regulatory region in the target genes. Butyrate induces retinoic acid production in gut dendritic cells, resulting in induction and stabilization of Foxp3 expression in regulatory T cells.

Active form of vitamin D3, generated through the enzymes produced in skin or in liver and kidney, binds to VDR, which makes heterodimers with RXR and binds to response element usually resides in distal area of target genes and exert its functions. Ultraviolet (UV) B and antimicrobial peptides, such as cathelicidin and S100 proteins, are inducers of active vitamin D3 production in epidermis. Active vitamin D3 systemically distribute through blood flow binding to vitamin D binding protein (DBP), enter target cells through binding to heat shock protein (HSP) 70 in cytoplasm, and finally transported to the nucleus binding to VDR [26]. VDR binds to its binding site in enhancer regions of Foxp3 gene, resulting in induction and stabilization of Foxp3 expression. Alternative receptors other than VDR have been reported, such as retinoid orphan receptor (ROR)α, RORγ [27], and aryl hydrocarbon receptor (AhR) [28]. By binding to these alternative receptors, vitamin D3 derivatives have been reported to suppress inflammatory reactions, such as Th17-type inflammation, through suppressing the transactivation function of these nuclear receptors [27].

pTregs are induced by CD103-positive dendritic cells (DCs) in mesenteric lymph nodes dependent on TGFβ and retinoic acid. Cutaneous CD103-positive DCs have also been reported to induce pTregs [29]. Recent report indicated that DCs in cervical lymph nodes induce Tregs, but are not CD103-positive DCs [30,31].

Recently, Gagliani et al. [32] reported intestinal Th17 can lose the ability to produce IL-17 and behave like regulatory T cells resembling CD4+Foxp3- Type 1 Tregs (Tr1). This functional reprogramming is irreversible, and these transdifferentiated Tr1 cells show anti-inflammatory properties and suppress Th17-mediated colitis.

Psoriasis patients have a decreased number of regulatory T cells with disturbed function. Several reports indicated that successful treatment of psoriasis restored the function and number of Tregs in peripheral blood [33,34]. Bovenschen [35] reported that Foxp3-positive regulatory T cells are easily converted into Foxp3-low, IL-17 producing, and RORγt-expressing cells. The plasticity of Treg/Th17 cells makes pathophysiology of the disease more complex (Figure 5).

6. Microbiome

Advancement in computer science and next generation sequencing (NGS) technique has enabled analysis of huge amounts of genetic data at once, revealing composition of microorganisms without culture. High throughput 16S rRNA sequencing of gut microbial populations or total genome sequencing and mass-spectrometry-based metabolomic analysis can characterize gut microbiome and metabolites. Gut microbiota is a dense and diverse microbial community composed of more than 100 trillion cells and 5 million genes over 3-fold and 100-fold more than host cells and genes. Gut microbiota is composed of thousands of species. However, the majority belong to six bacterial phyla: *Actinobacteria*, *Bacteroides*, *Firmicutes*, *Fusobacteria*, *Proteobacteria*, and *Verrucomicrobia*. Fungi, Archaea, protozoa, and viruses are also included in gut microbiota. The composition of microbiota is highly influenced by environmental factors such as food, drug, and hygiene conditions, and also dependent on age and genetic background. Microbiota functions as natural digestive organs, as they digest plant polysaccharides indigestible by the host, can biosynthesize essential amino acids and vitamins, and also detoxicate hazardous materials. Recent studies revealed they also have important roles in immune system development and resistance to pathogens. Biotransformation of drugs can occur through gut microbiota altering the effects of drugs expected in vitro studies or catalyzing them to cause undesirable effects. Human genome analysis has revealed genetic susceptibility to certain diseases, and analysis of microbiota as a "second genome" would reveal more important information for disease susceptibility and drug metabolism. Further studies on gut microbiota are needed to understand the precise mechanisms in disease susceptibility variance and drug effects and side effects profiles between individuals. Such research could enhance development of precision medicine [36].

Recent studies linked cardiac disease, insulin resistance, and metabolic syndrome to gut microbiota [37,38]. Several reports supported the contribution of gut microbiota in the production of TMA (trimethylamine), the precursor of TMAO (trimethylamine N-oxide), which is a known proatherogenic molecule independent of traditional cardiovascular disease (CVD) risk factors. TMAO is involved in host cholesterol metabolism and activates macrophages leading to increased risk of CVD, myocardial infarction, and stroke. Higher TMAO producers had more *Firmicutes* than *Bacteroides* within the stool. TMAO has also been suggested to be a candidate molecule of developing type 2 diabetes mellitus (DM). Dietary supplementation with TMAO in mice resulted in impaired glucose tolerance and adipose tissue inflammation promotion. Crasiun and Balskus reported that *cutC* gene expression by bacteria such as *Disulfovibrio* can cause increased conversion of choline to TMA. Compared to healthy controls, phyla *Bacteroides* and *Proteobacteria* were reduced and phyla *Firmicutes* and *Fusobacteria* were increased in coronary artery diseases (CAD) patients [39]. Similar results were reported revealing decrease in phylum *Bacteroides* and increase in phylum *Firmicutes* in CAD patients [40]. Sanchez-Alcoholado et al. [36] compared CAD patients with type 2 DM to CAD patients without type 2 DM and revealed these two groups had different composition of gut microbiota. CAD patients with type 2 DM had decreased phylum *Bacteroides* and increased phyla *Firmicutes* and *Proteobacteria*. They also revealed plasma TMAO levels were significantly higher in CAD with DM patients compared to CAD without DM patients, which correlated with the increase in phyla *Enterobacteriaceae* and *Desulfovibrio* and a decrease in phylum *Faecalibacterium*.

Obesity is related to gut dysbiosis and increased gut permeability, resulting in abnormal translocation of bacteria and bacterial component in blood circulation. The increase in gut barrier permeability caused increase in blood lipopolysaccharide (LPS) levels, resulting in systemic low-grade inflammation and metabolic disease including type 2 diabetes [41]. Glucagon-like protein (GLP) 2 is produced by L cells in the gut, which is regulated by the host nutritional status, and increases nutrient absorption. It induces gut epithelial cell proliferation and expression of tight junction proteins. It also regulates production of antimicrobial peptides by Paneth cells. Gut microbiota in lean individuals have been reported to induce endogenous GLP2 production, resulting in improvement in gut barrier function, while that of obese patients suppresses GLP2 production leading to gut barrier impairment and bacterial translocation in blood [42].

Zonulin is a protein modulating permeability of tight junctions in the digestive tract. It was originally discovered in patients with Celiac disease and type 1 diabetes. Zonulin binds to its receptor and activates the pathway of tight junction openings resulting in increased gut permeability. Increased permeability in gut epithelial tissues leads to increased passage of antigens, and triggers autoimmunity in susceptible individuals. Recent study reported gliadin binds to CXCR3 triggering the release of zonulin. Zonulin activates PKC and PLC resulting in actin poymelization and rearrangement of cytoskeleton inducing loosening of tight junctions in a reversible manner. Increased serum level and increased excretion in the feces of zonulin have been reported in patients with gut barrier disruption, such as patients with Celiac disease, as well as type-1 diabetes, obesity, and non-alcoholic fatty liver disease [43].

Activated effector cells are anabolic, consuming glucose as their carbon source, and utilizing glycolysis to obtain ATP. Memory and regulatory cells are catabolic, utilizing fatty acids, amino acids, as well as glucose for their energy source, and utilize oxidative phosphorylation to obtain ATP. Key molecules promoting the glycolytic and lipogenic pathway are mammalian target of Rapamycin (mTOR) and adenosine monophosphate-activated kinase (AMPK). AMPK and mTOR are energy sensors regulated by nutrients availability. Th17 cells depend on glycolytic-lipogenic pathway and fatty acid synthesis for their development, while Tregs depend on oxidative phosphorylation and consume exogenous fatty acids. HIF1α is the transcription factor which upregulates glycolytic pathway in Th17 cells binding to RORγt promoter and enhancing its expression, while also suppressing Foxp3 expression. It promotes differentiation of naïve T cells towards Th17 cells and inhibits differentiation into Treg cells under normoxic and hypoxic conditions. Inflammation sites are usually in hypoxic condition and show increased extracellular ATP concentration, which induces HIF1αactivation required for Th17 cell development, and AhR inactivation needed in Tr1 metabolism. Thus, metabolic factors have immune-modifying ability by skewing Th17/Treg balance resulting in skewed balance in inflammation or immune tolerance [44].

Gut microbiota profoundly affect T cell differentiation and response to immune stimuli. Segmented filamentous bacteria (SFB), a *Clostridia*-related species found mainly in rodents, specifically induces Th17 cells in the small intestine and other sites in autoimmune condition. SFB colonization is usually beneficial because it attenuates bacteria-induced colitis, while it also induces colitis in genetically susceptible mice strains. The abundance of SFB and the gut barrier function is regulated by IL-23R/IL-22 pathway. The disruption of gut barrier resulting in systemic distribution of bacteria or their components induces IL-23 pathway, initiating barrier repair, and Th17 responses in order to neutralize invading microbes. IL-23 induced by SFB stimulates production of IL-22 from ILC3 causing serum amyloid A production by epithelial cells [45] (Figure 6).

Psoriasis is considered a systemic and chronic inflammatory disease, involving skin, as well as the cardiovascular system, insulin homeostasis, psychomotor systems, and lipid metabolism. A recent study has detected bacterial DNA in blood in active psoriasis patients (bacterial translocation; BT), and those with bacterial DNA-positive psoriasis patients showed higher serum inflammatory cytokine levels, longer duration of disease and younger onset of disease. They suggested that psoriasis eruption may be related to bacterial DNA in blood originating in the gut [46]. Codoner et al. revealed phylum *Bacteroides* decreased and phylum *Faecalibacterium* increased in psoriasis patients. They compared the microbiome between BT-positive patients and BT-negative patients and did not find specific phyla of microbiome. They speculated that dysbiosis in psoriasis patient guts caused insufficient gut barrier permeability resulting in bacterial translocation into the blood stream [47]. Hidalgo-Cantabrana et al. reported recently the increase in *Bacteroides* and decrease in *Firmicutes* in psoriasis patients compared to healthy controls [48].

Bacteroides can produce short chain fatty acids (SCFA) such as propionates and butyrates. These SCFA bind to the G-protein-coupled receptor, GPR41 and GPR43, and induce GLP-1 and GLP-2 production in L cells, which influence the energy metabolism and improve gut barrier function [49]. *Akkermansia muciniphila* has also been suggested to produce SCFA to improve energy metabolism, which are decreased in obese patients compared to healthy controls. SCFA are also involved in the stabilization of Foxp3 expression as discussed above, resulting in improvement of regulatory T cell function. GPR41 and GPR43, the receptors for SCFA, are expressed on the surface of regulatory T cells distributed in the gut. The number of Tregs increased in mice supplemented with SCFA. Experimentally induced autoimmune encephalomyelitis was suppressed in mice supplemented with SCFA [49].

Scher et al. [50] reported gut microbiota composition was different in psoriatic arthritis patients and psoriasis without arthritis patients. They found that phylum *Actinobacteria* was significantly decreased in psoriatic arthritis patients. *Actinobacteria* phylum includes *Bifidobacterium* species, of which supplementation lowered the serum levels of CRP and TNFαa in psoriasis patients.

Another approach altering the gut microbial effect is to influence the pathway the microbiome uses. Farnesoid X receptor (FXR) is the essential nuclear receptor whose antagonist can inhibit high-fat diet-induced obesity in mice. FXR is involved in the metabolism of bile acid, lipid, and glucose. Intestine-specific FXR knockout mice were resistant to high-fat diet-induced obesity. However, contradictory results have been reported: FXR-null mice showed increased glucose intolerance on a chow diet, and FXR-agonist was effective in improving insulin sensitivity in genetically obese mice. Other studies presented that FXR-null mice showed increased glucose tolerance and FXR-agonist exacerbated insulin resistance and lipid metabolism in obese mice models. Li et al. speculated this discrepancy is due to differences in gut microbiota composition and the distinct roles of liver FXR and intestine FXR. Their study provided evidence that FXR inhibition in the intestine by antioxidant "tempol" or by genetic ablation of FXR is effective in suppressing diet-induced obesity and insulin resistance [51,52]. Other molecules in the context of microbiome signaling are peroxisome proliferator activated receptor (PPAR)s. Gut microbiota influence the expression of PPARs, and PPARs transduce signals to induce or suppress many molecules involved in inflammation, obesity, and insulin resistance [53].

7. Discussion and Conclusions

Many novel findings revealed the importance of innate immunity in psoriasis pathogenesis. The roles of skin resident cells and Tregs have been drawing attention in psoriasis pathogenesis. Epidemiological study revealed the relation between psoriasis and comorbid diseases such as cardiovascular diseases, diabetes mellitus and obesity, and the gut dysbiosis in psoriasis patients has recently been demonstrated. However, the underling mechanism and pathogenic roles of gut microbiome has to be clarified further. This review tried to hunt the findings in basic science and in metabolic diseases, and to combine them to be applied to future psoriasis research.

It is not clear whether dysbiosis in gut microbiota in psoriasis patients has the pathogenic roles or just the result of systemic inflammation in psoriasis. However, the recent study on gut microbiota and the immune regulatory mechanism suggests that dysbiosis in gut microbiota by inducing disfunction of Tregs and activation of Th17 and ILC3 could lead genetically susceptible individuals to develop psoriasis. It may also cause obesity, diabetes mellitus, and cardiovascular diseases, among individuals with distinct genetic backgrounds. The increase in number of psoriasis patients in Japan with westernization of life could be explained by the change of diet, resulting in a change in microbiota. Decrease of dietary fibers may reduce SCFA-producing phyla in gut microbiota, resulting in activation of gut dendritic cells to produce IL-23, which in turn may stimulate unstable Foxp3-positive Tregs to differentiate into IL-17-producing cells. Psoriasis has been recognized as a multifactorial genetic disease, not only depending on genetic background, but also on environmental factors including lifestyle habits, which could also be well-explained.

Skewed balance of skin resident cells may be generated by activation of epidermal keratinocytes producing slightly higher amount of CCL20 by commensal microbe stimulation in genetically susceptible individuals, which could be enhanced under the environment of disturbed Treg function and increased Th17 cytokines in individuals with dysbiosis.

In this review, the gut–skin axis is the main target of discussion, thus skin-specific cells, such as epidermal keratinocytes and dermal fibroblasts, are not discussed. The nuclear receptors such as RARs, VDR, and RORs are expressed not only in immune cells, but also in epidermal keratinocytes [26], making the epidermal keratinocytes another target of immune regulation. Skin has its own microbiome, through influencing the homeostasis of epidermis, it regulates the immune status of the whole body. The discussion on these issues have been left at another opportunity.

Systemic inflammation in psoriasis patients has led researchers to investigate the relation of psoriasis to metabolic diseases and has significantly deepened recent psoriasis investigation. A systemic approach to treat psoriasis has long been attempted with etretinate and cyclosporine, and recent biologics have shown remarkable therapeutic effects. Knowledge in skin resident cells are preferential to topical treatment, however, accumulating evidence in the gut–skin axis [54] would favor a nutritional approach or signal inhibition to change microbiome composition. Therefore, increasing therapeutic options may be available for future psoriasis treatment.

8. Figures, Tables, and Schemes

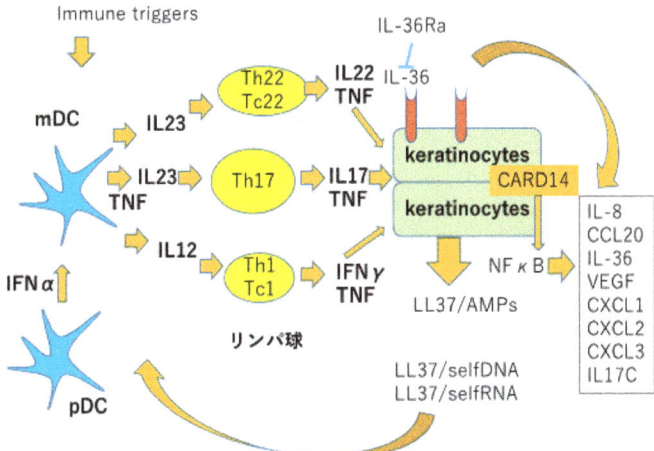

Figure 1. Pathogenesis of psoriasis. Modified from Lowes M.A. et al. Trends in Immunol 2016 [4].

External immune triggers, LL37 bound to self-DNA or RNA activate plasmacytoid and myeloid dendritic cells (pDC and mDC). Activated plasmacytoid cells produce type 1 interferons, and myeloid dendritic cells produce TNFα, iNOS, and IL-23, which activate Th17 cells to produce IL-17 and IL-22. IL-17 and IL-22 induce proliferation, production of cytokines, chemokines and antimicrobial peptides from epidermal keratinocytes, thus resulting in psoriatic phenotype.

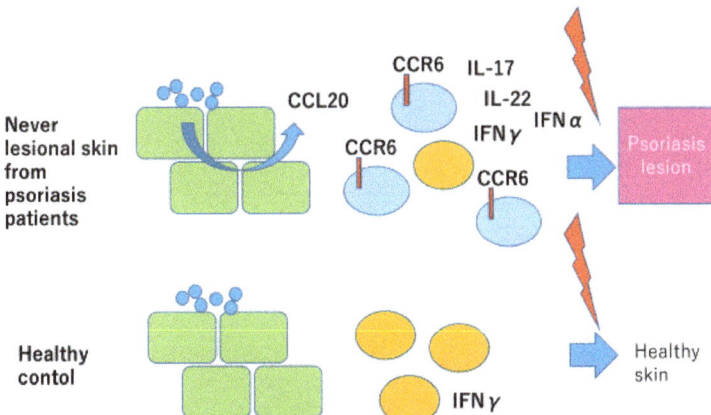

Figure 2. Skewed balance of tissue resident immune cells induces psoriasis in never-lesional skin of psoriasis patients. Modified from Gallais Sérézal I et al. J Allergy Clin Immunol 2018 [17].

Weak stimulation by commensal bacteria and fungi causes sparse production of CCL20 from the epidermal keratinocytes, resulting in skewed distribution of CCR6-positive, IL-17-producing cells in the never-lesional skin of psoriasis patients (NLP) over IFNγ-producing cells, which prepare conditions for psoriasis eruption when appropriate insults, such as bacterial or viral infection, or trauma occurs.

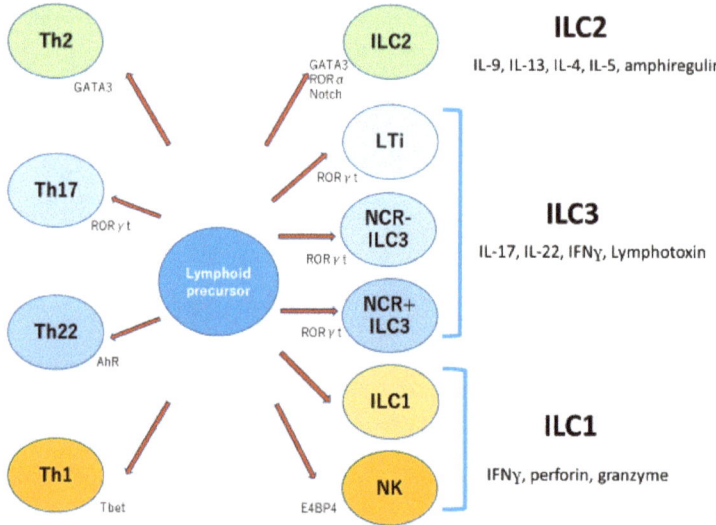

Figure 3. Three groups of innate lymphoid cells parallel three types of T helper cells. Modified from Walker JA et al. Nat Rev Immunol 2013 [18].

Innate lymphoid cells are divided into three groups; group 1, 2, and 3. Function and essential nuclear factors seem similar to those of corresponding T helper cells.

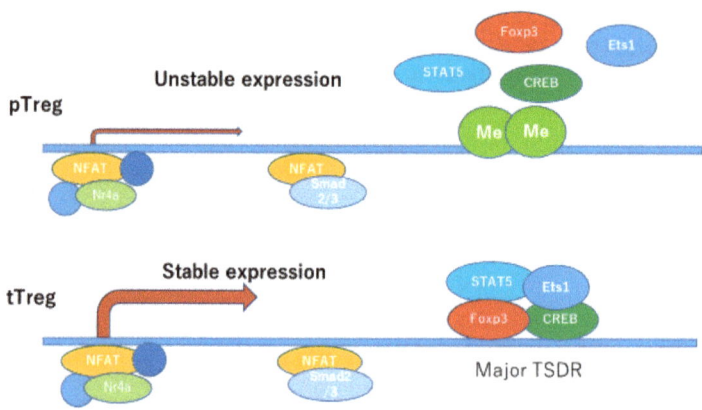

Figure 4. Expression of FOXP3 in pTreg is unstable. Modified from Kanamori M et al. Trends in Immunol 2016, and Iizuka-Koga et al. J Autoimmun 2017 [24,25].

Promoter lesion of FOXP3 gene contains major Treg-specific demethylated resion (TSDR), which binds transcription factors, such as FOXP3, CREB, Ets1, and STAT5 constitutively in tTregs, but just transiently in pTregs. TSDR in pTregs are partially methylated, which makes it difficult to bind transcription factors needed for the stable expression of FOXP3.

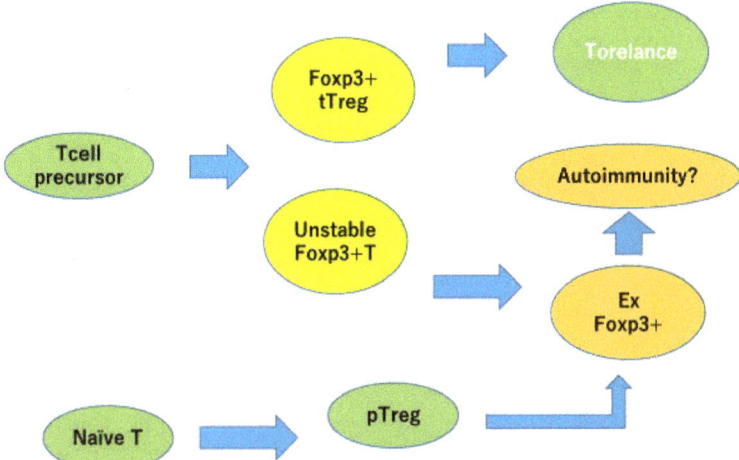

Figure 5. Foxp3-positive Tregs, but with unstable expression, would easily lose FOXP3 expression and become inflammatory. Modified from Iizuka-Koga M et al. J Autoimmun 2017 [25].

tTregs differentiated in thymus stably express FOXP3 and are involved in immune tolerance. Peripherally induced Tregs and Tregs with unstable FOXP3 expression can lose FOXP3 expression and become inflammatory cells, which may contribute to autoimmunity.

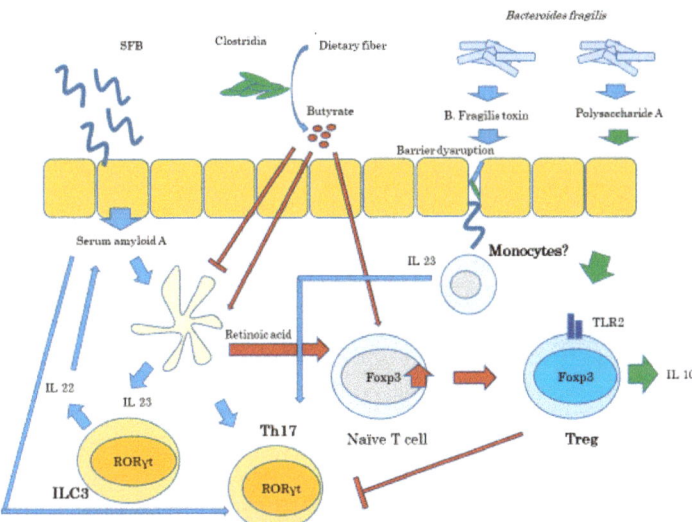

Figure 6. Gut microbiota regulates the balance of Th17 vs. Tregs. Modified from Omenetti S and Pizzaro TT. Frontiers Immuno 2015 [43].

Segmented filamentous bacteria (SFB) colonization allow them to closely contact to intestinal epithelium, which induce cytokines, such as serum amyloid A (SAA), and activate Th17. SAA also induces IL-23 production from dendritic cells, which indirectly activate Th17 and ILC3 to produce pro-inflammatory IL-17, and IL-22. IL-22 stimulate intestinal epithelial cells to produce SAA.

Clostridia is one of the commensal bacteria in the gut, which ferment dietary fibers and produce short chain fatty acids; butyrates. SCFA suppresses dendritic cell production of inflammatory cytokines, such as IL-6, and also induces retinoic acid (RA) production from dendritic cells, which induces and stabilizes FOXP3 expression in naïve Tcells. SCFA also directly act on naïve T cells to express FOXP3.

There are different strains of *Bacteroides fragilis*, one of which produces polysaccharide A (PSA) and induce IL-10 production from Treg cells, thereby inducing immune suppression. The other strain produces B. fragilis toxin (BFA), which causes impairment of tight junctions and disruption of intestinal barrier function. Recognition of microbial products from disseminated bacteria by microbe associated molecular patterns stimulates IL-23 production from monocytes and stimulates Th17 cells to produce IL-17 and exacerbates inflammation.

Author Contributions: M.K. contributed to reading and writing the whole manuscript and drawing the figures. All authors have read and agreed to the published version of the manuscript.

Funding: This research received no external funding.

Conflicts of Interest: The author declares no conflict of interest.

Abbreviations

IL	Interleukin
Th	T helper
DNA	Deoxy ribonucleic acid
RNA	Ribonucleic acid
CCL	CC chemokine ligand
CXCL	CXC chemokine ligand
CCR	CC chemokine receptor
CXCR	CXC chemokine receptor
TGFβ	Transforming growth factor beta
STAT	Signal transducers and activators of transcription
NFAT	Nuclear factor for activated T cells
AP-1	Activator protein 1
CREB	cAMP response element bunding protein
PKC	Protein kinase C
PLC	Phospholipase C
ATP	Adenosine triphosphate
HIF1	Hypoxia inducible factor
ROR	RAR-related orphan receptor
GATA	GATA binding protein
GPR	G-protein coupled receptor
CRP	C reactive protein
TCR	T cell receptor
CLA	Cutaneous lymphocyte associated antigen
IFN	Interferon
NK	Natural killer

References

1. Liang, Y.; Sarkar, M.K.; Tsoi, L.C.; Gudjonsson, J.E. Psoriasis: A mixed autoimmune and autoinflammatory disease. *Curr. Opin. Immunol.* **2017**, *49*, 1–8. [CrossRef] [PubMed]
2. Guttman-Yassky, E.; Krueger, J.G. Atopic dermatitis and psoriasis: Two different immune diseases or one spectrum? *Curr. Opin. Immunol.* **2017**, *48*, 68–73. [CrossRef] [PubMed]

3. Moy, A.P.; Murali, M.; Kroshinsky, D.; Horn, T.D.; Nazarian, R.M. T-helper immune phenotype may underlie 'paradoxical' tumour necrosis factor-α inhibitor therapy-related psoriasiform dermatitis. *Clin. Exp. Derm.* **2018**, *43*, 19–26. [CrossRef] [PubMed]
4. Lowes, M.A.; Russell, C.B.; Martin, D.A.; Towne, J.E.; Krueger, J.G. The IL-23/T17 pathogenic axis in psoriasis is amplified by keratinocyte responses. *Trends Immunol.* **2013**, *34*, 174–181. [CrossRef]
5. Jensen, P.; Skov, L. Psoriasis and Obesity. *Dermatology* **2016**, *232*, 633–639. [CrossRef]
6. Clark, R.A. Resident memory T cells in human health and disease. *Sci. Transl. Med.* **2015**, *7*, 269rv1. [CrossRef]
7. Boyman, O.; Hefti, H.P.; Conrad, C.; Nickoloff, B.J.; Suter, M.; Nestle, F.O. Spontaneous development of psoriasis in a new animal model shows an essential role for resident T cells and tumor necrosis factor-alpha. *J. Exp. Med.* **2004**, *199*, 731–736. [CrossRef]
8. Clark, R.A.; Chong, B.; Mirchandani, N.; Brinster, N.K.; Yamanaka, K.; Dowgiert, R.K.; Kupper, T.S. The vast majority of CLA+ T cells are resident in normal skin. *J. Immunol.* **2006**, *176*, 4431. [CrossRef]
9. Booth, J.S.; Toapanta, F.R.; Salerno-Goncalves, R.; Patil, S.; Kader, H.A.; Safta, A.M.; Czinn, S.J.; Greenwald, B.D.; Sztein, M.B. Characterization and functional properties of gastric tissue-resident memory T cells from children, adults, and the elderly. *Front. Immunol.* **2014**, *5*, 294. [CrossRef]
10. Okhrimenko, A.; Grün, J.R.; Westendorf, K.; Fang, Z.; Reinke, S.; von Roth, P.; Wassilew, G.; Kühl, A.A.; Kudernatsch, R.; Demski, S.; et al. Human memory T cells from the bone marrow are resting and maintain long-lasting systemic memory. *Proc. Nat. Acad. Sci.* **2014**, *111*, 9229–9234. [CrossRef]
11. Turner, D.L.; Bickham, K.L.; Thome, J.J.; Kim, C.Y.; D'Ovidio, F.; Wherry, E.J.; Farber, D.L. Lung niches for the generation and maintenance of tissue-resident memory T cells. *Mucosal Immunol.* **2014**, *7*, 501–510. [CrossRef] [PubMed]
12. Roberts, G.W.; Baird, D.; Gallagher, K.; Jones, R.E.; Pepper, C.J.; Williams, J.D.; Topley, N. Functional effector memory T cells enrich the peritoneal cavity of patients treated with peritoneal dialysis. *J. Am. Soc. Nephrol.* **2009**, *20*, 1895–1900. [CrossRef] [PubMed]
13. Purwar, R.; Campbell, J.; Murphy, G.; Richards, W.G.; Clark, R.A.; Kupper, T.S. Resident Memory T Cells (T(RM)) Are Abundant in Human Lung: Diversity, Function, and Antigen Specificity. *PLoS ONE* **2011**, *6*, e16245. [CrossRef] [PubMed]
14. Bhushan, M.; Bleiker, T.O.; Ballsdon, A.E.; Allen, M.H.; Sopwith, M.; Robinson, M.K.; Clarke, C.; Weller, R.P.; Graham-Brown, R.A.; Keefe, M.; et al. Anti-E-selectin is ineffective in the treatment of psoriasis: A randomized trial. *Br. J. Dermatol.* **2002**, *146*, 824–831. [CrossRef] [PubMed]
15. Cheuk, S.; Wikén, M.; Blomqvist, L.; Nylén, S.; Talme, T.; Ståhle, M.; Eidsmo, L. Epidermal Th22 and Tc17 cells form a localized disease memory in clinically healed psoriasis. *J. Immunol.* **2014**, *192*, 3111–3120. [CrossRef] [PubMed]
16. Matos, T.R.; O'Malley, J.T.; Lowry, E.L.; Hamm, D.; Kirsch, I.R.; Robins, H.S.; Kupper, T.S.; Krueger, J.G.; Clark, R.A. Clinically resolved psoriatic lesions contain psoriasis-specific IL-17-producing αβ T cell clones. *J. Clin. Invest.* **2017**, *127*, 4031–4041. [CrossRef] [PubMed]
17. Gallais Sérézal, I.; Hoffer, E.; Ignatov, B.; Martini, E.; Zitti, B.; Ehrström, M.; Eidsmo, L. A skewed pool of resident T cells triggers psoriasis-associated tissue responses in never-lesional skin from patients with psoriasis. *J. Allergy Clin. Immunol.* **2019**, *143*, 1444–1454. [CrossRef]
18. Walker, J.A.; Barlow, J.L.; McKenzie, A.N. Innate lymphoid cells–how did we miss them? *Nat. Rev. Immunol.* **2013**, *13*, 75–87. [CrossRef]
19. Bernink, J.H.; Peters, C.P.; Munneke, M.; te Velde, A.A.; Meijer, S.L.; Weijer, K.; Hreggvidsdottir, H.S.; Heinsbroek, S.E.; Legrand, N.; Buskens, C.J.; et al. Human type 1 lymphoid cells accumulate in inflamed mucosal tissues. *Nat. Immunol.* **2013**, *14*, 221–229. [CrossRef]
20. Villanova, F.; Flutter, B.; Tosi, I.; Grys, K.; Sreeneebus, H.; Perera, G.K.; Chapman, A.; Smith, C.H.; Di Meglio, P.; Nestle, F.O. Characterization of innate lymphoid cells in human skin and blood demonstrates increase of NKp44+ ILC3 in psoriasis. *J. Investig. Derm.* **2014**, *134*, 984–991. [CrossRef]
21. Zeng, B.; Shi, S.; Ashworth, G.; Dong, C.; Liu, J.; Xing, F. ILC3 function as a double-edged sword in inflammatory bowel diseases. *Cell Death Dis.* **2019**, *10*, 315. [CrossRef] [PubMed]
22. Soare, A.; Weber, S.; Maul, L.; Rauber, S.; Gheorghiu, A.M.; Luber, M.; Houssni, I.; Kleyer, A.; von Pickardt, G.; Gado, M.; et al. Cutting Edge: Homeostasis of Innate Lymphoid Cells Is Imbalanced in Psoriatic Arthritis. *J. Immunol.* **2018**, *200*, 1249–1254. [CrossRef] [PubMed]

23. Keren, A.; Shemer, A.; Ginzburg, A.; Ullmann, Y.; Schrum, A.G.; Paus, R.; Gilhar, A. Innate lymphoid cells 3 induce psoriasis in xenotransplanted healthy human skin. *J. Allergy Clin. Immunol.* **2018**, *142*, 305–308.e6. [CrossRef] [PubMed]

24. Kanamori, M.; Nakatsukasa, H.; Okada, M.; Lu, Q.; Yoshimura, A. Induced Regulatory T Cells: Their Development, Stability, and Applications. *Trends Immunol.* **2016**, *37*, 803–811. [CrossRef]

25. Iizuka-Koga, M.; Nakatsukasa, H.; Ito, M.; Akanuma, T.; Lu, Q.; Yoshimura, A. Induction and maintenance of regulatory T cells by transcription factors and epigenetic modifications. *J. Autoimmun.* **2017**, *83*, 113–121. [CrossRef]

26. Bikle, D.; Christakos, S. New aspects of vitamin D metabolism and action - addressing the skin as source and target. *Nat. Rev. Endocrinol.* **2020**, *16*, 234–252. [CrossRef]

27. Slominski, A.T.; Kim, T.K.; Takeda, Y.; Janjetovic, Z.; Brozyna, A.A.; Skobowiat, C.; Wang, J.; Postlethwaite, A.; Li, W.; Tuckey, R.C.; et al. RORα and ROR γ are expressed in human skin and serve as receptors for endogenously produced noncalcemic 20-hydroxy- and 20,23-dihydroxyvitamin D. *FASEB J.* **2014**, *28*, 2775–2789. [CrossRef]

28. Slominski, A.T.; Kim, T.K.; Janjetovic, Z.; Brożyna, A.A.; Żmijewski, M.A.; Xu, H.; Sutter, T.R.; Tuckey, R.C.; Jetten, A.M.; Crossman, D.K. Differential and Overlapping Effects of 20,23(OH)$_2$D3 and 1,25(OH)$_2$D3 on Gene Expression in Human Epidermal Keratinocytes: Identification of AhR as an Alternative Receptor for 20,23(OH)$_2$D3. *Int. J. Mol. Sci.* **2018**, *19*, 3072. [CrossRef]

29. Shiokawa, A.; Kotaki, R.; Takano, T.; Nakajima-Adachi, H.; Hachimura, S. Mesenteric lymph node CD11b$_-$CD103$_+$ PD-L1$_{High}$ dendritic cells highly induce regulatory T cells. *Immunology* **2017**, *152*, 52–64. [CrossRef]

30. Yamazaki, S.; Maruyama, A.; Okada, K.; Matsumoto, M.; Morita, A.; Seya, T. Dendritic cells from oral cavity induce Foxp3(+) regulatory T cells upon antigen stimulation. *PLoS ONE* **2012**, *7*, e51665. [CrossRef]

31. Yamazaki, S.; Odanaka, M.; Nishioka, A.; Kasuya, S.; Shime, H.; Hemmi, H.; Imai, M.; Riethmacher, D.; Kaisho, T.; Ohkura, N.; et al. Ultraviolet B-Induced Maturation of CD11b-Type Langerin$_-$ Dendritic Cells Controls the Expansion of Foxp3$_+$ Regulatory T Cells in the Skin. *J. Immunol.* **2018**, *200*, 119–129. [CrossRef] [PubMed]

32. Gagliani, N.; Vesely, M.C.A.; Iseppon, A.; Brockmann, L.; Xu, H.; Palm, N.W.; de Zoete, M.R.; Licona-Limón, P.; Paiva, R.S.; Ching, T.; et al. TH17 cells transdifferentiate into regulatory T cells during resolution of inflammation. *Nature* **2015**, *523*, 221–225. [CrossRef] [PubMed]

33. Quaglino, P.; Ortoncelli, M.; Comessatti, A.; Ponti, R.; Novelli, M.; Bergallo, M.; Costa, C.; Cicchelli, S.; Savoia, P.; Bernengo, M.G. Circulating CD4+CD25brightFOXP3+ T cells are up-regulated by biological therapies and correlate with the clinical response in psoriasis patients. *Dermatology* **2009**, *219*, 250–258. [CrossRef] [PubMed]

34. Saito, C.; Maeda, A.; Morita, A. Bath-PUVA therapy induces circulating regulatory T cells in patients with psoriasis. *J. Derm. Sci.* **2009**, *53*, 231–233. [CrossRef] [PubMed]

35. Bovenschen, H.J.; van de Kerkhof, P.C.; van Erp, P.E.; Woestenenk, R.; Joosten, I.; Koenen, H.J. Foxp3+ regulatory T cells of psoriasis patients easily differentiate into IL-17A-producing cells and are found in lesional skin. *J. Invest. Derm.* **2011**, *131*, 1853–1860. [CrossRef] [PubMed]

36. Spanogiannopoulos, P.; Bess, E.N.; Carmody, R.N.; Turnbaugh, P.J. The microbial pharmacists within us: A metagenomic view of xenobiotic metabolism. *Nat. Rev. Microbiol.* **2016**, *14*, 273–287. [CrossRef]

37. Sanchez-Alcoholado, L.; Castellano-Castillo, D.; Jordán-Martínez, L.; Moreno-Indias, I.; Cardila-Cruz, P.; Elena, D.; Muñoz-Garcia, A.J.; Queipo-Ortuño, M.I.; Jimenez-Navarro, M. Role of Gut Microbiota on Cardio-Metabolic Parameters and Immunity in Coronary Artery Disease Patients with and without Type-2 Diabetes Mellitus. *Front. Microbiol.* **2017**, *8*, 1936. [CrossRef]

38. Larsen, N.; Vogensen, F.K.; van den Berg, F.W.; Nielsen, D.S.; Andreasen, A.S.; Pedersen, B.K.; Al-Soud, W.A.; Sørensen, S.J.; Hansen, L.H.; Jakobsen, M. Gut microbiota in human adults with type 2 diabetes differs from non-diabetic adults. *PLoS ONE* **2010**, *5*, e9085. [CrossRef]

39. Cui, L.; Zhao, T.; Hu, H.; Zhang, W.; Hua, X. Association Study of Gut Flora in Coronary Heart Disease through High-Throughput Sequencing. *Biomed. Res. Int.* **2017**, *2017*, 3796359. [CrossRef]

40. Emoto, T.; Yamashita, T.; Kobayashi, T.; Sasaki, N.; Hirota, Y.; Hayashi, T.; So, A.; Kasahara, K.; Yodoi, K.; Matsumoto, T.; et al. Characterization of gut microbiota profiles in coronary artery disease patients using data mining analysis of terminal restriction fragment length polymorphism: Gut microbiota could be a diagnostic marker of coronary artery disease. *Heart Vessel.* **2017**, *32*, 39–46. [CrossRef]

41. Cani, P.D.; Everard, A.; Duparc, T. Gut microbiota, enteroendocrine functions and metabolism. *Curr. Opin. Pharm.* **2013**, *13*, 935–940. [CrossRef] [PubMed]
42. Cani, P.D.; Possemiers, S.; Van de Wiele, T.; Guiot, Y.; Everard, A.; Rottier, O.; Geurts, L.; Naslain, D.; Neyrinck, A.; Lambert, D.M.; et al. Changes in gut microbiota control inflammation in obese mice through a mechanism involving GLP-2-driven improvement of gut permeability. *Gut* **2009**, *58*, 1091–1103. [CrossRef] [PubMed]
43. Omenetti, S.; Pizarro, T.T. The Treg/Th17 Axis: A Dynamic Balance Regulated by the Gut Microbiome. *Front. Immunol.* **2015**, *6*, 639. [CrossRef] [PubMed]
44. Rahman, M.T.; Ghosh, C.; Hossain, M.; Linfield, D.; Rezaee, F.; Janigro, D.; Marchi, N.; van Boxel-Dezaire, A.H.H. IFN-γ, IL-17A, or zonulin rapidly increase the permeability of the blood-brain and small intestinal epithelial barriers: Relevance for neuro-inflammatory diseases. *Biochem. Biophys. Res. Commun.* **2018**, *507*, 274–279. [CrossRef] [PubMed]
45. Martin, A.M.; Sun, E.W.; Rogers, G.B.; Keating, D.J. The Influence of the Gut Microbiome on Host Metabolism Through the Regulation of Gut Hormone Release. *Front. Physiol.* **2019**, *10*, 428. [CrossRef]
46. Ramírez-Boscá, A.; Navarro-López, V.; Martínez-Andrés, A.; Such, J.; Francés, R.; Horga de la Parte, J.; Asín-Llorca, M. Identification of Bacterial DNA in the Peripheral Blood of Patients With Active Psoriasis. *Jama Derm.* **2015**, *151*, 670–671. [CrossRef]
47. Codoñer, F.M.; Ramírez-Bosca, A.; Climent, E.; Carrión-Gutierrez, M.; Guerrero, M.; Pérez-Orquín, J.M.; Horga de la Parte, J.; Genovés, S.; Ramón, D.; Navarro-López, V.; et al. Gut microbial composition in patients with psoriasis. *Sci. Rep.* **2018**, *8*, 3812. [CrossRef]
48. Hidalgo-Cantabrana, C.; Gómez, J.; Delgado, S.; Requena-López, S.; Queiro-Silva, R.; Margolles, A.; Coto, E.; Sánchez, B.; Coto-Segura, P. Gut microbiota dysbiosis in a cohort of patients with psoriasis. *Br. J. Dermatol.* **2019**, *181*, 1287–1295. [CrossRef]
49. Smith, P.M.; Howitt, M.R.; Panikov, N.; Michaud, M.; Gallini, C.A.; Bohlooly-Y., M.; Glickman, J.N.; Garrett, W.S. The microbial metabolites, short-chain fatty acids, regulate colonic Treg cell homeostasis. *Science* **2013**, *341*, 569–573. [CrossRef]
50. Scher, J.U.; Ubeda, C.; Artacho, A.; Attur, M.; Isaac, S.; Reddy, S.M.; Marmon, S.; Neimann, A.; Brusca, S.; Patel, T.; et al. Decreased bacterial diversity characterizes the altered gut microbiota in patients with psoriatic arthritis, resembling dysbiosis in inflammatory bowel disease. *Arthritis Rheumatol.* **2015**, *67*, 128–139. [CrossRef]
51. Jiang, C.; Xie, C.; Lv, Y.; Li, J.; Krausz, K.W.; Shi, J.; Brocker, C.N.; Desai, D.; Amin, S.G.; Bisson, W.H.; et al. Intestine-selective farnesoid X receptor inhibition improves obesity-related metabolic dysfunction. *Nat. Commun.* **2015**, *6*, 10166. [CrossRef] [PubMed]
52. Li, F.; Jiang, C.; Krausz, K.W.; Li, Y.; Albert, I.; Hao, H.; Fabre, K.M.; Mitchell, J.B.; Patterson, A.D.; Gonzalez, F.J. Microbiome remodelling leads to inhibition of intestinal farnesoid X receptor signalling and decreased obesity. *Nat Commun.* **2013**, *4*, 2384. [CrossRef] [PubMed]
53. den Besten, G.; Bleeker, A.; Gerding, A.; van Eunen, K.; Havinga, R.; van Dijk, T.H.; Oosterveer, M.H.; Jonker, J.W.; Groen, A.K.; Reijngoud, D.J.; et al. Short-Chain Fatty Acids Protect Against High-Fat Diet-Induced Obesity via a PPARγ-Dependent Switch From Lipogenesis to Fat Oxidation. *Diabetes* **2015**, *64*, 2398–2408. [CrossRef] [PubMed]
54. Salem, I.; Ramser, A.; Isham, N.; Ghannoum, M.A. The Gut Microbiome as a Major Regulator of the Gut-Skin Axis. *Front. Microbiol.* **2018**, *9*, 1459. [CrossRef]

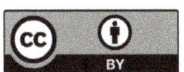

© 2020 by the author. Licensee MDPI, Basel, Switzerland. This article is an open access article distributed under the terms and conditions of the Creative Commons Attribution (CC BY) license (http://creativecommons.org/licenses/by/4.0/).

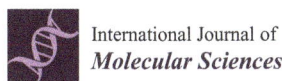

Review

Interleukin-17A and Keratinocytes in Psoriasis

Masutaka Furue [1,2,3,*], Kazuhisa Furue [1], Gaku Tsuji [1,2] and Takeshi Nakahara [1,3]

1. Department of Dermatology, Graduate School of Medical Sciences, Kyushu University, Maidashi 3-1-1, Higashiku, Fukuoka 812-8582, Japan; ffff5113@gmail.com (K.F.); gakku@dermatol.med.kyushu-u.ac.jp (G.T.); nakahara@dermatol.med.kyushu-u.ac.jp (T.N.)
2. Research and Clinical Center for Yusho and Dioxin, Kyushu University, Maidashi 3-1-1, Higashiku, Fukuoka 812-8582, Japan
3. Division of Skin Surface Sensing, Graduate School of Medical Sciences, Kyushu University, Maidashi 3-1-1, Higashiku, Fukuoka 812-8582, Japan
* Correspondence: furue@dermatol.med.kyushu-u.ac.jp; Tel.: +81-92-642-5581; Fax: +81-92-642-5600

Received: 22 January 2020; Accepted: 11 February 2020; Published: 13 February 2020

Abstract: The excellent clinical efficacy of anti-interleukin 17A (IL-17A) biologics on psoriasis indicates a crucial pathogenic role of IL-17A in this autoinflammatory skin disease. IL-17A accelerates the proliferation of epidermal keratinocytes. Keratinocytes produce a myriad of antimicrobial peptides and chemokines, such as CXCL1, CXCL2, CXCL8, and CCL20. Antimicrobial peptides enhance skin inflammation. IL-17A is capable of upregulating the production of these chemokines and antimicrobial peptides in keratinocytes. CXCL1, CXCL2, and CXCL8 recruit neutrophils and CCL20 chemoattracts IL-17A-producing CCR6$^+$ immune cells, which further contributes to forming an IL-17A-rich milieu. This feed-forward pathogenic process results in characteristic histopathological features, such as epidermal hyperproliferation, intraepidermal neutrophilic microabscess, and dermal CCR6$^+$ cell infiltration. In this review, we focus on IL-17A and keratinocyte interaction regarding psoriasis pathogenesis.

Keywords: psoriasis; keratinocytes; interleukin-17A; Th17; ILC3; CCL20; CXCL1; CXCL8; Koebner phenomenon; antimicrobial peptides

1. Introduction

Psoriasis is an immune-mediated chronic skin disease characterized by epidermal hyperproliferation, an intraepidermal accumulation of neutrophils, and dermal inflammatory cell infiltrates that are composed of dendritic cells and T cells [1]. It has an estimated global prevalence of 2–4% [1,2]. Males are twice as likely as females to be affected [3,4]. As desquamative erythema can affect any skin site, psoriasis profoundly impairs the patients' quality of life, treatment satisfaction and adherence, and socioeconomic stability [5–7]. The skin lesion usually appears on the sites with frequent trauma such as elbows and knees [8,9]. This injury-induced development of psoriasis is called Koebner phenomenon [8,9]. Environmental factors, such as smoking, also trigger or exacerbate psoriatic lesions [10,11]. Genetic factors are critically involved in the development of psoriasis [12,13]. In addition to skin eruption, approximately 30% of patients with psoriasis manifest psoriatic arthritis [14–19]. Psoriasis is also significantly comorbid with other autoimmune diseases, such as bullous pemphigoid [20–24]. Psoriasis is frequently associated with cardiovascular diseases, metabolic diseases, and renal disorders [25–36]. Cancer risk is slightly higher in patients with psoriasis [37]. The topical application of steroids and vitamin D3 analogues inhibits psoriatic inflammation and normalizes epidermal differentiation [38,39]. Systemic treatments, such as methotrexate, cyclosporine, phototherapy, and the phosphodiesterase 4 inhibitor apremilast, are useful for patients with extensive lesions [40–45].

That the tumor necrosis factor-α (TNF-α) and IL-23/IL-17A axes appear to be major drivers in the pathogenesis of psoriasis is underscored by the excellent response of psoriasis to biologics targeting

TNF-α, IL-23, and IL-17A, although a difference exists in their efficacy [46–61]. Anti-TNF-α/IL-23/IL-17A biologics successfully improve psoriatic arthritis [18,56,62–64]. Reductions in comorbid cardiovascular events and systemic inflammation have been reported in patients with psoriasis treated with anti-TNF/IL23/IL17 biologics [65,66].

As the clinical response to anti-IL-23/IL-17A biologics seems better than that to anti-TNF-α biologics in psoriasis, the IL-23/IL-17A axis likely plays a more crucial role than the TNF-α axis in the development of psoriasis [67–71]. Under the regulation of IL-23p19, IL-17A-producing CD4$^+$ helper T (Th17) cells create a self-amplifying, feed-forward inflammatory response that is markedly augmented in the presence of TNF-α [68,72,73]. In addition, Th17 cells produce high amounts of TNF-α [74,75]. Therefore, IL-17A inhibition by the anti-IL-17A biologic results in early clinical, histopathologic, and molecular resolution of psoriasis [69].

In addition, various murine psoriasis models stress a pivotal role of the IL-23/IL-17A axis in experimental psoriasis [76–80]. Multiple animal studies have indicated that the interaction between IL-17A and keratinocyte is the key issue in the development of psoriasis [76–79]. In parallel, the importance of IL-17A and keratinocyte interaction is reinforced in patients with psoriasis who are successfully treated with the anti-IL-17A biologic [69]. In this review, we will focus on the multifaceted biological response in keratinocytes stimulated by IL-17A with regard to psoriatic pathogenesis.

2. IL-17A Signaling System

The IL-17 family plays a critical role in the immune response in infectious, inflammatory, autoimmune, and neoplastic disorders [81,82]. The IL-17 family and its receptors are evolutionarily ancient, and they are present in species as early as lamprey and sea urchins [83,84]. IL-17 family members comprise IL-17A, IL-17B, IL-17C, IL-17D, IL-17E, IL-17F, and IL-17AF [81,82]. IL-17AF is a hybrid heterodimer of IL-17A and IL-17F. IL-17E is also called IL-25 and is related to the type 2 immune response and allergies [81,82,85]. Among IL-17 family members, IL-17A has been the most strongly implicated in human health and disease. IL-17A is produced from hematopoietic cells, including Th17, CD8+ cytotoxic T cell (Tc17), γδ T cell, natural killer cell, group 3 innate lymphoid cell (ILC3), and "natural" Th17 cell [86–89], but IL-17B, IL-17C, and IL-25 are preferentially produced from nonhematopoietic cells, including keratinocytes [81,82,90]. Both hematopoietic cells and keratinocytes produce IL-17F [81,82,90]. Keratinocyte-derived IL-17C is capable of stimulating Th17 cells to secrete more IL-17A [91].

The IL-17 receptor (IL-17R) is composed of five members: IL-17RA, IL-17RB, IL-17RC, IL-17RD, and IL-17RE [81,82,90]. IL-17A, IL-17F, and IL-17AF all share the same IL-17R comprising IL-17RA and IL-17RC heterodimers [81,82,90]. IL-17C binds to IL-17RA and IL-17RE heterodimers [92]. IL-25 ligates IL-17RA and IL-17RB [81,82,90]. A recent study showed that IL-17A also activates IL-17RA and IL-17RD heterodimers [93] (Figure 1). IL-17B binds IL-17RB, but another heterodimeric IL-17R member remains unidentified [82]. Keratinocytes express both IL-17RA/IL-17RC and IL-17RA/IL-17RD, and the binding of IL-17A induces the transcription of differential gene sets [93]. Initial subcellular events in the ligation of IL-17RA/RC by IL-17A are the recruitment and activation of ACT1 encoded by the *TRAF3IP2* gene, TRAF6 and CARMA2 complexes, and the downstream activation of nuclear factor kappa-light-chain-enhancer of activated B cells (NF-κB) and MAPKs [93–97]. The ligation of IL-17RA/IL-17RC by IL-17A induces the activation of NF-κB, ERK, p38 MAPK, and JNK, while that of IL-17RA/IL-17-RD mainly activates p38 MAPK and JNK and barely affects NF-κB and ERK [93]. In addition, IL-17RA physically and functionally interacts with and transactivates epidermal growth factor (EGFR) [98]. IL-17RD potentially interacts with and transactivates fibroblast growth factor 2 receptor [82,99].

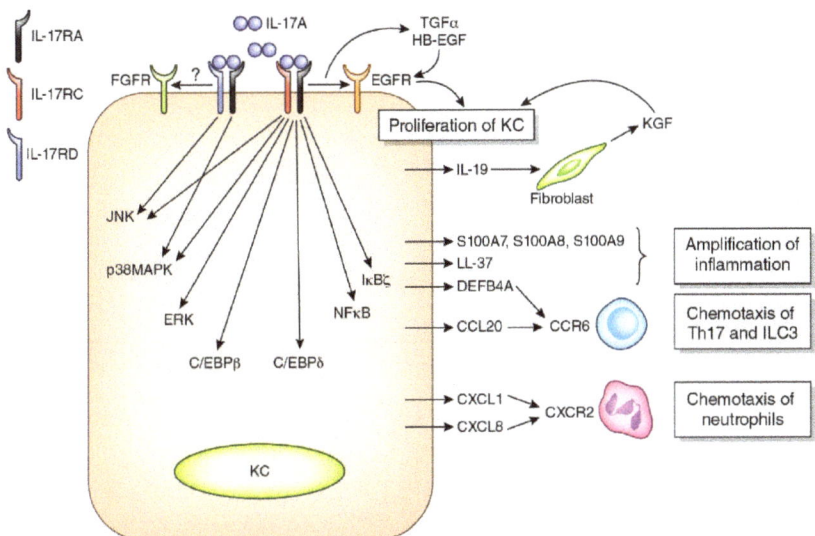

Figure 1. Simplified effects of anti-interleukin 17A (IL-17A) on keratinocyte (KC) with regard to psoriasis pathogenesis. IL-17A homodimers bind to IL-17 receptor A (IL-17RA) and IL-17RC or IL-17RA and IL-17RD heterodimers. The ligation of IL-17RA/IL-17RC activates epidermal growth factor receptor (EGFR) directly or by transforming growth factor-α (TGF-α) and heparin-binding EGF-like growth factor (HB-EGF) and promotes keratinocyte proliferation. The ligation of IL-17RA/IL-17RC activates various signal transduction molecules, including ERK, p38 MAPK, JNK, nuclear factor kappa-light-chain-enhancer of activated B cells (NFκB), IκBζ, C/CAAT-enhancer-binding protein β (C/EBPβ), and C/EBPδ. In contrast, the ligation of IL-17RA/IL-17RD preferentially activates JNK and p38 MAPK pathways. IL-17RA/IL-17RD is estimated to transactivate fibroblast growth factor receptor (FGFR); however, this is not conclusive. IL-17RA/IL-17RC signaling stimulates KCs to produce IL-19, which induces the production of keratinocyte growth factor (KGF) from fibroblasts. KGF also enhances the proliferation of KCs. IL-17A also induces the production of antimicrobial peptides, including S100A7, S100A8, S100A9, LL-37, and defensin β 4A (DEFB4A). These antimicrobial peptides amplify the local inflammatory process. Chemokines, such as CCL20, CXCL1, and CXCL8, are also produced from keratinocytes by IL-17RA/IL-17RC ligation. CCL20 is a key chemokine for the recruitment of CCR6[+] Th17 cells and group 3 innate lymphoid cells (ILC3). These CCR6[+] cells produce large amounts of IL-17A. DEFB4A also exhibits a chemotactic activity by binding to CCR6. CXCL1 and CXCL2 are potent chemoattractants for CXCR2[+] neutrophils. Therefore, IL-17A is associated with all of the histopathologic features of psoriasis.

In addition to the above-mentioned signaling cascades, IL-17A activates various other signal molecules including signal transducer and activator of transcription 3 (STAT3) in keratinocytes [100]. STAT3 is a very crucial signaling molecule in the development of psoriasis because transgenic mice with keratinocytes expressing a constitutively active Stat3 (K5.Stat3C mice) develop a skin phenotype either spontaneously, or in response to wounding, that closely resembles psoriasis [101]. Moreover, a STAT3 inhibitor STA-21 inhibits the generation of skin lesion in these psoriatic mice [102]. IL-17A is known to activate STAT3 via receptor-interacting protein 4 (RIP4) activation and upregulates the CCL20 expression [103]. IL-17A also upregulates keratin 17 expression via STAT1 and STAT3 activation [104]. IL-6 and IL-22 also play a synergistic role in development of psoriasis with IL-17A [68]. Notably, both IL-6 and IL-22 are potent STAT3 activators [105]. In accordance, biological or natural molecules such as indirubin and its derivatives useful for inactivating STAT3 exhibit therapeutic potential for psoriasis [106] (Figure 2). It reveals that IL-17 and IL-22 promote keratinocyte stemness and potentiate its regeneration [107]. IL-6 is produced from keratinocytes in response to IL-17A [108]. IL-22 is produced from Th17/22 cells, Th22 cells, and other immune cells [109,110].

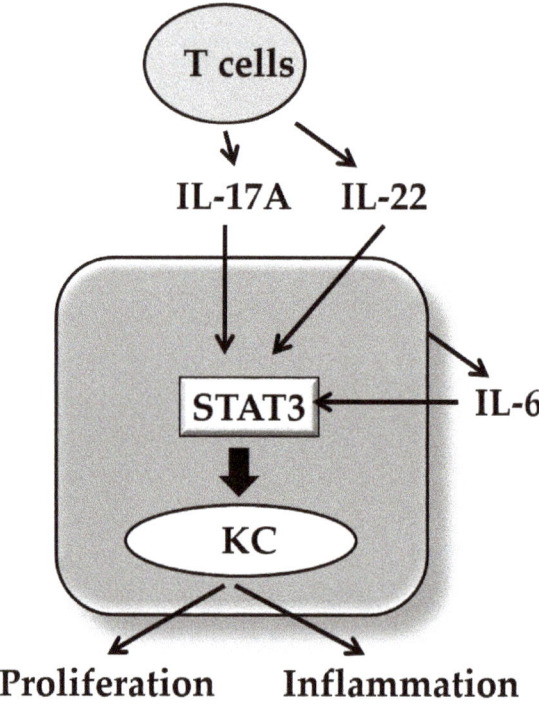

Figure 2. Pivotal role of signal transducer and activator of transcription 3 (STAT3) in psoriasis. The activation of STAT3 promotes keratinocyte (KC) proliferation and inflammatory response. IL-17A and IL-22 induce the STAT3 activation. IL-6 produced from KC also induces STAT3 activation.

In humans, impairment of the IL-17 signal causes infectious diseases, especially by *Candida albicans*, which is a ubiquitous fungus and commensal yeast of the intestines and skin [96]. Notably, deficiency of the *IL17RA*, *IL17RC*, *IL17F*, or *TRAF3IP2* genes is implicated in chronic mucocutaneous candidiasis disease (CMCD), which is characterized by recurrent or persistent infection affecting the nails, skin, and oral and genital mucosae caused by the *Candida* species, often *C. albicans* [96,111–113]. Impairment of the IL-17 signal is evident in other immunocompromised inborn errors, including autosomal-dominant hyper IgE syndrome, autosomal dominant *STAT1* gain-of-function, autosomal-recessive autoimmune polyendocrinopathy-candidiasis-ectodermal dystrophy (APECED), autosomal-recessive *CARD9* deficiency, *IL12RB1* deficiency, *IL12B* deficiency, and *RORC* deficiency [96]. However, these inborn errors seem to exhibit more complicated immune defects beyond IL-17 dysfunction and manifest CMCD together with other types of infection, including *Mycobacterium*, *Staphylococcus*, and viral disorders [96]. Of note, mice lacking *Traf3ip2* (*Act1*) or *Il17ra* manifest similar clinical phenotype as human CMCD patients lacking *IL17RA* or *IL17RC* [114–117]. A recent murine study by Sparber et al. also indicates that Malassezia infection selectively triggers the IL-17A-induced immune response [118]. These findings indicate a crucial role of IL-17A in anti-fungal immunity in humans and mice.

Mice overexpressing IL-17A in keratinocytes (K14-IL-17A$^{ind/+}$ mice) exhibit severe psoriasiform skin inflammation and vascular dysfunction in conjunction with infiltration of the vasculature by inflammatory myeloid cells [108]. The K14-IL-17A$^{ind/+}$ mice acquire the highest local and systemic IL-17A levels and exhibit a particularly severe psoriasis-like skin phenotype [108].

Homozygous CD11c-IL-17A$^{ind/ind}$ mice and heterozygous CD11c-IL-17A $^{ind/+}$ mice show a delayed onset of moderate to severe psoriasis-like skin disease associated with reduced amounts of cutaneous IL-17A compared with K14-IL-17A$^{ind/+}$ mice. In agreement with elevated skin and a stepwise increase in systemic IL-17A [119], homozygous CD11c-IL-17A $^{ind/ind}$ mice develop earlier and more severe skin lesions, as well as more pronounced vascular inflammation and dysfunction than heterozygous CD11c-IL-17A $^{ind/+}$ mice [76,119]. These experimental models indicate that IL-17A induces psoriasis-like lesions in a dose-dependent manner, irrespective of its cellular source [76,119].

3. IL-17A and Psoriasis

In the early 2000s, IL-23 was found to induce the production of IL-17A by activated CD4$^+$ T cells, which were later named Th17 cells [74,120]. These cells express RORγt (*RORC*) as the master transcription factor [121] and promoted the anti-infectious defense in the mucosa and skin [96], whereas excessive exposure to IL-23 induces their transformation into autoimmune or autoinflammatory immune cells [122,123]. Accordingly, the intradermal injection of IL-23 induces murine psoriasis-like dermatitis with epidermal acanthosis, neutrophil recruitment, and the infiltration of IL-17-producing T cells [78,79,124].

Psoriasis is one of the most typical IL-23/IL-17A-driven human diseases [68,72,73]. Th17 cells, Tc17 cells, IL-17-producing γδ T cells, and ILC3 can all be found in psoriatic skin [89,125,126]. IL-23 is composed of IL-23p40 and IL-23p19 subunits, and the expression of both is upregulated in the lesional skin compared to the nonlesional skin in psoriasis [127]. Dermal dendritic cells and monocytes are major sources of IL-23 production [128]. However, immunohistological staining also proves that IL23p40 and IL23p19 are expressed in normal and psoriatic keratinocytes [127–129]. Moreover, the epidermal expression of IL-23p40 and IL-23p19 is stronger in psoriasis lesions than in healthy controls [127–129]. Murine keratinocytes also produce biologically active IL-23 [130]. IL-23 can promote keratinocyte growth and histological acanthosis via the JAK2/AKT/STAT3/LMO4 signaling pathway [131]. LIM-domain only protein 4 (LMO4) is a LIM-domain protein that regulates keratinocyte proliferation and differentiation during embryogenesis [131]. In addition, TNF-α is an active stimulator of IL-23 production from keratinocytes in mice and possibly in humans [131]. In parallel, the anti-IL-23p40 antibody (Ustekinumab) [132,133] and anti-IL-23p19 antibodies (guselkumab, risankizumab, and tildrakizumab) [133–135] exhibit a high efficacy to psoriasis with a superiority of risankizumab over ustekinumab [133], and guselkumab over the anti-TNF-α antibody adalimumab [134].

The expression of *IL17A*, *IL17F*, and *IL17C* is upregulated in psoriatic lesional skin [136–138]. The intradermal injection of IL17C induces epidermal thickening and neutrophil infiltration [139]. As significant efficacy of the anti-IL17C antibody has recently been noted in murine psoriasis and atopic dermatitis [140], its human use has been suggested [141]. However, IL-17A is believed to be the most pathogenic IL-17 family member in psoriasis [68,69,72,73,142]. The lesional skin of psoriasis harbors IL-17A-producing immune cells [89,143], and transcriptomic analysis indicates a clear predominance of IL-17A signals [69,142]. Subsets of IL-17A-producing T cells are reactive to autoantigens, such as LL-37 (cathelicidin), a disintegrin and metalloprotease domain containing thrombospondin type 1 motif-like 5 (ADAMTSL5), keratin 17, and neolipid antigens generated by phospholipase A2 group IV D (PLA2G4D) [20,125,126,144–147]. IL-17A-dominant immune activation is also detected in the nonlesional skin of psoriasis [148].

There are three commercially available anti-IL17A biologics: secukinumab (fully human IgG1κ anti-IL17A antibody), ixekizumab (fully human IgG4 anti-IL17A antibody), and brodalumab (fully human IgG2 anti-IL17RA antibody). The severity of psoriatic skin lesions is generally evaluated by the Psoriasis Area and Severity Index (PASI) [149]. The efficacy of a therapeutic agent is assessed by the rate of responders who achieve 75%, 90%, and 100% reduction of PASI, namely, PASI75, PASI90, and PASI100, respectively. All three anti-IL-17A biologics exibit remarkable therapeutic efficacy for psoriasis. The PASI90 scores of secukinumab, ixekizumab, and brodalumab are reported to be as high as 60% to 70% at 12 weeks post treatment [150–152].

Regarding histology, the psoriatic epidermis is acanthotic and the proliferating capacity of keratinocyte is increased as determined by Ki67 positivity and cytokeratin 16 expression [68,153,154]. In accordance with the accumulation of neutrophils in psoriasis, the gene expression of neutrophilic cytochemokines CXCL1, CXCL2, CXCL8, and IL-36 is upregulated in the lesional skin of psoriasis [68,155–157]. Psoriatic keratinocytes produce a large amount of CCL20 [158,159], which is a potent chemoattractant for CCR6$^+$ IL-17A-producing Th17 [89,143,160], ILC3 [161,162], Tc17 [163,164], and γδ T cells [78,165]. Interestingly, IL-17A actively upregulates the production of these key cytochemokines as well as proliferative capacity in keratinocytes.

4. IL-17A and Keratinocyte Proliferation/Differentiation

Psoriatic keratinocytes simultaneously exhibit increased proliferation (Ki67$^+$ or cytokeratin 16$^+$ cell number) and differentiation [involucrin (IVL)$^+$ cell number] [69,166–168]. Accordingly, IL17A is an active promoter of keratinocyte proliferation and differentiation [168–171]. In psoriasis patients, the neutralization of IL-17A by ixekizumab [168] or secukinumab [69] significantly decreases histological acanthosis, the number of Ki-67$^+$-proliferating keratinocytes, and epidermal cytokeratin 16 expression. In the murine imiquimod-induced psoriasis model, topical imiquimod induces epidermal thickening that is significantly alleviated in *Traf3ip2* (*Act1*)-deficient mice in which IL-17 signaling is blocked [170]. The molecular mechanisms of the IL-17A-mediated acceleration of keratinocyte proliferation and differentiation are not yet fully understood.

IL-17A alone is likely to be insufficient to evoke a significant inflammatory response and may cooperatively or synergistically accelerate the proinflammatory cascade in combination with other cytokines, such as TNF-α, IL-23, IL-1β, IL-6, IL-22 and transforming growth factor-β (TGF-β) [68,172]. Transcriptomic analysis reveals a clear additive or synergistic gene regulation by IL-17A and TNF-α in human keratinocytes [173]. This gene regulation is likely attributable to two sets of transcription factors: NF-κB and the C/CAAT-enhancer-binding proteins (C/EBP), C/EBPβ, or C/EBPδ [169,173,174]. TNF-α is a strong inducer of active NF-κB, while IL-17A activates C/EBPβ or C/EBPδ and to a lesser extent NF-κB [169,173,174]. Therefore, the IL-17A blockade reduces the expression of these responsive genes to a greater extent than TNF-α inhibition [168].

The C/EBP family members are highly expressed transcription factors in epidermal keratinocytes and sebocytes in mice and humans and accelerate their differentiation [175]. The expression of C/EBPβ protein is located in the upper spinous layer and is strongly upregulated in the lesional skin of psoriasis [169]. Together with the elevated gene expression of *CEBPB*, the expression of keratinocyte-terminal differentiation genes, such as *IVL*, *FLG2*, and *TGM1*, is upregulated in the lesional skin of psoriasis [169]. In the promoter region of the *IVL* gene, there is a binding site for C/EBP, and the C/EBP transcription factor is necessary for the appropriate and continuous production of IVL protein [176]. These results suggest that IL-17A accelerates keratinocyte differentiation by increasing C/EBPβ protein in keratinocytes [168,169,173].

Regarding keratinocyte proliferation, IL-17A stimulates keratinocytes to produce IL-19 [173,177]. The combination of IL-17 and TNF-α results in the synergistic expression of IL-19 in keratinocytes. IL-17 alone promotes IL-19 expression by approximately 1.79-fold, and TNF-α alone slightly reduces IL-19 expression, whereas a combination of IL-17 and TNF-α promotes expression by 54.6-fold [173,177]. IL-19 itself promotes keratinocyte migration but not proliferation [178]. However, it activates fibroblasts to produce keratinocyte growth factor, which upregulates keratinocyte proliferation [178]. Additionally, the upregulation of cell cycle-related genes, such as CCNE1, CDCA5, and CDCA25A, suggests a direct contribution of IL-17 to epidermal KC proliferation [169]. The expression of cytokeratin 16 is upregulated in the lesional epidermis of psoriasis patients and in keratinocytes incubated with IL-17A [69,168,179]. The expression of cytokeratin 16 increases the proliferative capacity of keratinocytes via EGFR phosphorylation [180].

Other studies also underpin a possibility that IL-17A activates EGFR [98,181,182]. Chen et al. have demonstrated that IL-17A transactivates EGFR in keratinocyte stem cells [98]. IL-17A accelerates the enzymatic cleavage of amphiregulin, which activates EGFR in airway epithelial cells [181]. In the lesional skin of psoriasis, the expression of EGFR ligands, such as heparin-binding EGF, transforming growth factor-α, and amphiregulin, is overexpressed [183]. Consistent with these notions, the inhibition of EGFR by erlotinib or cetuximab successfully improves severe psoriasis [184–187]. These studies suggest that EGFR activation may partly explain the IL-17A-mediated upregulation of keratinocyte proliferation.

5. IL-17A and Cyto/Chemokines in Keratinocytes

In keratinocytes, IL-17A upregulates the expression of various psoriasis-related cyto/chemokines and antimicrobial peptides, such as CXCL1, CXCL8, IL-36G, CCL20, IL-19, IL-17C, S100A7, S100A8, S100A9, LL-37, and defensin β 4A (DEFB4A) [157,169,173,188–190]. The expression of these molecules is upregulated in the lesional skin of psoriasis and is downregulated to normal levels by biologics targeting TNF-α [128] or IL-17A [69,168]. Some are upregulated even in the nonlesional skin of patients with psoriasis [148]. The IL-17A-induced upregulation of these molecules is further amplified in the presence of TNF-α and IL-19 [173,177].

CXCL1 and CXCL8 are potent chemoattractants for neutrophils [191–193]. IL-36G induces CXCL1 and CXCL8 expression in an autocrine fashion in keratinocytes and recruits neutrophils [194]. Full-length IL-36G is cleaved by cathepsin G released from infiltrated neutrophils, and the cleaved IL-36G exhibits a more potent functional activity than the full-length one [192,195,196]. Moreover, IL-17A upregulates IL-36G production more potently in human psoriasis-derived keratinocytes than in healthy keratinocytes [197]. Therefore, the IL-17A, IL-36G, CXCL1/CXCL8, and neutrophils form a feed-forward vicious cycle, and an intraepidermal neutrophilic microabscess (Munro's microabscess or Kogoj's spongiform pustule) may develop [156,198,199]. The pathogenic significance of IL-36 is stressed more in pustular rather than plaque psoriasis [156,198,199]. In parallel, inhibition of the IL-36 pathway is efficacious for the treatment of pustular psoriasis [200].

While most chemokines redundantly bind to multiple receptors, CCL20 has only one known receptor, CCR6 [191]. CCR6 is expressed on dendritic cells [159] and IL-17-producing immune cells, including Th17 [89,143,201], ILC3 [161,162], Tc17 [163,164], and γδ T cells [78,165]. CCR6 is now considered a representative marker for Th17 cells [202,203]. The human psoriatic epidermis expresses abundant CCL20 with the dermal infiltration of CCR6$^+$ dendritic cells and skin-homing T cells [143,158,159]. Although dermal dendritic cells and T cells express CCL20 in the psoriatic dermis [159], the expression of CCL20 is largely confined to the psoriatic epidermis, suggesting that epidermal keratinocytes are the major source of CCL20 production in psoriatic lesions [158,159]. CCL20 is constitutively expressed in cultured keratinocytes [201,204], and its production is upregulated by TNF-α and IL-17A [182,204]. Scratch injury upregulates the gene expression of *CCL20*, *CXCL8*, and *IL36G*, which may be related to the scratch-induced Koebner phenomenon frequently observed in patients with psoriasis [201]. Preclinical studies have revealed that the humanized anti-CCR6 antibody efficiently inhibits the cutaneous infiltration of CCR6$^+$ T cells in human and murine models [205,206]. The development of small molecule inhibitors against CCR6 is also ongoing [207,208]. Targeting the CCL20/CCR6 axis may be a potential therapeutic strategy for the treatment of psoriasis.

6. IL-17A and Anti-Microbial Peptides in Keratinocytes

S100A7, S100A8, S100A9, LL-37, and DEFB4A are anti-microbial peptides, and their expression is upregulated by IL-17A in keratinocytes [189,209,210]. S100A7 (psoriasin) has a multifaceted role in keratinocyte pathophysiology, including wound healing, keratinocyte differentiation, nucleocytoplasmic transport, and chemotaxis for CD4$^+$ T cells, neutrophils, and monocytes [211]. The production of S100A7 is augmented in the presence of IL-19 [212], IL-36G [188], and TNF-α [213]. S100A8, S100A9, and S100A12 are alternatively known as calgranulin A, B, and C, respectively, and exhibit antimicrobial activity [214]. All are elevated in psoriatic plaque and decreased by treatment with anti-IL-17A antibody secukinumab [69,168,215]. The S100 family members primarily form homodimers or higher-order oligomers, but S100A8 and S100A9 uniquely form heterodimeric complexes, which are known as calprotectin [214]. The chelation of Zn^{2+} and Mn^{2+} by extracellular S100A8/A9 is a proposed mechanism of antimicrobial activity [214]. S100A12 also has a chemotactic activity for mast cells and monocytes [216]. Pure human S100A8/A9 has broad spectrum antimicrobial activities against microorganisms, including *Capnocytophaga sputigena*, *C. albicans*, *Escherichia coli*, *Staphylococcus aureus*, *S. epidermis*, *Borrelia burgdorferi*, and *Listeria monocytogenes*, in vitro, and S100A12 has antimicrobial activity against filarial parasites [214]. The receptor for advanced glycation end-products (RAGE) may serve as a common receptor for S100 proteins, including S100A7, S100A8, S100A9, and S100A12 [214]. S100A8/S100A9 augments the production of CXCL1, CXCL2, CXCL3, CXCL8, CCL20, IL-6, and TNF-α in keratinocytes [217], and it enhances keratinocyte proliferation [217]. The transcriptional co-activator IκBζ, encoded by the *NFKBIZ* gene, plays a critical role in IL-17A-, IL-17F-, and IL-17A/F-mediated signaling, such as the gene expression of *S100A7* and *CCL20* [218–220].

LL-37 is an antimicrobial peptide of human cathelicidin that is produced when keratinocytes are injured by a broad range of bacteria, viruses, and fungi [221,222]. In addition to antimicrobial peptide activity, LL-37 exhibits "alarmin" function, affects adenosine triphosphate-receptor P2X7 and Toll-like receptor (TLR) signaling, and EGFR transactivation or intracellular Ca^{2+} mobilization [223–225]. The released LL-37 binds to the infiltrated neutrophils [221]. Neutrophils are a rich source of extracellular DNA due to their neutrophil extracellular traps [226]. Upon stimulation with complexes of host DNA and LL-37, plasmacytoid dendritic cells produce large amounts of IFN-α [227]. Notably, LL-37 induced the proliferation of circulating $CD3^+$ T cells in 24 out of 52 patients with psoriasis (46%) [144]; therefore, LL-37 is effective for autoantigens. In total, 50 LL-37-reactive $CD3^+$ T cells, including both $CD4^+$ and $CD8^+$ T cells, express the skin-homing receptor cutaneous lymphocyte antigen [144]. LL-37 peptides bind to HLA-DR in dendritic cells and are presented to $CD4^+$ T cells, while LL-37 peptides and the HLA-C*0602 complex activate $CD8^+$ T cells [144,228]. The majority of LL-37-reactive $CD3^+$ T cells produce IL-17, and the capacity of their IL-17 production is associated with disease severity [144]. Interestingly, the LL-37-specific IL-17-producing T cells are exclusively $CD4^+$, whereas the LL-37-specific $CD8^+$ T cells do not produce IL-17 [144]. A recent study by Takahashi et al. revealed that LL-37 can bind to self-RNA and stimulate macrophages to produce IL-6 via a scavenger receptor [229].

DEFB4A is highly expressed in psoriasis plaques and is the most psoriasis-specific antimicrobial peptide [230,231]. In contrast, DEFB4A is expressed at negligible or low levels in normal skin and skin lesions of eczema [230–232]. The expression of DEFB4A is upregulated by IL-17A and synergistically by IL-17A and TNF-α [215,220]. The serum levels of DEFB4A are highly specific biomarkers for disease activity in patients with psoriasis [215]. The number of neutrophil extracellular traps increase in psoriasis and upregulate the expression of DEFB4A [226]. Notably, DEFB4A is a functional (non-chemokine) ligand for CCR6 and feasibly attracts Th17 cells [233,234].

Although the biological implications of increased antimicrobial peptides in psoriasis remain obscure, they are intimately associated with IL-17A-rich milieu. Therefore, the upregulated expression of these antimicrobial peptides is rapidly normalized by the neutralization of IL-17A by ixekizumab [168] or secukinumab [69].

7. Conclusions

IL-17A is a multifunctional cytokine produced from adaptive and innate immune cells, such as Th17 and ILC3s. It orchestrates and promotes the peripheral tissue defense system against microbial insult, especially fungal infection. Psoriasis is a major inflammatory skin disease in which the interaction between IL-17A and epidermal keratinocytes plays a critical pathogenic role. IL-17A stimulates the proliferation of keratinocytes. Keratinocytes also produce a variety of antimicrobial peptides and cytochemokines in response to IL-17A. The antimicrobial peptides further exacerbate skin inflammation. CCL20 produced from IL-17A-stimulated keratinocytes recruits IL-17A-producing Th17 cells and ILC3s and accelerates the feed-forward vicious cycle, which causes fully developed psoriasis. This pathogenetic scheme has been verified with a high clinical efficacy of anti-IL-17A biologics. Therefore, psoriasis is considered an excellent human model of how IL-17A works with target peripheral tissues, and it provides in-depth insight into human autoinflammatory diseases.

Author Contributions: M.F. wrote the first draft. K.F., G.T. and T.N. reviewed the draft. M.F. finalized the article. All authors have read and agreed to the published version of the manuscript.

Funding: This work was partly supported by a grant from The Ministry of Health, Labor, and Welfare in Japan (H30-Shokuhin-Shitei-005).

Conflicts of Interest: The authors have no conflicts of interest.

References

1. Boehncke, W.H.; Schön, M.P. Psoriasis. *Lancet* **2015**, *386*, 983–994. [CrossRef]
2. Michalek, I.M.; Loring, B.; John, S.M. A systematic review of worldwide epidemiology of psoriasis. *J. Eur. Acad. Dermatol. Venereol.* **2017**, *31*, 205–212. [CrossRef] [PubMed]
3. Ito, T.; Takahashi, H.; Kawada, A.; Iizuka, H.; Nakagawa, H. Epidemiological survey from 2009 to 2012 of psoriatic patients in Japanese Society for Psoriasis Research. *J. Dermatol.* **2018**, *45*, 293–301. [CrossRef] [PubMed]
4. Ogawa, E.; Okuyama, R.; Seki, T.; Kobayashi, A.; Oiso, N.; Muto, M.; Nakagawa, H.; Kawada, A. Epidemiological survey of patients with psoriasis in Matsumoto city, Nagano Prefecture, Japan. *J. Dermatol.* **2018**, *45*, 314–317. [CrossRef] [PubMed]
5. Ichiyama, S.; Ito, M.; Funasaka, Y.; Abe, M.; Nishida, E.; Muramatsu, S.; Nishihara, H.; Kato, H.; Morita, A.; Imafuku, S.; et al. Assessment of medication adherence and treatment satisfaction in Japanese patients with psoriasis of various severities. *J. Dermatol.* **2018**, *45*, 727–731. [CrossRef]
6. Souza, C.S.; de Castro, C.C.S.; Carneiro, F.R.O.; Pinto, J.M.N.; Fabricio, L.H.Z.; Azulay-Abulafia, L.; Romiti, R.; Cestari, T.F.; Suzuki, C.E.; Biegun, P.M.; et al. Metabolic syndrome and psoriatic arthritis among patients with psoriasis vulgaris: Quality of life and prevalence. *J. Dermatol.* **2019**, *46*, 3–10. [CrossRef]
7. Takahashi, H.; Satoh, K.; Takagi, A.; Iizuka, H. Cost-efficacy and pharmacoeconomics of psoriatic patients in Japan: Analysis from a single outpatient clinic. *J. Dermatol.* **2019**, *46*, 478–481. [CrossRef]
8. Miller, R.A. The Koebner phenomenon. *Int. J. Dermatol.* **1982**, *21*, 192–197. [CrossRef]
9. Weiss, G.; Shemer, A.; Trau, H. The Koebner phenomenon: Review of the literature. *J. Eur. Acad. Dermatol. Venereol.* **2002**, *16*, 241–248. [CrossRef]
10. Dai, Y.X.; Wang, S.C.; Chou, Y.J.; Chang, Y.T.; Chen, T.J.; Li, C.P.; Wu, C.Y. Smoking, but not alcohol, is associated with risk of psoriasis in a Taiwanese population-based cohort study. *J. Am. Acad. Dermatol.* **2019**, *80*, 727–734. [CrossRef]
11. Kamiya, K.; Kishimoto, M.; Sugai, J.; Komine, M.; Ohtsuki, M. Risk factors for the development of psoriasis. *Int. J. Mol. Sci.* **2019**, *20*, 4347. [CrossRef] [PubMed]
12. O'Rielly, D.D.; Jani, M.; Rahman, P.; Elder, J.T. The Genetics of Psoriasis and Psoriatic Arthritis. *J. Rheumatol Suppl.* **2019**, *95*, 46–50. [PubMed]
13. Elder, J.T. Expanded genome-wide association study meta-analysis of psoriasis expands the catalog of common psoriasis-associated variants. *J. Investig. Dermatol. Symp. Proc.* **2018**, *19*, S77–S78. [CrossRef] [PubMed]
14. Diani, M.; Perego, S.; Sansoni, V.; Bertino, L.; Gomarasca, M.; Faraldi, M.; Pigatto, P.D.M.; Damiani, G.; Banfi, G.; Altomare, G.; et al. Differences in osteoimmunological biomarkers predictive of psoriatic arthritis among a large Italian cohort of psoriatic patients. *Int. J. Mol. Sci.* **2019**, *20*, 5617. [CrossRef] [PubMed]
15. Mease, P.J.; Palmer, J.B.; Hur, P.; Strober, B.E.; Lebwohl, M.; Karki, C.; Reed, G.W.; Etzel, C.J.; Greenberg, J.D.; Helliwell, P.S. Utilization of the validated psoriasis epidemiology screening tool to identify signs and symptoms of psoriatic arthritis among those with psoriasis: A cross-sectional analysis from the US-based Corrona Psoriasis Registry. *J. Eur. Acad. Dermatol. Venereol.* **2019**, *33*, 886–892. [CrossRef] [PubMed]
16. Yamamoto, T.; Kawada, A. Clinical characteristics of Japanese patients with psoriatic arthritis: Comparison with East Asian countries. *J. Dermatol.* **2018**, *45*, 273–278. [CrossRef]

17. Yamamoto, T.; Ohtsuki, M.; Sano, S.; Morita, A.; Igarashi, A.; Okuyama, R.; Kawada, A. Late-onset psoriatic arthritis in Japanese patients. *J. Dermatol.* **2019**, *46*, 169–170. [CrossRef]
18. Yamamoto, T.; Ohtsuki, M.; Sano, S.; Morita, A.; Igarashi, A.; Okuyama, R.; Kawada, A. Switching biologics in the treatment of psoriatic arthritis in Japan. *J. Dermatol.* **2019**, *46*, e113–e114. [CrossRef]
19. Umezawa, Y.; Yanaba, K.; Asahina, A.; Nakagawa, H.; Fukuda, T.; Fukuda, K. Usefulness of dual-energy computed tomography for the evaluation of psoriatic arthritis accompanied by knee osteoarthritis. *J. Dermatol.* **2019**, *46*, e30–e32. [CrossRef]
20. Furue, K.; Ito, T.; Tsuji, G.; Kadono, T.; Nakahara, T.; Furue, M. Autoimmunity and autoimmune co-morbidities in psoriasis. *Immunology* **2018**, *154*, 21–27. [CrossRef]
21. Ho, Y.H.; Hu, H.Y.; Chang, Y.T.; Li, C.P.; Wu, C.Y. Psoriasis is associated with increased risk of bullous pemphigoid: A nationwide population-based cohort study in Taiwan. *J. Dermatol.* **2019**, *46*, 604–609. [CrossRef] [PubMed]
22. Ichiyama, S.; Hoashi, T.; Kanda, N.; Hashimoto, H.; Matsushita, M.; Nozawa, K.; Ueno, T.; Saeki, H. Psoriasis vulgaris associated with systemic lupus erythematosus successfully treated with apremilast. *J. Dermatol.* **2019**, *46*, e219–e221. [CrossRef] [PubMed]
23. Chujo, S.; Asahina, A.; Itoh, Y.; Kobayashi, K.; Sueki, H.; Ishiji, T.; Umezawa, Y.; Nakagawa, H. New onset of psoriasis during nivolumab treatment for lung cancer. *J. Dermatol.* **2018**, *45*, e55–e56. [CrossRef] [PubMed]
24. Kamata, M.; Asano, Y.; Shida, R.; Maeda, N.; Yoshizaki, A.; Miyagaki, T.; Kawashima, T.; Tada, Y.; Sato, S. Secukinumab decreased circulating anti-BP180-NC16a autoantibodies in a patient with coexisting psoriasis vulgaris and bullous pemphigoid. *J. Dermatol.* **2019**, *46*, e216–e217. [CrossRef]
25. Bayaraa, B.; Imafuku, S. Relationship between environmental factors, age of onset and familial history in Japanese patients with psoriasis. *J. Dermatol.* **2018**, *45*, 715–718. [CrossRef] [PubMed]
26. Chiu, H.Y.; Chang, W.L.; Shiu, M.N.; Huang, W.F.; Tsai, T.F. Psoriasis is associated with a greater risk for cardiovascular procedure and surgery in patients with hypertension: A nationwide cohort study. *J. Dermatol.* **2018**, *45*, 1381–1388. [CrossRef]
27. Furue, M.; Kadono, T. "Inflammatory skin march" in atopic dermatitis and psoriasis. *Inflamm. Res.* **2017**, *66*, 833–842. [CrossRef]
28. Momose, M.; Asahina, A.; Fukuda, T.; Sakuma, T.; Umezawa, Y.; Nakagawa, H. Evaluation of epicardial adipose tissue volume and coronary artery calcification in Japanese patients with psoriasis vulgaris. *J. Dermatol.* **2018**, *45*, 1349–1352. [CrossRef]
29. Takamura, S.; Takahashi, A.; Inoue, Y.; Teraki, Y. Effects of tumor necrosis factor-α, interleukin-23 and interleukin-17A inhibitors on bodyweight and body mass index in patients with psoriasis. *J. Dermatol.* **2018**, *45*, 1130–1134. [CrossRef]
30. Wang, C.C.; Tang, C.H.; Huang, K.C.; Huang, S.Y.; Sue, Y.M. Increased risk of incident psoriasis in end-stage renal disease patients on chronic hemodialysis: A nationwide population-based cohort study. *J. Dermatol.* **2018**, *45*, 1063–1070. [CrossRef]
31. Han, J.H.; Lee, J.H.; Han, K.D.; Kim, H.N.; Bang, C.H.; Park, Y.M.; Lee, J.Y.; Kim, T.Y. Increased risk of psoriasis in subjects with abdominal obesity: A nationwide population-based study. *J. Dermatol.* **2019**, *46*, 695–701. [CrossRef] [PubMed]
32. Jung, K.J.; Kim, T.G.; Lee, J.W.; Lee, M.; Oh, J.; Lee, S.E.; Chang, H.J.; Jee, S.H.; Lee, M.G. Increased risk of atherosclerotic cardiovascular disease among patients with psoriasis in Korea: A 15-year nationwide population-based cohort study. *J. Dermatol.* **2019**, *46*, 859–866. [CrossRef] [PubMed]
33. Masaki, S.; Bayaraa, B.; Imafuku, S. Prevalence of inflammatory bowel disease in Japanese psoriatic patients. *J. Dermatol.* **2019**, *46*, 590–594. [CrossRef] [PubMed]
34. Tokuyama, M.; Shimizu, T.; Yamada, T.; Kondoh, A.; Mabuchi, T. Case of psoriasis vulgaris with atrial fibrillation, heart failure and chronic kidney disease which were found accidentally through blood examination during apremilast treatment. *J. Dermatol.* **2019**, *46*, e239–e240. [CrossRef]
35. Yamazaki, F.; Takehana, K.; Tamashima, M.; Okamoto, H. Improvement in abnormal coronary arteries estimated by coronary computed tomography angiography after secukinumab treatment in a Japanese psoriatic patient. *J. Dermatol.* **2019**, *46*, e51–e52. [CrossRef]
36. Wójcik, P.; Biernacki, M.; Wroński, A.; Łuczaj, W.; Waeg, G.; Žarković, N.; Skrzydlewska, E. Altered lipid metabolism in blood mononuclear cells of psoriatic patients indicates differential changes in psoriasis vulgaris and psoriatic arthritis. *Int. J. Mol. Sci.* **2019**, *20*, 4249.

37. Lee, J.H.; Kim, H.J.; Han, K.D.; Kim, H.N.; Park, Y.M.; Lee, J.Y.; Park, Y.G.; Lee, Y.B. Cancer risk in 892089 patients with psoriasis in Korea: A nationwide population-based cohort study. *J. Dermatol.* **2019**, *46*, 95–102. [CrossRef]
38. Hsu, S.; Papp, K.A.; Lebwohl, M.G.; Bagel, J.; Blauvelt, A.; Duffin, K.C.; Crowley, J.; Eichenfield, L.F.; Feldman, S.R.; Fiorentino, D.F.; et al. Consensus guidelines for the management of plaque psoriasis. *Arch. Dermatol.* **2012**, *148*, 95–102. [CrossRef]
39. Imafuku, S.; Zheng, M.; Tada, Y.; Zhang, X.; Theng, C.; Thevarajah, S.; Zhao, Y.; Song, H.J. Asian consensus on assessment and management of mild to moderate plaque psoriasis with topical therapy. *J. Dermatol.* **2018**, *45*, 805–811. [CrossRef]
40. Meephansan, J.; Subpayasarn, U.; Ponnikorn, S.; Chakkavittumrong, P.; Juntongjin, P.; Komine, M.; Ohtsuki, M.; Poovorawan, Y. Methotrexate, but not narrowband ultraviolet B radiation, suppresses interleukin-33 mRNA levels in psoriatic plaques and protein levels in serum of patients with psoriasis. *J. Dermatol.* **2018**, *45*, 322–325. [CrossRef]
41. Kishimoto, M.; Komine, M.; Hioki, T.; Kamiya, K.; Sugai, J.; Ohtsuki, M. Real-world use of apremilast for patients with psoriasis in Japan. *J. Dermatol.* **2018**, *45*, 1345–1348. [CrossRef] [PubMed]
42. Morita, A. Current developments in phototherapy for psoriasis. *J. Dermatol.* **2018**, *45*, 287–292. [CrossRef] [PubMed]
43. Oh, E.H.; Koh, W.S.; Shin, J.M.; Kim, J.E.; Ko, J.Y.; Ro, Y.S. Clinical experience of cyclosporin treatment in patients with psoriasis and psoriatic arthritis. *J. Dermatol.* **2018**, *45*, 329–330. [CrossRef] [PubMed]
44. Pongparit, K.; Chularojanamontri, L.; Limphoka, P.; Silpa-Archa, N.; Wongpraparat, C. Effectiveness of and factors associated with clinical response to methotrexate under daily life conditions in Asian patients with psoriasis: A retrospective cohort study. *J. Dermatol.* **2018**, *45*, 540–545. [CrossRef] [PubMed]
45. Okazaki, S.; Osawa, R.; Nakajima, H.; Nakajima, K.; Sano, S. Favorable response to apremilast in a patient with refractory psoriasis verrucosa. *J. Dermatol.* **2019**, *46*, 544–547. [CrossRef]
46. Furue, K.; Ito, T.; Furue, M. Differential efficacy of biologic treatments targeting the TNF-α/IL-23/IL-17 axis in psoriasis and psoriatic arthritis. *Cytokine* **2018**, *111*, 182–188. [CrossRef]
47. Furue, K.; Ito, T.; Tsuji, G.; Kadono, T.; Furue, M. Psoriasis and the TNF/IL23/IL17 axis. *G. Ital. Dermatol. Venereol.* **2019**, *154*, 418–424. [CrossRef]
48. Sawyer, L.M.; Malottki, K.; Sabry-Grant, C.; Yasmeen, N.; Wright, E.; Sohrt, A.; Borg, E.; Warren, R.B. Assessing the relative efficacy of interleukin-17 and interleukin-23 targeted treatments for moderate-to-severe plaque psoriasis: A systematic review and network meta-analysis of PASI response. *PLoS ONE* **2019**, *14*, e0220868. [CrossRef]
49. Kamata, M.; Tada, Y. Safety of biologics in psoriasis. *J. Dermatol.* **2018**, *45*, 279–286. [CrossRef]
50. Momose, M.; Asahina, A.; Umezawa, Y.; Nakagawa, H. Long-term clinical efficacy and safety of secukinumab for Japanese patients with psoriasis: A single-center experience. *J. Dermatol.* **2018**, *45*, 318–321.
51. Ogawa, E.; Sato, Y.; Minagawa, A.; Okuyama, R. Pathogenesis of psoriasis and development of treatment. *J. Dermatol.* **2018**, *45*, 264–272. [CrossRef] [PubMed]
52. Ohtsuki, M.; Kubo, H.; Morishima, H.; Goto, R.; Zheng, R.; Nakagawa, H. Guselkumab, an anti-interleukin-23 monoclonal antibody, for the treatment of moderate to severe plaque-type psoriasis in Japanese patients: Efficacy and safety results from a phase 3, randomized, double-blind, placebo-controlled study. *J. Dermatol.* **2018**, *45*, 1053–1062. [CrossRef] [PubMed]
53. Bayaraa, B.; Imafuku, S. Sustainability and switching of biologics for psoriasis and psoriatic arthritis at Fukuoka University Psoriasis Registry. *J. Dermatol.* **2019**, *46*, 389–398. [CrossRef] [PubMed]
54. Kamiya, K.; Karakawa, M.; Komine, M.; Kishimoto, M.; Sugai, J.; Ohtsuki, M. Results of a retrospective study on the efficacy and safety of adalimumab 80 mg administrated every other week in patients with psoriasis at a single Japanese institution. *J. Dermatol.* **2019**, *46*, 199–205. [CrossRef]
55. Komatsu-Fujii, T.; Honda, T.; Otsuka, A.; Kabashima, K. Inverse responses of the skin and nail lesions of psoriatic arthritis to an anti-interleukin-17A antibody and an anti-tumor necrosis factor-α antibody. *J. Dermatol.* **2019**, *46*, e440–e441. [CrossRef]
56. Komatsu-Fujii, T.; Honda, T.; Otsuka, A.; Kabashima, K. Improvement of nail lesions in a patient with psoriatic arthritis by switching the treatment from an anti-interleukin-17A antibody to an anti-tumor necrosis factor-α antibody. *J. Dermatol.* **2019**, *46*, e158–e160. [CrossRef]

57. Lee, M.G.; Huang, Y.H.; Lee, J.H.; Lee, S.C.; Kim, T.G.; Aw, D.C.; Bao, W.; Dee, C.M.A.; Guana, A.; Tsai, T.F. Secukinumab demonstrates superior efficacy and a faster response in clearing skin in Asian subjects with moderate to severe plaque psoriasis compared with ustekinumab: Subgroup analysis from the CLEAR study. *J. Dermatol.* **2019**, *46*, 752–758. [CrossRef]
58. Okubo, Y.; Ohtsuki, M.; Morita, A.; Yamaguchi, M.; Shima, T.; Tani, Y.; Nakagawa, H. Long-term efficacy and safety of secukinumab in Japanese patients with moderate to severe plaque psoriasis: 3-year results of a double-blind extension study. *J. Dermatol.* **2019**, *46*, 186–192. [CrossRef]
59. Shibata, T.; Muto, J.; Takama, H.; Yanagishita, T.; Ito, T.; Watanabe, D. Case of psoriatic erythroderma induced by the discontinuation of the chronic use of topical steroid after dialysis initiation and successfully treated with secukinumab. *J. Dermatol.* **2019**, *46*, e119–e120. [CrossRef]
60. Tada, Y.; Ishii, K.; Kimura, J.; Hanada, K.; Kawaguchi, I. Patient preference for biologic treatments of psoriasis in Japan. *J. Dermatol.* **2019**, *46*, 466–477. [CrossRef]
61. Tsuruta, N.; Narisawa, Y.; Imafuku, S.; Ito, K.; Yamaguchi, K.; Miyagi, T.; Takahashi, K.; Fukamatsu, H.; Morizane, S.; Koketsu, H.; et al. Cross-sectional multicenter observational study of psoriatic arthritis in Japanese patients: Relationship between skin and joint symptoms and results of treatment with tumor necrosis factor-α inhibitors. *J. Dermatol.* **2019**, *46*, 193–198. [CrossRef]
62. Veale, D.J.; Fearon, U. The pathogenesis of psoriatic arthritis. *Lancet* **2018**, *391*, 2273–2284. [CrossRef]
63. Assefa, G.T.; Kaneko, S.; Oguro, H.; Morita, E. Treatment of psoriasis and psoriatic arthritis with secukinumab after unsatisfactory response to ustekinumab in multiple sclerosis patient. *J. Dermatol.* **2019**, *46*, e112–e113. [CrossRef] [PubMed]
64. Mourad, A.; Gniadecki, R. Treatment of dactylitis and enthesitis in psoriatic arthritis with biologic agents: A systematic review and metaanalysis. *J. Rheumatol.* **2019**, *47*, 59–65. [CrossRef] [PubMed]
65. Korman, N.J. Management of psoriasis as a systemic disease: What is the evidence? *Br. J. Dermatol.* **2019**. [CrossRef]
66. Lockshin, B.; Balagula, Y.; Merola, J.F. Interleukin 17, inflammation, and cardiovascular risk in patients with psoriasis. *J. Am. Acad. Dermatol.* **2018**, *79*, 345–352. [CrossRef]
67. Erichsen, C.Y.; Jensen, P.; Kofoed, K. Biologic therapies targeting the interleukin (IL)-23/IL-17 immune axis for the treatment of moderate-to-severe plaque psoriasis: A systematic review and meta-analysis. *J. Eur. Acad. Dermatol. Venereol.* **2020**, *34*, 30–38. [CrossRef]
68. Krueger, J.G.; Brunner, P.M. Interleukin-17 alters the biology of many cell types involved in the genesis of psoriasis, systemic inflammation and associated comorbidities. *Exp. Dermatol.* **2018**, *27*, 115–123. [CrossRef]
69. Krueger, J.G.; Wharton, K.A., Jr.; Schlitt, T.; Suprun, M.; Torene, R.I.; Jiang, X.; Wang, C.Q.; Fuentes-Duculan, J.; Hartmann, N.; Peters, T.; et al. IL-17A inhibition by secukinumab induces early clinical, histopathologic, and molecular resolution of psoriasis. *J. Allergy Clin. Immunol.* **2019**, *144*, 750–763. [CrossRef]
70. Mease, P.J.; Smolen, J.S.; Behrens, F.; Nash, P.; Liu Leage, S.; Li, L.; Tahir, H.; Gooderham, M.; Krishnan, E.; Liu-Seifert, H.; et al. A head-to-head comparison of the efficacy and safety of ixekizumab and adalimumab in biological-naïve patients with active psoriatic arthritis: 24-week results of a randomised, open-label, blinded-assessor trial. *Ann. Rheum. Dis.* **2020**, *79*, 123–131. [CrossRef]
71. Warren, R.B.; Barker, J.; Finlay, A.Y.; Burden, A.D.; Kirby, B.; Armendariz, Y.; Williams, R.; Hatchard, C.; Khare, S.; Griffiths, C.E.M. Secukinumab for patients failing previous TNFα-inhibitor therapy: Results of a randomised open-label study (Signature). *Br. J. Dermatol.* **2019**. [CrossRef] [PubMed]
72. Hawkes, J.E.; Chan, T.C.; Krueger, J.G. Psoriasis pathogenesis and the development of novel targeted immune therapies. *J. Allergy Clin. Immunol.* **2017**, *140*, 645–653. [CrossRef] [PubMed]
73. Hawkes, J.E.; Yan, B.Y.; Chan, T.C.; Krueger, J.G. Discovery of the IL-23/IL-17 signaling pathway and the treatment of psoriasis. *J. Immunol.* **2018**, *201*, 1605–1613. [CrossRef] [PubMed]
74. Langrish, C.L.; Chen, Y.; Blumenschein, W.M.; Mattson, J.; Basham, B.; Sedgwick, J.D.; McClanahan, T.; Kastelein, R.A.; Cua, D.J. IL-23 drives a pathogenic T cell population that induces autoimmune inflammation. *J. Exp. Med.* **2005**, *201*, 233–240. [CrossRef]
75. Shiga, T.; Sato, K.; Kataoka, S.; Sano, S. TNF inhibitors directly target Th17 cells via attenuation of autonomous TNF/TNFR2 signalling in psoriasis. *J. Dermatol. Sci.* **2015**, *77*, 79–81. [CrossRef]
76. Schüler, R.; Brand, A.; Klebow, S.; Wild, J.; Veras, F.P.; Ullmann, E.; Roohani, S.; Kolbinger, F.; Kossmann, S.; Wohn, C.; et al. Antagonization of IL-17A attenuates skin inflammation and vascular dysfunction in mouse models of psoriasis. *J. Investig. Dermatol.* **2019**, *139*, 638–647. [CrossRef]

77. Moos, S.; Mohebiany, A.N.; Waisman, A.; Kurschus, F.C. Imiquimod-induced psoriasis in mice depends on the IL-17 signaling of keratinocytes. *J. Investig. Dermatol.* **2019**, *139*, 1110–1117. [CrossRef]
78. Mabuchi, T.; Takekoshi, T.; Hwang, S.T. Epidermal CCR6+ γδ T cells are major producers of IL-22 and IL-17 in a murine model of psoriasiform dermatitis. *J. Immunol.* **2011**, *187*, 5026–5031. [CrossRef]
79. Mabuchi, T.; Singh, T.P.; Takekoshi, T.; Jia, G.F.; Wu, X.; Kao, M.C.; Weiss, I.; Farber, J.M.; Hwang, S.T. CCR6 is required for epidermal trafficking of γδ-T cells in an IL-23-induced model of psoriasiform dermatitis. *J. Investig. Dermatol.* **2013**, *133*, 164–171. [CrossRef]
80. Nakajima, K.; Sano, S. Mouse models of psoriasis and their relevance. *J. Dermatol.* **2018**, *45*, 252–263. [CrossRef]
81. Brembilla, N.C.; Senra, L.; Boehncke, W.H. The IL-17 family of cytokines in psoriasis: IL-17A and beyond. *Front. Immunol.* **2018**, *9*, 1682. [CrossRef] [PubMed]
82. McGeachy, M.J.; Cua, D.J.; Gaffen, S.L. The IL-17 family of cytokines in health and disease. *Immunity* **2019**, *50*, 892–906. [CrossRef] [PubMed]
83. Buckley, K.M.; Ho, E.C.H.; Hibino, T.; Schrankel, C.S.; Schuh, N.W.; Wang, G.; Rast, J.P. IL17 factors are early regulators in the gut epithelium during inflammatory response to Vibrio in the sea urchin larva. *Elife* **2017**, *6*. [CrossRef] [PubMed]
84. Han, Q.; Das, S.; Hirano, M.; Holland, S.J.; McCurley, N.; Guo, P.; Rosenberg, C.S.; Boehm, T.; Cooper, M.D. Characterization of lamprey IL-17 family members and their receptors. *J. Immunol.* **2015**, *195*, 5440–5451. [CrossRef] [PubMed]
85. Aktar, M.K.; Kido-Nakahara, M.; Furue, M.; Nakahara, T. Mutual upregulation of endothelin-1 and IL-25 in atopic dermatitis. *Allergy* **2015**, *70*, 846–854. [CrossRef]
86. Cua, D.J.; Tato, C.M. Innate IL-17-producing cells: The sentinels of the immune system. *Nat. Rev. Immunol.* **2010**, *10*, 479–489. [CrossRef] [PubMed]
87. Chen, L.; He, Z.; Slinger, E.; Bongers, G.; Lapenda, T.L.S.; Pacer, M.E.; Jiao, J.; Beltrao, M.F.; Soto, A.J.; Harpaz, N.; et al. IL-23 activates innate lymphoid cells to promote neonatal intestinal pathology. *Mucosal Immunol.* **2015**, *8*, 390–402. [CrossRef]
88. Cai, Y.; Shen, X.; Ding, C.; Qi, C.; Li, K.; Li, X.; Jala, V.R.; Zhang, H.G.; Wang, T.; Zheng, J.; et al. Pivotal role of dermal IL-17-producing γδ T cells in skin inflammation. *Immunity* **2011**, *35*, 596–610. [CrossRef]
89. Villanova, F.; Flutter, B.; Tosi, I.; Grys, K.; Sreeneebus, H.; Perera, G.K.; Chapman, A.; Smith, C.H.; Di Meglio, P.; Nestle, F.O. Characterization of innate lymphoid cells in human skin and blood demonstrates increase of NKp44+ ILC3 in psoriasis. *J. Investig. Dermatol.* **2014**, *134*, 984–991. [CrossRef]
90. Matsuzaki, G.; Umemura, M. Interleukin-17 family cytokines in protective immunity against infections: Role of hematopoietic cell-derived and non-hematopoietic cell-derived interleukin-17s. *Microbiol. Immunol.* **2018**, *62*, 1–13. [CrossRef]
91. Chang, S.H.; Reynolds, J.M.; Pappu, B.P.; Chen, G.; Martinez, G.J.; Dong, C. Interleukin-17C promotes Th17 cell responses and autoimmune disease via interleukin-17 receptor E. *Immunity* **2011**, *35*, 611–621. [CrossRef] [PubMed]
92. Hu, Y.; Ota, N.; Peng, I.; Refino, C.J.; Danilenko, D.M.; Caplazi, P.; Ouyang, W. IL-17RC is required for IL-17A- and IL-17F-dependent signaling and the pathogenesis of experimental autoimmune encephalomyelitis. *J. Immunol.* **2010**, *184*, 4307–4316. [CrossRef] [PubMed]
93. Su, Y.; Huang, J.; Zhao, X.; Lu, H.; Wang, W.; Yang, X.O.; Shi, Y.; Wang, X.; Lai, Y.; Dong, C. Interleukin-17 receptor D constitutes an alternative receptor for interleukin-17A important in psoriasis-like skin inflammation. *Sci. Immunol.* **2019**, *4*. [CrossRef]
94. Liu, C.; Swaidani, S.; Qian, W.; Kang, Z.; Sun, P.; Han, Y.; Wang, C.; Gulen, M.F.; Yin, W.; Zhang, C.; et al. A CC′ loop decoy peptide blocks the interaction between Act1 and IL-17RA to attenuate IL-17- and IL-25-induced inflammation. *Sci.Signal* **2011**, *4*, ra72. [CrossRef] [PubMed]
95. Sønder, S.U.; Saret, S.; Tang, W.; Sturdevant, D.E.; Porcella, S.F.; Siebenlist, U. IL-17-induced NF-kappaB activation via CIKS/Act1: Physiologic significance and signaling mechanisms. *J. Biol. Chem.* **2011**, *286*, 12881–12890. [CrossRef] [PubMed]
96. Okada, S.; Puel, A.; Casanova, J.L.; Kobayashi, M. Chronic mucocutaneous candidiasis disease associated with inborn errors of IL-17 immunity. *Clin. Transl. Immunology* **2016**, *5*, e114. [CrossRef] [PubMed]

97. Wang, M.; Zhang, S.; Zheng, G.; Huang, J.; Songyang, Z.; Zhao, X.; Lin, X. Gain-of-function mutation of Card14 leads to spontaneous psoriasis-like skin inflammation through enhanced keratinocyte response to IL-17A. *Immunity* **2018**, *49*, 66–79. [CrossRef] [PubMed]
98. Chen, X.; Cai, G.; Liu, C.; Zhao, J.; Gu, C.; Wu, L.; Hamilton, T.A.; Zhang, C.J.; Ko, J.; Zhu, L.; et al. IL-17R-EGFR axis links wound healing to tumorigenesis in Lrig1(+) stem cells. *J. Exp. Med.* **2019**, *216*, 195–214. [CrossRef]
99. Tsang, M.; Friesel, R.; Kudoh, T.; Dawid, I.B. Identification of Sef, a novel modulator of FGF signalling. *Nat. Cell Biol.* **2002**, *4*, 165–169. [CrossRef]
100. Calautti, E.; Avalle, L.; Poli, V. Psoriasis: A STAT3-centric view. *Int. J. Mol. Sci.* **2018**, *19*, 171. [CrossRef]
101. Sano, S.; Chan, K.S.; Carbajal, S.; Clifford, J.; Peavey, M.; Kiguchi, K.; Itami, S.; Nickoloff, B.J.; DiGiovanni, J. Stat3 links activated keratinocytes and immunocytes required for development of psoriasis in a novel transgenic mouse model. *Nat. Med.* **2005**, *11*, 43–49. [CrossRef] [PubMed]
102. Miyoshi, K.; Takaishi, M.; Nakajima, K.; Ikeda, M.; Kanda, T.; Tarutani, M.; Iiyama, T.; Asao, N.; DiGiovanni, J.; Sano, S. Stat3 as a therapeutic target for the treatment of psoriasis: A clinical feasibility study with STA-21, a Stat3 inhibitor. *J. Investig. Dermatol.* **2011**, *131*, 108–117. [CrossRef] [PubMed]
103. Bae, H.C.; Jeong, S.H.; Kim, J.H.; Lee, H.; Ryu, W.I.; Kim, M.G.; Son, E.D.; Lee, T.R.; Son, S.W. RIP4 upregulates CCL20 expression through STAT3 signalling in cultured keratinocytes. *Exp. Dermatol.* **2018**, *27*, 1126–1133. [CrossRef] [PubMed]
104. Shi, X.; Jin, L.; Dang, E.; Chang, T.; Feng, Z.; Liu, Y.; Wang, G. IL-17A upregulates keratin 17 expression in keratinocytes through STAT1- and STAT3-dependent mechanisms. *J. Investig. Dermatol.* **2011**, *131*, 2401–2408. [CrossRef]
105. Honma, M.; Minami-Hori, M.; Takahashi, H.; Iizuka, H. Podoplanin expression in wound and hyperproliferative psoriatic epidermis: Regulation by TGF-β and STAT-3 activating cytokines, IFN-γ, IL-6, and IL-22. *J. Dermatol. Sci.* **2012**, *65*, 134–140. [CrossRef]
106. Miyoshi, K.; Takaishi, M.; Digiovanni, J.; Sano, S. Attenuation of psoriasis-like skin lesion in a mouse model by topical treatment with indirubin and its derivastive E804. *J. Dermatol. Sci.* **2012**, *65*, 70–72. [CrossRef]
107. Ekman, A.K.; Bivik Eding, C.; Rundquist, I.; Enerbäck, C. IL-17 and IL-22 promote keratinocyte stemness in the germinative compartment in psoriasis. *J. Investig. Dermatol.* **2019**, *139*, 1564–1573. [CrossRef]
108. Karbach, S.; Croxford, A.L.; Oelze, M.; Schüler, R.; Minwegen, D.; Wegner, J.; Koukes, L.; Yogev, N.; Nikolaev, A.; Reißig, S.; et al. Interleukin 17 drives vascular inflammation, endothelial dysfunction, and arterial hypertension in psoriasis-like skin disease. *Arterioscler. Thromb. Vasc. Biol.* **2014**, *34*, 2658–2668. [CrossRef]
109. Cordoro, K.M.; Hitraya-Low, M.; Taravati, K.; Sandoval, P.M.; Kim, E.; Sugarman, J.; Pauli, M.L.; Liao, W.; Rosenblum, M.D. Skin-infiltrating, interleukin-22-producing T cells differentiate pediatric psoriasis from adult psoriasis. *J. Am. Acad. Dermatol.* **2017**, *77*, 417–424. [CrossRef]
110. Diani, M.; Altomare, G.; Reali, E. T cell responses in psoriasis and psoriatic arthritis. *Autoimmun. Rev.* **2015**, *14*, 286–292. [CrossRef]
111. Puel, A.; Cypowyj, S.; Bustamante, J.; Wright, J.F.; Liu, L.; Lim, H.K.; Migaud, M.; Israel, L.; Chrabieh, M.; Audry, M.; et al. Chronic mucocutaneous candidiasis in humans with inborn errors of interleukin-17 immunity. *Science* **2011**, *332*, 65–68. [CrossRef] [PubMed]
112. Boisson, B.; Wang, C.; Pedergnana, V.; Wu, L.; Cypowyj, S.; Rybojad, M.; Belkadi, A.; Picard, C.; Abel, L.; Fieschi, C.; et al. An ACT1 mutation selectively abolishes interleukin-17 responses in humans with chronic mucocutaneous candidiasis. *Immunity* **2013**, *39*, 676–686. [CrossRef] [PubMed]
113. Ling, Y.; Cypowyj, S.; Aytekin, C.; Galicchio, M.; Camcioglu, Y.; Nepesov, S.; Ikinciogullari, A.; Dogu, F.; Belkadi, A.; Levy, R.; et al. Inherited IL-17RC deficiency in patients with chronic mucocutaneous candidiasis. *J. Exp. Med.* **2015**, *212*, 619–631. [CrossRef] [PubMed]
114. Ferreira, M.C.; Whibley, N.; Mamo, A.J.; Siebenlist, U.; Chan, Y.R.; Gaffen, S.L. Interleukin-17-induced protein lipocalin 2 is dispensable for immunity to oral candidiasis. *Infect. Immun.* **2014**, *82*, 1030–1035. [CrossRef]
115. Conti, H.R.; Shen, F.; Nayyar, N.; Stocum, E.; Sun, J.N.; Lindemann, M.J.; Ho, A.W.; Hai, J.H.; Yu, J.J.; Jung, J.W.; et al. Th17 cells and IL-17 receptor signaling are essential for mucosal host defense against oral candidiasis. *J. Exp. Med.* **2009**, *206*, 299–311. [CrossRef]
116. Conti, H.R.; Gaffen, S.L. IL-17-mediated immunity to the opportunistic fungal pathogen Candida albicans. *J. Immunol.* **2015**, *195*, 780–788. [CrossRef]

117. Li, J.; Vinh, D.C.; Casanova, J.L.; Puel, A. Inborn errors of immunity underlying fungal diseases in otherwise healthy individuals. *Curr. Opin. Microbiol.* **2017**, *40*, 46–57. [CrossRef]
118. Sparber, F.; De Gregorio, C.; Steckholzer, S.; Ferreira, F.M.; Dolowschiak, T.; Ruchti, F.; Kirchner, F.R.; Mertens, S.; Prinz, I.; Joller, N.; et al. The skin commensal yeast Malassezia triggers a type 17 response that coordinates anti-fungal immunity and exacerbates skin inflammation. *Cell Host Microbe* **2019**, *25*, 389–403. [CrossRef]
119. Wohn, C.; Brand, A.; van Ettinger, K.; Brouwers-Haspels, I.; Waisman, A.; Laman, J.D.; Clausen, B.E. Gradual development of psoriatic skin lesions by constitutive low-level expression of IL-17A. *Cell. Immunol.* **2016**, *308*, 57–65. [CrossRef]
120. Aggarwal, S.; Ghilardi, N.; Xie, M.H.; de Sauvage, F.J.; Gurney, A.L. Interleukin-23 promotes a distinct CD4 T cell activation state characterized by the production of interleukin-17. *J. Biol. Chem.* **2003**, *278*, 1910–1914. [CrossRef]
121. Ivanov, I.I.; McKenzie, B.S.; Zhou, L.; Tadokoro, C.E.; Lepelley, A.; Lafaille, J.J.; Cua, D.J.; Littman, D.R. The orphan nuclear receptor RORgammat directs the differentiation program of proinflammatory IL-17+ T helper cells. *Cell* **2006**, *126*, 1121–1133. [CrossRef] [PubMed]
122. Gaffen, S.L. Structure and signalling in the IL-17 receptor family. *Nat. Rev. Immunol.* **2009**, *9*, 556–567. [CrossRef] [PubMed]
123. Villegas, J.A.; Bayer, A.C.; Ider, K.; Bismuth, J.; Truffault, F.; Roussin, R.; Santelmo, N.; Le Panse, R.; Berrih-Aknin, S.; Dragin, N. Il-23/Th17 cell pathway: A promising target to alleviate thymic inflammation maintenance in myasthenia gravis. *J. Autoimmun.* **2019**, *98*, 59–73. [CrossRef] [PubMed]
124. Chan, J.R.; Blumenschein, W.; Murphy, E.; Diveu, C.; Wiekowski, M.; Abbondanzo, S.; Lucian, L.; Geissler, R.; Brodie, S.; Kimball, A.B.; et al. IL-23 stimulates epidermal hyperplasia via TNF and IL-20R2-dependent mechanisms with implications for psoriasis pathogenesis. *J. Exp. Med.* **2006**, *203*, 2577–2587. [CrossRef]
125. Furue, M.; Kadono, T. The contribution of IL-17 to the development of autoimmunity in psoriasis. *Innate Immun.* **2019**, *25*, 337–343. [CrossRef]
126. Arakawa, A.; Siewert, K.; Stöhr, J.; Besgen, P.; Kim, S.M.; Rühl, G.; Nickel, J.; Vollmer, S.; Thomas, P.; Krebs, S.; et al. Melanocyte antigen triggers autoimmunity in human psoriasis. *J. Exp. Med.* **2015**, *212*, 2203–2212. [CrossRef]
127. Lee, E.; Trepicchio, W.L.; Oestreicher, J.L.; Pittman, D.; Wang, F.; Chamian, F.; Dhodapkar, M.; Krueger, J.G. Increased expression of interleukin 23 p19 and p40 in lesional skin of patients with psoriasis vulgaris. *J. Exp. Med.* **2004**, *199*, 125–130. [CrossRef]
128. Zaba, L.C.; Cardinale, I.; Gilleaudeau, P.; Sullivan-Whalen, M.; Suárez-Fariñas, M.; Fuentes-Duculan, J.; Novitskaya, I.; Khatcherian, A.; Bluth, M.J.; Lowes, M.A.; et al. Amelioration of epidermal hyperplasia by TNF inhibition is associated with reduced Th17 responses. *J. Exp. Med.* **2007**, *204*, 3183–3194. [CrossRef]
129. Piskin, G.; Sylva-Steenland, R.M.; Bos, J.D.; Teunissen, M.B. In vitro and in situ expression of IL-23 by keratinocytes in healthy skin and psoriasis lesions: Enhanced expression in psoriatic skin. *J. Immunol.* **2006**, *176*, 1908–1915. [CrossRef]
130. Li, H.; Yao, Q.; Mariscal, A.G.; Wu, X.; Hülse, J.; Pedersen, E.; Helin, K.; Waisman, A.; Vinkel, C.; Thomsen, S.F.; et al. Epigenetic control of IL-23 expression in keratinocytes is important for chronic skin inflammation. *Nat. Commun.* **2018**, *9*, 1420. [CrossRef]
131. Tu, Z.; Zhang, S.; Zhou, G.; Zhou, L.; Xiang, Q.; Chen, Q.; Zhao, P.; Zhan, H.; Zhou, H.; Sun, L. LMO4 is a disease-provocative transcription coregulator activated by IL-23 in psoriatic keratinocytes. *J. Investig. Dermatol.* **2018**, *138*, 1078–1087. [CrossRef] [PubMed]
132. McInnes, I.B.; Kavanaugh, A.; Gottlieb, A.B.; Puig, L.; Rahman, P.; Ritchlin, C.; Brodmerkel, C.; Li, S.; Wang, Y.; Mendelsohn, A.M.; et al. Efficacy and safety of ustekinumab in patients with active psoriatic arthritis: 1 year results of the phase 3, multicentre, double-blind, placebo-controlled PSUMMIT 1 trial. *Lancet* **2013**, *382*, 780–789. [CrossRef]
133. Papp, K.A.; Blauvelt, A.; Bukhalo, M.; Gooderham, M.; Krueger, J.G.; Lacour, J.P.; Menter, A.; Philipp, S.; Sofen, H.; Tyring, S.; et al. Risankizumab versus ustekinumab for moderate-to-severe plaque psoriasis. *N. Engl. J. Med.* **2017**, *376*, 1551–1560. [CrossRef] [PubMed]

134. Blauvelt, A.; Papp, K.A.; Griffiths, C.E.; Randazzo, B.; Wasfi, Y.; Shen, Y.K.; Li, S.; Kimball, A.B. Efficacy and safety of guselkumab, an anti-interleukin-23 monoclonal antibody, compared with adalimumab for the continuous treatment of patients with moderate to severe psoriasis: Results from the phase III, double-blinded, placebo- and active comparator-controlled VOYAGE 1 trial. *J. Am. Acad. Dermatol.* **2017**, *76*, 405–417.

135. Reich, K.; Papp, K.A.; Blauvelt, A.; Tyring, S.K.; Sinclair, R.; Thaçi, D.; Nograles, K.; Mehta, A.; Cichanowitz, N.; Li, Q.; et al. Tildrakizumab versus placebo or etanercept for chronic plaque psoriasis (reSURFACE 1 and reSURFACE 2): Results from two randomised controlled, phase 3 trials. *Lancet* **2017**, *390*, 276–288. [CrossRef]

136. Johansen, C.; Usher, P.A.; Kellerup, R.B.; Lundsgaard, D.; Iversen, L.; Kragballe, K. Characterization of the interleukin-17 isoforms and receptors in lesional psoriatic skin. *Br. J. Dermatol.* **2009**, *160*, 319–324. [CrossRef]

137. Johnston, A.; Fritz, Y.; Dawes, S.M.; Diaconu, D.; Al-Attar, P.M.; Guzman, A.M.; Chen, C.S.; Fu, W.; Gudjonsson, J.E.; McCormick, T.S.; et al. Keratinocyte overexpression of IL-17C promotes psoriasiform skin inflammation. *J. Immunol.* **2013**, *190*, 2252–2262. [CrossRef]

138. Martin, D.A.; Towne, J.E.; Kricorian, G.; Klekotka, P.; Gudjonsson, J.E.; Krueger, J.G.; Russell, C.B. The emerging role of IL-17 in the pathogenesis of psoriasis: Preclinical and clinical findings. *J. Investig. Dermatol.* **2013**, *133*, 17–26. [CrossRef]

139. Ramirez-Carrozzi, V.; Sambandam, A.; Luis, E.; Lin, Z.; Jeet, S.; Lesch, J.; Hackney, J.; Kim, J.; Zhou, M.; Lai, J.; et al. IL-17C regulates the innate immune function of epithelial cells in an autocrine manner. *Nat. Immunol.* **2011**, *12*, 1159–1166. [CrossRef]

140. Vandeghinste, N.; Klattig, J.; Jagerschmidt, C.; Lavazais, S.; Marsais, F.; Haas, J.D.; Auberval, M.; Lauffer, F.; Moran, T.; Ongenaert, M.; et al. Neutralization of IL-17C reduces skin inflammation in mouse models of psoriasis and atopic dermatitis. *J. Investig. Dermatol.* **2018**, *138*, 1555–1563. [CrossRef]

141. Guttman-Yassky, E.; Krueger, J.G. IL-17C: A unique epithelial cytokine with potential for targeting across the spectrum of atopic dermatitis and psoriasis. *J. Investig. Dermatol.* **2018**, *138*, 1467–1469. [CrossRef] [PubMed]

142. Tsoi, L.C.; Rodriguez, E.; Degenhardt, F.; Baurecht, H.; Wehkamp, U.; Volks, N.; Szymczak, S.; Swindell, W.R.; Sarkar, M.K.; Raja, K.; et al. Atopic dermatitis is an IL-13-dominant disease with greater molecular heterogeneity compared to psoriasis. *J. Investig. Dermatol.* **2019**, *139*, 1480–1489. [CrossRef] [PubMed]

143. Pène, J.; Chevalier, S.; Preisser, L.; Vénéreau, E.; Guilleux, M.H.; Ghannam, S.; Molès, J.P.; Danger, Y.; Ravon, E.; Lesaux, S.; et al. Chronically inflamed human tissues are infiltrated by highly differentiated Th17 lymphocytes. *J. Immunol.* **2008**, *180*, 7423–7430. [CrossRef]

144. Lande, R.; Botti, E.; Jandus, C.; Dojcinovic, D.; Fanelli, G.; Conrad, C.; Chamilos, G.; Feldmeyer, L.; Marinari, B.; Chon, S.; et al. The antimicrobial peptide LL37 is a T-cell autoantigen in psoriasis. *Nat. Commun.* **2014**, *5*, 5621. [CrossRef] [PubMed]

145. Fuentes-Duculan, J.; Bonifacio, K.M.; Hawkes, J.E.; Kunjravia, N.; Cueto, I.; Li, X.; Gonzalez, J.; Garcet, S.; Krueger, J.G. Autoantigens ADAMTSL5 and LL37 are significantly upregulated in active Psoriasis and localized with keratinocytes, dendritic cells and other leukocytes. *Exp. Dermatol.* **2017**, *26*, 1075–1082. [CrossRef] [PubMed]

146. Yunusbaeva, M.; Valiev, R.; Bilalov, F.; Sultanova, Z.; Sharipova, L.; Yunusbayev, B. Psoriasis patients demonstrate HLA-Cw*06:02 allele dosage-dependent T cell proliferation when treated with hair follicle-derived keratin 17 protein. *Sci. Rep.* **2018**, *8*, 6098. [CrossRef] [PubMed]

147. Cheung, K.L.; Jarrett, R.; Subramaniam, S.; Salimi, M.; Gutowska-Owsiak, D.; Chen, Y.L.; Hardman, C.; Xue, L.; Cerundolo, V.; Ogg, G. Psoriatic T cells recognize neolipid antigens generated by mast cell phospholipase delivered by exosomes and presented by CD1a. *J. Exp. Med.* **2016**, *213*, 2399–2412. [CrossRef] [PubMed]

148. Chiricozzi, A.; Suárez-Fariñas, M.; Fuentes-Duculan, J.; Cueto, I.; Li, K.; Tian, S.; Brodmerkel, C.; Krueger, J.G. Increased expression of interleukin-17 pathway genes in nonlesional skin of moderate-to-severe psoriasis vulgaris. *Br. J. Dermatol.* **2016**, *174*, 136–145. [CrossRef] [PubMed]

149. Weisman, S.; Pollack, C.R.; Gottschalk, R.W. Psoriasis disease severity measures: Comparing efficacy of treatments for severe psoriasis. *J. Dermatolog. Treat.* **2003**, *14*, 158–165. [CrossRef] [PubMed]

150. Langley, R.G.; Elewski, B.E.; Lebwohl, M.; Reich, K.; Griffiths, C.E.; Papp, K.; Puig, L.; Nakagawa, H.; Spelman, L.; Sigurgeirsson, B.; et al. Secukinumab in plaque psoriasis–results of two phase 3 trials. *N. Engl. J. Med.* **2014**, *371*, 326–338. [CrossRef] [PubMed]

151. Gordon, K.B.; Blauvelt, A.; Papp, K.A.; Langley, R.G.; Luger, T.; Ohtsuki, M.; Reich, K.; Amato, D.; Ball, S.G.; Braun, D.K.; et al. Phase 3 trials of ixekizumab in moderate-to-severe plaque psoriasis. *N. Engl. J. Med.* **2016**, *375*, 345–356. [CrossRef] [PubMed]

152. Lebwohl, M.; Strober, B.; Menter, A.; Gordon, K.; Weglowska, J.; Puig, L.; Papp, K.; Spelman, L.; Toth, D.; Kerdel, F.; et al. Phase 3 studies comparing brodalumab with ustekinumab in psoriasis. *N. Engl. J. Med.* **2015**, *373*, 1318–1328. [CrossRef] [PubMed]
153. Paramio, J.M.; Casanova, M.L.; Segrelles, C.; Mittnacht, S.; Lane, E.B.; Jorcano, J.L. Modulation of cell proliferation by cytokeratins K10 and K16. *Mol. Cell Biol.* **1999**, *19*, 3086–3094. [CrossRef] [PubMed]
154. Krueger, J.G.; Ferris, L.K.; Menter, A.; Wagner, F.; White, A.; Visvanathan, S.; Lalovic, B.; Aslanyan, S.; Wang, E.E.; Hall, D.; et al. Anti-IL-23A mAb BI 655066 for treatment of moderate-to-severe psoriasis: Safety, efficacy, pharmacokinetics, and biomarker results of a single-rising-dose, randomized, double-blind, placebo-controlled trial. *J. Allergy Clin. Immunol.* **2015**, *136*, 116–124. [CrossRef] [PubMed]
155. Kulke, R.; Tödt-Pingel, I.; Rademacher, D.; Röwert, J.; Schröder, J.M.; Christophers, E. Co-localized overexpression of GRO-alpha and IL-8 mRNA is restricted to the suprapapillary layers of psoriatic lesions. *J. Investig. Dermatol.* **1996**, *106*, 526–530. [CrossRef] [PubMed]
156. Furue, K.; Yamamura, K.; Tsuji, G.; Mitoma, C.; Uchi, H.; Nakahara, T.; Kido-Nakahara, M.; Kadono, T.; Furue, M. Highlighting interleukin-36 signalling in plaque psoriasis and pustular psoriasis. *Acta Derm. Venereol.* **2018**, *98*, 5–13. [CrossRef] [PubMed]
157. Johnston, A.; Xing, X.; Guzman, A.M.; Riblett, M.; Loyd, C.M.; Ward, N.L.; Wohn, C.; Prens, E.P.; Wang, F.; Maier, L.E.; et al. IL-1F5, -F6, -F8, and -F9: A novel IL-1 family signaling system that is active in psoriasis and promotes keratinocyte antimicrobial peptide expression. *J. Immunol.* **2011**, *186*, 2613–2622. [CrossRef]
158. Homey, B.; Dieu-Nosjean, M.C.; Wiesenborn, A.; Massacrier, C.; Pin, J.J.; Oldham, E.; Catron, D.; Buchanan, M.E.; Müller, A.; de Waal Malefyt, R.; et al. Up-regulation of macrophage inflammatory protein-3 alpha/CCL20 and CC chemokine receptor 6 in psoriasis. *J. Immunol.* **2000**, *164*, 6621–6632. [CrossRef]
159. Kim, T.G.; Jee, H.; Fuentes-Duculan, J.; Wu, W.H.; Byamba, D.; Kim, D.S.; Kim, D.Y.; Lew, D.H.; Yang, W.I.; Krueger, J.G.; et al. Dermal clusters of mature dendritic cells and T cells are associated with the CCL20/CCR6 chemokine system in chronic psoriasis. *J. Investig. Dermatol.* **2014**, *134*, 1462–1465. [CrossRef]
160. Furue, K.; Ito, T.; Tsuji, G.; Nakahara, T.; Furue, M. The CCL20 and CCR6 axis in psoriasis. *Scand. J. Immunol.* **2019**. [CrossRef]
161. Bando, J.K.; Gilfillan, S.; Song, C.; McDonald, K.G.; Huang, S.C.; Newberry, R.D.; Kobayashi, Y.; Allan, D.S.J.; Carlyle, J.R.; Cella, M.; et al. The tumor necrosis factor superfamily member RANKL suppresses effector cytokine production in group 3 innate lymphoid cells. *Immunity* **2018**, *48*, 1208–1219. [CrossRef]
162. Talayero, P.; Mancebo, E.; Calvo-Pulido, J.; Rodríguez-Muñoz, S.; Bernardo, I.; Laguna-Goya, R.; Cano-Romero, F.L.; García-Sesma, A.; Loinaz, C.; Jiménez, C.; et al. Innate lymphoid cells groups 1 and 3 in the epithelial compartment of functional human intestinal allografts. *Am. J. Transplant.* **2016**, *16*, 72–82. [CrossRef]
163. Diani, M.; Casciano, F.; Marongiu, L.; Longhi, M.; Altomare, A.; Pigatto, P.D.; Secchiero, P.; Gambari, R.; Banfi, G.; Manfredi, A.A.; et al. Increased frequency of activated CD8(+) T cell effectors in patients with psoriatic arthritis. *Sci. Rep.* **2019**, *9*, 10870. [CrossRef]
164. Steel, K.J.A.; Srenathan, U.; Ridley, M.; Durham, L.E.; Wu, S.Y.; Ryan, S.E.; Hughes, C.D.; Chan, E.; Kirkham, B.W.; Taams, L.S. Synovial IL-17A+ CD8+ T cells display a polyfunctional, pro-inflammatory and tissue-resident memory phenotype and function in psoriatic arthritis. *Arthritis Rheumatol.* **2019**. [CrossRef]
165. Campbell, J.J.; Ebsworth, K.; Ertl, L.S.; McMahon, J.P.; Newland, D.; Wang, Y.; Liu, S.; Miao, Z.; Dang, T.; Zhang, P.; et al. IL-17-secreting γδ T Cells are completely dependent upon CCR6 for homing to inflamed skin. *J. Immunol.* **2017**, *199*, 3129–3136. [CrossRef]
166. Ishida-Yamamoto, A.; Iizuka, H. Differences in involucrin immunolabeling within cornified cell envelopes in normal and psoriatic epidermis. *J. Investig. Dermatol.* **1995**, *104*, 391–395. [CrossRef]
167. Caldwell, C.J.; Hobbs, C.; McKee, P.H. The relationship of Ki67 and involucrin expression in proliferative, pre-neoplastic and neoplastic skin. *Clin. Exp. Dermatol.* **1997**, *22*, 11–16. [CrossRef]
168. Krueger, J.G.; Fretzin, S.; Suárez-Fariñas, M.; Haslett, P.A.; Phipps, K.M.; Cameron, G.S.; McColm, J.; Katcherian, A.; Cueto, I.; White, T.; et al. IL-17A is essential for cell activation and inflammatory gene circuits in subjects with psoriasis. *J. Allergy Clin. Immunol.* **2012**, *130*, 145–154.e9. [CrossRef] [PubMed]

169. Chiricozzi, A.; Nograles, K.E.; Johnson-Huang, L.M.; Fuentes-Duculan, J.; Cardinale, I.; Bonifacio, K.M.; Gulati, N.; Mitsui, H.; Guttman-Yassky, E.; Suárez-Fariñas, M.; et al. IL-17 induces an expanded range of downstream genes in reconstituted human epidermis model. *PLoS ONE* **2014**, *9*, e90284. [CrossRef] [PubMed]
170. Ha, H.L.; Wang, H.; Pisitkun, P.; Kim, J.C.; Tassi, I.; Tang, W.; Morasso, M.I.; Udey, M.C.; Siebenlist, U. IL-17 drives psoriatic inflammation via distinct, target cell-specific mechanisms. *Proc. Natl. Acad. Sci. USA* **2014**, *111*, E3422–E3431. [CrossRef] [PubMed]
171. Ma, W.Y.; Jia, K.; Zhang, Y. IL-17 promotes keratinocyte proliferation via the downregulation of C/EBPα. *Exp. Ther. Med.* **2016**, *11*, 631–636. [CrossRef] [PubMed]
172. Zenobia, C.; Hajishengallis, G. Basic biology and role of interleukin-17 in immunity and inflammation. *Periodontol. 2000* **2015**, *69*, 142–159. [CrossRef] [PubMed]
173. Chiricozzi, A.; Guttman-Yassky, E.; Suárez-Fariñas, M.; Nograles, K.E.; Tian, S.; Cardinale, I.; Chimenti, S.; Krueger, J.G. Integrative responses to IL-17 and TNF-α in human keratinocytes account for key inflammatory pathogenic circuits in psoriasis. *J. Investig. Dermatol.* **2011**, *131*, 677–687. [CrossRef] [PubMed]
174. Lawrence, T. The nuclear factor NF-kappaB pathway in inflammation. *Cold Spring Harb. Perspect. Biol.* **2009**, *1*, a001651. [CrossRef] [PubMed]
175. House, J.S.; Zhu, S.; Ranjan, R.; Linder, K.; Smart, R.C. C/EBPalpha and C/EBPbeta are required for Sebocyte differentiation and stratified squamous differentiation in adult mouse skin. *PLoS ONE* **2010**, *5*, e9837. [CrossRef] [PubMed]
176. Crish, J.F.; Gopalakrishnan, R.; Bone, F.; Gilliam, A.C.; Eckert, R.L. The distal and proximal regulatory regions of the involucrin gene promoter have distinct functions and are required for in vivo involucrin expression. *J. Investig. Dermatol.* **2006**, *126*, 305–314. [CrossRef] [PubMed]
177. Witte, E.; Kokolakis, G.; Witte, K.; Philipp, S.; Doecke, W.D.; Babel, N.; Wittig, B.M.; Warszawska, K.; Kurek, A.; Erdmann-Keding, M.; et al. IL-19 is a component of the pathogenetic IL-23/IL-17 cascade in psoriasis. *J. Investig. Dermatol.* **2014**, *134*, 2757–2767. [CrossRef]
178. Sun, D.P.; Yeh, C.H.; So, E.; Wang, L.Y.; Wei, T.S.; Chang, M.S.; Hsing, C.H. Interleukin (IL)-19 promoted skin wound healing by increasing fibroblast keratinocyte growth factor expression. *Cytokine* **2013**, *62*, 360–368. [CrossRef]
179. Yang, L.; Fan, X.; Cui, T.; Dang, E.; Wang, G. Nrf2 promotes keratinocyte proliferation in psoriasis through up-regulation of keratin 6, keratin 16, and keratin 17. *J. Investig. Dermatol.* **2017**, *137*, 2168–2176. [CrossRef]
180. Paladini, R.D.; Coulombe, P.A. Directed expression of keratin 16 to the progenitor basal cells of transgenic mouse skin delays skin maturation. *J. Cell Biol.* **1998**, *142*, 1035–1051. [CrossRef]
181. Acciani, T.H.; Suzuki, T.; Trapnell, B.C.; Le Cras, T.D. Epidermal growth factor receptor signalling regulates granulocyte-macrophage colony-stimulating factor production by airway epithelial cells and established allergic airway disease. *Clin. Exp. Allergy* **2016**, *46*, 317–328. [CrossRef] [PubMed]
182. Furue, K.; Ito, T.; Tanaka, Y.; Hashimoto-Hachiya, A.; Takemura, M.; Murata, M.; Kido-Nakahara, M.; Tsuji, G.; Nakahara, T.; Furue, M. The EGFR-ERK/JNK-CCL20 pathway in scratched keratinocytes may underpin koebnerization in psoriasis atients. *Int. J. Mol. Sci.* **2020**, *21*, 434. [CrossRef] [PubMed]
183. Johnston, A.; Gudjonsson, J.E.; Aphale, A.; Guzman, A.M.; Stoll, S.W.; Elder, J.T. EGFR and IL-1 signaling synergistically promote keratinocyte antimicrobial defenses in a differentiation-dependent manner. *J. Investig. Dermatol.* **2011**, *131*, 329–337. [CrossRef] [PubMed]
184. Goepel, L.; Jacobi, A.; Augustin, M.; Radtke, M.A. Rapid improvement of psoriasis in a patient with lung cancer after treatment with erlotinib. *J. Eur. Acad. Dermatol. Venereol.* **2018**, *32*, e311–e313. [CrossRef] [PubMed]
185. Overbeck, T.R.; Griesinger, F. Two cases of psoriasis responding to erlotinib: Time to revisiting inhibition of epidermal growth factor receptor in psoriasis therapy? *Dermatology* **2012**, *225*, 179–182. [CrossRef]
186. Trivin, F.; Boucher, E.; Raoul, J.L. Complete sustained regression of extensive psoriasis with cetuximab combination chemotherapy. *Acta Oncol.* **2004**, *43*, 592–593. [CrossRef]
187. Neyns, B.; Meert, V.; Vandenbroucke, F. Cetuximab treatment in a patient with metastatic colorectal cancer and psoriasis. *Curr. Oncol.* **2008**, *15*, 196–197. [CrossRef]
188. Carrier, Y.; Ma, H.L.; Ramon, H.E.; Napierata, L.; Small, C.; O'Toole, M.; Young, D.A.; Fouser, L.A.; Nickerson-Nutter, C.; Collins, M.; et al. Inter-regulation of Th17 cytokines and the IL-36 cytokines in vitro and in vivo: Implications in psoriasis pathogenesis. *J. Investig. Dermatol.* **2011**, *131*, 2428–2437. [CrossRef]

189. Gläser, R.; Meyer-Hoffert, U.; Harder, J.; Cordes, J.; Wittersheim, M.; Kobliakova, J.; Fölster-Holst, R.; Proksch, E.; Schröder, J.M.; Schwarz, T. The antimicrobial protein psoriasin (S100A7) is upregulated in atopic dermatitis and after experimental skin barrier disruption. *J. Investig. Dermatol.* **2009**, *129*, 641–649. [CrossRef]
190. Nograles, K.E.; Zaba, L.C.; Guttman-Yassky, E.; Fuentes-Duculan, J.; Suárez-Fariñas, M.; Cardinale, I.; Khatcherian, A.; Gonzalez, J.; Pierson, K.C.; White, T.R.; et al. Th17 cytokines interleukin (IL)-17 and IL-22 modulate distinct inflammatory and keratinocyte-response pathways. *Br. J. Dermatol.* **2008**, *159*, 1092–1102. [CrossRef]
191. Baggiolini, M. Chemokines in pathology and medicine. *J. Intern. Med.* **2001**, *250*, 91–104. [CrossRef] [PubMed]
192. Johnston, A.; Xing, X.; Wolterink, L.; Barnes, D.H.; Yin, Z.; Reingold, L.; Kahlenberg, J.M.; Harms, P.W.; Gudjonsson, J.E. IL-1 and IL-36 are dominant cytokines in generalized pustular psoriasis. *J. Allergy Clin. Immunol.* **2017**, *140*, 109–120. [CrossRef] [PubMed]
193. Nedoszytko, B.; Sokołowska-Wojdyło, M.; Ruckemann-Dziurdzińska, K.; Roszkiewicz, J.; Nowicki, R.J. Chemokines and cytokines network in the pathogenesis of the inflammatory skin diseases: Atopic dermatitis, psoriasis and skin mastocytosis. *Postepy. Dermatol. Alergol.* **2014**, *31*, 84–91. [CrossRef] [PubMed]
194. Li, N.; Yamasaki, K.; Saito, R.; Fukushi-Takahashi, S.; Shimada-Omori, R.; Asano, M.; Aiba, S. Alarmin function of cathelicidin antimicrobial peptide LL37 through IL-36γ induction in human epidermal keratinocytes. *J. Immunol.* **2014**, *193*, 5140–5148. [CrossRef] [PubMed]
195. Henry, C.M.; Sullivan, G.P.; Clancy, D.M.; Afonina, I.S.; Kulms, D.; Martin, S.J. Neutrophil-derived proteases escalate inflammation through activation of IL-36 family cytokines. *Cell Rep.* **2016**, *14*, 708–722. [CrossRef]
196. Pfaff, C.M.; Marquardt, Y.; Fietkau, K.; Baron, J.M.; Lüscher, B. The psoriasis-associated IL-17A induces and cooperates with IL-36 cytokines to control keratinocyte differentiation and function. *Sci. Rep.* **2017**, *7*, 15631. [CrossRef]
197. Muhr, P.; Zeitvogel, J.; Heitland, I.; Werfel, T.; Wittmann, M. Expression of interleukin (IL)-1 family members upon stimulation with IL-17 differs in keratinocytes derived from patients with psoriasis and healthy donors. *Br. J. Dermatol.* **2011**, *165*, 189–193. [CrossRef]
198. Gabay, C.; Towne, J.E. Regulation and function of interleukin-36 cytokines in homeostasis and pathological conditions. *J. Leukoc. Biol.* **2015**, *97*, 645–652. [CrossRef]
199. Madonna, S.; Girolomoni, G.; Dinarello, C.A.; Albanesi, C. The significance of IL-36 hyperactivation and IL-36R targeting in psoriasis. *Int. J. Mol. Sci.* **2019**, *20*, 3318. [CrossRef]
200. Bachelez, H.; Choon, S.E.; Marrakchi, S.; Burden, A.D.; Tsai, T.F.; Morita, A.; Turki, H.; Hall, D.B.; Shear, M.; Baum, P.; et al. Inhibition of the interleukin-36 pathway for the treatment of generalized pustular psoriasis. *N. Engl. J. Med.* **2019**, *380*, 981–983. [CrossRef]
201. Furue, K.; Ito, T.; Tanaka, Y.; Yumine, A.; Hashimoto-Hachiya, A.; Takemura, M.; Murata, M.; Yamamura, K.; Tsuji, G.; Furue, M. Cyto/chemokine profile of in vitro scratched keratinocyte model: Implications of significant upregulation of CCL20, CXCL8 and IL36G in Koebner phenomenon. *J. Dermatol. Sci.* **2019**, *94*, 244–251. [CrossRef] [PubMed]
202. Maecker, H.T.; McCoy, J.P.; Nussenblatt, R. Standardizing immunophenotyping for the Human Immunology Project. *Nat. Rev. Immunol.* **2012**, *12*, 191–200. [CrossRef]
203. Singh, S.P.; Zhang, H.H.; Foley, J.F.; Hedrick, M.N.; Farber, J.M. Human T cells that are able to produce IL-17 express the chemokine receptor CCR6. *J. Immunol.* **2008**, *180*, 214–221. [CrossRef] [PubMed]
204. Harper, E.G.; Guo, C.; Rizzo, H.; Lillis, J.V.; Kurtz, S.E.; Skorcheva, I.; Purdy, D.; Fitch, E.; Iordanov, M.; Blauvelt, A. Th17 cytokines stimulate CCL20 expression in keratinocytes in vitro and in vivo: Implications for psoriasis pathogenesis. *J. Investig. Dermatol.* **2009**, *129*, 2175–2183. [CrossRef] [PubMed]
205. Bouma, G.; Zamuner, S.; Hicks, K.; Want, A.; Oliveira, J.; Choudhury, A.; Brett, S.; Robertson, D.; Felton, L.; Norris, V.; et al. CCL20 neutralization by a monoclonal antibody in healthy subjects selectively inhibits recruitment of CCR6(+) cells in an experimental suction blister. *Br. J. Clin. Pharmacol.* **2017**, *83*, 1976–1990. [CrossRef] [PubMed]
206. Robert, R.; Ang, C.; Sun, G.; Juglair, L.; Lim, E.X.; Mason, L.J.; Payne, N.L.; Bernard, C.C.; Mackay, C.R. Essential role for CCR6 in certain inflammatory diseases demonstrated using specific antagonist and knockin mice. *JCI Insight* **2017**, *2*. [CrossRef]

207. Tawaraishi, T.; Sakauchi, N.; Hidaka, K.; Yoshikawa, K.; Okui, T.; Kuno, H.; Chisaki, I.; Aso, K. Identification of a novel series of potent and selective CCR6 inhibitors as biological probes. *Bioorg. Med. Chem. Lett.* **2018**, *28*, 3067–3072. [CrossRef]
208. Campbell, J.J.; Ebsworth, K.; Ertl, L.S.; McMahon, J.P.; Wang, Y.; Yau, S.; Mali, V.R.; Chhina, V.; Kumamoto, A.; Liu, S.; et al. Efficacy of chemokine receptor inhibition in treating IL-36α-induced psoriasiform inflammation. *J. Immunol.* **2019**, *202*, 1687–1692. [CrossRef]
209. Mose, M.; Kang, Z.; Raaby, L.; Iversen, L.; Johansen, C. TNFα- and IL-17A-mediated S100A8 expression is regulated by p38 MAPK. *Exp. Dermatol.* **2013**, *22*, 476–481. [CrossRef]
210. Liang, S.C.; Tan, X.Y.; Luxenberg, D.P.; Karim, R.; Dunussi-Joannopoulos, K.; Collins, M.; Fouser, L.A. Interleukin (IL)-22 and IL-17 are coexpressed by Th17 cells and cooperatively enhance expression of antimicrobial peptides. *J. Exp. Med.* **2006**, *203*, 2271–2279. [CrossRef]
211. D'Amico, F.; Skarmoutsou, E.; Granata, M.; Trovato, C.; Rossi, G.A.; Mazzarino, M.C. S100A7: A rAMPing up AMP molecule in psoriasis. *Cytokine Growth Factor Rev.* **2016**, *32*, 97–104. [CrossRef] [PubMed]
212. Sa, S.M.; Valdez, P.A.; Wu, J.; Jung, K.; Zhong, F.; Hall, L.; Kasman, I.; Winer, J.; Modrusan, Z.; Danilenko, D.M.; et al. The effects of IL-20 subfamily cytokines on reconstituted human epidermis suggest potential roles in cutaneous innate defense and pathogenic adaptive immunity in psoriasis. *J. Immunol.* **2007**, *178*, 2229–2240. [CrossRef] [PubMed]
213. Hegyi, Z.; Zwicker, S.; Bureik, D.; Peric, M.; Koglin, S.; Batycka-Baran, A.; Prinz, J.C.; Ruzicka, T.; Schauber, J.; Wolf, R. Vitamin D analog calcipotriol suppresses the Th17 cytokine-induced proinflammatory S100 "alarmins" psoriasin (S100A7) and koebnerisin (S100A15) in psoriasis. *J. Investig. Dermatol.* **2012**, *132*, 1416–1424. [CrossRef] [PubMed]
214. Hsu, K.; Champaiboon, C.; Guenther, B.D.; Sorenson, B.S.; Khammanivong, A.; Ross, K.F.; Geczy, C.L.; Herzberg, M.C. Anti-infective protective properties of S100 calgranulins. *Antiinflamm. Antiallergy Agents Med. Chem.* **2009**, *8*, 290–305. [CrossRef]
215. Kolbinger, F.; Loesche, C.; Valentin, M.A.; Jiang, X.; Cheng, Y.; Jarvis, P.; Peters, T.; Calonder, C.; Bruin, G.; Polus, F.; et al. β-Defensin 2 is a responsive biomarker of IL-17A-driven skin pathology in patients with psoriasis. *J. Allergy Clin. Immunol.* **2017**, *139*, 923–932. [CrossRef]
216. Yan, W.X.; Armishaw, C.; Goyette, J.; Yang, Z.; Cai, H.; Alewood, P.; Geczy, C.L. Mast cell and monocyte recruitment by S100A12 and its hinge domain. *J. Biol. Chem.* **2008**, *283*, 13035–13043. [CrossRef]
217. Nukui, T.; Ehama, R.; Sakaguchi, M.; Sonegawa, H.; Katagiri, C.; Hibino, T.; Huh, N.H. S100A8/A9, a key mediator for positive feedback growth stimulation of normal human keratinocytes. *J. Cell Biochem.* **2008**, *104*, 453–464. [CrossRef]
218. Muta, T. IkappaB-zeta: An inducible regulator of nuclear factor-kappaB. *Vitam. Horm.* **2006**, *74*, 301–316.
219. Bertelsen, T.; Iversen, L.; Johansen, C. The human IL-17A/F heterodimer regulates psoriasis-associated genes through IκBζ. *Exp. Dermatol.* **2018**, *27*, 1048–1052. [CrossRef]
220. Muromoto, R.; Hirao, T.; Tawa, K.; Hirashima, K.; Kon, S.; Kitai, Y.; Matsuda, T. IL-17A plays a central role in the expression of psoriasis signature genes through the induction of IκB-ζ in keratinocytes. *Int. Immunol.* **2016**, *28*, 443–452. [CrossRef]
221. Dorschner, R.A.; Pestonjamasp, V.K.; Tamakuwala, S.; Ohtake, T.; Rudisill, J.; Nizet, V.; Agerberth, B.; Gudmundsson, G.H.; Gallo, R.L. Cutaneous injury induces the release of cathelicidin anti-microbial peptides active against group A Streptococcus. *J. Investig. Dermatol.* **2001**, *117*, 91–97. [CrossRef] [PubMed]
222. Reinholz, M.; Ruzicka, T.; Schauber, J. Cathelicidin LL-37: An antimicrobial peptide with a role in inflammatory skin disease. *Ann. Dermatol.* **2012**, *24*, 126–135. [CrossRef] [PubMed]
223. Tomasinsig, L.; Pizzirani, C.; Skerlavaj, B.; Pellegatti, P.; Gulinelli, S.; Tossi, A.; Di Virgilio, F.; Zanetti, M. The human cathelicidin LL-37 modulates the activities of the P2X7 receptor in a structure-dependent manner. *J. Biol. Chem.* **2008**, *283*, 30471–30481. [CrossRef] [PubMed]
224. Di Nardo, A.; Braff, M.H.; Taylor, K.R.; Na, C.; Granstein, R.D.; McInturff, J.E.; Krutzik, S.; Modlin, R.L.; Gallo, R.L. Cathelicidin antimicrobial peptides block dendritic cell TLR4 activation and allergic contact sensitization. *J. Immunol.* **2007**, *178*, 1829–1834. [CrossRef]
225. Tokumaru, S.; Sayama, K.; Shirakata, Y.; Komatsuzawa, H.; Ouhara, K.; Hanakawa, Y.; Yahata, Y.; Dai, X.; Tohyama, M.; Nagai, H.; et al. Induction of keratinocyte migration via transactivation of the epidermal growth factor receptor by the antimicrobial peptide LL-37. *J. Immunol.* **2005**, *175*, 4662–4668. [CrossRef]

226. Hu, S.C.; Yu, H.S.; Yen, F.L.; Lin, C.L.; Chen, G.S.; Lan, C.C. Neutrophil extracellular trap formation is increased in psoriasis and induces human β-defensin-2 production in epidermal keratinocytes. *Sci. Rep.* **2016**, *6*, 31119. [CrossRef]
227. Lande, R.; Gregorio, J.; Facchinetti, V.; Chatterjee, B.; Wang, Y.H.; Homey, B.; Cao, W.; Wang, Y.H.; Su, B.; Nestle, F.O.; et al. Plasmacytoid dendritic cells sense self-DNA coupled with antimicrobial peptide. *Nature* **2007**, *449*, 564–569. [CrossRef]
228. Mabuchi, T.; Hirayama, N. Binding affinity and interaction of LL-37 with HLA-C*06:02 in psoriasis. *J. Investig. Dermatol.* **2016**, *136*, 1901–1903. [CrossRef]
229. Takahashi, T.; Kulkarni, N.N.; Lee, E.Y.; Zhang, L.J.; Wong, G.C.L.; Gallo, R.L. Cathelicidin promotes inflammation by enabling binding of self-RNA to cell surface scavenger receptors. *Sci. Rep.* **2018**, *8*, 4032. [CrossRef]
230. Ong, P.Y.; Ohtake, T.; Brandt, C.; Strickland, I.; Boguniewicz, M.; Ganz, T.; Gallo, R.L.; Leung, D.Y. Endogenous antimicrobial peptides and skin infections in atopic dermatitis. *N. Engl. J. Med.* **2002**, *347*, 1151–1160. [CrossRef]
231. de Jongh, G.J.; Zeeuwen, P.L.; Kucharekova, M.; Pfundt, R.; van der Valk, P.G.; Blokx, W.; Dogan, A.; Hiemstra, P.S.; van de Kerkhof, P.C.; Schalkwijk, J. High expression levels of keratinocyte antimicrobial proteins in psoriasis compared with atopic dermatitis. *J. Investig. Dermatol.* **2005**, *125*, 1163–1173. [CrossRef] [PubMed]
232. Nomura, I.; Goleva, E.; Howell, M.D.; Hamid, Q.A.; Ong, P.Y.; Hall, C.F.; Darst, M.A.; Gao, B.; Boguniewicz, M.; Travers, J.B.; et al. Cytokine milieu of atopic dermatitis, as compared to psoriasis, skin prevents induction of innate immune response genes. *J. Immunol.* **2003**, *171*, 3262–3269. [CrossRef] [PubMed]
233. Yang, D.; Chertov, O.; Bykovskaia, S.N.; Chen, Q.; Buffo, M.J.; Shogan, J.; Anderson, M.; Schröder, J.M.; Wang, J.M.; Howard, O.M.; et al. Beta-defensins: Linking innate and adaptive immunity through dendritic and T cell CCR6. *Science* **1999**, *286*, 525–528. [CrossRef] [PubMed]
234. Ghannam, S.; Dejou, C.; Pedretti, N.; Giot, J.P.; Dorgham, K.; Boukhaddaoui, H.; Deleuze, V.; Bernard, F.X.; Jorgensen, C.; Yssel, H.; et al. CCL20 and β-defensin-2 induce arrest of human Th17 cells on inflamed endothelium in vitro under flow conditions. *J. Immunol.* **2011**, *186*, 1411–1420. [CrossRef] [PubMed]

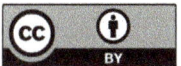 © 2020 by the authors. Licensee MDPI, Basel, Switzerland. This article is an open access article distributed under the terms and conditions of the Creative Commons Attribution (CC BY) license (http://creativecommons.org/licenses/by/4.0/).

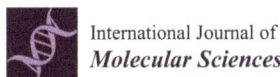

Review

Efficacy and Safety of Biologics for Psoriasis and Psoriatic Arthritis and Their Impact on Comorbidities: A Literature Review

Masahiro Kamata and Yayoi Tada *

Department of Dermatology, Teikyo University School of Medicine, 2-11-1 Kaga, Itabashi-ku, Tokyo 173-8605, Japan; mkamata-tky@umin.ac.jp
* Correspondence: ytada-tky@umin.ac.jp; Tel.: +81-3-3964-1211; Fax: +81-3-3814-1503

Received: 13 February 2020; Accepted: 26 February 2020; Published: 1 March 2020

Abstract: Psoriasis is a chronic inflammatory skin disease characterized by scaly indurated erythema. It impairs patients' quality of life enormously. It has been recognized not only as a skin disease but as a systemic disease, since it also causes arthritis (psoriatic arthritis) and mental disorders. Furthermore, an association with cardiovascular events is indicated. With the advent of biologics, treatment of psoriasis dramatically changed due to its high efficacy and tolerable safety. A variety of biologic agents are available for the treatment of psoriasis nowadays. However, characteristics such as rapidity of onset, long-term efficacy, safety profile, and effects on comorbidities are different. Better understanding of those characteristic leads to the right choice for individual patients, resulting in higher persistence, longer drug survival, higher patient satisfaction, and minimizing the disease impact of psoriasis. In this paper, we focus on the efficacy and safety profile of biologics in psoriasis patients, including plaque psoriasis and psoriatic arthritis. In addition, we discuss the impact of biologics on comorbidities caused by psoriasis.

Keywords: biologics; psoriasis; psoriatic arthritis; tumor necrosis factor-α; inteleukin-23; interluekin-17

1. Introduction

Psoriasis is a chronic inflammatory skin disease characterized by scaly indurated erythema. The prevalence of psoriasis in children ranges from 0% (Taiwan) to 2.1% (Italy), and in adults it varies from 0.91% (United States) to 8.5% (Norway) [1]. It impairs patients' quality of life enormously. It has been recognized not only as a skin disease but as a systemic disease, since it also causes arthritis (psoriatic arthritis; PsA) and mental disorders. Furthermore, an association with cardiovascular events is indicated [2]. With the advent of biologics, treatment of psoriasis dramatically changed due to its high efficacy and tolerable safety. In addition, the efficacy of biologics helps us to understand the pathogenesis of psoriasis. Whereas biologics have shown dramatically excellent efficacy, their safety has been a concern. To date, data on their efficacy and safety have been accumulated. In this paper, we focus on the efficacy and safety profile of biologics in psoriasis patients, including plaque psoriasis and PsA. In addition, we discuss the impact of biologics on comorbidities caused by psoriasis.

2. Efficacy and Safety of Biologics

Although approved biologic agents differ by countries, biologic agents commonly used for the treatment of psoriasis are categorized into three groups, tumor necrosis factor (TNF)-α inhibitors, interleukin (IL)-23 inhibitors, and IL-17 inhibitors, as shown in Table 1. Infliximab, adalimumab, etanercept, certolizumab-pegol, and golimumab are TNF-α inhibitors. Golimumab is used only for PsA. Ustekinumab is an anti-IL-12/23p40 antibody. Guselkumab, risankizumab, tildrakizumab, and mirikizumab are anti-IL-23p19 antibodies. Secukinumab, and ixekizumab are anti-IL-17A antibodies. Brodalumab is an anti-IL-17RA antibody. Bimekizumab is an anti-IL-17A/F antibody, which blocks both IL-17A and IL-17F. Many randomized controlled trials (RCTs) were conducted, and they demonstrated that the drugs are efficacious for moderate-to-severe plaque psoriasis. Recently, network meta-analyses enabled indirect comparison among those agents.

Table 1. Target of biologics.

Target of biologics	Drug
TNF-α inhibitors	Infliximab Adalimumab Golimumab (for psoriatic arthritis) Certolizumab-pegol Etanercept
IL-12/23 inhibitor	Ustekinumab
IL-23 inhibitors	Guselkumab Risankizumab Tildrakizumab (not approved yet) Mirikizumab (not approved yet)
IL-17 inhibitors	Secukinumab Ixekizumab Brodalumab Bimekizumab (not approved yet)
CTLA4-Ig	Abatacept (for psoriatic arthritis)

2.1. Plaque Psoriasis

Since previous review articles have illustrated the pathogenesis of psoriasis, we do not refer to the details [3,4]. Briefly, various triggers activate plasmacytoid dendritic cells, which are important in early-phase psoriasis. Meanwhile, TNF-α/iNOS-producing dendritic cells (TIP-DCs) play a pivotal role in maintaining psoriasis. TIP-DC activated by TNF-α secrete TNF-α, which activate themselves in an autocrine way. TIP-DCs also produce IL-23, which maintains and proliferates Th-17 cells. IL-23-stimulated Th17 cells are pathogenic and produce excessive IL-17A, F, and IL-22. Those cytokines drive keratinocytes to abnormal differentiation and proliferation, which forms psoriasis plaque. Activated keratinocytes also work as immune cells. They produce anti-microbial peptides and TNF-α, which activate dendritic cells including TIP-DC. This vicious inflammatory cycle makes the plaque remain and deteriorate. Activated keratinocytes secrete IL-17C, which activates keratinocytes in an autocrine way. Recently, the contribution of resident memory T cells [5–8], epidermal dendritic cells [9] in the epidermis, and type 3 innate lymphoid cells [8,10] to the development of psoriasis and recurrent plaque has attracted attention.

New biologic agents such as risankizumab [11], guselkumab [12–16], ixekizumab [17–23], and brodalumab [24,25] demonstrated high efficacy for patients with moderate-to-severe psoriasis. The percentage of patients who achieved more than a 90% reduction in the Psoriasis Area Severity Index (PASI) score at 16 weeks after initiating each treatment (PASI 90) was about 70%–80%, and that at 52 weeks was about 80%–90% in respective clinical trials. PASI 100 was about 50%–60% at 52 weeks. Those biologic agents showed high efficacy.

Ellis et al. appraised two network-meta analyses that assessed systemic therapies for moderate-to-severe psoriasis [26]. They concluded that newer biologics targeting theIL-12/23 and IL-17 axes appear to be more effective than older biologics and oral agents.

Sawyer et al. analyzed 17 studies reporting outcomes at 40-64 weeks in order to evaluate long-term efficacy [27]. Four 52-week RCTs revealed that brodalumab was significantly more efficacious than secukinumab, ustekinumab, and etanercept. Secukinumab was also more efficacious than ustekinumab, and both outperformed etanercept. Evidence from 13 additional studies and four further therapies (adalimumab, apremilast, infliximab and ixekizumab) revealed that brodalumab was most effective, followed by ixekizumab and secukinumab, then ustekinumab, infliximab and adalimumab. Etanercept had the lowest expected long-term efficacy. They concluded that brodalumab is associated with a higher likelihood of sustained PASI response, including complete clearance, at week 52 than comparators.

Sawyer et al. performed a network meta-analysis including 77 trials (34,816 patients) [28]. They revealed the superiority of brodalumab, ixekizumab, secukinumab, guselkumab and risankizumab to tildrakizumab, ustekinumab, all TNF-α inhibitors, and non-biologic systemic treatments in efficacy for plaque psoriasis. Furthermore, brodalumab, ixekizumab, and risankizumab showed higher efficacy than secukinumab, but did not significantly compared with guselkumab. In terms of PASI 90 and PASI 100 response, brodalumab, ixekizumab, guselkumab, and risankizumab demonstrated the greatest benefits.

According to the meta-analysis of 140 studies reported by Shidian et al. [29], in terms of the percentage of patients who attained PASI 90, infliximab, ixekizumab, secukinumab, bimekizumab, brodalumab, risankizumab, and guselkumab showed higher efficacy than ustekinumab, adalimumab, certolizumab, and etanercept. Moreover, adalimumab and ustekinumab were more efficacious than certolizumab and etanercept. No significant difference was observed between any of the interventions and the placebo for the risk of severe adverse events.

Generally, we can expect a rapid onset of efficacy on IL-17 inhibitors, especially brodalumab [30,31] and ixekizumab [32–34]. IL-17 inhibitors and IL-23 inhibitors, especially brodalumab, ixekizumab, and risankizumab showed high efficacy in the long-term [28,29].

2.2. Psoriatic Arthritis

A systematic review revealed 14.0%–22.7% of psoriasis patients having arthritis PsA in psoriasis patients [35]. PsA is characterized by enthesitis and arthritis in peripheral and axial involvement with bone proliferation and erosion [36,37]. PsA patients show distal interphalangeal joint involvement, which is usually asymmetric. In the pathogenesis of PsA, it is advocated that inflammation occurs in entheses in the early phase, and that the progression of enthesitis results in accompaniment with synovitis. In the initiation phase of enthesitis, innate immune cells are thought to play a key role. Thereafter, once certain entheseal cells are stimulated with IL-23, they secrete inflammatory cytokines such as IL-17A, IL-22 and TNF-α, consequently augmenting inflammation [36]. Focusing on enthesitis which is characteristic of PsA, Araujo et al. reported that ustekinumab, an anti-IL-12/IL-23p40 antibody, was superior to TNF-α inhibitors in the clearance of enthesitis [38], which underscores the importance of IL-23 in enthesitis. With regard to the contributions of TNF-α to the development of PsA [39,40], TNF-α increases the number of osteoclast precursor cells. TNF-α promotes differentiation into osteoclasts through RANKL-dependent pathways and promotes bone resorption. TNF-α inhibits Wnt signaling and induces apoptosis of osteoblasts, thereby reducing bone repair capacity. Recently, IL-23-independent IL-17-producing cells have drawn attention, especially in the pathogenesis of axial involvement of PsA. PsA and ankylosing spondylitis (AS) are recognized as one of spondyloarthritis (SpA) characterized by enthesitis, peripheral and axial arthritis, and negative laboratory results of rheumatoid factor and anti-cyclic citrullinated peptide antibody [41]. It indicates that the responsiveness of a certain drug for AS reflects its responsiveness for axial involvement of PsA. Anti-IL-17 antibodies, secukinumab [42] and ixekizumab [43], demonstrated efficacy for AS, but anti-IL-23 antibody, risankizumab [44], did not. Those results of clinical trials suggest the importance of IL-23-independent IL-17-producing cells in the axial involvement of PsA. iNKT and γδ-T cells are candidates of IL-23-independent IL-17-producing cells in SpA joints. Venken et al. reported that iNKT and γδ-T cells were a major source of T-cell-derived IL-17 in SpA joints and that those cells produced abundant IL-17 with anti-CD3 antibody/anti-CD28 antibody stimulation even in the absence of IL-23 [45]. Those data suggest that PsA patients with axial involvement would be better to be treated with IL-17 inhibitors such as ixekizumab and secukinumab, or TNF-α inhibitors, instead of anti-IL-23 antibodies such as risankizumab. Although the prevalence of having axial involvement in PsA patients differs by diagnosis criteria, it is reported to be from 23.6% to 55.4% [46,47]. In treating PsA patients, we should consider the considerable percentage of PsA patients having axial involvement and choose the right biologic agent. Mease et al. found the clinical characteristics of 192 PsA patients with axial involvement by comparing them with 1338 PsA patients without it [48]. Axial involvement was defined as physician-reported presence of spinal involvement at enrollment, and/or radiograph or MRI showing sacroiliitis. Patients with axial involvement showed a higher likelihood of moderate-to-severe psoriasis(body surface area ≥ 3%, 42.5% vs. 31.5%), lower prevalence of minimal disease activity (30.1% vs. 46.2%), higher nail psoriasis scores (visual analog scale; VAS 11.4 vs. 6.5), enthesitis counts (5.1 vs. 3.4), serum C-reactive protein levels (4.1 vs. 2.4 mg/L), and scores for physical function (Health Assessment Questionnaire, 0.9 vs. 0.6), pain (VAS, 47.7 vs. 36.2), and fatigue (VAS, 50.2 vs. 38.6) than patients without axial involvement. The American College of Rheumatology (ACR) and the National Psoriasis Foundation (NPF) published guidelines for PsA in 2019 [49], although nearly all recommendations were conditional since the quality of evidence was most often low or very low, and occasionally moderate.

Kawalec et al. conducted the network meta-analysis with eight eligible RCTs for efficacy (ACR 20 and ACR 50, PASI 75) and safety outcomes [50]. RCTs for abatacept, apremilast, secukinumab, or ustekinumab in adults with moderate-to-severe PsA were included. There were significant differences in the ACR20 response rate between secukinumab 150 mg and apremilast 20 mg, and between secukinumab 300 mg and apremilast 20 or 30 mg. Any adverse events occurred more often in apremilast 20 and 30 mg compared with the placebo and compared with secukinumab 150 mg. No significant differences were revealed for severe adverse events among biologics and between biologics and the placebo. In the overall population, as well as in the anti-TNF-α-naive subpopulation, secukinumab at a dose of 300 and 150 mg was ranked the highest for the ACR20 endpoint, while in the anti-TNF-α-experienced subpopulation, secukinumab 300 mg and apremilast 30 mg revealed the highest rank. For severe adverse events, the safest was ustekinumab 90 mg.

Dressler et al. also conducted a systematic review of approved systemic treatments for PsA [51]. Data were extracted from 20 trials for ACR 20, ACR 50, and adverse events after 16–24 weeks. Results for ACR 20 were infliximab + methotrexate vs. methotrexate: relative risk (RR) 1.40 (95% CI 1.07–1.84), very low-quality evidence; ixekizumab Q2W vs. adalimumab Q2W: RR 1.08 (95% CI 0.86–1.36), very low quality. In three placebo-controlled comparisons, leflunomide, methotrexate (MTX), and sulfasalazine failed to show statistical superiority for ACR. Besides the established treatment of anti-TNF antibodies and ustekinumab for psoriatic arthritis, the newer treatment options of anti-IL-17 antibodies and apremilast are also effective for the treatment of PsA. Based on just one comparative trial and one drug each, the new class of anti-IL 17 antibodies appears to be equally effective compared to the group of anti-TNF antibodies; for apremilast, this is yet unclear.

Lu et al., RCTs evaluated the efficacy and safety of targeted synthetic disease modifying anti-rheumatic drugs (DMARDs: tofacitinib, apremilast), as well as biological DMARDs (guselkumab, ustekinumab, secukinumab, ixekizumab, brodalumab, abatacept, adalimumab, etanercept, infliximab, certolizumab, and golimumab) for active PsA by a systemic literature review of 29 RCTs, including 10,204 participants and 17 treatments [52]. All treatments showed efficacy in ACR 20 and PASI 75 at 12–16 weeks in comparison with a placebo. As for safety, tofacitinib, apremilast, and ixekizumab 80 mg every 2 weeks demonstrated a higher rate of adverse events; however, in severe adverse events no significant difference was observed among all treatments. Network meta-analysis revealed that infliximab, golimumab, etanercept, adalimumab, guselkumab, and secukinumab 300 mg showed superiority to other drugs in both ACR 20 and PASI 75. Focusing on biologic-naïve patients, the results were similar to those above. Among biologic-experienced/failed patients, ustekinumab, secukinumab (300 mg and 150 mg), ixekizumab, abatacept, certolizumab pegol, tofacitinib, and apremilast still demonstrated higher ACR 20 then placebo, whereas only ustekinumab, secukinumab (300 mg), ixekizumab and tofacitinib were still associated with higher PASI 75.

In interpreting these systematic reviews, we should be aware that most clinical trials only assessed peripheral arthritis and did not assess enthesitis, dactylitis, or even axial involvement. As written above, it would be better to treat PsA with axial involvement with TNF-α inhibitors or IL-17 inhibitors instead of IL-23 inhibitors. When deciding on a treatment for PsA, we should not focus only on efficacy for arthritis, but also take skin manifestation into consideration. The safety profile should be also considered.

2.3. Safety Concerns of Biologics

As written above, biologic agents demonstrated tolerable safety profiles in the clinical trials. However, accumulating evidence revealed drug-specific concerns. We have already discussed the safety concerns of biologics in the previous literature [53]. Therefore, we refer to this issue in brief. It has been reported that TNF-α inhibitors are associated with serious infection (slightly increased risk), tuberculosis, paradoxical reaction, lupus, and infusion reaction (only infliximab). IL-17 inhibitors are associated with candidiasis, neutropenia, and inflammatory bowel disease. As of now, there have never been IL-23 inhibitor-specific adverse events reported. Safety concerns common in biologics include hepatitis B virus reactivation and interstitial pneumonia. Those concerns were raised during use of TNF-α inhibitors. Evidence of newer drugs such as IL-17 inhibitors and IL-23 inhibitors are insufficient. Accumulation of evidence is needed. Regarding immunogenicity, generally, predispositions of higher immunogenicity are observed in humanized monoclonal antibodies rather than in human monoclonal antibodies. The effect of immunogenicity on efficacy and safety seems limited in new biologic agents. However, since psoriasis is a chronic disease and some patients need to receive biologics for a long period of time, it might affect effectiveness and safety in the long-term. Longer observation is necessary to clarify this. With respect to malignancy, its rates are higher in psoriasis patients than the adult general population, but these treatments do not appear to increase malignancy risk.

Kaushik and Lebwohl focus on pregnant and pediatric patients with moderate-to-severe psoriasis, and those with chronic infections, such as hepatitis, HIV, and latent tuberculosis, and describe appropriate systematic treatment for them [54].

3. Impact of Biologics on Comorbidities

Psoriasis imposes a psychological burden on patients. The prevalence of having depression or anxiety is higher in psoriasis patients than in controls [55–57]. A systematic review and meta-analysis investigating 18 studies including a total of 1,767,583 participants, of whom 330,207 had psoriasis, reported that patients with psoriasis had a significantly higher likelihood of suicidal ideation, suicide attempts, and completed suicides [58]. Strober et al. evaluated the effect of biologic therapy (ustekinumab, infliximab, etanercept, and adalimumab) on depression in psoriasis patients utilizing Psoriasis Longitudinal Assessment and Registry (PSOLAR). The incidence rates of depressive symptoms were 3.01 (95% CI, 2.73–3.32), 5.85 (95% CI, 4.29–7.97), and 5.70 (95% CI, 4.58–7.10) per 100 patient-years for biologics, phototherapy, and conventional therapy, respectively. Compared with conventional therapy, biologics reduced the risk for depressive symptoms (hazard ratio, 0.76; 95% CI, 0.59–0.98), whereas phototherapy did not (hazard ratio, 1.05; 95% CI, 0.71–1.54) [59].

Cohen et al. investigated 12,502 psoriasis patients aged 20 years and above and 24,287 age- and sex-matched controls utilizing Clalit Health Services, the largest healthcare provider organization in Israel, and revealed that psoriasis was associated with Crohn's disease (CD; odds ratio, 2.49; 95% CI, 1.71–3.62) as well as ulcerative colitis (UC; odds ratio, 1.64; 95% CI, 1.15–2.33) [60]. Focusing on the effect of biologics, randomized control trials for CD with secukinumab and brodalumab resulted in a disproportionate number of cases of worsening and no evidence of efficacy [61,62]. In addition, exacerbations of inflammatory disease have been reported in psoriasis patients receiving IL-17 inhibitors [22,25,60]. Lee et al. found that IL-17A-dependent regulation of the tight junction protein occludin in the intestinal mucosa during epithelial injury limits excessive permeability and maintains barrier integrity, and revealed that IL-23-independent IL-17 production by $\gamma\delta$ T cells was important for the maintenance and protection of epithelial barriers in the intestinal mucosa. Whereas IL-17 inhibition exacerbates inflammatory bowel disease, TNF-α inhibitors are approved for the treatment of CD and UC, and IL-23 inhibitors demonstrated clinical improvement [63,64].

Recently, "psoriatic march", the concept of a causal link between psoriasis and cardiovascular disease, has been widely recognized. Systemic inflammation may cause insulin resistance, which in turn triggers endothelial cell dysfunction, leading to atherosclerosis and finally myocardial infarction or stroke [65,66]. Systematic review and meta-analysis analyzing 14 papers, including a total of 25,042 patients with psoriasis, revealed the association of psoriasis with metabolic syndrome. They reported that metabolic syndrome was present in 31.4% of patients with psoriasis (odds ratio, 1.42; 95% CI, 1.28–1.65) [67]. Other articles indicated that obesity is associated with the onset, exacerbation, and intractability of psoriasis [68–72]. As for hyperglycemia, Ikumi et al. revealed that hyperglycemia is highly associated with psoriasis, mainly through IL-17. In patients, the severity of psoriasis correlated with high blood glucose levels, and anti-IL-17A monoclonal antibody therapy reduced HbA1c levels significantly in these patients. In imiquimod-induced psoriasiform dermatitis, treatment with anti-IL-17A monoclonal antibody decreased fasting blood glucose levels [73]. Concerning endothelial cell dysfunction, flow-mediated dilation (FMD) is a marker that reflects endothelial cell dysfunction. Avgerinou et al. investigated FMD in 14 psoriasis patients before and 12 weeks after treatment with adalimumab, and reported that it improved after treatment with adalimumab [74]. von Stebut et al. conducted a 52-week, randomized, double-blind, placebo-controlled, exploratory trial in patients with moderate-to-severe plaque psoriasis without clinical cardiovascular disease, named Evaluation of Cardiovascular Risk Markers in Psoriasis Patients Treated with Secukinumab (CARIMA) [75]. Although a statistical difference was not observed in the baseline-adjusted mean FMD between patients receiving secukinumab and those receiving placebo at week 12, FMD was significantly higher than baseline in patients receiving the label dose of 300 mg secukinumab for 52 weeks. Regarding atherosclerosis, Hjuler et al. examined calcified coronary plaque, utilizing cardiac computed tomography angiography in severe psoriasis patients, severe atopic dermatitis patients, and retrospectively matched controls [76]. They demonstrated that psoriasis patients showed an increased prevalence of severe coronary stenosis (stenosis >70%) (psoriasis 14.6%, controls 0%; $p = 0.02$) and 3-vessel coronary affection or left main artery disease (psoriasis 20%, controls 3%; $p = 0.02$), whereas AD patients showed an increased prevalence of mild single-vessel affection (AD 40.7%, controls 9.1%; $p = 0.005$). Elnabawi et al. conducted a prospective, observational study in order to investigate the effect of biologic therapy on coronary artery plaque [77]. Analysis of 121 participants who were biologics-naïve at baseline and received biologic therapy for one year revealed that biologic therapy was associated with a 6% reduction in non-calcified plaque burden ($p = 0.005$) reduction in necrotic core ($p = 0.03$), with no effect on fibrous burden ($p = 0.71$), indicating that biologic therapy in severe psoriasis was associated with favorable modulation of coronary plaque indices. After one-year of biologic therapy, non-calcified plaque burden decreased by 5% in patients treated with TNF-α inhibitors ($p = 0.06$), by 2% in patients treated with anti-IL12/23 antibody ($p = 0.36$), and by 12% in patients treated with IL-17 inhibitors ($p < 0.001$). Patients treated with IL-17 inhibitors demonstrated a significantly greater reduction in non-calcified coronary plaque burden compared with those treated with anti-IL12/23 antibody and those with no biologic treatment. Patients treated with TNF-α inhibitors showed a significantly greater reduction in non-calcified coronary plaque burden only compared those with non-biologic treatment ($p < 0.01$). Regarding cardiovascular events, a systemic review and meta-analysis demonstrated that mild and severe psoriasis are associated with an increased risk of myocardial infarction and stroke, and that severe psoriasis is also associated with an increased risk of cardiovascular mortality [78]. Yang et al. conducted a meta-analysis on the effect of TNF-α inhibitors on cardiovascular events in psoriasis and psoriatic arthritis, analyzing five studies (49,795 patients). Compared with topical/photo treatment, TNF-α inhibitors were associated with a significant lower risk of cardiovascular events (RR, 0.58; 95% confidence interval; CI, 0.43 to 0.77; $p < 0.001$). Additionally, compared with MTX treatment, risk of cardiovascular events was also markedly decreased in the

TNF-α inhibitor group (RR, 0.67; 95% CI, 0.52 to 0.88; $p = 0.003$). Wu et al. also examined patients receiving TNF-α inhibitors ($n = 9148$) and patients receiving MTX ($n = 8581$). Psoriasis patients receiving TNF-α inhibitors had a lower major cardiovascular event risk compared to those receiving MTX (Kaplan–Meier rates: 1.45% vs. 4.09%: $p < 0.01$. Hazard ratio = 0.55; $p < 0.01$) [79]. The direct effect of IL-17 inhibitors or IL-23 inhibitors on cardiovascular events has not been reported yet.

Kaushik and Lebwohl also described specific comorbidities and insights to choose the appropriate systemic treatment in patients with moderate-to-severe psoriasis [80]. The choice of appropriate biologic therapy for a patient is often determined by the presence of comorbidities.

4. Conclusions

Evidence of new drugs on long-term efficacy, safety, and impacts on comorbidities is relatively low. Further accumulation is needed to clarify them. Currently, a variety of biologic agents are available for the treatment of psoriasis. However, characteristics such as rapidity of onset, long-term efficacy, safety profile, and effects on comorbidities are different. Better understanding those characteristics leads to the right choice for individual patients, resulting in higher persistence, longer drug survival, higher patient satisfaction, and minimizing the disease impact of psoriasis.

Funding: This research received no external funding.

Conflicts of Interest: M.K. received grants for research from Torii Pharmaceutical, Eisai, Maruho, and Novartis Pharma, and honoraria for lectures from Maruho, LEO Pharma, Eisai, AbbVie, Kyowa Kirin, Eli Lilly, Taiho Pharmaceutical, Mitsubishi Tanabe Pharma, and Janssen Pharmaceutical. Y.T. received grants for research from Maruho, LEO Pharma, Eisai, AbbVie, Kyowa Hakko Kirin, Taiho Pharmaceutical, Celgene, and Eli Lilly, and honoraria for lectures from Maruho, LEO Pharma, Eisai, AbbVie, Kyowa Kirin, Eli Lilly, Taiho Pharmaceutical, Mitsubishi Tanabe Pharma, and Janssen Pharmaceutical.

References

1. Parisi, R.; Symmons, D.P.; Griffiths, C.E.; Ashcroft, D.M. Global epidemiology of psoriasis: a systematic review of incidence and prevalence. *J. Invest. Dermatol.* **2013**, *133*, 377–385. [CrossRef] [PubMed]
2. Takeshita, J.; Grewal, S.; Langan, S.M.; Mehta, N.N.; Ogdie, A.; Van Voorhees, A.S.; Gelfand, J.M. Psoriasis and comorbid diseases: Epidemiology. *J. Am. Acad. Dermatol.* **2017**, *76*, 377–390. [CrossRef] [PubMed]
3. Lynde, C.W.; Poulin, Y.; Vender, R.; Bourcier, M.; Khalil, S. Interleukin 17A: toward a new understanding of psoriasis pathogenesis. *J. Am. Acad. Dermatol.* **2014**, *71*, 141–150. [CrossRef] [PubMed]
4. Ogawa, E.; Sato, Y.; Minagawa, A.; Okuyama, R. Pathogenesis of psoriasis and development of treatment. *J. Dermatol.* **2018**, *45*, 264–272. [CrossRef]
5. Cheuk, S.; Wiken, M.; Blomqvist, L.; Nylen, S.; Talme, T.; Stahle, M.; Eidsmo, L. Epidermal Th22 and Tc17 cells form a localized disease memory in clinically healed psoriasis. *J. Immunol.* **2014**, *192*, 3111–3120. [CrossRef]
6. Cheuk, S.; Schlums, H.; Gallais Serezal, I.; Martini, E.; Chiang, S.C.; Marquardt, N.; Gibbs, A.; Detlofsson, E.; Introini, A.; Forkel, M.; et al. CD49a Expression Defines Tissue-Resident CD8(+) T Cells Poised for Cytotoxic Function in Human Skin. *Immunity* **2017**, *46*, 287–300. [CrossRef]
7. Gallais Serezal, I.; Classon, C.; Cheuk, S.; Barrientos-Somarribas, M.; Wadman, E.; Martini, E.; Chang, D.; Xu Landen, N.; Ehrstrom, M.; Nylen, S.; et al. Resident T Cells in Resolved Psoriasis Steer Tissue Responses that Stratify Clinical Outcome. *J. Invest. Dermatol.* **2018**, *138*, 1754–1763. [CrossRef]
8. Villanova, F.; Flutter, B.; Tosi, I.; Grys, K.; Sreeneebus, H.; Perera, G.K.; Chapman, A.; Smith, C.H.; Di Meglio, P.; Nestle, F.O. Characterization of innate lymphoid cells in human skin and blood demonstrates increase of NKp44+ ILC3 in psoriasis. *J. Invest. Dermatol.* **2014**, *134*, 984–991. [CrossRef]
9. Martini, E.; Wiken, M.; Cheuk, S.; Gallais Serezal, I.; Baharom, F.; Stahle, M.; Smed-Sorensen, A.; Eidsmo, L. Dynamic Changes in Resident and Infiltrating Epidermal Dendritic Cells in Active and Resolved Psoriasis. *J. Invest. Dermatol.* **2017**, *137*, 865–873. [CrossRef]
10. Dyring-Andersen, B.; Geisler, C.; Agerbeck, C.; Lauritsen, J.P.; Gudjonsdottir, S.D.; Skov, L.; Bonefeld, C.M. Increased number and frequency of group 3 innate lymphoid cells in nonlesional psoriatic skin. *Br. J. Dermatol.* **2014**, *170*, 609–616. [CrossRef]

11. Gordon, K.B.; Strober, B.; Lebwohl, M.; Augustin, M.; Blauvelt, A.; Poulin, Y.; Papp, K.A.; Sofen, H.; Puig, L.; Foley, P.; et al. Efficacy and safety of risankizumab in moderate-to-severe plaque psoriasis (UltIMMa-1 and UltIMMa-2): results from two double-blind, randomised, placebo-controlled and ustekinumab-controlled phase 3 trials. *Lancet* **2018**, *392*, 650–661. [CrossRef]
12. Reich, K.; Griffiths, C.E.M.; Gordon, K.B.; Papp, K.A.; Song, M.; Randazzo, B.; Li, S.; Shen, Y.K.; Han, C.; Kimball, A.B.; et al. Maintenance of clinical response and consistent safety profile with up to 3 years of continuous treatment with guselkumab: Results from the VOYAGE 1 and VOYAGE 2 trials. *J. Am. Acad. Dermatol.* **2019**. [CrossRef] [PubMed]
13. Reich, K.; Armstrong, A.W.; Langley, R.G.; Flavin, S.; Randazzo, B.; Li, S.; Hsu, M.C.; Branigan, P.; Blauvelt, A. Guselkumab versus secukinumab for the treatment of moderate-to-severe psoriasis (ECLIPSE): results from a phase 3, randomised controlled trial. *Lancet* **2019**, *394*, 831–839. [CrossRef]
14. Blauvelt, A.; Papp, K.A.; Griffiths, C.E.; Randazzo, B.; Wasfi, Y.; Shen, Y.K.; Li, S.; Kimball, A.B. Efficacy and safety of guselkumab, an anti-interleukin-23 monoclonal antibody, compared with adalimumab for the continuous treatment of patients with moderate to severe psoriasis: Results from the phase III, double-blinded, placebo- and active comparator-controlled VOYAGE 1 trial. *J. Am. Acad. Dermatol.* **2017**, *76*, 405–417.
15. Gordon, K.B.; Blauvelt, A.; Foley, P.; Song, M.; Wasfi, Y.; Randazzo, B.; Shen, Y.K.; You, Y.; Griffiths, C.E.M. Efficacy of guselkumab in subpopulations of patients with moderate-to-severe plaque psoriasis: A pooled analysis of the phase III VOYAGE 1 and VOYAGE 2 studies. *Br. J. Dermatol.* **2018**, *178*, 132–139. [CrossRef]
16. Foley, P.; Gordon, K.; Griffiths, C.E.M.; Wasfi, Y.; Randazzo, B.; Song, M.; Li, S.; Shen, Y.K.; Blauvelt, A. Efficacy of Guselkumab Compared With Adalimumab and Placebo for Psoriasis in Specific Body Regions: A Secondary Analysis of 2 Randomized Clinical Trials. *JAMA Dermatol* **2018**, *154*, 676–683. [CrossRef]
17. Paul, C.; Griffiths, C.E.M.; van de Kerkhof, P.C.M.; Puig, L.; Dutronc, Y.; Henneges, C.; Dossenbach, M.; Hollister, K.; Reich, K. Ixekizumab provides superior efficacy compared with ustekinumab over 52 weeks of treatment: Results from IXORA-S, a phase 3 study. *J. Am. Acad. Dermatol.* **2019**, *80*, 70–79. [CrossRef]
18. Blauvelt, A.; Gooderham, M.; Iversen, L.; Ball, S.; Zhang, L.; Agada, N.O.; Reich, K. Efficacy and safety of ixekizumab for the treatment of moderate-to-severe plaque psoriasis: Results through 108 weeks of a randomized, controlled phase 3 clinical trial (UNCOVER-3). *J. Am. Acad. Dermatol.* **2017**, *77*, 855–862. [CrossRef]
19. Imafuku, S.; Torisu-Itakura, H.; Nishikawa, A.; Zhao, F.; Cameron, G.S. Efficacy and safety of ixekizumab treatment in Japanese patients with moderate-to-severe plaque psoriasis: Subgroup analysis of a placebo-controlled, phase 3 study (UNCOVER-1). *J. Dermatol.* **2017**, *44*, 1285–1290. [CrossRef]
20. Nash, P.; Kirkham, B.; Okada, M.; Rahman, P.; Combe, B.; Burmester, G.R.; Adams, D.H.; Kerr, L.; Lee, C.; Shuler, C.L.; et al. Ixekizumab for the treatment of patients with active psoriatic arthritis and an inadequate response to tumour necrosis factor inhibitors: results from the 24-week randomised, double-blind, placebo-controlled period of the SPIRIT-P2 phase 3 trial. *Lancet* **2017**, *389*, 2317–2327. [CrossRef]
21. Saeki, H.; Nakagawa, H.; Nakajo, K.; Ishii, T.; Morisaki, Y.; Aoki, T.; Cameron, G.S.; Osuntokun, O.O. Efficacy and safety of ixekizumab treatment for Japanese patients with moderate to severe plaque psoriasis, erythrodermic psoriasis and generalized pustular psoriasis: Results from a 52-week, open-label, phase 3 study (UNCOVER-J). *J. Dermatol.* **2017**, *44*, 355–362. [CrossRef] [PubMed]
22. Gordon, K.B.; Blauvelt, A.; Papp, K.A.; Langley, R.G.; Luger, T.; Ohtsuki, M.; Reich, K.; Amato, D.; Ball, S.G.; Braun, D.K.; et al. Phase 3 Trials of Ixekizumab in Moderate-to-Severe Plaque Psoriasis. *N. Engl. J. Med.* **2016**, *375*, 345–356. [CrossRef] [PubMed]
23. Griffiths, C.E.; Reich, K.; Lebwohl, M.; van de Kerkhof, P.; Paul, C.; Menter, A.; Cameron, G.S.; Erickson, J.; Zhang, L.; Secrest, R.J.; et al. Comparison of ixekizumab with etanercept or placebo in moderate-to-severe psoriasis (UNCOVER-2 and UNCOVER-3): results from two phase 3 randomised trials. *Lancet* **2015**, *386*, 541–551. [CrossRef]
24. Puig, L.; Lebwohl, M.; Bachelez, H.; Sobell, J.; Jacobson, A.A. Long-term efficacy and safety of brodalumab in the treatment of psoriasis: 120-week results from the randomized, double-blind, placebo- and active comparator-controlled phase 3 AMAGINE-2 trial. *J. Am. Acad. Dermatol.* **2020**, *82*, 352–359. [CrossRef]
25. Lebwohl, M.; Strober, B.; Menter, A.; Gordon, K.; Weglowska, J.; Puig, L.; Papp, K.; Spelman, L.; Toth, D.; Kerdel, F.; et al. Phase 3 Studies Comparing Brodalumab with Ustekinumab in Psoriasis. *N. Engl. J. Med.* **2015**, *373*, 1318–1328. [CrossRef]

26. Ellis, A.G.; Flohr, C.; Drucker, A.M. Network meta-analyses of systemic treatments for psoriasis: a critical appraisal: Original Articles: Jabbar-Lopez ZK, Yiu ZZN, Ward V et al. Quantitative evaluation of biologic therapy options for psoriasis: a systematic review and network meta-analysis. J Invest Dermatol 2017; 137:1646-54. Sbidian E, Chaimani A, Garcia-Doval I et al. Systemic pharmacological treatments for chronic plaque psoriasis: a network meta-analysis. Cochrane Database Syst Rev 2017; 12:CD011535. *Br. J. Dermatol.* **2019**, *180*, 282–288.
27. Sawyer, L.M.; Cornic, L.; Levin, L.A.; Gibbons, C.; Moller, A.H.; Jemec, G.B. Long-term efficacy of novel therapies in moderate-to-severe plaque psoriasis: a systematic review and network meta-analysis of PASI response. *J. Eur Acad Dermatol Venereol* **2019**, *33*, 355–366. [CrossRef]
28. Sawyer, L.M.; Malottki, K.; Sabry-Grant, C.; Yasmeen, N.; Wright, E.; Sohrt, A.; Borg, E.; Warren, R.B. Assessing the relative efficacy of interleukin-17 and interleukin-23 targeted treatments for moderate-to-severe plaque psoriasis: A systematic review and network meta-analysis of PASI response. *PLoS ONE* **2019**, *14*, e0220868-10. [CrossRef]
29. Sbidian, E.; Chaimani, A.; Afach, S.; Doney, L.; Dressler, C.; Hua, C.; Mazaud, C.; Phan, C.; Hughes, C.; Riddle, D.; et al. Systemic pharmacological treatments for chronic plaque psoriasis: a network meta-analysis. *Cochrane Database Syst. Rev.* **2020**, *1*, Cd011535-10. [CrossRef]
30. Papp, K.A.; Lebwohl, M.G. Onset of Action of Biologics in Patients with Moderate-to-Severe Psoriasis. *J. Drugs Dermatol.* **2017**, *17*, 247–250.
31. Yao, C.J.; Lebwohl, M.G. Onset of Action of Antipsoriatic Drugs for Moderate-to-Severe Plaque Psoriasis: An Update. *J. Drugs Dermatol.* **2019**, *18*, 229–233. [PubMed]
32. Blauvelt, A.; Papp, K.; Gottlieb, A.; Jarell, A.; Reich, K.; Maari, C.; Gordon, K.B.; Ferris, L.K.; Langley, R.G.; Tada, Y.; et al. A head-to-head comparison of ixekizumab vs. guselkumab in patients with moderate-to-severe plaque psoriasis: 12-week efficacy, safety and speed of response from a randomized, double-blinded trial. *Br. J. Dermatol.* **2019**. [CrossRef] [PubMed]
33. Khattri, S.; Goldblum, O.; Solotkin, K.; Amir, Y.; Min, M.S.; Ridenour, T.; Yang, F.E.; Lebwohl, M. Early Onset of Clinical Improvement with Ixekizumab in a Randomized, Open-label Study of Patients with Moderate-to-severe Plaque Psoriasis. *J. Clin. Aesthet Dermatol.* **2018**, *11*, 33–37. [PubMed]
34. Blauvelt, A.; Papp, K.A.; Lebwohl, M.G.; Green, L.J.; Hsu, S.; Bhatt, V.; Rastogi, S.; Pillai, R.; Israel, R. Rapid onset of action in patients with moderate-to-severe psoriasis treated with brodalumab: A pooled analysis of data from two phase 3 randomized clinical trials (AMAGINE-2 and AMAGINE-3). *J. Am. Acad. Dermatol.* **2017**, *77*, 372–374. [CrossRef]
35. Alinaghi, F.; Calov, M.; Kristensen, L.E.; Gladman, D.D.; Coates, L.C.; Jullien, D.; Gottlieb, A.B.; Gisondi, P.; Wu, J.J.; Thyssen, J.P.; et al. Prevalence of psoriatic arthritis in patients with psoriasis: A systematic review and meta-analysis of observational and clinical studies. *J. Am. Acad. Dermatol.* **2019**, *80*, 251–265. [CrossRef]
36. Schett, G.; Lories, R.J.; D'Agostino, M.A.; Elewaut, D.; Kirkham, B.; Soriano, E.R.; McGonagle, D. Enthesitis: from pathophysiology to treatment. *Nat. Rev. Rheumatol* **2017**, *13*, 731–741. [CrossRef]
37. Merola, J.F.; Espinoza, L.R.; Fleischmann, R. Distinguishing rheumatoid arthritis from psoriatic arthritis. *RMD Open* **2018**, *4*, e000656-10. [CrossRef]
38. Araujo, E.G.; Englbrecht, M.; Hoepken, S.; Finzel, S.; Kampylafka, E.; Kleyer, A.; Bayat, S.; Schoenau, V.; Hueber, A.; Rech, J.; et al. Effects of ustekinumab versus tumor necrosis factor inhibition on enthesitis: Results from the enthesial clearance in psoriatic arthritis (ECLIPSA) study. *Semin Arthritis Rheum* **2019**, *48*, 632–637. [CrossRef]
39. Ritchlin, C.T.; Colbert, R.A.; Gladman, D.D. Psoriatic Arthritis. *N. Engl. J. Med.* **2017**, *376*, 957–970. [CrossRef]
40. Heiland, G.R.; Zwerina, K.; Baum, W.; Kireva, T.; Distler, J.H.; Grisanti, M.; Asuncion, F.; Li, X.; Ominsky, M.; Richards, W.; et al. Neutralisation of Dkk-1 protects from systemic bone loss during inflammation and reduces sclerostin expression. *Ann. Rheum Dis.* **2010**, *69*, 2152–2159. [CrossRef]
41. van Tubergen, A.; Weber, U. Diagnosis and classification in spondyloarthritis: identifying a chameleon. *Nat. Rev. Rheumatol.* **2012**, *8*, 253–261. [CrossRef] [PubMed]
42. Baeten, D.; Sieper, J.; Braun, J.; Baraliakos, X.; Dougados, M.; Emery, P.; Deodhar, A.; Porter, B.; Martin, R.; Andersson, M.; et al. Secukinumab, an Interleukin-17A Inhibitor, in Ankylosing Spondylitis. *N. Engl. J. Med.* **2015**, *373*, 2534–2548. [CrossRef] [PubMed]

43. Dougados, M.; Wei, J.C.; Landewe, R.; Sieper, J.; Baraliakos, X.; Van den Bosch, F.; Maksymowych, W.P.; Ermann, J.; Walsh, J.A.; Tomita, T.; et al. Efficacy and safety of ixekizumab through 52 weeks in two phase 3, randomised, controlled clinical trials in patients with active radiographic axial spondyloarthritis (COAST-V and COAST-W). *Ann. Rheum Dis.* **2020**, *79*, 176–185. [CrossRef] [PubMed]
44. Baeten, D.; Ostergaard, M.; Wei, J.C.; Sieper, J.; Jarvinen, P.; Tam, L.S.; Salvarani, C.; Kim, T.H.; Solinger, A.; Datsenko, Y.; et al. Risankizumab, an IL-23 inhibitor, for ankylosing spondylitis: results of a randomised, double-blind, placebo-controlled, proof-of-concept, dose-finding phase 2 study. *Ann. Rheum Dis.* **2018**, *77*, 1295–1302. [CrossRef] [PubMed]
45. Venken, K.; Jacques, P.; Mortier, C.; Labadia, M.E.; Decruy, T.; Coudenys, J.; Hoyt, K.; Wayne, A.L.; Hughes, R.; Turner, M.; et al. RORgammat inhibition selectively targets IL-17 producing iNKT and gammadelta-T cells enriched in Spondyloarthritis patients. *Nat. Commun.* **2019**, *10*, 9–10. [CrossRef] [PubMed]
46. Hanly, J.G.; Russell, M.L.; Gladman, D.D. Psoriatic spondyloarthropathy: a long term prospective study. *Ann. Rheum Dis.* **1988**, *47*, 386–393. [CrossRef] [PubMed]
47. Battistone, M.J.; Manaster, B.J.; Reda, D.J.; Clegg, D.O. The prevalence of sacroilitis in psoriatic arthritis: new perspectives from a large, multicenter cohort. A Department of Veterans Affairs Cooperative Study. *Skeletal Radiol.* **1999**, *28*, 196–201. [CrossRef]
48. Mease, P.J.; Palmer, J.B.; Liu, M.; Kavanaugh, A.; Pandurengan, R.; Ritchlin, C.T.; Karki, C.; Greenberg, J.D. Influence of Axial Involvement on Clinical Characteristics of Psoriatic Arthritis: Analysis from the Corrona Psoriatic Arthritis/Spondyloarthritis Registry. *J. Rheumatol.* **2018**, *45*, 1389–1396. [CrossRef]
49. Singh, J.A.; Guyatt, G.; Ogdie, A.; Gladman, D.D.; Deal, C.; Deodhar, A.; Dubreuil, M.; Dunham, J.; Husni, M.E.; Kenny, S.; et al. Special Article: 2018 American College of Rheumatology/National Psoriasis Foundation Guideline for the Treatment of Psoriatic Arthritis. *Arthritis Rheumatol.* **2019**, *71*, 5–32. [CrossRef]
50. Kawalec, P.; Holko, P.; Mocko, P.; Pilc, A. Comparative effectiveness of abatacept, apremilast, secukinumab and ustekinumab treatment of psoriatic arthritis: a systematic review and network meta-analysis. *Rheumatol. Int.* **2018**, *38*, 189–201. [CrossRef]
51. Dressler, C.; Eisert, L.; Pham, P.A.; Nast, A. Efficacy and safety of systemic treatments in psoriatic arthritis: a systematic review, meta-analysis and GRADE evaluation. *J. Eur. Acad. Dermatol. Venereol.* **2019**, *33*, 1249–1260. [CrossRef] [PubMed]
52. Lu, C.; Wallace, B.I.; Waljee, A.K.; Fu, W.; Zhang, Q.; Liu, Y. Comparative efficacy and safety of targeted DMARDs for active psoriatic arthritis during induction therapy: A systematic review and network meta-analysis. *Semin Arthritis Rheum* **2019**, *49*, 381–388. [CrossRef] [PubMed]
53. Kamata, M.; Tada, Y. Safety of biologics in psoriasis. *J. Dermatol.* **2018**, *45*, 279–286. [CrossRef] [PubMed]
54. Kaushik, S.B.; Lebwohl, M.G. Psoriasis: Which therapy for which patient: Focus on special populations and chronic infections. *J. Am. Acad. Dermatol.* **2019**, *80*, 43–53. [CrossRef]
55. Dalgard, F.J.; Gieler, U.; Tomas-Aragones, L.; Lien, L.; Poot, F.; Jemec, G.B.E.; Misery, L.; Szabo, C.; Linder, D.; Sampogna, F.; et al. The psychological burden of skin diseases: a cross-sectional multicenter study among dermatological out-patients in 13 European countries. *J. Invest. Dermatol.* **2015**, *135*, 984–991. [CrossRef]
56. Kurd, S.K.; Troxel, A.B.; Crits-Christoph, P.; Gelfand, J.M. The risk of depression, anxiety, and suicidality in patients with psoriasis: a population-based cohort study. *Arch. Dermatol.* **2010**, *146*, 891–895.
57. Dowlatshahi, E.A.; Wakkee, M.; Arends, L.R.; Nijsten, T. The prevalence and odds of depressive symptoms and clinical depression in psoriasis patients: a systematic review and meta-analysis. *J. Invest. Dermatol.* **2014**, *134*, 1542–1551. [CrossRef]
58. Singh, S.; Taylor, C.; Kornmehl, H.; Armstrong, A.W. Psoriasis and suicidality: A systematic review and meta-analysis. *J. Am. Acad. Dermatol.* **2017**, *77*, 425–440. [CrossRef]
59. Strober, B.; Gooderham, M.; de Jong, E.; Kimball, A.B.; Langley, R.G.; Lakdawala, N.; Goyal, K.; Lawson, F.; Langholff, W.; Hopkins, L.; et al. Depressive symptoms, depression, and the effect of biologic therapy among patients in Psoriasis Longitudinal Assessment and Registry (PSOLAR). *J. Am. Acad. Dermatol.* **2018**, *78*, 70–80. [CrossRef]
60. Cohen, A.D.; Dreiher, J.; Birkenfeld, S. Psoriasis associated with ulcerative colitis and Crohn's disease. *J. Eur. Acad. Dermatol. Venereol.* **2009**, *23*, 561–565. [CrossRef]
61. Hueber, W.; Sands, B.E.; Lewitzky, S.; Vandemeulebroecke, M.; Reinisch, W.; Higgins, P.D.; Wehkamp, J.; Feagan, B.G.; Yao, M.D.; Karczewski, M.; et al. Secukinumab, a human anti-IL-17A monoclonal antibody,

for moderate to severe Crohn's disease: unexpected results of a randomised, double-blind placebo-controlled trial. *Gut* **2012**, *61*, 1693–1700. [CrossRef] [PubMed]
62. Targan, S.R.; Feagan, B.; Vermeire, S.; Panaccione, R.; Melmed, G.Y.; Landers, C.; Li, D.; Russell, C.; Newmark, R.; Zhang, N.; et al. A Randomized, Double-Blind, Placebo-Controlled Phase 2 Study of Brodalumab in Patients With Moderate-to-Severe Crohn's Disease. *Am. J. Gastroenterol.* **2016**, *111*, 1599–1607. [CrossRef] [PubMed]
63. Feagan, B.G.; Sandborn, W.J.; Gasink, C.; Jacobstein, D.; Lang, Y.; Friedman, J.R.; Blank, M.A.; Johanns, J.; Gao, L.L.; Miao, Y.; et al. Ustekinumab as Induction and Maintenance Therapy for Crohn's Disease. *N. Engl. J. Med.* **2016**, *375*, 1946–1960. [CrossRef] [PubMed]
64. Sands, B.E.; Chen, J.; Feagan, B.G.; Penney, M.; Rees, W.A.; Danese, S.; Higgins, P.D.R.; Newbold, P.; Faggioni, R.; Patra, K.; et al. Efficacy and Safety of MEDI2070, an Antibody Against Interleukin 23, in Patients With Moderate to Severe Crohn's Disease: A Phase 2a Study. *Gastroenterology* **2017**, *153*, 77–86. [CrossRef]
65. Boehncke, W.H.; Boehncke, S.; Tobin, A.M.; Kirby, B. The 'psoriatic march': a concept of how severe psoriasis may drive cardiovascular comorbidity. *Exp. Dermatol.* **2011**, *20*, 303–307. [CrossRef]
66. Furue, M.; Kadono, T. "Inflammatory skin march" in atopic dermatitis and psoriasis. *Inflamm. Res.* **2017**, *66*, 833–842. [CrossRef]
67. Rodriguez-Zuniga, M.J.M.; Garcia-Perdomo, H.A. Systematic review and meta-analysis of the association between psoriasis and metabolic syndrome. *J. Am. Acad. Dermatol.* **2017**, *77*, 657–666. [CrossRef]
68. Naldi, L.; Chatenoud, L.; Linder, D.; Belloni Fortina, A.; Peserico, A.; Virgili, A.R.; Bruni, P.L.; Ingordo, V.; Lo Scocco, G.; Solaroli, C.; et al. Cigarette smoking, body mass index, and stressful life events as risk factors for psoriasis: results from an Italian case-control study. *J. Invest. Dermatol.* **2005**, *125*, 61–67. [CrossRef]
69. Sterry, W.; Strober, B.E.; Menter, A. Obesity in psoriasis: the metabolic, clinical and therapeutic implications. Report of an interdisciplinary conference and review. *Br. J. Dermatol.* **2007**, *157*, 649–655. [CrossRef]
70. Naldi, L.; Addis, A.; Chimenti, S.; Giannetti, A.; Picardo, M.; Tomino, C.; Maccarone, M.; Chatenoud, L.; Bertuccio, P.; Caggese, E.; et al. Impact of body mass index and obesity on clinical response to systemic treatment for psoriasis. Evidence from the Psocare project. *Dermatology (Basel, Switzerland)* **2008**, *217*, 365–373. [CrossRef]
71. Tobin, A.M.; Hackett, C.B.; Rogers, S.; Collins, P.; Richards, H.L.; O'Shea, D.; Kirby, B. Body mass index, waist circumference and HOMA-IR correlate with the Psoriasis Area and Severity Index in patients with psoriasis receiving phototherapy. *Br. J. Dermatol.* **2014**, *171*, 436–438. [CrossRef] [PubMed]
72. Gisondi, P.; Del Giglio, M.; Di Francesco, V.; Zamboni, M.; Girolomoni, G. Weight loss improves the response of obese patients with moderate-to-severe chronic plaque psoriasis to low-dose cyclosporine therapy: a randomized, controlled, investigator-blinded clinical trial. *Am. J. Clin Nutr* **2008**, *88*, 1242–1247. [PubMed]
73. Ikumi, K.; Odanaka, M.; Shime, H.; Imai, M.; Osaga, S.; Taguchi, O.; Nishida, E.; Hemmi, H.; Kaisho, T.; Morita, A.; et al. Hyperglycemia Is Associated with Psoriatic Inflammation in Both Humans and Mice. *J. Invest. Dermatol.* **2019**, *139*, 1329–1338. [CrossRef] [PubMed]
74. Avgerinou, G.; Tousoulis, D.; Siasos, G.; Oikonomou, E.; Maniatis, K.; Papageorgiou, N.; Paraskevopoulos, T.; Miliou, A.; Koumaki, D.; Latsios, G.; et al. Anti-tumor necrosis factor alpha treatment with adalimumab improves significantly endothelial function and decreases inflammatory process in patients with chronic psoriasis. *Int. J. Cardiol.* **2011**, *151*, 382–383. [CrossRef]
75. von Stebut, E.; Reich, K.; Thaci, D.; Koenig, W.; Pinter, A.; Korber, A.; Rassaf, T.; Waisman, A.; Mani, V.; Yates, D.; et al. Impact of Secukinumab on Endothelial Dysfunction and Other Cardiovascular Disease Parameters in Psoriasis Patients over 52 Weeks. *J. Invest. Dermatol.* **2019**, *139*, 1054–1062. [CrossRef]
76. Hjuler, K.F.; Bottcher, M.; Vestergaard, C.; Deleuran, M.; Raaby, L.; Botker, H.E.; Iversen, L.; Kragballe, K. Increased Prevalence of Coronary Artery Disease in Severe Psoriasis and Severe Atopic Dermatitis. *Am. J. Med.* **2015**, *128*, 1325–1334. [CrossRef]
77. Elnabawi, Y.A.; Dey, A.K.; Goyal, A.; Groenendyk, J.W.; Chung, J.H.; Belur, A.D.; Rodante, J.; Harrington, C.L.; Teague, H.L.; Baumer, Y.; et al. Coronary artery plaque characteristics and treatment with biologic therapy in severe psoriasis: results from a prospective observational study. *Cardiovasc. Res.* **2019**, *115*, 721–728. [CrossRef]
78. Armstrong, E.J.; Harskamp, C.T.; Armstrong, A.W. Psoriasis and major adverse cardiovascular events: a systematic review and meta-analysis of observational studies. *J. Am. Heart Assoc.* **2013**, *2*, e000062-10. [CrossRef]

79. Wu, J.J.; Guerin, A.; Sundaram, M.; Dea, K.; Cloutier, M.; Mulani, P. Cardiovascular event risk assessment in psoriasis patients treated with tumor necrosis factor-alpha inhibitors versus methotrexate. *J. Am. Acad. Dermatol.* **2017**, *76*, 81–90. [CrossRef]
80. Kaushik, S.B.; Lebwohl, M.G. Psoriasis: Which therapy for which patient: Psoriasis comorbidities and preferred systemic agents. *J. Am. Acad. Dermatol.* **2019**, *80*, 27–40. [CrossRef]

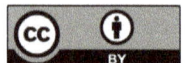

© 2020 by the authors. Licensee MDPI, Basel, Switzerland. This article is an open access article distributed under the terms and conditions of the Creative Commons Attribution (CC BY) license (http://creativecommons.org/licenses/by/4.0/).

MDPI
St. Alban-Anlage 66
4052 Basel
Switzerland
Tel. +41 61 683 77 34
Fax +41 61 302 89 18
www.mdpi.com

International Journal of Molecular Sciences Editorial Office
E-mail: ijms@mdpi.com
www.mdpi.com/journal/ijms

www.ingramcontent.com/pod-product-compliance
Lightning Source LLC
LaVergne TN
LVHW070508100526
838202LV00014B/1810